W9-AKW-374

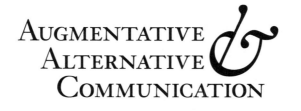

AUGMENTATIVE & ALTERNATIVE COMMUNICATION

SUPPORTING
CHILDREN
& ADULTS
WITH COMPLEX
COMMUNICATION
NEEDS

THIRD EDITION

by

David R. Beukelman, Ph.D.
University of Nebraska
Lincoln, Nebraska

Pat Mirenda, Ph.D.
University of British Columbia
Vancouver, British Columbia

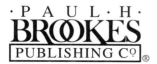
·P A U L ·H·
BROOKES
PUBLISHING Cº®

BALTIMORE • LONDON • SYDNEY

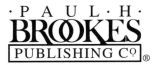

Paul H. Brookes Publishing Co.
Post Office Box 10624
Baltimore, Maryland 21285-0624

www.brookespublishing.com

Copyright © 2005 by Paul H. Brookes Publishing Co., Inc.
All rights reserved.

"Paul H. Brookes Publishing Co." is a registered trademark
of Paul H. Brookes Publishing Co., Inc.

Typeset by Integrated Publishing Services, Inc., Grand Rapids, Michigan.
Manufactured in the United States of America by
The Maple Press Co., York, Pennsylvania.

The individuals described in this book are composites or real people whose situations are masked and are based on the authors' experiences. In all instances, names and identifying details have been changed to protect confidentiality.

Purchasers of *Augmentative and Alternative Communication: Supporting Children and Adults with Complex Communication Needs, Third Edition,* are granted permission to photocopy forms for educational purposes. Although photocopying for educational purposes is unlimited, none of the forms may be reproduced to generate revenue for any program or individual. Photocopies may only be made from an original book. *Unauthorized use beyond this privilege is prosecutable under federal law.* You will see the copyright protection notice at the bottom of each photocopiable page.

Second printing, February 2006.

Library of Congress Cataloging-in-Publication Data

Beukelman, David R., 1943–
    Augmentative and alternative communication : supporting children and adults
    with complex communication needs / by David R. Beukelman and Pat Mirenda.
    —3rd ed.
        p.   ;   cm.
    Includes bibliographical references and index.
    ISBN-13: 978-1-55766-684-0 (hardcover)
    ISBN-10: 1-55766-684-9 (hardcover)
    1. People with disabilities—Means of communication.   2. Communication
    devices for people with disabilities.
    [DNLM: 1. Communication Disorders—rehabilitation.   2. Communication
    Aids for Disabled. WL 340.2 B566a   2005]   I. Mirenda, Pat.   II. Title.
    RC423.B477   2005
    616.85′503—dc22   2005011941

British Library Cataloguing in Publication data are available from the British Library.

Contents

About the Authors. vii
About the Contributors ix
Preface. xi
Acknowledgments xv

Part I   Augmentative and Alternative Communication Processes

  1   Augmentative and Alternative Communication Processes. 3
  2   Message Management: Vocabulary, Small Talk, and Storytelling 15
  3   Symbols and Rate Enhancement 35
  4   Alternative Access 81
  5   Team Building for AAC Assessment and Intervention 111
  6   Principles of Assessment 133
  7   Assessment of Specific Capabilities 159
  8   Principles of Decision Making, Intervention, and Evaluation 219

**Part II   Augmentative and Alternative Communication Interventions for
          Individuals with Developmental Disabilities**

  9   AAC Issues for People with Developmental Disabilities 235
10   AAC Strategies for Beginning Communicators: Opportunity
      and Nonsymbolic Interventions 255
11   AAC Strategies for Beginning Communicators:
      Symbolic Approaches. 287
12   Language Learning and Development 327
13   Literacy Development of Children Who Use AAC 351
      with Janet Sturm
14   Educational Inclusion of Students Who Use AAC. 391

**Part III Augmentative and Alternative Communication Interventions for
          Individuals with Acquired Disabilities**

15   Adults with Acquired Physical Disabilities 435
      with Laura J. Ball
16   Adults with Severe Aphasia 467
      Kathryn L. Garrett and Joanne P. Lasker
17   Adults with Degenerative Cognitive/Linguistic Disorders 505
      with Elizabeth K. Hanson
18   Individuals with Traumatic Brain Injury. 517
      with Susan Fager
19   AAC in Intensive and Acute Medical Settings 533

References 547

Appendix: Resources and Web Links 607

Index 611

ABOUT THE AUTHORS

David R. Beukelman, Ph.D., Professor, Department of Special Education and Communication Disorders, University of Nebraska–Lincoln, 118 Barkley Memorial Center, Lincoln, NE 68583

Dr. Beukelman specializes in the areas of augmentative communication and motor speech disorders of children and adults. He is the Barkley Professor of Communication Disorders at the University of Nebraska–Lincoln and Director of Research and Education of the Speech and Language Pathology Division of the Munroe-Meyer Institute of Genetics and Rehabilitation, Omaha, Nebraska. He is a senior researcher in the Institute for Rehabilitation Science and Engineering at Madonna Rehabilitation Hospital. He is a partner in the Rehabilitation Engineering and Research Center for Communication Enhancement. Previously, Dr. Beukelman was Director of the Augmentative Communication Program, University of Washington Hospital, and Associate Professor in the Department of Rehabilitation Medicine of the University of Washington–Seattle. He teaches courses in augmentative and alternative communication, motor speech disorders, and cleft palate. From 1994 to 1997, he was editor of the journal *Augmentative and Alternative Communication*. He currently serves as a series editor for the *Augmentative and Alternative Communication Series* published by Paul H. Brookes Publishing Co.

Pat Mirenda, Ph.D., Professor, Faculty of Education, University of British Columbia, 2125 Main Mall, Vancouver, British Columbia V6T 1Z4, CANADA

Dr. Mirenda earned her doctorate in behavioral disabilities from the University of Wisconsin–Madison. For 8 years, she was a faculty member in the Department of Special Education and Communication Disorders, University of Nebraska–Lincoln. From 1992 to 1996, she provided a variety of training, research, and support services to individuals with severe disabilities through CBI Consultants, Ltd., in Vancouver, British Columbia. She is now Professor in the Department of Educational and Counseling Psychology and Special Education at the University of British Columbia. From 1998 to 2001, she was editor of the journal *Augmentative and Alternative Communication.* In 2004, she was named a Fellow of the American Speech-Language-Hearing Association and was awarded the Killiam Teaching Prize at the University of British Columbia. Dr. Mirenda is the author of numerous book chapters and research publications; she lectures widely and teaches courses on augmentative and alternative communication, inclusive education, developmental disabilities, autism, and positive behavior support. Her current research focuses on describing the developmental trajectories of young children with autism and factors that predict the outcomes of early intervention.

About the Contributors

Laura J. Ball, Ph.D., CCC-SLP, Associate Professor, University of Nebraska Medical Center, 985450 Nebraska Medical Center, Omaha, NE 68198

Dr. Ball is a faculty member of Rehabilitation Medicine in the Department of Pediatrics at the University of Nebraska Medical Center. She coordinates the AAC program at the Munroe-Meyer Institute for Genetics and Rehabilitation. She specializes in motor speech disorders and AAC for children with developmental apraxia of speech and for adults with amyotrophic lateral sclerosis.

Susan Fager, M.S., CCC-SLP, Assistive Technology Program Coordinator, Madonna Rehabilitation Hospital, 5401 South Street, Lincoln, NE 68506

Ms. Fager is the AAC specialist and coordinator for the Assistive Technology Program at Madonna Rehabilitation Hospital. She also is a researcher in the Institute for Rehabilitation Science and Engineering at Madonna and a doctoral student at the University of Nebraska–Lincoln. She specializes in AAC and adult acquired communication disabilities.

Kathryn L. Garrett, Ph.D., CCC-SLP, Associate Professor, Department of Speech-Language Pathology, Duquesne University, 600 Forbes Avenue, Pittsburgh, PA 15282

Dr. Garrett received her B.S. degree from Penn State and her M.S. and Ph.D. degrees from the University of Nebraska–Lincoln in 1985 and 1993, respectively. She has co-authored numerous articles and chapters in the area of augmentative communication and aphasia and has also presented on the topic at regional, national, and international conferences. She currently directs a comprehensive treatment program for individuals with chronic aphasia and other neurologically based communication disorders at the Duquesne University Speech-Language-Hearing Clinic. She also teaches and conducts research on how alternative communication strategies affect the interactional competence of communicators with aphasia. Dr. Garrett is co-investigator (with University of Pittsburgh colleagues from the School of Nursing) on an NIH grant investigating how AAC and communication strategy training affects interactions between nurse caregivers and nonspeaking ICU patients.

Elizabeth K. Hanson, Ph.D., CCC-SLP, Assistant Professor, Communication Disorders Department, University of South Dakota, 414 East Clark Street, Vermillion, SD 57069

Dr. Hanson received her Ph.D. from the University of Nebraska–Lincoln. She received her M.S. from the University of Wisconsin–Madison and practiced as an AAC specialist at the Communication Development Program/Communication Aids & Systems Clinic at the Waisman Center at University of Wisconsin–Madison. While at Nebraska, Dr. Hanson supervised masters students working with clients requiring AAC services. Her professional interests include augmentative and alternative communication, motor speech disorders, and cleft lip and palate.

Joanne P. Lasker, Ph.D., CCC-SLP, Assistant Professor, Department of Communication Disorders, Florida State University, 305 Regional Rehabilitation Center, Tallahassee, FL 32306

Dr. Lasker received her doctorate at the University of Nebraska–Lincoln and was a faculty member at Western Michigan University. Currently, she is an Assistant Professor in the Department of Communication Disorders at Florida State University. As a clinician, researcher, and teacher, she has specialized in aphasia and augmentative and alternative communication. She is the author of several articles and book chapters. Her research has explored issues pertaining to AAC assessment protocols, context-based intervention practices, partner training, and the acceptance of AAC approaches by adults with aphasia and their communication partners.

Janet Sturm, Ph.D., CCC-SLP, Associate Professor, Communication Disorders, Central Michigan University, 2167 Health Prof., Mount Pleasant, MI 48859

Dr. Sturm received her doctorate at the University of Nebraska–Lincoln and completed a postdoctoral fellowship at the Munroe-Meyer Institute of Genetics and Rehabilitation in Omaha, Nebraska. Dr. Sturm's professional interests include communication in classroom environments and literacy development.

Preface

Augmentative and Alternative Communication: Supporting Children and Adults with Complex Communication Needs, Third Edition, is an introductory text written for practicing professionals, preprofessional students, and facilitators who are interested in learning more about communication options for people who are unable to meet their daily communication needs through natural modes such as speech, gestures, or handwriting. Because severe communication disorders can result from a variety of conditions, diseases, and syndromes that affect people of all ages, many individuals may be interested in these approaches. Several characteristics of the augmentative and alternative communication (AAC) field have shaped the format, content, and organization of this book.

First, AAC is a multidisciplinary field in which individuals who use AAC and their families, along with computer programmers, educators, engineers, linguists, occupational therapists, physical therapists, psychologists, speech-language pathologists, and many other professionals, have contributed to the knowledge and practice base. We have attempted to be sensitive to these multiple perspectives and contributions by directly citing pertinent information from a wide variety of sources and by guiding the reader to appropriate additional resources when necessary. In particular, we wish to acknowledge the work of Melanie Fried-Oken and Hank A. Bersani, Jr., who edited *Speaking Up and Spelling It Out: Personal Essays on Augmentative and Alternative Communication* (Paul H. Brookes Publishing Co., 2000), a book that documents the experiences of several individuals who rely on AAC, as well as the writings contained in *Beneath the Surface: Creative Expressions of Augmented Communicators* (Williams & Krezman, 2000).

Second, the AAC field has developed in many countries over the past five decades. For example, in 2005, individuals from more than 50 countries were members of the International Society for Augmentative and Alternative Communication (ISAAC). Although we are both from North America, we have made an effort to offer an international perspective in this book by including information about the contributions of AAC users, researchers, and clinicians from around the world. Unfortunately, within the constraints of an introductory textbook, only a limited number of these contributions can be cited specifically. Thus, we acknowledge that our primary sources of material have come from North America and hope that our AAC colleagues in other countries will tolerate our inability to represent multinational efforts more comprehensively.

Third, AAC interventions involve both electronic and nonelectronic systems. AAC technology changes very rapidly—products are being upgraded continually, and new products are always being introduced. Such product information presented in book form would be outdated very quickly. Therefore, we refer our readers to the AAC web site hosted by the Barkley AAC Center at the University of Nebraska–Lincoln (http://aac.unl.edu), which provides links to the web sites of manufacturers and publishers in the AAC field. Information on this web site is updated regularly. In addition, readers may refer to the resources and links in the Appendix for more information about the companies providing the AAC products and services that are mentioned in this book.

A fourth characteristic of the AAC field is that it incorporates three general areas of information. The first area relates to the processes of AAC: messages, symbols, alternative access, assessment, and intervention planning. The second area describes procedures that have been developed to serve individuals with developmental disabilities who require AAC services. The third area focuses on people with disabilities that are acquired later in life. In an effort to cover these areas, we have divided the book into three sections.

The eight chapters in Part I are organized to introduce readers to AAC processes. Chapter 1 introduces the reader to AAC in general and to people with complex communication needs in particular. Often using these individuals' own words, we attempt to convey what it means to communicate using AAC systems. Chapter 2 reviews the message types that are frequently communicated by AAC users and thus are stored in their systems. Chapter 3 is a detailed presentation of the most common aided and unaided symbol systems used to represent messages, as well as an introduction to the most common message encoding and rate enhancement strategies. Chapter 4 discusses a range of alternative access options that are designed to accommodate a variety of motor, language, and cognitive impairments. Chapter 5 focuses on team building to support AAC assessment and intervention. Chapters 6 and 7 discuss assessment, and Chapter 8 considers AAC intervention decision making. The latter three chapters also discuss in detail the interaction, participation, and consensus management frameworks that we have utilized extensively.

Part II contains six chapters that review AAC interventions for individuals with developmental disabilities. Specifically, Chapter 9 introduces AAC concerns unique to people with cerebral palsy, intellectual disabilities, autism spectrum disorders, and developmental apraxia of speech. Chapter 10 describes opportunity interventions as well as AAC strategies for individuals who communicate through nonsymbolic means. Chapter 11 focuses on techniques and strategies for beginning communicators who use symbolic approaches. Chapter 12 deals with the language development of individuals who use AAC; and Chapter 13, written with Janet Sturm, focuses on literacy development. Chapter 14 describes a framework for the educational integration and inclusion of students with AAC systems in schools.

Part III, composed of the last five chapters of the book, focuses on individuals with acquired communication disorders. Chapter 15, written with Laura J. Ball, reviews AAC interventions for adults with acquired physical disabilities, including amyotrophic lateral sclerosis, multiple sclerosis, Parkinson's disease, and brain-stem stroke. Chapter 16, written by Kathryn L. Garrett and Joanne P. Lasker, describes a functional classification scheme for people with severe aphasia and contains related intervention strategies and techniques. Chapter 17, written with Elizabeth K. Hanson, introduces AAC strategies for people with degenerative language and cognitive disorders, including primary progressive aphasia and dementia. Chapter 18, written with Susan Fager, addresses AAC assessment and intervention techniques that are organized according to the cognitive levels of people with traumatic brain injury. Finally, Chapter 19 reviews a wide range of AAC interventions for people in intensive and acute care medical settings.

We note that this third edition of this book, along with the previous two editions, were collaborative efforts, with both of us completing those tasks that fit our areas of expertise and skills. Because we shared these tasks so completely, it was difficult to order the authorship for the first edition, and we had hoped to reverse the order for subsequent editions. We have not done so, however, in order not to confuse the status of this book as a third edition.

REFERENCES

Fried-Oken, M., & Bersani, H.A., Jr. (Eds.). (2000). *Speaking up and spelling it out: Personal essays on augmentative and alternative communication*. Baltimore: Paul H. Brookes Publishing Co.

Williams, M.B., & Krezman, C.J. (Eds.). (2000). *Beneath the surface: Creative expressions of augmented communicators*. Toronto: ISAAC Press.

ACKNOWLEDGMENTS

As we revised this book, we remained keenly aware of our dependence on those who have documented their experiences in the augmentative and alternative communication field. In order to tell the "AAC story," we cited traditional documents—professional research papers, scholarly books, and manuals. We also made extensive use of the perspectives of AAC users, as documented in a variety of magazines, videotapes, and other popular sources. AAC facilitators have also contributed to this book by giving their conclusions about the AAC experience through formal and informal case studies. Thus, we wish to thank those publishers, editors, associations, manufacturers, and institutions that supported the newsletters, bulletins, books, videotapes, magazines, and journals that now contain the historical record of the AAC field. Without these resources, we simply would have been unable to compile our book.

We also want to acknowledge the role of the Barkley Trust in supporting AAC efforts at the University of Nebraska–Lincoln through the years. While we were revising this book, David R. Beukelman also served as Director of Research and Education of the Speech and Language Pathology Division of the Munroe-Meyer Institute of Genetics and Rehabilitation.

Special appreciation is also due to a number of individuals with whom we have been fortunate to work before and during the production of this book. These include the students, families, staff, and administrators of the public school system in Lincoln, Nebraska; the Institute for Rehabilitation Science and Engineering at Madonna Rehabilitation Hospital, Lincoln; the Munroe-Meyer Institute of Genetics and Rehabilitation, Omaha; the Educational Center for Students with Disabilities at the University of Nebraska–Lincoln; CBI Consultants, Ltd., Vancouver; Sunny Hill Health Centre for Children, Vancouver; Special Education Technology–British Columbia (SET-BC); and Richmond School District #38 and Surrey School District #36 in British Columbia. These individuals have collaborated with us through the years and have thus greatly contributed to our AAC experiences and knowledge. Laura Hayes and Kristin Maassen managed the composite reference list. They also organized, typed, proofed, checked, and rechecked the manuscript, and we are truly grateful for their support. We have appreciated the support, encouragement, and assistance from the people at Paul H. Brookes Publishing Co., especially Melissa Behm, Elaine Niefeld, Janet Krejci, and Tara Gebhardt. Finally, we thank those individuals who rely on AAC and their families who, through the years, have taught us about the AAC field and who have allowed us to use their stories. May their voices grow ever stronger.

To Roxy Bullock and the staffs at Meadowlane School and Lincoln East Middle/High Schools, who taught us so much about how to integrate students who relied on AAC into regular schools.

To Bill Rush, who used AAC to engage his community by writing books, newspaper columns, and personal letters. Through his writings, he taught us much about the needs and aspirations of individuals with disabilities.

To Tom Rutz and his family, who showed us how to remain fully engaged in family and community life even as amyotrophic lateral sclerosis took his natural speech and he came to rely on AAC.

To Alan Koenig, who taught us about hope, tenacity, friendship, and the power of being part of an AAC network, as he worked to regain his ability to communicate following a stroke.

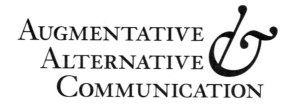

PART I

Augmentative & Alternative Communication Processes

CHAPTER 1

AUGMENTATIVE AND ALTERNATIVE COMMUNICATION PROCESSES

> The silence of speechlessness is never golden. We all need to communicate and connect with each other—not just in one way, but also in as many ways as possible. It is a basic human need, a basic human right. And much more than this, it is a basic human power. (Williams, 2000, p. 248)

Approximately 1.3% of all individuals (i.e., more than 3.5 million Americans) have such significant communication disabilities that they cannot rely on their natural speech to meet their daily communication needs. Without access to speech, these individuals are severely restricted in their communication and participation in all aspects of life—education, employment, family, and community. The development of augmentative and alternative communication (AAC) strategies offers great potential to enhance the communication of individuals with complex communication needs. However, to date, this potential has not been fully realized. There is an urgent need for people to assist those who rely on AAC strategies. In addition to helping individuals who rely on AAC and their families and caregivers, there is a continuing need to develop a range of competent AAC stakeholders. These include people who design new technologies; teachers; speech-language pathologists; physical therapists; occupational therapists; rehabilitation engineers and technicians who provide AAC intervention services; people who shape public policy and funding; and researchers who document AAC use and acceptance patterns as well as investigate communication processes when AAC strategies are used.

WHAT IS AUGMENTATIVE AND ALTERNATIVE COMMUNICATION?

A document produced by Augmentative and Alternative Communication Special Interest Division 12 of the American Speech-Language-Hearing Association (ASHA) defined AAC as follows:

> . . . AAC refers to an area of research, clinical and educational practice. AAC involves attempts to study and when necessary compensate for temporary or permanent im-

pairments, activity limitations, and participation restrictions of persons with severe disorders of speech-language production and/or comprehension, including spoken and written modes of communication. (2005, p. 1)

ASHA (2004, 2005) has defined several terms commonly used in the AAC field. AAC should be thought of as a system with four primary components: symbols, aids, strategies, and techniques. An AAC system involves the use of multiple components or modes for communication. A variety of symbol types are available for inclusion in AAC systems. These include graphic, auditory, gestural, and textured or tactile symbols, which can be unaided (such as signs, gestures, and facial expression) or aided (such as real objects, pictures, line drawings, or orthography). This means that interventions designed to increase the ability of individuals with the most severe intellectual disabilities (i.e., those requiring pervasive support) to communicate through gestures and other natural modes fall within the domain of the AAC intervention specialist.

The term *AAC aid* refers to "a device, either electronic or non-electronic, that is used to transmit or receive messages." In this text, we use the terms *aid* and *device* interchangeably. The term *technique* refers to the ways that messages can be transmitted. (See Chapter 4 for more detailed information about access techniques such as direct selection of symbol choices or scanning through choices.) Finally, an AAC *strategy* refers to the ways in which messages can be conveyed most effectively and efficiently. Strategies can have three different purposes: to enhance message timing, to assist grammatical formulation of messages, and to enhance communication rate. These four components—symbol, aid, technique, and strategy—are the critical elements that comprise all AAC interventions (ASHA, 2004, pp. 1–2).

WHO RELIES ON AUGMENTATIVE AND ALTERNATIVE COMMUNICATION?

There is no typical person who relies on AAC. People who use or need to have access to AAC come from all age groups, socioeconomic groups, and ethnic and racial backgrounds. Their only unifying characteristic is the fact that, for whatever reason, they require adaptive assistance for speaking and/or writing, because their gestural, speech, and/or written communication is temporarily or permanently inadequate to meet all of their communication needs. Although some individuals may be able to produce a limited amount of speech, it alone is inadequate to meet their varied communication needs.

A variety of congenital or acquired conditions can cause the inability to speak or write without adaptive assistance. The most common congenital causes of such severe communication disorders include intellectual disability, cerebral palsy, autism, and developmental apraxia of speech. Acquired impairments that most often result in the need for AAC assistance include amyotrophic lateral sclerosis, multiple sclerosis, traumatic brain injury, stroke, and spinal cord injury. (See Parts II and III of this book for prevalence figures and demographic information related to each of these impairments.)

Published prevalence estimates of the number of people with severe speech and/or writing impairments vary widely, depending on the country, age group, and type(s) of disability surveyed. In Canada, data from the 2001 Participation and Activity Limitation Survey (PALS) suggested that approximately 318,000 Canadians older than age 4 years have difficulty speaking and being understood (Cossette & Duclos, 2003); this represents approximately 1.5% of the total population older than age 4 years. The United States Census Bureau has estimated that 1.3% of the population (older than age 15 years) experiences difficulty in having their speech understood. Extending this percentage to the population of 281.4 million people, one might assume that approximately 3.5 million people in the United States experience complex communication needs.

Outside North America, demographic estimates of the AAC population are more variable. Paralleling the North American estimates, a study by Enderby and Philipp (1986) suggested that 800,000 individuals (1.4% of the total population) in the United Kingdom have a severe communication disorder that makes it difficult for them to be understood by anyone outside their immediate family. An Australian survey of the province of Victoria, which has more than 4 million residents, however, identified approximately 5,000 individuals who were unable to speak adequately for communication; this represents only 0.12% of the population (Bloomberg & Johnson, 1990). Similarly, a nationwide survey in Hungary conducted from 1988 to 1989 suggested that 0.06% of the population had severe speech disorders; however, this did not include people with autism spectrum disorders or with acquired disorders such as aphasia (Kalman & Pajor, 1996). The wide variations found in these studies are probably due more to the definitions and sampling techniques used than to actual differences in prevalence rates.

The prevalence of severe communication disorders also appears to vary considerably with age. Based on the results of several studies, Blackstone (1990) suggested that 0.2%–0.6% of the total school-age population worldwide has a severe speech impairment. A Canadian study suggested that the prevalence rate increases to 0.8% of individuals from age 45 to 54 years and reaches a high of 4.2% for people age 85 years and older (Hirdes, Ellis-Hale, & Pearson Hirdes, 1993).

WHAT IS IT LIKE TO RELY ON AAC STRATEGIES?

Perhaps more relevant (certainly, more interesting) than demographic figures are the stories and experiences of people who rely on AAC. In Table 1.1, we provide a number of resources that contain the writings of people who rely on AAC, as they provide first-person accounts. From these and other accounts, we can sense what it is like to be unable to communicate through traditional speech or writing and to rely on AAC. Rick Creech, a young man with cerebral palsy, provides us with a pretty stark description of being unable to speak:

> If you want to know what it is like to be unable to speak, there is a way. Go to a party and don't talk. Play mute. Use your hands if you wish but don't use paper and pencil. Paper and pencil are not always handy for a mute person. Here is what you will find: people talking; talking behind, beside, around, over, under, through, and even for you. But never with you. You are ignored until finally you feel like a piece of furniture. (Musselwhite & St. Louis, 1988, p. 104)

Table 1.1.   Selected first-person accounts by individuals who rely on augmentative and alternative communication

Blackstone, S. (Ed.). (2000). *Beneath the surface: Creative expression of augmented communicators.* Toronto: ISAAC.

Brown, C. (1954). *My left foot.* London: Secker & Warburg.

Fried-Oken, M., & Bersani, H.A., Jr. (Eds.) (2000). *Speaking up and spelling it out: Personal essays on augmentative and alternative communication.* Baltimore: Paul H. Brookes Publishing Co.

Fried-Oken, M., Howard, J., & Stewart, S. (1991). Feedback on AAC intervention from adults who are temporarily unable to speak. *Augmentative and Alternative Communication, 8,* 41–56.

Mirenda, P., & Bopp, K. (2003). "Playing the game": Strategic competence in AAC. In J.C. Light, D.R. Beukelman, & J. Reichle (Eds.), *Communicative competence for individuals who use AAC: From research to effective practice* (pp. 401–437). Baltimore: Paul H. Brookes Publishing Co.

Nolan, C. (1987). *Under the eye of the clock.* New York: St. Martin's Press.

A woman with motor neuron disease (a progressive disorder) wrote about what it was like for her and her family:

> Our lives were being turned upside down; frustration, anger, exasperation, and exhaustion were very evident. No one knew what to do for the best and the family felt helpless. . . . I have tried—and to some extent succeeded—to keep calm, because with the amount of communicating I have to do to cope each day, I would be in a permanent state of frustration. If, however, I do show some signs of frustration, I am told repeatedly to keep calm! (Easton, 1989, pp. 16–17)

In an early AAC account, Christy Brown, who first communicated by writing with chalk held in his left foot, recounted the day when he printed his first letter:

> I drew it—the letter "A." There it was on the floor before me. . . . I looked up. I saw my mother's face for a moment, tears on her cheeks . . . . I had done it! It had started—the thing that was to give my mind its chance of expressing itself. . . . That one letter, scrawled on the floor with a broken bit of yellow chalk gripped between my toes, was my road to a new world, my key to mental freedom. (1954, p. 17)

Janice Staehely comments eloquently on the limitations of one-way communication, as she writes:

> One day I was listening to a song on the radio, the song "Life is a dance; you'll learn as you go" played. The words sounded so profound to me. Just as a dance couldn't possibly be a dance unless people moved to it, so language doesn't become communication until people grow to express it back. It has to be a two-way exchange. (2000, p. 3)

Beyond having an interactive form, communication allows people to participate in activities that are important to them. Gus Estrella and Janice Staehely provide insight into how their ability to use AAC affected their family relationships:

> So how important is an augmentative communication device to a person who has a severe speech disability? And when does the importance of an augmentative communication device become more evident to the person and to their family and friends? This may vary from person to person, and it could occur during different stages in a person's life. In my personal life, the importance became more evident at different points in my life. One was definitely when my father and I started talking and sharing things that

we couldn't before. We would talk about baseball, the Los Angeles Dodgers in particular. And who can forget basketball and the Arizona Wildcats? We were finally having father and son conversations, just like the other fathers and sons were having since the beginning of time. (Estrella, 2000, p. 40)

With my new voice, my world began to open up. Cautiously at first, I went to work learning the [AAC device]. I didn't want another costly communication device collecting dust. However, my positive outlook of finally connecting with people by spoken words gave me the extra push I needed. Soon even my family's skepticism toward [my AAC device] vanished as they saw my communication with people increase. I will never forget the time when my sister was so pleased that she could keep a conversation with me going while tending her garden. (Staehely, 2000, p. 3)

AAC technology also allows people to develop social networks beyond their immediate families and those who are in face-to-face relationships with them. Sharon Price and Gordon Cardona both describe the expansion of their social networks and social roles:

When I got my new computer, I also got hooked up to the Internet and to e-mail. My world changed overnight! At the time, I was very much involved with the local Disability Services Advisory Council. With my speech problem, they had a very hard time understanding me. When I got e-mail, I had no problems. When there were questions that the council wanted my input on, all they had to do was send an e-mail, and they would get an answer right back from me. (Price, 2000, p. 114)

Currently, I use my [AAC device] to communicate at work, in meetings, and on the phone. At home, I usually communicate by facial expressions, letter signing, and typing notes on my computer. Usually when people get to know me and my communication methods, they have no trouble understanding me. Of course, some people learn faster than others. Also, e-mail plays a heavy role in my communication methods. There are many people to whom I only e-mail instead of picking up the phone and calling them. I feel e-mail is the most effective way for me to communicate. (Cardona, 2000, p. 244)

Although employment has been an illusive goal for many with complex communication needs, AAC strategies support efforts to enter or to maintain involvement in the employment arena. David Chapple, an individual with developmental disability, and Stephen Hawking, the Nobel Prize–winning scientist who has an acquired disability, both provide some insight as they write:

With the help of augmentative and alternative communication (AAC), I have achieved my goal of starting my career as a software engineer. Although I have the strong computer skills to get a job and to work competitively, AAC has helped me with all the other facets of my job: my interview, my programming work, and my relationships with peers. At my interview, I was able to respond to the questions quickly and intelligently. With my voice output communication aid (VOCA), I can store programming commands under icon sequences so I can type a programming line within seconds. Finally, AAC has helped me to express my sense of humor and technical ideas to my coworkers. (Chapple, 2000, p. 155)

Without my computer, I cannot communicate . . . . [It] has provided me with the means to continue working and researching . . . . [It] also allows me to keep in touch with my family and friends; I can e-mail and make phone calls at any time using the mobile technology. . . .It is vital for my security and safety that I can make calls for myself should the need arise. (Stephen Hawking, in an Internet interview, Intel Worldwide Employee Communications, 2003)

PURPOSES OF COMMUNICATION INTERACTIONS

The ultimate goal of an AAC intervention is not to find a technological solution to communication problems but to enable individuals to efficiently and effectively engage in a variety of interactions and participate in activities of their choice. Light (1988), in an extensive review of AAC interaction research, identified four agendas or purposes that communicative interactions fulfill: 1) communication of needs/wants, 2) information transfer, 3) social closeness, and 4) social etiquette (see Table 1.2). To Light's list, we would add a fifth purpose—to communicate with oneself or conduct an internal dialogue.

As shown in Table 1.2, the goal of expressing one's needs and wants is to regulate the behavior of the listener toward an action-oriented response. Examples include asking for help or ordering food in a restaurant. Here, the content of the message is important, the vocabulary is relatively predictable, and the accuracy and rate of message production are critical. It is likely that the high degree of predictability and concreteness inherent in these messages explains why needs/wants vocabulary often tends to predominate in many communication systems. In fact, it is not unusual to see communication books or boards that consist almost entirely of such vocabulary, regardless of how motivating or relevant the person using the AAC system finds the messages.

The second area of interaction, information transfer, involves messages that are much more complex and difficult to convey because the goal is to share information rather than to regulate behavior. Examples of people engaging in this kind of interaction include a child telling teachers what she did over the weekend, an adolescent talking with friends about the upcoming senior prom, and an adult answering questions during a job interview. As is the case with needs/wants, the content of the message is quite important. Information transfer messages, however, are likely to be composed of novel (rather than predictable) words and sentences that allow the speaker to communicate about a wide variety of topics. Accuracy and rate of message production again remain paramount.

Communication related to social closeness greatly differs from the expression of needs and wants or the transfer of information. The goal of this type of interaction relates to establishing, maintaining, or developing personal relationships. Thus, the content of the message is less important than the interaction itself. Examples of people interacting in this way include a child telling a joke to classmates, a group of teenagers cheering for their team at a basketball game, and a woman expressing her feelings of sympathy to a friend whose mother recently died. In such interactions, the rate, accuracy, and content of the message, as well as the independence of the person communicating, are secondary to the feelings achieved through the interaction, which are connectedness and, to a greater or lesser extent, intimacy.

The goal of the fourth type of interaction listed in Table 1.2, social etiquette, is to conform to social conventions of politeness through interactions that are often brief and contain predictable vocabulary. Examples of people practicing social etiquette include a child saying "please" and "thank you" to his or her grandmother and an adult expressing appreciation to a caregiver. These messages closely resemble messages that express needs

Table 1.2.   Characteristics of interactions intended to meet various social purposes

Characteristics	Social purpose of the interaction			
	Expression of needs/wants	Information transfer	Social closeness	Social etiquette
Goal of the interaction	To regulate the behavior of another as a means to fulfill needs/wants	To share information	To establish, maintain, and/or develop personal relationships	To conform to social conventions of politeness
Focus of interaction	Desired object or action	Information	Interpersonal relationship	Social convention
Duration of the interaction	Limited. Emphasis is on initiating interaction.	May be lengthy. Emphasis is on developing interaction.	May be lengthy. Emphasis is on maintaining interaction.	Limited. Emphasis is on fulfilling designated turns.
Content of communication	Important	Important	Not important	Not important
Predictability of communication	Highly predictable	Not predictable	May be somewhat predictable	Highly predictable
Scope of communication	Limited scope	Wide scope	Wide scope	Very limited scope
Rate of communication	Important	Important	May not be important	Important
Tolerance for communication breakdown	Little tolerance	Little tolerance	Some tolerance	Little tolerance
Number of participants	Usually dyadic	Dyadic, small or large group	Usually dyadic or small group	Dyadic, small or large group
Independence of the communicator	Important	Important	Not important	Important
Partner	Familiar or unfamiliar	Familiar or unfamiliar	Usually familiar	Familiar or unfamiliar

From Light, J. (1988). Interaction involving individuals using augmentative and alternative communication systems: State of the art and future directions. *Augmentative and Alternative Communication, 4,* 76; reprinted by permission of Taylor & Francis Ltd, http://www.tandf.co.uk/journals.

and wants because rate, accuracy, and communicative independence all are important factors for success.

The fifth type of interaction is to communicate with one's self or conduct an internal dialogue. In order to remain organized on a day-to-day basis, most of us make lists, enter information into our calendars, and prepare daily activity schedules. We also keep diaries, journals of our insights, lists of future plans, and record personal reflections.

Typically, there are multiple functional goals involved in any single communication interaction. In the context of AAC interventions, the intervention team must identify these goals for each person who uses AAC, so that team members can make appropriate systems and vocabulary available. One wonders how many times communication interventions have "failed" (e.g., "She has a wonderful communication system but refuses to use it") because of a discrepancy between the communication agenda of the person who uses the AAC device and an AAC specialist or parent. For example, some people who use AAC prefer to use low-technology systems that require ongoing interaction and turn taking with their communication partners (e.g., alphabet boards with messages spelled out) because they enjoy the social closeness achieved through such approaches (see Haaf, 1994, for an example). Anne McDonald, who uses such a board in addition to technology, noted that "if using the computer means I . . . [have] less personal contact then it [is not] worthwhile. I don't like using a machine if there's a person available to help me . . . . The message, not the medium, is what matters for people who cannot use their own voices" (McDonald, 1994, p. 15). Similarly, when an individual using an AAC system wants to achieve social closeness but the available vocabulary of the communication system is primarily related to needs/wants and social etiquette, problems are bound to occur. Careful attention to the needs and priorities of people who use AAC and their partners is critically important in order to maximize competence.

Communicative competence from the perspective of the person who uses AAC involves the ability to efficiently and effectively transmit messages in all four of the interaction categories, based on individual interests, circumstances, and abilities. Communication partners report that AAC users who are judged to be competent communicators also possess an additional set of skills. The research of Light (1988) and Light and Binger (1998) suggested that competent communicators are able to do the following:

- Portray a positive self-image to their communication partners

- Show interest in others and draw others into interactions

- Actively participate and take turns in a symmetrical fashion

- Be responsive to their communication partners by, for example, making relevant comments, asking partner-focused questions, and negotiating shared topics

- Put their partners at ease with their AAC system through the use of, for example, an introductory strategy (e.g., a card that says, HI, MY NAME IS GORDON; I USE THIS MACHINE TO COMMUNICATE. I WILL TOUCH THE PICTURES OF WHAT I WANT TO SAY); humor and predictable, readable nonverbal signals might also serve this purpose.

AAC teams should be aware of the fact that different types of partners might perceive the importance of various strategies related to communicative competence differently. For example, Light, Binger, Bailey, and Millar (1997) found evidence that for both adults without prior AAC experience and professionals with prior AAC experience, nonverbal feedback from those who use AAC during conversational interactions was positively related to their perceptions of communicative competence. However, adolescents without experience did not find this factor to be critical. Clearly, part of every AAC intervention should involve 1) identification of critical skills for communicative competence from the perspective of relevant listeners and 2) strategic instruction to support the highest level of communicative competence possible. Such strategies are described in detail in Chapter 11.

ASSISTIVE TECHNOLOGY IS ONLY PART OF THE ANSWER

The personal accounts of the lived experiences of persons who rely on AAC are encouraging. Certainly, assistive communicate technology can change people's lives. However,

AAC technology is not magic. We remind you that a piano alone doesn't make a pianist, nor does a basketball make an athlete. Likewise, an AAC device alone doesn't make one a competent, proficient communicator (Beukelman, 1991). Those who rely on AAC strategies begin as AAC novices and evolve in competence to become AAC experts with appropriate support, instruction, practice, and encouragement.

Light and colleagues (Light, 1989b; Light, Arnold, & Clark, 2003; Light, Roberts, Dimarco, & Greiner, 1998) described in detail the components of communicative competence for those who rely on AAC. They identify four components: linguistic, operational, social, and strategic competence.

Linguistic Competence

Linguistic competence refers to the receptive and expressive language skills of one's native language(s). It also involves knowledge of the linguistic code unique to one's AAC system, such as line drawings, words, signs, and so forth. Equally important, the people who use AAC must learn the language spoken by communication partners in order to receive messages. For the bilingual individual, this may mean learning his or her family's native language as well as that of the community at large (Light, 1989b). For individuals with acquired disabilities, much of this learning may be in place at the time of intervention, leaving only AAC-specific tasks to be mastered. For people with congenital disabilities, however, all of these skills must be learned within the accompanying physical, sensory, or cognitive constraints.

Parents, communication specialists, friends, and other facilitators can play a major role in assisting those who use AAC to master this formidable set of tasks. First, facilitators can offer ongoing opportunities for practicing expressive language (both native and augmentative) in natural contexts (Romski & Sevcik, 1996). In some cases, this may be simply helping the person to learn the augmentative symbol system or code. In other cases, especially if the individual has a history of poor generalization, facilitators may themselves have to learn the symbol system in order to provide sufficient opportunities for practice (e.g., manual signing [Loeding, Zangari, & Lloyd, 1990; Spragale & Micucci, 1990]). It is also important for facilitators to provide augmented input models in the language of the community and family as well as in the symbols or codes used in the AAC display. Receptive language input strategies may include aided language stimulation vests or boards (Goossens', 1989), symbol song strips used with music (Musselwhite & St. Louis, 1988), joint use of the AAC user's display by the facilitator (Romski & Sevcik, 1996), or key-word input provided through manual signing (see Blackstone, Cassatt-James, & Bruskin, 1988, for additional strategies). Specific strategies for encouraging linguistic competence in relation to the AAC system are discussed in greater detail in Chapter 12. Blockberger and Sutton (2003) published a summary of research related to the development of linguistic competence by those who rely on AAC.

Operational Competence

Operational competence refers to the technical skills needed to operate the AAC system accurately and efficiently. The most immediate need for people who rely on AAC and those who support them is to acquire operational competence as quickly as possible when an AAC system is introduced. This requires instruction in all operational and maintenance aspects of the device or system (see Lee & Thomas, 1990, for details). Often, the person who relies on AAC is not the primary recipient of much of this instruction, and facilitators may take on much of the responsibility for operational competence. These facilitators may be parents, spouses, or other family members; educational, residential, or vocational staff; friends; and other people who are involved in and committed to the communicative well-being of the individual who relies on AAC. In school settings, new facilitators may have to be trained in AAC operation each school year to keep pace with staff turnover and teacher and staff rotations. For example, one fourth-grade student who has worked with the same speech-language pathologist and paraprofessional since kindergarten has nonetheless had 16 people trained in operational aspects of her system over a 5-year period (Beukelman, 1991). Specifically, the needs are to 1) keep the vocabulary in the device up to date; 2) construct overlays or other displays as needed; 3) protect the device against breakage, damage, or other problems; 4) secure necessary repairs; 5) modify the system for tomorrow's needs; and 6) generally ensure day-to-day availability and operation of the device. Generally, unaided or low-tech devices require less operational competence, which is one reason why they may be preferable when capable facilitators are not available.

Social Competence

Social competence refers to skills of social interaction such as initiating, maintaining, developing, and terminating communication interactions. Of the four areas identified by Light (1989b), social competence has been the focus of most of the research in the AAC field (e.g., Kraat, 1985; Light, 1988). Social competence requires the person who relies on AAC to have knowledge, judgment, and skills in both the sociolinguistic and sociorelational aspects of communication or "competence as to when to speak, when not [to], and as to what to talk about, with whom, when, where, in what manner" (Hymes, 1972, p. 277). For example, sociolinguistic skills include abilities to 1) initiate, maintain, and terminate conversations; 2) give and take turns; 3) communicate a variety of functions (e.g., requesting, rejecting); and 4) engage in a variety of coherent and cohesive interactions. Light (1988) suggested that some sociorelational skills that are important for persons who rely on AAC to learn include 1) a positive self-image, 2) an interest in others and a desire to communicate, 3) active participation in conversation, 4) responsiveness to partners, and 5) the ability to put partners at ease.

Opportunities to practice social competence skills in natural contexts are critical for AAC users and facilitators. A number of facilitator training manuals and approaches have been developed for AAC users who have a variety of backgrounds and AAC system needs (e.g., Blackstone et al., 1988; Culp & Carlisle, 1988; Light & Binger, 1998; Light, Dattilo, English, Gutierrez, & Hartz, 1992; Light, McNaughton, & Parnes, 1986; MacDonald & Gillette, 1986; McNaughton & Light, 1989; Pepper & Weitzman, 2004; Reichle et al., 1991; Siegel-Causey & Guess, 1989). Both the number and the quality of such efforts are indicative of the importance of providing extensive training in social competence skills to both AAC users and their facilitators.

Information, training, and support efforts related to social competence must often go beyond specific training. In many cases, it is also important for AAC teams to work directly with communication partners who encounter the person who uses AAC only on social occasions. For example, friends and peers may need information about how to adjust their interactions to accommodate the requirements of the AAC system (e.g., allowing sufficient pauses for message composition). The AAC team may need to explain how to interact with someone who uses a low-tech display (e.g., echoing messages as they are indicated, in order to provide feedback). Brief in-service training to an entire school class may help to demystify the AAC system, and in many cases the individual who uses AAC can participate in or conduct these sessions. Whatever the content and however brief, communication partner interventions such as these are often just as critical as more extensive facilitator training endeavors.

Strategic Competence

Strategic competence involves the compensatory strategies that people who rely on AAC use to deal with functional limitations associated with AAC use. These may include interacting with persons unfamiliar with AAC, resolving communication breakdowns, and compensating for a slow speaking rate. Because even the most flexible AAC systems impose some interactive limitations on their users, people who use AAC need the knowledge, judgment, and skills that allow them to "communicate effectively within restrictions" (Light, 1989b, p. 141). Instruction in strategic competence involves teaching various adaptive or coping strategies to use when communication breakdowns occur. For example, the person who relies on AAC may learn to transmit the message "Please slow down and wait for me to finish," or learn to use a gesture that means "No, you misunderstood." This is another area of training from which both facilitators and those who use AAC can benefit. For example, many times those who rely on AAC appreciate the increased efficiency that results if the communication partner helps to co-construct messages by guessing. In order for this to occur, however, a facilitator or the person who uses AAC him- or herself must teach the partner how to guess accurately. Mirenda and Bopp (2003) published a summary of the research related to strategic competence in AAC.

The evolution toward expertise requires that key stakeholders are and remain AAC competent so that appropriate assessment, intervention, and mentoring can occur. It also assumes that the stakeholders are properly prepared and that the standards and guidelines of AAC practice are increasingly understood and implemented (ASHA, 2004, 2005). Unfortunately, this is not always the case. Yet, there are encouraging signs for the future. First, current research in AAC focuses on both the processes and the outcomes of AAC interventions (Schlosser, 2003b). The relatively recent emphasis on evidence-based practice in AAC will hopefully increase the information base on which AAC practice guidelines can be developed. Such guidelines will clarify appropriate intervention practices that will guide AAC service providers. The development of practice guidelines is an evolutionary process, based on the best information that the field has at any given time. Second, there is a growing awareness of the need for mentoring (or coaching) of those who rely on AAC so that they can become increasingly competent communicators. People who rely on AAC strategies face a daunting challenge to become proficient communicators when those around them typically do not use AAC techniques. In other words, they simply cannot do what typically developing children do, which is to observe their parents, family members, and peers and learn from them. Usually, AAC intervention experts provide the only coaching and mentoring for someone new to AAC technology. Unfortunately, as of 2005 the quality and availability of such mentoring varies considerably. Several efforts have been described that support mentor–protégé relationships among expert and novice AAC users (Cohen & Light, 2000; Light, McNaughton, Krezman, Williams, & Gulens, 2000).

PREPARING FOR THE FUTURE

The future success of the AAC effort depends on the preparation and development of competent AAC stakeholders. The capability of universities to prepare graduates with AAC competence is expanding. However, there are still training programs that prepare professionals to assist people with disabilities but provide little or no systematic training in AAC. This book is written in the hope that university programs that train special educators, physical therapists, occupational therapists, rehabilitation engineers, and speech-language pathologists will provide assistive technology and AAC training to their graduates.

The need is ongoing to provide continuing education to other AAC stakeholders, so they remain competent technology developers, researchers, interventionists, and public policy advocates. Because people who rely on AAC are not limited to an age category, etiology, location, or situation, and because they need ongoing support at least at some level, the need for competent AAC personnel remains urgent. It is our purpose to provide a text that will initiate the reader on a path toward AAC competence and expertise to serve individuals with complex communication needs.

OVERVIEW OF CHAPTERS

The organization of this book reflects our experiences while teaching AAC classes together at the University of Nebraska–Lincoln, as well as our solo experiences since that time. We realize that individuals from a wide range of disciplines will be introduced to AAC through this text; therefore, the chapters in Part I provide specific information about the concepts, strategies, and techniques that are unique to the AAC field. In Part II, we shift our focus to the AAC needs of people with developmental disabilities by emphasizing nonsymbolic and symbolic strategies for beginning communicators, language learning, literacy, and inclusion in school. In Part III, we deal with individuals who were at one time able to speak and write but now require AAC systems because of an acquired injury, disease, or condition.

CHAPTER 2

MESSAGE MANAGEMENT

Vocabulary, Small Talk, and Storytelling

Message management is the formulation, storage, and retrieval of messages in AAC applications (Stuart, Lasker, & Beukelman, 2000). You might consider how it would feel to be restricted to the words, phrases, and stories selected for you by someone else. Even if you could spell out all of your messages at a rate of about five to seven words per minute, you would still need complete phrases to communicate urgent messages, break into a conversation, engage in small talk, or tell a joke or a lengthy story. Obviously, the appropriateness of the messages stored in your augmentative and alternative communication (AAC) system would be very important to you. If you could pick a few people to select your messages for you, who would they be—people who know a lot about language or people who know a lot about *you?* What do you think?

AAC is about helping individuals who cannot speak well enough to meet their daily communication needs to interact with others. To that end, this book contains extensive information about symbols, communication boards, switches, displays, and speech output. However, because the central goal of AAC is to provide individuals with the opportunity and capability 1) to communicate messages so that they can interact in conversations; 2) to participate at home, in school, at work, and during recreational activities; 3) to learn their native language; 4) to establish and maintain their social roles (e.g., friend, student, spouse, mentor, and employee); and 5) to meet their personal needs, we designed this chapter to introduce the factors that influence message selection in AAC in such contexts. Because the message selection process in AAC is unique and is influenced by such a wide range of factors, this chapter provides an overview to supplement information that is included in Chapters 9–19, which cover specific interventions.

The Barkley AAC Center's World Wide Web site (http://aac.unl.edu) provides extensive messaging resources across the age span.

FACTORS THAT INFLUENCE AAC MESSAGE SELECTION

Because word selection and message formulation are such efficient processes for most typical speakers, people usually enter communication situations without giving much consideration beforehand to the words, phrases, and stories they will use. Of course, there are times when we plan our messages and even rehearse them, such as when we make marriage proposals, participate in employment interviews, and appear in court. However, message selection during natural speech interactions and written communication is usually so automatic that even most AAC specialists themselves have little experience selecting vocabulary items in advance of the acts of speaking or writing. Even interventionists who have regular contact with individuals who experience communication disorders such as stuttering, voice problems, articulation problems, and cleft palate rarely need to preselect messages to support conversational or written communication.

As we write this book, I have been assisting a close friend of mine to communicate effectively in a range of situations. He has amyotrophic lateral sclerosis and uses AAC technology. Each Tuesday evening, Tom and his wife invite members of their social and professional networks to drop by a local restaurant for "Time with Tom." They do not know who will attend or if they will visit with the usual 25–50 guests or the approximately 200 that appeared on his birthday. Of course, we have the usual "small talk" messages entered into his talking AAC device. Each week we prepare for this event by predicting the messages Tom will use and then programming pages of personal news, jokes, thoughts for the week, comments on events in the local and national news, and sports, as well as personal comments for specific individuals with special health, family or personal issues who might attend. Tom spells out novel messages as well, but with the crowd of changing guests, he doesn't have much time to prepare complex, novel messages. (D. Beukelman, personal communication, August 2004)

In addition to the lack of experience with which most AAC facilitators (i.e., people who assume or are assigned responsibility for supporting an individual's communicative efforts) approach message selection, a variety of other factors influence the types of messages used by different communicators. Differences in age, gender, and social role exert powerful influences on both natural speakers and those who rely on AAC. Children use different messages than adults. Older adults speak about different topics and use different small-talk phrases than younger adults. Men and women tend to talk about different topics. When those who rely on AAC and their facilitators represent different age, gender, and social cohorts, message selection becomes even more complicated.

In addition to generic differences in message use, individuals vary with regard to their message needs and preferences. The environments in which they live influence the ways in which they wish to communicate. Communication at home is different from that in nursing centers, community living facilities, schools, and hospitals. The type of disability experienced influences people's interactions with caregivers, medical staff, education personnel, and family. The messages included in AAC systems must reflect individual differences related to the names of family members, streets, stores, pets, and interests. Finally, differing life experiences leave individuals with different stories to tell.

For a person who experiences a disabling event or condition, the transition from being a nondisabled individual to one with a chronic disability is an evolutionary journey (Stuart et al., 2000). As one passes through the stages of awareness, loss, accommodation, and regaining of self, the need for unique vocabulary is necessary but (as of yet) poorly understood. In time, individuals with chronic disability often go on to mentor others and teach others about their journey. This also requires specialized vocabulary from that commonly available in most AAC systems.

Fortunately, the futures of individuals with lifelong disabilities are not nearly as limited as they once were (Miranda, 1993). At one time, people with lifelong disabilities lived segregated lives at home or in institutions; thus, their communication needs were quite restricted and predictable. Since the 1970s, however, societal involvement of people with disabilities has increased dramatically. As people with disabilities are included more successfully in the educational, social, religious, recreational, volunteer, and vocational realms of our communities, their communication needs change dramatically (McNaughton, Light, & Arnold, 2002). As their opportunities and choices continue to increase, their communication needs expand. Unfortunately, as persons who rely on AAC become more involved in a variety of contexts and situations, their potential for victimization also increases. Bryen, Carey, and Frantz (2003) reported that nearly half of the individuals (ages 18–39 years) who rely on AAC and participated in their survey experienced some type of crime during their lifetime. These results support the need for vocabulary that is necessary to report victimization for legal and counseling purposes.

Changes in technology have also had an extensive impact on the communication patterns of individuals with severe communication disorders. Early in the development of the AAC field, the memory and display capabilities of AAC systems were so limited that these devices could store only relatively small message sets. With new electronic designs and inexpensive computer memory, the storage and computing capacity of electronic communication devices has expanded dramatically; many now have a nearly limitless capacity for message storage. Thus, AAC devices can now include an unrestricted number of messages including those related to small talk, scripts, and stories that earlier systems could not manage. In addition, with the advent of dynamic display devices (i.e., computer screens that change like the pages of a book and use lights to signal available message options), AAC facilitators can organize and symbolize huge message pools using strategies that do not rely solely on the memory capabilities of those who rely on AAC (see Chapter 3). Finally, the voice output options available in modern AAC devices are intelligible enough to allow AAC use in a wide range of social contexts. Together, these technological advances permit the use of message sets to support communication with strangers as well as with friends and before large or small groups as well as on a one-to-one basis.

As the 21st century begins, debates over the "best" way to manage messages in AAC devices continue . . . . [D]iscussions regarding the relative merits of word-based versus phrase-based message formulation [are] recurrent themes . . . . Those who [support] word-based strategies [stress] the generative flexibility of this approach as compared with the phrase-based approach. Those who [support] phrase-based strategies [cite] improved communication rate and timing as compared with the word-based approach. AAC device designers have responded to this debate by developing a range of AAC products that utilize a variety of message management strategies . . . . It is our impression that these arguments changed little during the 1990s. Unfortunately, the debate focuses on the "best" way to design AAC devices rather than on approaches that adjust message management in response to specific concerns influencing AAC users as they participate in all avenues of life. (Stuart et al., 2000, pp. 25–26)

THE MESSAGES OF CONVERSATION

Most conversations have a rather predictable structure. Usually, a person initiates a conversation with a greeting followed by a segment of small talk. Some conversations then progress to an information-sharing segment, whereas others do not. The shared information can take a variety of forms, including stories (i.e., narratives), procedural descriptions, or content-specific conversations. Most conversations close with some wrap-up remarks and a final farewell. To provide the messages needed to support conversation, it is useful to select and organize messages with this conversational contour in mind.

Greetings

Greetings are essential to initiating social interactions. Greetings can be rather generic in that they do not usually convey specific information. Rather, they signal awareness of someone's presence, communicate the speaker's intention to be friendly, and often include a bid to start a conversation. Despite the apparent simplicity of greetings, however, AAC teams must have some awareness of the social status or ages of the individuals involved when selecting appropriate greetings. This awareness is generally communicated by the degree of formality used for the greeting. Usually, a younger person does not greet an older person or a person of higher status (e.g., an employer, a teacher) with an excessively informal or familiar message. However, at least in middle-class North American culture, it is permissible to use informal messages that may contain personal references (e.g., "Hey! Big guy!") or even mild profanity (e.g., "How ya doing, you old *&#?") with close friends or peers. Although specific greeting conventions may change from culture to culture, there is always a need for variety in this type of message. Thus, greeting messages should include a range of message options that are culturally sensitive so that individuals are able to signal their awareness of social conventions. In addition, the availability of a range of different messages discourages the overuse of the same greetings.

This week, pay attention to how you greet others. Notice that you use a variety of different greetings. Try to determine whether you understand the social rules that you use. Pay careful attention to those around you, and note the age, familiarity, and gender of individuals who say things such as "Well, hello, dear!" "Hi there!" "Goodness gracious, it's been a long time!" "Good morning!" and "What's up?"

Small Talk

Small talk is a type of conversational exchange used for initiating and maintaining conversational interactions. Small-talk scripts provide for the incremental sequence of social engagement and disengagement messages that seem necessary when people attempt to interact in a social setting. Some conversations may never progress past the small-talk stage, such as often occurs at cocktail parties. Often, however, it seems as though small talk is used as a transition between the greeting and the information-sharing stage, especially when the communication partners do not know each other well or do not possess a lot of shared information.

Adults who rely on AAC frequently report that social situations are very difficult for them. The following are remarks we have collected through the years:

"Dinner parties with my spouse kill me. Eating, talking, smiling, and small talk—it is too much to handle."

"My fiancée told me that she wouldn't go to a party with me again until I learned something about small talk!"

"I didn't get serious about learning small talk until I was 45 years old. I thought it was a total waste of time. Why should I work so hard to say nothing of content? But I was wrong."

One type of small talk in particular can be quite effective for AAC use. We call it *generic small talk* or small talk that people can use with a variety of different conversational partners because it does not refer to specific shared information. Table 2.1 contains some examples of generic and specific small talk.

In an effort to determine the relative frequency and types of generic small talk used by speakers of various ages without disabilities, several groups of researchers at the University of Nebraska–Lincoln recorded everyday conversations using portable, voice-activated tape recorders. Nearly half of the utterances of preschool children (3–5 years of age) in both home and school settings were classified as generic small talk. For young adults (20–30 years of age), 39% of all utterances were generic small talk (Ball, Marvin, Beukelman, Lasker, & Rupp, 1997; King, Spoeneman, Stuart, & Beukelman, 1995; Lasker,

Table 2.1.   Examples of generic and specific small talk

Generic	Specific
How is your family?	How is your wife?
What's happening?	What are you doing?
Isn't that beautiful!	That is a beautiful flower!
Good story!	Good story about your vacation!
She is great.	She is a great teacher.

Ball, Bringewatt, Stuart, & Marvin, 1996). Older men and women used somewhat less small talk than the young adults; 31% of the utterances of 65–74-year-olds and 26% of the utterances of 75–85-year-olds were small talk. These results confirm the extensive role of small talk in everyday communicative interactions for individuals across the age range. To interact in integrated social contexts, access to small talk and the ability to use it seems essential.

Overall, preschool children produced more utterances classified as confirmation/negation messages (26%) than any other type of small talk. They used continuers and environmental control utterances with similar frequencies. This high level of use of environmental control phrases is highly unique to preschool children, because none of the adult groups used these phrases more than 1% of the time. The young children also commented quite frequently about internal and external evaluations. For all of the adult groups, continuers were the most commonly used type of generic small-talk utterance.

The messages used during small talk vary somewhat across the age span. Those who use AAC should have opportunities to select the messages that they prefer from detailed resource lists and other sources. Detailed information about small-talk use patterns is now available on the Barkley AAC Center's World Wide Web site.

Storytelling

For adults, storytelling is a rather common communication form. Older adults in particular use stories to entertain, teach, and establish social closeness with their peers. Storytelling remains an important communication form even for adults who are unable to speak. This is particularly true as older adults begin to focus more and more of their social time on acquaintances and friends rather than on families. As these individuals lose their spouses and move to retirement or care facilities, the need to socially connect with individuals their own age becomes important, and storytelling provides a vehicle for this.

In his very interesting book, *Tell Me a Story: A New Look at Real and Artificial Memory*, Schank (1990) discussed story formulation, refinement, and storage in detail. He pointed out that we use stories from a variety of sources. *First-person stories* are those that have occurred to the speaker personally. *Second-person stories* are those that a speaker has learned from others through listening or reading. It is permissible to tell a second-person story, as long as we give credit to the source. *Official stories* are those that are used to teach a lesson or explain a phenomenon and are frequently used by families, schools, and religious groups. Finally, *fantasy stories* are those that are "made up." Marvin and her colleagues studied the communication patterns of typically developing preschool children and found that, on average, 9% of what they talked about at home and 11% of their conversations at school involved some type of fantasy (Marvin, Beukelman, & Bilyeu, 1994).

As the memory capacity of electronic AAC devices has increased and the intelligibility of speech synthesis has improved, storytelling with AAC systems has become much more practical. AAC facilitators play an important role in storytelling by assisting people who use AAC to capture stories for this type of communication. First, the facilitator must understand the story that the individual wishes to include in his or her AAC system. This is critical because storytelling is very personal and must be individualized to reflect personal experiences (e.g., through first-person stories), interests (e.g., through second-person stories), and affiliations (e.g., through official stories). Next, the facilitator can help to program the AAC device by dividing the story into segments (usually of sentence length) that the device can release sequentially with synthetic speech to tell the story, one sentence at a time. Finally, opportunities to practice telling the story should be provided. As the number of stories included in an AAC system increases, AAC facilitators also need to assist by indexing them according to the main topics, key participants, or major life events they represent so that stories can be retrieved efficiently. Of course, facilitators can also use nonelectronic AAC strategies to store and retrieve stories. For example, a man with aphasia due to stroke used to tell the story of how he got his unusual name, Roderick, by guiding his communication partner through his communication book one segment at a time, indicating the line of the story that the partner should read aloud. Other individuals may tell stories using line-drawing symbols arranged in sequential order with the written story underneath each symbol.

Procedural Descriptions

Procedural descriptions provide detailed information about processes or procedures. Usually, they 1) are rich in detail, 2) contain information that must be related sequentially, and 3) require communication that is both timely and efficient. Examples include giving someone directions about how to drive to your house for the first time or telling someone your recipe for a favorite cake. In addition to the kinds of procedures that most speakers may need to describe, many individuals with disabilities need to instruct family members and attendants about the procedures required for personal care and other specific needs. Typically, these descriptions are unique to the individual communicator.

Content-Specific Conversations

Content-specific conversations contain the informational give-and-take with which we all are familiar. Typically, these conversations are not scripted and the vocabulary in them varies widely depending on many different factors, including the communication partners themselves, the topic, the context, and so forth. To participate successfully in such conversations, unique and novel messages usually need to be able to be generated. Most individuals do so by constructing messages on a letter-by-letter or word-by-word basis.

Wrap-Up Remarks and Farewell Statements

Most communicators use wrap-up remarks to signal their desire or intent to end an interaction. Then they terminate conversations with farewell statements. Phrases such as "Nice to talk with you," "We need to talk again some time," "I have to go now," "I have work to do," "The kids need me," and "The phone is ringing" are typical wrap-up remarks in conversations. Phrases such as "See ya," "Good-bye," "So long," and "See you later" are typically used as farewell statements, at least in North America. The Barkley AAC Center's World Wide Web site contains extensive information about wrap-up remarks and farewell statements used by people of different ages.

VOCABULARY NEEDS FOR DIFFERENT COMMUNICATION MODES AND CONTEXTS

The words with which we communicate are greatly influenced by different communication contexts and modalities. For example, we speak more colloquially and casually when conversing with friends than we do when presenting a formal report to a class, business meeting, or professional group. When adults speak to young children, they use different words and grammatical structures than when they speak to other adults. Furthermore, written communication is somewhat different from spoken communication. It is important for the AAC team to have a general knowledge of these different vocabulary-use patterns when selecting vocabulary items for AAC systems.

Spoken and Written Communication

Although speaking and writing may seem to be different but equivalent ways of communicating, there are actually inherent differences between these two modes of communication that may not be immediately apparent (Barritt & Kroll, 1978). In general, spoken communication involves the use of more personal references and more first- and second-person pronouns (e.g., *I, we, you*) than does written communication. Less lexical (i.e., vocabulary) diversity is present in speech than in writing because speakers tend to repeat words more often. Speech also tends to contain shorter thought units, more monosyllabic and familiar words, and more subordinate ideas than writing.

In a study that compared spoken and written language in the classroom, McGinnis (1991) collected 1,000-word spoken and written samples from 34 third-grade students in a general education setting. She found that the students' written vocabulary was considerably more diverse than their spoken vocabulary. For example, the type-to-token ratio (TTR, the number of different words divided by the total number of words in a sample) was lower for spoken (TTR = 0.30) than for written language samples (TTR = 0.46). This indicates that the children repeated more spoken words than written words because fewer spoken words represented a greater proportion of the total language sample than did a similar sample of written words.

School Talk and Home Talk

Vocabulary use also varies for spoken communication, depending on the communication context. For example, "school talk" can be quite different from "home talk." Children do not use language in school for the same purposes, such as to meet immediate needs and achieve social closeness with familiar partners, as they do at home. Instead, children talk primarily with relatively unfamiliar adults in school in order to build a theory of reality, share their understanding of actions and situations, and acquire knowledge (Westby, 1985).

In doing so, they must "shift away from the expectation of shared assumptions (implicit meaning) to interpreting overtly lexicalized intentions (explicit meaning)" (1985, p. 187).

Few investigations have documented in detail the vocabulary-use patterns of children or adults at home and in school. One exception is the work of Marvin and colleagues (1994), which recorded the vocabulary spoken by five typically developing preschool-age children at home and in school. Approximately one third of the words produced by these children were spoken only at school, one third were spoken only at home, and one third were spoken both at home and at school. Beukelman, Jones, and Rowan (1989) reported that 100 words accounted for 60% of those produced at school by six typically developing children (3–4 years of age) when 3,000-word samples from each child were analyzed. In addition, in a related study, Fried-Oken and More (1992) reported a vocabulary core list for preschoolers based on development and environmental language sources.

Differences across specific school environments might also be expected to have dramatic effects on the words that children communicate in classrooms. The content of elementary and secondary school curricula in various subject areas requires students to have access to vocabulary items that may change daily or weekly. For example, as the topics in a student's science unit shift from plants, to planets, to prehistoric animals, to rocks, the extent to which he or she can communicate successfully in the classroom will depend largely on the availability of appropriate vocabulary. The vocabulary set designed to support a student's conversational interactions, which are relatively stable and predictable, is unlikely to be useful in meeting frequently changing curricular communication needs. (For a more complete discussion of communication patterns in school settings, see Chapter 14.)

Age Variables

Research reports suggest that age, gender, and cultural (e.g., ethnic) differences may affect the topics and vocabulary words that an individual uses during interactions. For example, researchers have investigated the communication patterns of older adults from at least two different perspectives. One perspective has been to study and document the language differences between older adults and younger people in order to describe the language impairments that people experience as they grow older. Studies from this perspective have suggested that people produce fewer proper nouns, more general nouns, and more ambiguous references as they age. In addition, the lexical variety of their nominal and syntactic structures decreases (Kemper, 1988; Kynette & Kemper, 1986; Ulatowska, Cannito, Hayashi, & Fleming, 1985). Goodglass (1980) reported that the size of individuals' active expressive vocabularies decreases quite markedly during their seventies.

A second perspective has been to view aging in terms of a model of human cognitive development, in which the performance of older adults is seen as a legitimate, adaptive stage of development (Mergler & Goldstein, 1983). Viewed from this perspective, older adults appear to tailor their communicative interactions to the unique task of "telling," that is, information sharing. In their role as "tellers," older adults relate to the past as a resource for assigning meaning to the present (Boden & Bielby, 1983). For example, Stuart, Vanderhoof, and Beukelman (1993) examined the topical references that five older women, ranging in age from 63 to 79 years, made during conversational exchanges. The younger women made more "present-oriented" comments and referred much more frequently to topics related to family life than did the older women. In contrast, the older women referred to their social networks outside the family much more often than did their younger counterparts.

Balandin and Iacono (1998a, 1998b) studied vocabulary use by adults during meal-break conversations in an employment setting. This investigation was completed in Australia. Tonsing and Alant (2004) documented the topics of social conversation in the workplace. This study was completed in South Africa. These authors reported a relatively high degree of overlap among these studies.

Gender Variables

A number of researchers have written about the influence of gender on language and word use. For example, men and women appear to use parts of speech differently. Men use fewer pronouns and more adjectives, unusual adverbs, and prepositions than do women. Women use more auxiliary words and negations than do men (Gleser, Gottschalk, & John, 1959; Poole, 1979). Men also appear to speak about different topics than women. Gleser and colleagues (1959) found that women refer to motivations, feelings, emotions, and themselves more often than do men. Men tend to refer to time, space, quantity, and destructive actions more often than do women.

Stuart (1991) summarized the work of a number of different researchers who examined the differences between "male talk" and "female talk" as follows: The studies were conducted in a Spanish village; in a traditional working-class family in England; among !Kung bushmen in Africa; during sidewalk conversations in New York City; Columbus, Ohio; and London; among women working in a telephone company in Somerville, Massachusetts; between blue-collar couples in New York; and among participants in the draft resistance movement in the United States. The results were impressively similar and can be reported collectively. Female topics were found to be people (themselves, other women, men), personal lives/interpersonal matters (age, lifestyles, life's troubles), household needs, books, food, clothes, and decorations. Male topics were found to be work (land, crops, weather, animals, prices, business, money, wages, machinery, and carpentry), legal matters, taxes, army experience, and sports or amusements (baseball, motorcycles, sailing, hunting, mountain climbing, and cockfighting). (1991, pp. 43–44)

Information about the vocabulary-use patterns of those who rely on AAC of different genders and ages is still very limited. Until such information is available, AAC specialists must be sensitive to how these factors and others (e.g., cultural differences) may affect the vocabulary selection process. Peer informants are perhaps the best source of knowledge about an individual's specific vocabulary needs, and AAC teams should use their insights as a resource to guard against the selection of inappropriate vocabulary. We have found that the summary list provided on the Barkley AAC Center's World Wide Web site provides excellent resource material from which personalized vocabulary lists can be developed.

VOCABULARY NEEDS OF PEOPLE WITH DIFFERENT COMMUNICATION CAPABILITIES

The overall communication capability of individuals who use an AAC system is another important factor that AAC teams should consider as they select vocabulary. This section discusses three types of individuals: 1) those who are preliterate, such as young children who have not yet learned to write and read; 2) those who are nonliterate, such as individuals who are not able to learn to read or write and people who have lost these abilities because of their impairments; and 3) those who are literate.

> They [people who use AAC] are unable to create spontaneously their own lexicon and must operate with a vocabulary selected by someone else or preselected, not spontaneously chosen by themselves. (Carlson, 1981, p. 140)

Vocabulary Selection for Preliterate Individuals

Individuals who are preliterate have not yet developed reading and writing skills. These individuals are often young children, but they may also be older individuals or even adults who never received the instruction needed to become literate. Thus, their AAC systems represent vocabulary items with one or more of the symbols or codes discussed in Chapter 3. Generally, the vocabulary requirements of preliterate individuals can be divided into two categories: vocabulary that is needed to communicate essential messages and vocabulary that is needed to develop their language skills.

Coverage Vocabulary

Vanderheiden and Kelso (1987) referred to vocabulary that is needed to communicate essential messages as *coverage vocabulary* because it contains messages that are necessary to cover an individual's basic communication needs. Because preliterate individuals are unable to spell out unique messages on a letter-by-letter basis, AAC teams must take care to include as many such messages as these individuals will require, regardless of how frequently they will use the messages. For example, a person may use a message such as I AM HAVING TROUBLE BREATHING very rarely, but if this could be even an occasional occurrence, it should be included in the coverage vocabulary.

Coverage vocabulary is highly dependent on the communication needs of an individual. As noted previously, these needs are likely to change, depending on an individual's age and the communicative context. For example, the coverage vocabulary needed at a birthday party would be very different from that required during a physical therapy session. Coverage vocabularies for preliterate individuals are selected through careful analyses of their environmental and communication needs. (The details of these processes are discussed later in this chapter.)

Coverage vocabularies for preliterate individuals are commonly organized by context (environment or activity) so that the words are available when needed. Thus, AAC teams may design separate communication activity displays to contain the vocabulary items that an individual needs while eating, dressing, bathing, playing a specific game, participating in specific school activities, and so forth. Team members or facilitators may situate these activity boards strategically in the environment where a particular activity takes place, such as in the kitchen, bathroom, or specific classroom area, so that they are available when needed. At other times, the individual may store activity displays in a carrying case or notebook so that the appropriate board is available for a specific communication context. (Additional activity board strategies are discussed in detail in Chapters 9, 11, and 12.) Alternatively, the AAC team may program vocabulary items into an electronic speech-generating device (SGD), using "themes" or "levels" that are contextually relevant to the individual.

Developmental Vocabulary

The vocabulary set for an AAC system may also include words that the individual does not yet know and that are selected not so much for "functional" purposes but to encourage language and vocabulary growth. At least some developmental vocabulary words should be provided to people across the age range, because language growth is an ongoing process (Romski & Sevcik, 1996). For example, if a preliterate child is about to experience something for the first time, such as a circus, then his or her AAC team may include vocabulary items associated with the new context on the communication display even though the child has never before used them. During the circus, the child's parent or friend may point to various vocabulary items on the display that are associated with the circus events such as CLOWN, LION, FUNNY, and SCARY. This gives the child opportunities to develop language and learn new vocabulary items through exposure, just as children who speak learn new words by hearing people say them over and over again.

For beginning communicators of any age, developmental vocabulary items should include words or messages that encourage them to use various language structures and combinations. For example, beginning communicators should have access to words such as *more* to indicate continuation, *no* to indicate negation, and *there* to indicate location. AAC teams might include a variety of nouns, verbs, and adjectives to support the individual's use of word combinations (e.g., *more car, no eat*). As the person's language abilities expand, team members should select vocabulary to encourage the use of combinations of two, three, and four words or more. Lahey and Bloom (1977) suggested that developmental vocabulary should include words from at least the following semantic categories:

- Substantive words (i.e., people, places, things)

- Relational words (e.g., *big, little*)

- Generic verbs (e.g., *give, get, make*)

- Specific verbs (e.g., *eat, drink, sleep*)

- Emotional state words (e.g., *happy, scared*)

- Affirmation/negation words (e.g., *yes, no, not*)

- Recurrence/discontinuation words (e.g., *more, all gone*)

- Proper names for people first and personal pronouns later; initially, proper names can be used instead of pronouns for possessives (e.g., *Mike car* instead of *his car*) as well as object–agent relations (e.g., *Pat want* instead of *I want*)

- Single adjectives first (e.g., *hot, dirty*) and their polar opposites later (e.g., *cold, clean*); initially, *not* + adjective can be used for a polar opposite (e.g., *not + hot = cold*)

- Relevant colors

- Relevant prepositions

In one study, Banajee, Decarlo, and Stricklin (2003) investigated the core vocabulary of 50 toddlers in preschool settings. They reported that all 50 children used nine common words (*I, no, yes/yeah, want, it, that, my, you, more*). Other commonly used words included *mine, the, is, on, in, here, out, off, a, go, who, some, help,* and *all done/finished.* These words represented different pragmatic functions such as requesting, affirming, and negating. No nouns were included in the list. Rescorla, Alley, and Christine (2001) studied the frequency of word use in the lexicons of toddlers. These authors provided extensive information about frequency of word use in the appendix of their article.

Vocabulary Selection for Nonliterate Individuals

Nonliterate individuals are unable to spell well enough to formulate their messages on a letter-by-letter basis and are not expected to develop or regain these spontaneous spelling skills. Most of these individuals are also unable to read, except perhaps for functional sight words that they have memorized. The vocabulary selection process for nonliterate individuals primarily aims to meet their daily, ongoing communication needs in a variety of environments. Nevertheless, the messages selected for these individuals may differ in a number of ways from those selected for preliterate individuals.

First, messages selected for nonliterate individuals are nearly always chosen from a functional rather than a developmental perspective. Single words or, more often, whole messages are selected to meet individual communication needs. These messages are represented by one or more types of symbols, as discussed in Chapter 3. Second, it is very important that the coverage vocabulary selected for nonliterate individuals is age and gender appropriate. Many of these individuals, especially those with intellectual disability or other developmental disabilities, may be adolescents or adults; special care must be taken not to select words and messages for them that are appropriate only for infants or young children. For example, a symbol of a happy face may be used for a young child to represent the word *happy,* whereas for an adolescent this same symbol might be translated to mean *awesome.* Even better, a THUMBS UP symbol might be used to represent *awesome* or *way to go* on an adolescent's display.

It is also appropriate to include at least some developmental vocabulary in the AAC systems of nonliterate individuals. For example, new messages should be added whenever new environments or participation opportunities are included in the individual's life. However, the goal is to expand the words and concepts about which the individual can communicate rather than to increase his or her use of complex syntactic forms. Again, efficient, functional communication in a variety of age-appropriate contexts is of paramount importance for these individuals.

Vocabulary Selection for Literate Individuals

Individuals who are able to read and spell have access to a greater variety of message preparation options. Literate individuals are able to formulate messages on a letter-by-letter and word-by-word basis and to retrieve complete messages, with appropriate AAC equipment, once they have been stored. Depending on the communication needs of an individual, AAC teams may prepare three different types of messages for quick retrieval: those related to timing enhancement, those related to message acceleration, and those related to fatigue reduction.

Timing Enhancement

Some messages require careful timing in order to be appropriate. Although a literate person may have the ability to spell timely messages, their meanings may be lost if they are not communicated quickly. For example, if the message PLEASE PICK UP MY FEET BEFORE YOU ROLL MY WHEELCHAIR FORWARD is not delivered in a timely manner, then it loses its relevance when the wheelchair is moved while the person is formulating the message. Thus, messages that have important timing requirements are usually stored and retrieved in their entirety. Additional examples of such messages include WAIT JUST A MINUTE, I'M NOT FINISHED YET; BEFORE YOU GO, WOULD YOU HELP ME WITH THIS?; and WHEN WILL WE MEET AGAIN? Those who rely on AAC and their facilitators are the best sources for identifying unique messages related to timing enhancement.

Message Acceleration

In addition to timing enhancement, AAC teams often select vocabulary items to accelerate overall communication rate. Vanderheiden and Kelso (1987) introduced the term *acceleration vocabulary* to refer to words or messages that occur so frequently and are so lengthy that the use of an encoding strategy to retrieve them results in substantial keystroke savings (see Chapter 3 for a more complete discussion of message encoding and communication rate enhancement). Thus, the AAC team chooses words for a message acceleration vocabulary set not to allow an individual to communicate particular ideas but rather to speed up the rate at which he or she can communicate them.

Fatigue Reduction

The third type of vocabulary set that AAC teams typically select for people who are literate is one that will result in reduced fatigue. In many cases, words and phrases that compose the acceleration vocabulary set are the same as those that are encoded to reduce fatigue. In certain situations, however, selecting vocabulary to reduce fatigue requires a slightly different approach than when selecting other kinds of vocabulary. For example, fatigue is a cumulative problem for some individuals. Early in the morning, they may be able to use their AAC systems with more physical efficiency than later in the day or the evening. In such cases, AAC teams should select fatigue reduction vocabulary items to cover these individuals' communication needs during the portion of the day when their fatigue levels are highest (e.g., the evening). In this way, they can avoid having to spell out words when they are tired. Analyses of communication patterns during periods of high fatigue can guide the selection of words and messages that will be most helpful to reduce fatigue.

VOCABULARY RESOURCES

Rarely does one individual have enough knowledge and experience to select all the vocabulary items needed in a specific environment. Rather, it is necessary to obtain this vocabulary information from a variety of sources. This section summarizes the sources that AAC teams commonly use during vocabulary selection and includes indications of the situations in which particular sources are most useful.

Core Vocabulary

Core vocabulary refers to words and messages that are commonly used by a variety of individuals and occur very frequently. Empirical research or intervention reports that assess vocabulary-use patterns of a number of individuals generally identify core vocabulary items. AAC teams have used three sources to identify core vocabularies for specific individuals: 1) word lists based on the vocabulary-use patterns of other individuals who successfully use AAC systems, 2) word lists based on the use patterns of the specific individual, and 3) word lists based on the performance of natural speakers or writers in similar contexts.

Vocabulary-Use Patterns of People Who Communicate Through AAC

Of particular interest in developing core vocabulary lists is the performance of individuals who are operationally and socially competent with their AAC systems. Researchers collected communication samples from these individuals over extended periods of time and analyzed their word-use patterns. The first of these studies involved the entire body of words produced on a letter-by-letter basis over 14 days by five young adults with disabilities who used Canon Communicators (Beukelman, Yorkston, Poblete, & Naranjo, 1984). From a composite list that consisted of all words produced by all five individuals, see Vocabulary Resources on the Barkley AAC Web site. Approximately 80% of the words communicated by the five individuals were represented by these 500 most frequently occurring words.

In subsequent research, Yorkston, Smith, and Beukelman (1990) compared the vocabulary lists produced by people who used AAC strategies during communicative interactions with six different composite word lists selected from published vocabulary sources. The 10 individuals all used spelling to express their messages. The results indicated that the individuals actually used between 27% and 60% of the words included in the various published lists.

A manual entitled *See What We Say: Situational Vocabulary for Adults Who Use Augmentative and Alternative Communication* (Collier, 2000) was developed with input from 15 adults who rely on AAC. The manual contains suggested vocabulary items for numerous situations including directing personal care; interviewing service providers; communicating about one's AAC system; communicating about seating, transportation, advocacy, banking, finances, eating out, and using the telephone; participating at a conference; sexuality; and death and bereavement.

Vocabulary-Use Patterns of a Specific Individual

Individualized word lists, which are word lists compiled from the past performance of the specific individual for whom an AAC system is being developed, are even more efficient vocabulary sources than composite lists (Yorkston et al., 1990). This is not unexpected, because it could be assumed that the past performance of an individual would be the best predictor of his or her future performance. In the past, it was difficult to obtain and analyze communication samples from an individual in order to develop an individualized word list. More recently, performance measurement and analysis technology is included in many AAC devices to help monitor vocabulary-use patterns of an individual. The privacy of such technology has been a concern, so the person who relies on AAC technology needs to be involved in any decision to monitor performance in this way (Blackstone, Williams, & Joyce, 2002). See Chapter 3 for more information.

Vocabulary-Use Patterns of Typically Developing Speakers or Writers

A considerable number of studies have examined vocabulary-use patterns of typical natural speakers and writers. These composite lists provide a rich source of core vocabulary information and can be useful when developing vocabulary lists for specific individuals. As noted previously, Yorkston and colleagues (1990) indicated that vocabulary selection for individuals who rely on AAC is quite complex because a composite vocabulary list contains only a fraction of the total words that will be needed. These authors summarized their views about the role of core vocabularies in AAC applications in the following statement:

> Our data . . . suggest that [standard word lists] are an excellent source of potential words to be included in an AAC application. The inclusion of standard word lists in the memory of an AAC device is a great timesaving for augmented communicators and their facilitators. However, these standard lists must not be taught without careful consideration. Systematic strategies are required to eliminate unnecessary or "costly" words from the standard vocabulary lists as an AAC device is individualized for a given client. (1990, p. 223)

Fringe Vocabulary

Fringe vocabulary refers to vocabulary words and messages that are specific or unique to the individual. For example, these might include names of specific people, locations, and activities, as well as preferred expressions. Such words serve to personalize the vocabulary included in an AAC system and to allow expression of ideas and messages that do not appear in core vocabulary lists. By their very nature, fringe vocabulary items must be recommended by those who use AAC or by informants who know them or their communicative situations quite well. The most important potential informant is the individual who will be using the AAC system. Their ability to serve as informants about their own vocabulary and message needs depends on numerous factors including age, cognitive and language abilities, and the level of facilitator support provided.

One type of fringe vocabulary relates to the special interests of people who rely on AAC. Through face-to-face interaction and electronic mail, they have increasing opportunities to develop and maintain these interests and to communicate with others about them. Interests—such as pets, art, gardening, sports, politics, religion, advocacy, music, technology, and investments—are associated with specialized vocabulary. To effectively support communication about these topics, specialized vocabulary must be available in one's AAC system. Higginbotham (J. Higginbotham, personal communication, November 2003) suggested that the Internet can be a useful source of specialized vocabulary and information to support special interest communication.

Informants

When selecting fringe vocabulary items, one or two AAC team members, often professionals, can have a tendency to select items without consulting a sufficient number of informants. A study by Yorkston, Fried-Oken, and Beukelman (1988) indicated that only about half of the top 100 fringe vocabulary words selected by two types of informants were the same for those who use AAC. Thus, it is clear that AAC teams should consult multiple informants to obtain the best possible list of fringe words. The most obvious informants are spouses, parents, siblings, teachers, and other caregivers. Informants such as employers, co-workers, peers, and friends often offer valuable vocabulary suggestions as well. Of course, whenever possible, those who rely on AAC should identify potential informants as well as suggest words and messages to be included or retained in the vocabulary.

Little research has examined the performance or role of informants in vocabulary selection. Morrow, Beukelman, Mirenda, and Yorkston (1993) studied three types of informants—parents, speech-language pathologists, and teachers—who often select vocabulary. Their results indicated that each of the informants contributed an important number of fringe words to the composite vocabularies for the child participants and that none of the informants could be eliminated from the vocabulary selection process. Specifically, for three of the six children involved in the study, their mothers contributed the most fringe words. For the other three children, their speech-language pathologists offered the most fringe words. Fringe words contributed by teachers, although fewer in number, were particularly crucial to classroom participation. Fallon, Light, and Paige (2001) developed and field tested a vocabulary selection questionnaire. A copy of the questionnaire is included in the appendix of their article.

Vocabulary Selection Processes

Although very little research has been done regarding how to select fringe vocabularies, important suggestions to guide this process have been made. Musselwhite and St. Louis (1988) suggested that initial vocabulary items should be of high interest to the individual, have potential for frequent use, denote a range of semantic notions and pragmatic functions, reflect the "here and now" for ease of learning, have potential for later multiword use, and provide ease of production or interpretation. In addition to the questionnaire mentioned above, several other processes have been widely used in the AAC field to facilitate achievement of these criteria, including environmental or ecological inventories and communication diaries and checklists.

Environmental or Ecological Inventories   In an effort to personalize vocabulary, several authors presented environmental or ecological inventory processes that AAC teams can use to document how the individual participates in and observes various activities (Carlson, 1981; Mirenda, 1985; Reichle, York, & Sigafoos, 1991). Carlson stated, "By discriminating between observation and participation events, it is possible to gain a better picture of the [individual's] actual experiences within the area rather than the [facilitator's] perception of the experience" (1981, p. 142). During an environmental inventory, the AAC team observes and documents the vocabulary words used by peers both with and without disabilities during frequently occurring activities. The team then reduces this pool of vocabulary items to a list of the most critical words that the student who uses AAC can manage.

> Parental vocabulary diaries . . . are invaluable supplements to professional observations. I find it is not possible to rely on such diaries for information about pronunciation or grammar, but most parents have little trouble learning how to keep a list of words used by the child during the day. (Crystal, 1987, p. 41)

Communication Diaries and Checklists   Vocabulary diaries are records of the words or phrases needed in a variety of contexts. Usually, communication diaries are kept by informants who simply record the needed vocabulary on a blank piece of paper throughout the day. Carefully constructed vocabulary checklists such as the MacArthur-Bates Communicative Development Inventory: Words and Sentences (Fenson et al., 1993) can also be useful as a shortcut to vocabulary selection, as they provide informants with ideas about potential vocabulary words from which to choose. Morrow and colleagues (1993) studied informants' reactions to the communication diary, environmental inventory (after Carlson, 1981), and vocabulary checklist processes (Bristow & Fristoe, 1984). Parents, teachers, and speech-language pathologists all rated the communication diary and environmental inventory methods as being moderately easy to use and rated the vocabulary checklist as slightly more satisfactory.

CONCLUSIONS

Various aspects of the initial vocabulary selection process have been discussed in this chapter. It is important to emphasize that vocabulary selection also involves the ongoing process of vocabulary *maintenance*. Individuals employ some words and phrases so commonly that it is easy for them and their facilitators to decide to retain them in the system. Other words and phrases may be used less frequently, either because they were poorly chosen in the first place or because they have outlived their usefulness. The latter applies particularly to vocabulary items that AAC teams selected for specific contexts, such as a particular unit of study in the classroom, or for special events, such as Thanksgiving or other holidays. Items for use in special contexts should be eliminated from the available lexicon once they are not needed, to make space for other, more important words and to reduce the cognitive load for users, who must scan many items prior to selection. Although there is no research about systematic vocabulary maintenance processes and the decision making involved in these processes, such research is sorely needed.

CHAPTER 3

Symbols and Rate Enhancement

It's summertime, and you're in the car on the way home. The light turns red, so you stop; then it turns green, and you begin driving again. While you drive, you think about the chapter you just read on messaging and find yourself wondering, "What is the relationship between messages and symbols?" As you ponder this, you notice a "detour" sign pointing to a side street because of construction, and you follow the detour. You pass by an ice cream store and decide to stop for a treat. When you walk into the store, the clerk asks for your order, and you say "I want that" and point to a full color picture of a hot fudge sundae. The clerk gives you your sundae and your change, and you smile and wave as you leave. As you begin driving again, you continue to wonder, "Messages? Symbols? How are they related?" Little do you realize that you've just experienced five examples of this relationship. *Can you find all five in the story?*

The relationship between symbols and messages is actually quite simple. All of us—not just people who use augmentative and alternative communication (AAC)—communicate messages and represent those messages with symbols. Symbols can be used both with and without communication aids such as speech-generating devices (SGDs). As illustrated in the previous example, symbols can convey whole messages such as *Stop, Go, Turn here, Thanks,* and *Good-bye,* as well as partial messages such as *(I want a) hot fudge sundae.* Even those of us who can speak use symbols every single day to both receive and send messages. Without symbols, we would not be able to communicate in writing or send nonverbal messages conveying empathy, warmth, and approval. There would be no golden arches! No mouse ears! No labels, no warning signs, no newspapers, and no textbooks! Without the ability to send messages via gestures, body language, written words, and other symbols, communication as we now know it would be a vastly different—and much less rich—experience.

Nothing so distinguishes humans from other species as the creative and flexible use of symbols. (DeLoache, Pierroutsakos, & Troseth, 1997, p. 38)

Much of the power of AAC lies in the vast array of symbols and signals, other than those used in speech, that people can employ to send messages. Especially for individuals who cannot read or write, the ability to represent messages and concepts in alternative ways is central to communication. Acknowledgment of the importance of symbols has prompted much of the research and clinical effort devoted to studying and developing comprehensive symbol systems that are easy to use and learn. In this chapter, we review many of the most commonly used types of symbols and discuss their usefulness for various individuals.

OVERVIEW OF SYMBOLS

A number of definitions and taxonomies have been used to describe symbols and their various forms (see Fuller, Lloyd, & Schlosser, 1992). Basically, a *symbol* is "something that stands for or represents something else" (Vanderheiden & Yoder, 1986, p. 15). This "something else" is termed its *referent*.

Symbols can be described in terms of many characteristics, including realism, iconicity, ambiguity, complexity, figure–ground differential, perceptual distinctness, acceptability, efficiency, and size (see Fuller, Lloyd, & Stratton, 1997; Schlosser, 2003f; and Schlosser & Sigafoos, 2002, for a review of these issues). Of these, iconicity has received the most attention from both researchers and clinicians. The term *iconicity* refers to "any association that an individual forms between a symbol and its referent" (Schlosser, 2003f, p. 350). This relationship may be based on a visual–perceptual relationship or on any idiosyncratic association made by the viewer (Robinson & Griffith, 1979). At one end of the iconicity continuum are *transparent* symbols, in which "the shape, motion, or function of the referent is depicted to such an extent that meaning of the symbol can be readily guessed in the absence of the referent" (Fuller & Lloyd, 1991, p. 217). At the other end are *opaque* symbols, "in which no [symbol–referent] relationship is perceived even when the meaning of the symbol is known" (Fuller & Lloyd, 1991, p. 217). For example, a color photograph of a shoe is transparent, whereas the written word *shoe* is opaque. Between the two extremes are *translucent* symbols, "in which the meaning of the referent may or may not be obvious but a relationship can be perceived between the symbol and the referent once the meaning is provided" (Fuller & Lloyd, 1991, p. 217). For example, one gesture commonly used in North America for *Stop!* involves moving a flat hand or finger quickly across the throat, often accompanied by a distressed facial expression. One needs to understand that this gesture of "cutting one's throat" refers to the Hollywood film industry expression *Cut!* (which also means *Stop!*). Translucent symbols are often defined by numerical ratings of the amount of relationship to a referent perceived to be present in the symbol (Lloyd & Blischak, 1992).

Symbols can be divided into those that are *aided*, which require some type of external assistance such as a device for production, and those that are *unaided*, which require no external device for production (Lloyd & Fuller, 1986). Aided symbols include real objects and black-and-white line drawings, and unaided symbols include facial expressions, manual signs, and natural speech and vocalizations. In addition, some symbol sets incorporate the use of aided and unaided elements; we refer to these as *combined symbol sets* (e.g., the Makaton Vocabulary [Grove & Walker, 1990]).

The Development of Symbol Understanding

As noted previously, the meaning of any given symbol is mediated by various factors that are intrinsic to the viewer, including his or her motivation, neurological status, age, sensory abilities, cognitive skills, communication/language abilities, and world experience (Mineo Mollica, 2003). For example, iconicity and symbol learning appear to be, at least to some extent, "culture-bound, time-bound, and, in general, experience-bound" (Brown, 1977, p. 29). Thus, Dunham (1989) found that adults with and without mental retardation differed in their abilities to guess the meanings of manual signs that adults without disabilities rated low in "guessability." The different cultural and experiential backgrounds of these two groups are among the factors likely to have influenced the results. In addition, the longitudinal work of Romski and Sevcik (1996) suggested that spoken language comprehension plays a critical role in the symbol learning process. In their work with youth with severe cognitive disabilities, these researchers found that those who understood the meanings of specific referents learned to recognize the referents' abstract symbols more readily than did individuals without such comprehension skills. Several researchers have also suggested that the reinforcement value of a referent is also likely to affect its learnability (Schlosser & Sigafoos, 2002). Thus, a very abstract symbol representing a highly desired item such as a candy bar might be more readily learned than a highly guessable symbol for a less desired item such as water. Finally, instructional factors such as the availability of voice output (Schlosser, Belfiore, Nigam, Blischak, & Hetzroni, 1995) and the teaching strategies used during instruction (Mineo Mollica, 2003) also appear to influence both initial and generalized symbol learning.

> One can never assume that young children will detect a given symbol–referent relation, no matter how transparent that relation seems to adults or older children. (DeLoache, Miller, & Rosengren, 1997, p. 312)

It is also clear that numerous developmental factors influence the ability to learn to recognize, use, and understand various types of relationships between symbols (specifically, pictures) and their referents (Stephenson & Linfoot, 1996). Developmental age appears to be one of the most salient of such factors. It is quite clear from studies of children without disabilities that the development of "pictorial competence"—the ability to perceive, interpret, understand, and use pictures communicatively—develops gradually over the first few years of life (DeLoache, Pierroutsakos, & Uttal, 2003, p. 114). Until some time in the second year, typically developing children respond to pictures as they would objects, by trying to grasp them (i.e., they perceive pictures to be *the same as* their referents) (Callaghan, 1999; DeLoache, Pierroutsakos, & Troseth, 1997). Toward the end of the second year, they begin to understand that pictures are two-dimensional objects in their own right (i.e., they perceive pictures as objects *separate from* their referents). Finally, around the middle of the third year of life, young children begin to understand that pictures can stand for objects (i.e., they perceive pictures as symbols). There is also a predictable pattern for the acquisition of graphic symbol production. In Western culture, the ability to produce simple representational drawings "from scratch" begins to emerge sometime after the third birthday and improves with regard to both accuracy and quality as children grow older (Callaghan, 1999).

In order to examine how children of different ages represent abstract language concepts across cultures, Light and her colleagues asked young children (2–7 years old) to draw pictures (i.e., symbols) of early emerging language concepts such as *what's that, who's that, more,* and *all gone* (Light & Drager, 2002; Lund, Millar, Herman, Hinds, & Light, 1998). They found the children's drawings to be very different from those depicted in commercially available AAC symbol sets. For example, the children's drawings often embedded concepts within the contexts in which they occurred, rather than depicting them generically. Thus, their drawings for the word *who* typically included a small person standing with a larger person, with a third person depicted some distance away. When asked to explain their drawings, the children said that they were the small person, standing with their parent (the large person), asking "Who's that?" when viewing someone they didn't know. This contrasts dramatically with the symbol for *who* that is featured in some AAC symbol sets, which consists of an outline of a person's head with a question mark in the middle. In several studies, these researchers have found considerable consistency in the drawings of children with disabilities (Light, Drager, Haley, & Hartnett, 2004) and those from different cultural and linguistic backgrounds as well (e.g., African American, Hispanic, Russian, Indian, and Norwegian children) (Light, Drager, D'Silva, et al., 2004). These studies suggest that typical AAC symbols may be less transparent to the children who use them than intended by their adult inventors, and this may place more learning demands on the children than is optimal.

> In European countries, the term *sign* is used instead of *symbol* as a generic term for "linguistic forms that are not speech, [including] all kinds of manual and graphic forms. (von Tetzchner & Jensen, 1996, p. 10)

UNAIDED SYMBOLS: GESTURES AND VOCALIZATIONS

> There's language in her eye, her cheek, her lip,
> Nay, her foot speaks; her wanton spirits look out
> At every joint and motive of her body.
> (Shakespeare, *Troilus and Cressida,* Act IV, Scene V)

Nonverbal behavior can repeat, contradict, substitute for, complement, accent, or regulate verbal behavior (Knapp, 1980). Nonverbal behavior includes gestures, vocalizations, and other paralinguistic elements; physical characteristics (e.g., physique, body and breath odor); proxemics (e.g., seating arrangements, personal space requirements); artifacts (e.g., clothes, perfume, makeup); and environmental factors that may influence impressions and interactions (e.g., the neatness or disorder of a room may affect how one interacts with the person who lives there). Although all of these are important elements of communication, gestures and vocalizations are perhaps the most extensive forms of non-verbal behavior and are therefore discussed in more detail in the following sections.

> At 20 months, Amy conveyed the message "You [one of several adults present in the room] give me that [a glass of water]," by orienting toward her potential partner, staring intently at her and then, once the communicative channel was open, pointing with one hand to the agent, the other to the object. (Adamson & Dunbar, 1991, p. 279, describing the communication of a young child with a tracheostomy)

Gestures

Gestural behavior includes fine and gross motor body movements, facial expressions, eye behaviors, and postures. Ekman and Friesen (1969) developed a classification system for describing these behaviors in terms of the communicative and adaptive purposes they generally serve. According to this system, *emblems* are gestural behaviors that can be translated, or defined, by a few words or a phrase and that can be used without speech to convey messages. There is usually a high level of agreement about the meaning of emblems among members of the same culture. For example, in North America, head shaking is generally understood as an emblem for *no*, whereas head nodding is an emblem meaning *yes*. People usually produce emblems with their hands, although they may use their entire bodies, as in pantomime. As is the case for verbal speech, people interpret emblems differently depending on circumstances; for example, a nose wrinkle may mean *I'm disgusted* or *Phew! That smells bad!* depending on the context.

Comprehension of some emblems may depend on a person's cognitive and language abilities. For example, individuals with Angelman syndrome (AS), a genetic disorder that results in significant cognitive/communication/motor impairments, often experience difficulty using even idiosyncratic (i.e., "natural") gestural emblems for communication (Jolleff & Ryan, 1993). In response to this dilemma, Calculator (2002) successfully taught the families of 10 children with AS to encourage the children to use gestures that were already in their repertoires but were not used communicatively; he referred to these as "enhanced natural gestures."

> Ruth talks through her eyes, facial expressions, grunts and sighs and other sounds, and selects two or three words/messages/fragments/clues from her word board to germinate the conversation. . . . Ruth's communication is, in the most fundamental sense, pure poetry. (Steve Kaplan, describing the communication skills of his co-author for the book *I Raise My Eyes to Say Yes*; Sienkiewicz-Mercer & Kaplan, 1989, pp. xii–xiii)

Illustrators are nonverbal behaviors that accompany speech and illustrate what is being said (Knapp, 1980). Among other functions, illustrators 1) emphasize a word or a phrase (e.g., pointing emphatically to a chair while saying "Sit down"), 2) depict a referent or a spatial relationship (e.g., spreading the hands far apart while saying "You should have seen the size of the one that got away"), 3) depict the pacing of an event (e.g., snapping the fingers rapidly while saying "It was over with before I knew it"), or 4) illustrate a verbal statement through repetition or substitution of a word or a phrase (e.g., miming the action of writing while saying "Where's my pencil?"). Knapp (1980) suggested that people use illustrators less consciously and less deliberately than emblems and that speakers use them most frequently in face-to-face interactions when they are excited, when the receiver is not paying attention or does not comprehend the message, or when the interaction is generally difficult.

Affect displays are facial expressions or body movements that display emotional states. Affect displays differ from emblems in that they are more subtle, less stylized, and less intentional (Knapp, 1980); in fact, in many cases, an affect display may contradict a concurrent verbal statement. The person using these subtle gestures may be largely unaware of them, although the gestures may be obvious to the receiver of the message. Affect displays that convey happiness, surprise, fear, sadness, anger, and disgust or contempt may occur cross-culturally, although their contextual appropriateness is governed by specific social rules regarding age, sex, and role position (Ekman & Friesen, 1969).

> Saying "I agree completely" while shaking the head "no" and crossing the arms in front of the body is an example of an affect display that contradicts a concurrent verbal statement.

Regulators are nonverbal behaviors that maintain and regulate conversational speaking and listening between two or more people. Regulators may function to initiate or terminate interactions or to tell the speaker to continue, repeat, elaborate, hurry up, talk about something more interesting, or give the listener a chance to talk, among other functions (Ekman & Friesen, 1969). Similar to emblems, regulators tend to be quite culturally bound (Hetzroni & Harris, 1996). In North America, head nods and eye behaviors are the most common regulators of turn-taking interactions for most people. For example, when one wishes to terminate an interaction, the amount of eye contact often decreases markedly, whereas nodding accompanied by wide-eyed gazing can urge a speaker to continue. Like illustrators, regulators are thought to be learned from watching others interact, but, unlike illustrators, they are emitted almost involuntarily. However, we are usually aware of these behaviors when they are sent by those with whom we interact.

The final category of gestures, *adaptors*, are learned behaviors that a person generally uses more often when he or she is alone; adaptors are not intentionally used in communication. Nevertheless, their use may be triggered by verbal interactions that produce emotional responses, particularly those associated with anxiety of some sort (Knapp, 1980). Adaptors can be divided into three types: self, object, and alter adaptors. *Self-adaptors* refer to manipulations of one's own body and include holding, rubbing, scratching, or pinching oneself. People often use self-adaptors with little conscious effort and with no intention to communicate, and these behaviors receive little external feedback from others; in fact, other people rarely wish to be caught looking at them. Rubbing one's nose when feeling stress and wiping around the corners of the eyes when feeling sad are two examples of this type of self-adaptor. *Object adaptors* involve the manipulation of objects, are often learned later in life, and have less social stigma associated with them. Often, the person producing these gestures is aware of them and may intend to communicate a message with them. Chewing on a pencil instead of smoking a cigarette when anxious is an example of an object adaptor. *Alter adaptors* are thought to be learned early in life in conjunction with interpersonal experiences such as giving and taking or protecting oneself against impending harm. Ekman (1976) distinguished these learned behaviors by their adaptability. For example, a child who has been physically abused may react to an adult's sudden advance by crouching and moving his or her hands toward his or her face in a protective motion. Later in life, this alter adaptor may be manifest as a step backward with a slight hand movement toward the body when a stranger approaches; this is an alteration of the initial self-protective behavior.

Some questions to ask during AAC assessment that acknowledge the differences across cultures with regard to nonverbal communication:

- Is eye contact expected when listening? When talking? For children? For adults? Does eye contact (or a lack thereof) have social significance, e.g., sign of respect? Disrespect? Insincerity?
- Is touching/hand holding a norm? Are there gender differences? What are the norms related to personal space? Displaying particular body parts?
- Is silence expected when listening? When learning? As a respect signal? Does it indicate lack of interest? Is laughter a communication device?
- Are gestures acceptable? What do they mean?
- What types of nonverbal cues are used to assist communication? To commence and terminate communication? Is turn taking consecutive or coexisting?

(Adapted from Harris, cited in Blackstone, 1993; and Hetzroni & Harris, 1996)

Vocalizations and Speech

People who have difficulty with speech often produce vocalizations that are communicative in nature. These may range from involuntary sounds, such as sneezing, coughing, hiccupping, and snoring, to voluntary vocalizations, such as yawning, laughing, crying, moaning, yelling, and belching, that often signify physical or emotional states. Some individuals are also able to produce vocalizations that substitute for speech, such as "uh-huh" for *yes* or "uh-uh" for *no*. Such vocalizations may be idiosyncratic and may require interpretation by people who are familiar with these individuals' repertoires of vocal signals.

Communication partners may also use vocalizations and speech as all or part of a communication or message display. For example, auditory scanning, either unaided or aided, can be particularly appropriate for those who rely on AAC with severe visual impairments who understand spoken language (Kovach & Kenyon, 2003). Beukelman, Yorkston, and Dowden (1985) described the use of auditory scanning by a young man who sustained a traumatic brain injury in an automobile accident. Because of the resulting impairments, he was unable to speak and was cortically blind. He communicated by having his partner verbally recite numbers corresponding to "chunks" of the alphabet, for example, 1 = *abcdef* and 2 = *ghijkl*. When his partner gave the number of the chunk he desired, he indicated his choice by making a predetermined motor movement. His partner then began to recite individual letters in the chunk until he signaled that the letter he desired had been announced. This laborious process continued until he spelled out the entire message. Similarly, Shane and Cohen (1981) described a commonly used process they called "20 questions," in which the communication partner asks questions and the person who uses AAC responds with "yes" or "no" answers. Many SGDs and software programs provide an aided form of this technique, in which the options are announced via digitized or synthesized speech (see Blackstone, 1994a, for a review).

Toni can say one word. She can raise her hand to say "yes." Kerry will say, "Some juice please, Mom." As soon as she says that, Toni will make loud noises. So I'll ask her if she wants some juice, and she'll raise her hand. A couple of months ago, we had supper and we got done eating and Kerry said, "More spaghetti please." As soon as Kerry said that, Toni, who was sitting between Dad and me, made loud noises. I said, "You want more spaghetti?" Then she shot up her hand. Now, when Toni gets off the school bus (or is taken off in her wheelchair), and the minute I pick up my teacup, she'll start with the noises. That's your cue to ask if she wants a drink. So she's figuring out ways to get her point across. (A mother describing the communication of her foster daughter, Toni, in Biklen, 1992, p. 56)

UNAIDED SYMBOLS: GESTURAL CODES

In addition to common nonverbal signals, formalized gestural codes have been developed for use by people who have communication impairments. These codes differ from sign languages because they do not have a linguistic base. Formalized gestural codes have been developed as idiosyncratic systems for individuals in nursing homes, hospitals, and residential centers (Musselwhite & St. Louis, 1988). The only gestural code that is used and disseminated in North America is Amer-Ind.

Amer-Ind

Amer-Ind is based on American Indian Hand Talk, a system used by a variety of Native American tribes to communicate across intertribal language barriers. Developed by a communication specialist who was taught Hand Talk by her Iroquois relatives (Skelly, 1979), the system consists of 250 concept labels that are equivalent to approximately 2,500 English words because each signal has multiple meanings (Musselwhite & St. Louis, 1988).

Additional meanings can be achieved through a process called agglutination, in which words can be combined to create new concepts (e.g., garage = *place* + *drive* + *shelter*). Skelly and her colleagues (Skelly, 1979; Skelly, Schinsky, Smith, Donaldson, & Griffin, 1975) reported that untrained observers accurately recognized between 80% and 88% of the hand signals. Later studies suggested that adults who do not have disabilities can guess between 50% and 60% of the signals when the signals are presented without reference to their conceptual categories (Campbell & Jackson, 1995; Daniloff, Lloyd, & Fristoe, 1983; Doherty, Daniloff, & Lloyd, 1985). Nonetheless, these signals are still considerably more guessable than American Sign Language (ASL), which has reported guessability levels between 10% and 30% (Daniloff et al., 1983).

Amer-Ind has been used with some success by children who have severe to profound cognitive disabilities (e.g., Daniloff & Shafer, 1981) as well as by adults who have aphasia, apraxia, dysarthria, dysphonia, early-stage Alzheimer's dementia, laryngectomies, and glossectomies (Bonvillian & Friedman, 1978; Daniloff, Noll, Fristoe, & Lloyd, 1982; Rosenbek, LaPointe, & Wertz, 1989; Skelly, 1979; Skelly et al., 1975; Skelly, Schinsky, Smith, & Fust, 1974; Welland, 1999). It appears that the average Amer-Ind signal can be produced at an earlier stage in motor development and requires less complex motor coordination than does the average ASL sign (Daniloff & Vergara, 1984). Therefore, this system might have advantages for people with upper extremity impairments.

UNAIDED SYMBOLS: MANUAL SIGN SYSTEMS

A number of manual sign systems, the majority of which were originally designed for and used by people who have hearing impairments, also have been used by people with severe communication disorders who are able to hear. Prior to 1990, manual signing, used alone or combined with speech, was the form of augmentative communication used most often with people diagnosed as having autism or cognitive disabilities in the United States (Matas, Mathy-Laikko, Beukelman, & Legresley, 1985), the United Kingdom (Kiernan, 1983; Kiernan, Reid, & Jones, 1982), and Australia (Iacono & Parsons, 1986). This approach has also been used to some extent in the remediation of developmental apraxia (Culp, 1989). However, controlled research studies with people with cognitive disabilities have reported mixed success, with many reports indicating that self-initiated spontaneous use of learned signs or structures often does not occur (see Bryen & Joyce, 1985, and Goldstein, 2002, for reviews). Failure to implement recommended practice strategies in manual sign assessment and intervention appears to be the primary reason for such poor clinical results (Bryen & Joyce, 1985).

Regardless of concerns related to efficacy with certain populations, manual signs continue to be useful with a wide variety of people with severe communication disorders. Lloyd and Karlan (1984) suggested six reasons why manual sign approaches might be appropriate alternatives to speech-only approaches. First, language input is simplified and the rate of presentation is slowed when manual signs are combined with speech (Wilbur & Peterson, 1998). Second, expressive responding is facilitated by reduction in the physical demands and psychological pressure for speech and by the enhancement of the interventionist's ability to shape gradual approximations and provide physical guidance. Third, vocabulary that is limited yet functional can be taught while maintaining the individual's attention. Fourth, manual signs allow simplified language input while minimizing auditory short-term memory and processing requirements. Fifth, stimulus processing is facilitated with the use of the visual mode, which has temporal and referential advantages over the speech mode. Sixth, manual signs have the advantage over speech or symbolic representation because signs are closer visually to their referents than are spoken words.

Considerations for Use

As noted previously, manual sign languages permit the coding of an essentially infinite number of messages; they also allow nuances of meaning to be added through accompanying body language. Some of the considerations relevant to the effective use of manual signs include intelligibility, motoric complexity and other considerations, and combining signs and speech or other AAC techniques, as discussed briefly in the sections that follow.

Intelligibility

The majority of ASL and Signed English signs cannot be guessed by unfamiliar individuals such as those who might be encountered on buses or in stores, recreational facilities, and other community environments (Lloyd & Karlan, 1984). This concern was illustrated in a study of two adolescents with autism who were taught to use both manual signs and the Picture Communication Symbols (PCS) system (Johnson, 1994) to order food in a restaurant (Rotholz, Berkowitz, & Burberry, 1989). Almost none of the youths' manual sign requests were understood by the restaurant counterperson without assistance from a teacher. In contrast, successful request rates of 80%–100% were reported when the PCS system was used in the students' communication books. Although the conclusions that can be drawn from this study are preliminary, it illustrates clearly the intelligibility limitations of manual signing when it is used with untrained community members and suggests that multimodal systems (e.g., manual signing plus a pictorial communication book) may be necessary.

Iconicity

Some research has shown that signs that are high in iconicity are both easier to learn and easier to recognize (e.g., Konstantareas, Oxman, & Webster, 1978; Kozleski, 1991b). Thus, facilitators who are teaching single, functional signs to beginning communicators may find it advantageous to select individual vocabulary items from several different manual sign systems (e.g., ASL, Signed English) to maximize learnability. Of course, if manual signing is being taught as a language system, such selective use of signs across systems is inadvisable.

Motoric Complexity and Other Considerations

Studies of manual sign acquisition suggest that the signs generally acquired first by young children of deaf parents are those that 1) require contact between the hands (Bonvillian & Siedlecki, 1998); 2) are produced in the "neutral space" in front of the signer's body or against the chin, mouth, forehead, or trunk (Bonvillian & Siedlecki, 1996); 3) require a single, simple manual alphabet handshape such as 5 (spread hand), G (index finger points), A (fist), or B (flat hand) (Bonvillian & Siedlecki, 1998); and 4) require bidirectional movements (e.g., to-and-fro, up-and-down) (Bonvillian & Siedlecki, 1998). Because signs with these characteristics are acquired earliest and produced most accurately by typical children, one can surmise that such signs are among the "easiest" to learn.

In addition, Doherty (1985) noted that, ideally, signs taught in the same environment or time frame should be dissimilar from other signs being taught; for example, teaching the signs for both EAT and DRINK during lunch in the school cafeteria is probably not a good idea because these signs are both motorically and conceptually similar. Finally, and most important, manual signs selected for instruction should be motivating and functional. Selecting signs for initial instruction that meet all of these requirements is a formidable task because it appears that functionality and learnability may be at least somewhat incompatible (Luftig, 1984). Nonetheless, Musselwhite and St. Louis (1988) provided a useful matrix to make decisions about signs to be included in an initial lexicon. A modified form of the matrix is presented in Table 3.1.

Combining Signs and Speech or Other AAC Techniques

Simultaneous or total communication requires that manual signs be presented at the same time as words are spoken, usually in the context of a telegraphic or key-word signing approach (see Bonvillian & Nelson, 1978; Casey, 1978; Konstantareas, 1984; and Schaeffer, 1980). Multiple research studies have found a combined manual sign plus speech intervention to be more effective in establishing production and/or comprehension skills than either mode taught singly (e.g., Barrera, Lobato-Barrera, & Sulzer-Azaroff, 1980; Brady & Smouse, 1978). However, some individuals may be more apt to attend to the manual sign component than the speech component when the two modes are combined (Carr, Binkoff, Kologinsky, & Eddy, 1978). Furthermore, some research has suggested that the usefulness of simultaneous instruction may depend on whether the individual has mastered generalized imitation at the point of intervention (Carr & Dores, 1981; Carr, Pridal, & Dores, 1984).

Interventions combining manual signs, speech, and other AAC techniques may also be useful for some individuals for reasons other than enhanced intelligibility to unfamiliar partners. For example, a series of studies by Iacono and her colleagues demonstrated that instruction with manual signs plus line-drawing symbols on an SGD appeared to have advantages over sign-alone instruction in teaching the use of two-word utterances (Iacono & Duncum, 1995; Iacono, Mirenda, & Beukelman, 1993; Iacono & Waring, 1996). In addition, the use of a multimodal system has the advantage of "covering all the bases" in instances in which it is not clear which symbol system might be best (Reichle, York, & Sigafoos, 1991). Finally, for some individuals, such as children with developmental apraxia of speech (DAS), a multimodal AAC system might well be the system of choice (Cumley & Swanson, 1999).

A videotape, *Early Use of Total Communication: Parents' Perspectives on Using Sign Language with Young Children with Down Syndrome,* and an accompanying booklet by Gibbs and Springer, are available from Paul H. Brookes Publishing Co. The videotape illustrates how total communication, an approach in which speech and sign language are used simultaneously, creates an avenue for children with Down syndrome to communicate successfully.

Table 3.1. Decision-making matrix for selecting manual signs for initial instruction

Code: Numbers in parentheses in each category indicate weightings that reflect the relative importance of the factor. For example, "preference" has a weighting of 3, compared with "contact," which has a weighting of 1. This means that learner preference is considerably more important than physical contact between the two hands when selecting the sign (although both have been found to be related to the rate of acquisition). A plus sign (+) indicates that a sign meets the requirement (assign 1 point × weighting) and a minus sign (−) indicates that it does not (0 points). AAC teams can use this matrix to decide which signs to teach first (i.e., those with higher overall scores from a potential pool of signs).

According to this example, the signs to teach first to this learner should include MORE and EAT, followed by PLAY and MUSIC, with TOILET lowest on the list of five potential signs.

Sign	Learner and representational factors			Motoric factors				Total score
	(3) Preference	(2) Used frequently	(1) Transparent	(1) Contact between hands	(1) Produced in neutral space	(1) Single, simple hand shape	(1) Simple bidirectional movement	
MORE	+++	++	0	+	+	+	+	10
TOILET	0	++	0	0	0	+	+	4
EAT	+++	++	+	0	+	+	+	9
MUSIC	+++	+	0	0	0	+	+	6
PLAY	+++	++	0	0	+	0	+	7

Source: Musselwhite & St. Louis (1988).

Augmentative and Alternative Communication: Supporting Children and Adults with Complex Communication Needs, Third Edition, by David R. Beukelman and Pat Mirenda. Copyright © 2005 Paul H. Brookes Publishing Co., Inc. All rights reserved.

There simply are no clear, empirically validated guidelines to use when making decisions about when and with whom to use manual signs in combination with other techniques. Thus, facilitators must make such decisions based largely on experience and logic. The available evidence suggests that multimodal instruction does not appear to reduce an individual's motivation to speak and may in fact enhance it (e.g., Cregan, 1993; Silverman, 1995).

Types of Manual Sign Systems

The term *manual sign system* actually refers to three main types of systems: 1) those that are alternatives to the spoken language of a particular country (e.g., ASL, Swedish Sign Language), 2) those that parallel the spoken language (manually coded English [MCE]), and 3) those that interact with or supplement another means of transmitting a spoken language (e.g., fingerspelling). We review the primary manual sign systems used in North America in the sections that follow, with particular reference to their applicability to AAC interventions.

National Sign Languages

In most countries, national sign languages have been developed through use by the Deaf community for many years. In the United States and most of Canada, ASL or Ameslan is used within the Deaf community for face-to-face interactions. In the province of Quebec, Canada, a distinctly different system, Langue des Signes Québécoises (LSQ), is used by people who are deaf.

ASL is related neither to English nor to the sign languages of other countries, so Deaf communities in China, France, Great Britain, Japan, Norway, Sweden, and many other countries have their own distinct languages. Only a few teachers of people with hearing impairments in the United States appear to use ASL with their students; thus, it is not a pedagogical language, although it is the predominant language of the Deaf community (Hoffmeister, 1990). Because ASL does not follow or approximate English word order, it is not used concurrently with speech.

"Sign It" is a game that teaches more than 800 ASL signs as players move their markers to complete a treacherous journey on the board. An accompanying book *Signing Illustrated,* illustrates over 1,350 ASL signs and expressions. The game is available from Permanent Reflections in Toronto, Ontario, Canada.

Pure-form ASL is rarely used with people who have communication difficulties not primarily due to a hearing impairment. Instead, an invented manual signing approach, in which ASL signs are combined with speech and produced in English word order, is often used. This technique is termed *key-word signing* (KWS) and is discussed in a following section in this chapter.

Manual Sign Parallel Systems (Manually Coded English)

In North America, a number of manual sign systems that code English word order, syntax, and grammar have been developed for educational use with individuals with hearing and other communicative impairments. These systems have been referred to as educational sign systems (Musselwhite & St. Louis, 1988), pedagogical signs (Vanderheiden & Lloyd, 1986), and MCE (Karlan, 1990; Vanderheiden & Lloyd, 1986). We use the term *MCE* in acknowledgment of its common use in the Deaf community (Stedt & Moores, 1990).

Outside North America, many manual sign parallel systems have been developed for use by persons with severe communication disorders. For example, in Ireland, Lámh (the Communication Augmentation Sign System) is used widely by children with intellectual disabilities (Kearns, 1990). Similarly, simplified sign lexica based on Finnish Sign Language (Pulli & Jaroma, 1990) and Swedish Sign Language (Granlund, Ström, & Olsson, 1989) have been used in Scandinavia.

The three most commonly used MCE systems in North America are Pidgin Sign English (Woodward, 1990), Signed English (Bornstein, Saulnier, & Hamilton, 1983), and Signing Exact English (SEE-2) (Gustason, Pfetzing, & Zawolkow, 1980). All three of these can be used in conjunction with tactual reception of signing by individuals with deaf-blindness who learned to sign before becoming blind (Reed, Delhorne, Durlach, & Fischer, 1990). In addition, KWS, a type of MCE, has been developed primarily for use with people who have communication disorders and cognitive disabilities but can hear. We discuss these four MCE systems in the sections that follow.

Pidgin Sign English   Pidgin Sign English (PSE) is perhaps best described as ASL-like English when used by people who can hear and English-like ASL when used by people who have hearing impairments (Woodward, 1990). Many versions of PSE have evolved from interactions between skilled deaf and hearing signers. One of the most common varieties is Conceptually Accurate Signed English (CASE), which combines English grammatical order with ASL signs, invented signs, and fingerspelling. Because of the considerable geographical variability in PSE dialects, few studies have described the grammatical characteristics of this MCE system. PSE appears to be used extensively in the education of students who have hearing impairments in a total communication context, in conjunction with speech or extensive mouthing of English words (Woodward, 1990).

Signs of the Times (Shroyer, 1982) presents 1,185 CASE signs organized into 41 lessons that contain clear illustrations of all vocabulary, English glosses and synonyms, sample sentences to define vocabulary context, and practice sentences to clarify sign language usage. The book also includes suggestions for teachers, an appendix of conceptual signs, an extensive index, and a reading reference list. It is available from Gallaudet University Press.

Signed English   Signed English was designed in the early 1970s as a simple and flexible alternative to existing manual English systems. Although originally designed for preschoolers with hearing impairments, it has been expanded and adapted so that it can be used by older students as well (Bornstein, 1990). Signed English consists of more than 3,100 signs and uses 14 sign markers (e.g., *-ed, -ing*).

Signed English has been used for many years in conjunction with speech with students with cognitive disabilities, and it was the first manual sign system reported to be successfully implemented with children with autism (Creedon, 1973). Bryen and Joyce (1985) reported that Signed English was identified in the majority of studies of students with cognitive disabilities that named a specific manual sign system.

A wide variety of support materials are available for classroom and community use of Signed English, including the *Comprehensive Signed English Dictionary* (Bornstein et al., 1983), texts, storybooks, flash cards, videotapes, coloring books, songbooks and records, poems, and posters. These are available through Gallaudet University Press.

Signing Exact English   Signing Exact English (SEE) was first made available in 1972 and uses modified and supplemented ASL signs to give a clear and complete visual presentation of English. It consists of approximately 4,000 signs and more than 70 word ending, tense, and affix signs (e.g., *-est, -ed, -ing, -ment, un-*). The system was developed around 10 basic grammatical principles that ensure internal consistency and provide guidelines for adding new signs (see Gustason, 1990). SEE is motorically and linguistically more complex than Signed English and may, therefore, be less useful for people with severe communication disorders not due primarily to hearing impairments (Musselwhite & St. Louis, 1988). However, it is widely used in Deaf communities around the world, and is believed to enhance the ability to learn English and to acquire English literacy skills (S.E.E. Center for the Advancement of Deaf Children Web site: http://www.seecenter.org/).

Numerous SEE support materials, including articles, story books, videotapes, illustrated dictionaries, flash cards, songs, and posters are available for parents, teachers, and others through the Modern Signs Press (Los Alamitos, CA; http://www.modsigns.com/).

Tactual Reception of Signing   Tactual reception of signing is commonly used by individuals with deafblindness who acquire their knowledge of sign language before becoming blind (Reed et al., 1990). In this method, the deafblind person places one or two hands on the dominant hand of the signer and passively traces the motion of the signing hand. Thus, the various formational properties of signs are received tactually by the deafblind person, who then communicates expressively using conventional sign language. Tactual signing can be used in conjunction with ASL, PSE, or Signed English. Research suggests that individuals with experience in the tactual reception of signing can receive approximately 1.5 signs per second; this compares favorably with typical signing rates of 2.5 signs per second for visual reception of signs by individuals who can see (Bellugi & Fischer, 1972; Reed, Delhorne, Durlach, & Fischer, 1995).

Key-Word Signing   With KWS (Grove & Walker, 1990; Windsor & Fristoe, 1989), spoken English is used simultaneously with manual signs for the critical words in a sentence, such as base nouns, base verbs, prepositions, adjectives, and adverbs. Thus, the sentence *Go get the cup and put it on the table* might involve the use of the signs GET, CUP, PUT, ON, and TABLE while the entire sentence is spoken.

The term *key-word signing* probably most accurately describes the majority of interventions that use manual signs in English word order and that have been used with people with disabilities other than hearing impairments. Because these interventions almost always include the use of speech in addition to manual signs, they have been referred to as total communication or simultaneous communication approaches. Bryen and Joyce (1985) reported that of 25 studies they reviewed in which some type of manual sign system was used with students with severe cognitive disabilities, 4 purported to have used ASL, 6 used Signed English, 2 used what is now referred to as SEE, and 13 used other or unspecified systems. It is quite likely that KWS, using signs from the other named systems, was the approach actually used in the majority of these studies.

> The distinction between ASL, Signing Exact English, key-word signing, and other MCE systems is important in order to respect the legitimacy of ASL as the language of the Deaf culture as well as to be precise in sharing empirical and clinical results of interventions.

Manual Supplements to Spoken Language

Manual systems that interact with or supplement spoken English have been used with children who have hearing impairments and, to a limited extent, with individuals with communicative disorders to support the development of speech and literacy skills. Nevertheless, most of these techniques (including gestural or eye-blink codes) have not achieved widespread use in the field of AAC. One exception is Cued Speech (Kipila & Williams-Scott, 1990), a system of eight hand shapes that represent groups of consonant sounds plus four positions around the face that represent groups of vowel sounds and diphthongs. Combinations of these hand configurations show the exact pronunciation of words in concurrent speech. Cued Speech has been adapted to approximately 60 other spoken language and dialects around the world (Caldwell, 1997). Like SEE, Cued Speech is primarily used to improve the early English language development of children who are deaf and to provide them with a foundation for English reading and spelling. However, it has also been used in combination with other techniques to support communication development in individuals with autism, Down syndrome, cerebral palsy, and other disorders (Caldwell, 1997).

AIDED SYMBOLS: TANGIBLE SYMBOLS

Rowland and Schweigert (1989, 2000a) coined the term *tangible symbol* to refer to two- or three-dimensional aided symbols that are permanent, manipulable with a simple motor behavior, tactually discriminable, and highly iconic. We use the term in a more restricted sense to refer to symbols that can be discriminated based on tangible properties (e.g., shape, texture, consistency); thus, we do not include two-dimensional (i.e., pictorial) symbols in this category. Tangible symbols are typically used with individuals with visual or dual sensory impairments and severe cognitive disabilities, but they may also be appropriate for other populations (e.g., as beginning communication symbols for children with visual impairments; see Chen, 1999). Tangible symbols discussed in the following sections are real objects, miniature objects, partial objects, artificially associated and textured symbols, and other tangible symbols.

Real Objects

Real object symbols may be identical to, similar to, or associated with their referents. For example, an identical symbol for *brush your teeth* might be a toothbrush that is the same color and type as the individual's actual toothbrush. A similar symbol might be a toothbrush of a different color and type, whereas an associated symbol might be a tube of toothpaste or container of dental floss. Other examples of associated symbols include a sponge that represents *cleaning the kitchen counter* or an audiocassette that represents *music time* in the preschool classroom. Associated symbols may also include remnants of activities—items such as a ticket stub from the movies or a hamburger wrapper from a fast-food restaurant.

Many people with cognitive disabilities are able to match identical and nonidentical (i.e., similar) object symbols with similar accuracy (Mirenda & Locke, 1989). This suggests that both types of object symbols may be equal in enabling recognition of their referent; however, it is important to be cautious in this assumption, especially with beginning communicators. It is also important to consider the individual sensory input needs of individuals with visual impairments when selecting real objects for them to use. Rowland and Schweigert (1989, 1990, 2000b) reported numerous examples of successful use of real object symbols with individuals who have visual and dual sensory impairments.

Miniature Objects

Miniature objects may be more practical than real objects in some situations but need to be selected carefully to maximize effectiveness (Vanderheiden & Lloyd, 1986). For example, miniatures that are much smaller than their referents may be more difficult for students with cognitive disabilities to recognize than some types of two-dimensional symbols (Mineo Mollica, 2003; Mirenda & Locke, 1989). Nevertheless, miniature objects that are reasonably smaller than their referents have been used successfully with individuals with cerebral palsy (Landman & Schaeffler, 1986); dual sensory impairments (Rowland & Schweigert, 1989, 2000b); and a wide variety of cognitive, sensory, and/or motor impairments (Rowland & Schweigert, 2000b).

In addition to size, tactile similarity is also critical when using miniature objects with people who cannot see. It is unlikely that an individual with visual impairments will readily recognize the relationship between a miniature plastic toilet and a real toilet because they feel different with respect to size, shape, and texture. In this case, a real object associated with the toilet (e.g., a small roll of toilet paper) might be more appropriate as a bathroom symbol.

People with visual impairments "see" with their fingers and hands, so the tangible symbols they use should be tactually similar to or associated with their referents. For example, Catherine, a woman with dual sensory impairments, wears a pair of leather half-gloves (i.e., gloves with the fingers cut off) whenever she goes horseback riding. She uses the same gloves as tangible symbols for horseback riding in her schedule system at home, because they remind her of (and smell like!) this activity.

Partial Objects

In some situations, particularly those that involve referents that are large, partial objects may be useful symbols. For example, the top of a spray bottle of window cleaner may be used to represent *washing the windows* at a vocational site. Also included in this category are "symbols with one or two shared features" (Rowland & Schweigert, 1989, p. 229), such as thermoform symbols that are the same size and shape as their referents. The use of partial objects may be a good alternative when tactile similarity cannot be met with miniature objects.

Artificially Associated and Textured Symbols

Tangible symbols may also be constructed by selecting shapes and textures that can be artificially associated with a referent. For example, if a wooden apple is attached to a cafeteria door, then a similar apple could be used to signify *lunchtime* (Rowland & Schweigert, 1989, 2000a). Textured symbols, a subtype of artificial symbols, may be either logically or arbitrarily associated with their referents. For example, a piece of spandex material would be a logically associated textured symbol to represent a bathing suit because many suits are made of this material. Alternatively, a square of velvet could be arbitrarily selected to represent a favorite snack. Several case studies have documented the successful use of textured symbols with individuals with one or more sensory impairments in addition to severe cognitive disabilities (Locke & Mirenda, 1988; Mathy-Laikko et al., 1989; Murray-Branch, Udvari-Solner, & Bailey, 1991).

Other Tangible Symbols

Case study reports have documented the usefulness of adapting line-drawing symbols, such as Blissymbols, for use with people with visual impairments (Edman, 1991; Garrett, 1986). This approach creates a tactually discriminable relief symbol using a thermoform process, photoengraving, or other method. The individual then learns to associate the raised outline of the symbol with its referent.

> Instructional materials and videotapes developed by Rowland and Schweigert related to the use of tangible symbols are available through Design to Learn. A manual for using tangible symbols with individuals with autism (Vicker, 1996) is available from the Indiana Resource Center for Autism.

AIDED SYMBOLS: REPRESENTATIONAL SYMBOLS

Many types of two-dimensional symbols can be used to represent various concepts. These representational symbols include photographs, line drawings, and abstract symbols. We review the major representational symbol types used in North America in terms of their relative iconicity, as well as in terms of those individuals with whom they have been used successfully.

Photographs

High-quality color or black-and-white photographs may be used to represent objects, verbs, people, places, and activities. Photographs may be produced with a camera or obtained from catalogs, magazines, coupons, product labels, or advertisements (Mirenda, 1985). A research study found that people with cognitive disabilities matched color photographs to their referents somewhat more accurately than black-and-white photographs (Mirenda & Locke, 1989). Another study found that people with intellectual disabilities matched black-and-white photographs to their referents more accurately than line drawings (Sevcik & Romski, 1986). Dixon (1981) found that students with severe disabilities were more able to associate objects with their color photographs when the photographic objects were cut out than when they were not. Reichle and colleagues (1991) suggested that the context in which a photograph appears might affect an individual's ability to recognize it; for example, a photograph of a watering can may become more recognizable when it appears next to a photograph of a plant.

> Digital or printed sets of high-quality color or black-and-white photographs are available from companies such as the Attainment Company, Early Learning Images, Mayer-Johnson, Inc., Silver Lining Multimedia, and Speechmark Publishing.

Line-Drawing Symbols

Over the years, many sets of line-drawing symbols have been developed in North America and elsewhere to meet the needs of individuals with complex communication needs. Some, such as Picsyms (Carlson, 1985) and Self-Talk symbols (Johnson, 1986), are no longer commercially available but are mentioned briefly in this section in comparison with other symbol sets. The primary sets that are used in North America are highlighted in more detail.

Picture Communication Symbols (PCS)

Figure 3.1 illustrates PCS, a widely used system of more than 7,000 clear, simple black-and-white or color line drawings (Johnson, 1994). The PCS system can be purchased in a variety of printed formats, including stamps and photocopiable symbol books. Both Windows- and Macintosh-based versions of a software program called Boardmaker (Mayer-Johnson, Inc.) can generate communication displays made of either black-and-white or color PCS in 24 languages, including several that use non-Roman alphabets (e.g., He-

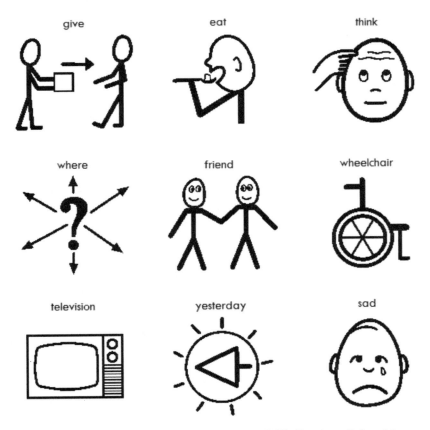

Figure 3.1.   Examples of Picture Communication Symbols (PCS). (From Lynne E. Bernstein, Ed. *The Vocally Impaired: Clinical Practice and Research* published by Allyn & Bacon, Boston, MA. Copyright © 1988 by Pearson Education. Reprinted by permission of the publisher. The Picture Communication Symbols™ © 1981–2004 by Mayer-Johnson LLC. All Rights Reserved Worldwide. Used with permission.)

brew, Korean, Japanese, Russian, and Hmong [Vietnam]). In addition, the PCS for more than 500 verbs have been animated and are available in color. In addition, a wide variety of PCS teaching materials are also available.

Three research studies (Mirenda & Locke, 1989; Mizuko, 1987; Mizuko & Reichle, 1989) indicated that both PCS and Picsyms are more transparent than Blissymbols for preschoolers without disabilities and for school-age and adult individuals with cognitive disabilities. In a comparative study of Blissymbols, PCS, Pictogram symbols, Picsyms, and rebus symbols, PCS and rebuses were learned more easily across nouns, verbs, and modifiers (Bloomberg, Karlan, & Lloyd, 1990). One study found that PCS for concrete nouns (e.g., APPLE) were learned more readily by children with cerebral palsy than those for abstract nouns (e.g., DIRECTION) (Hochstein, McDaniel, Nettleton, & Neufeld, 2003). In a cross-cultural study, 147 adults whose first language was either English (both European Americans and African Americans), Chinese, or Mexican Spanish agreed that PCS representing nouns, verbs, and adjectives were more closely related to their word meanings than either DynaSyms or Blissymbols (Huer, 2000; see also Huer, 2003, and Nigam, 2003). Research studies on the learnability of PCS indicated that preschoolers without disabilities learned more PCS over three trials than either Picsyms or Blissymbols (Mizuko, 1987), whereas adults with cognitive disabilities appeared to find PCS and Picsyms equally learnable (Mizuko & Reichle, 1989). AAC teams have used PCS successfully in AAC interventions with people with cognitive disabilities (Heller, Allgood, Ware, Arnold, & Castelle, 1996; Mirenda & Santogrossi, 1985), cerebral palsy (Goossens', 1989), deaf-blindness (Rowland & Schweigert, 2000b), and autism (Hamilton & Snell, 1993; Rotholz et al., 1989), among other impairments.

An extensive catalog of Picture Communication Symbols and related products can be obtained from Mayer-Johnson, Inc. (Solana Beach, CA). In addition, PCS greeting cards are available from Giving Greetings (Sudbury, MA).

Rebus Symbols

A *rebus* is a picture that visually or nominally represents a word or a syllable. For example, a rebus of a knot could be used to symbolize either *knot* or *not*. There are many types of rebuses (Vanderheiden & Lloyd, 1986), but the most common collection of these in North America was developed as a mechanism for teaching young children without disabilities to read (Woodcock, Clark, & Davies, 1968). This work was adapted and expanded as a system of communication symbols for people with communication impairments (Van Oosterum & Devereux, 1985). The Rebus Symbol Development Project in the United Kingdom has expanded on this work and developed numerous software and other products that incorporate rebuses. Figure 3.2 depicts several Widgit rebuses.

Dictionaries and software products that utilize the Widgit Rebus Symbols are available in the United Kingdom and many other countries from Widgit Software

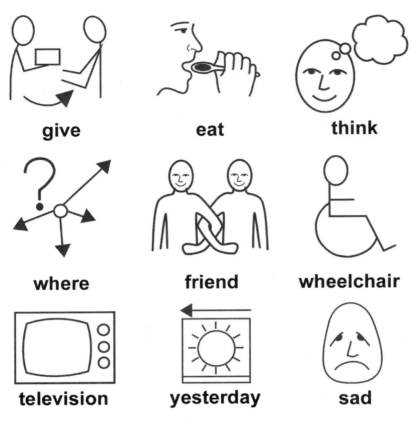

give eat think

where friend wheelchair

television yesterday sad

Figure 3.2. Examples of Widgit Rebus Symbols. (Widgit Rebus Symbols used with permission from Widgit Software Ltd. Tel: 01223 425558.)

Ltd. In addition, *Writing with Symbols 2000,* a symbol-supported reading and writing software product from Don Johnston, Inc., incorporates both 4,000 Widgit Rebuses and 3,800 PCS. It is available in English as well as several other languages, including Turkish, Hebrew, and Welsh.

DynaSyms

DynaSyms are a set of over 3,000 symbols that are currently available on the Dynamo and the DynaVox 4 Series of dedicated communication devices (see Figure 3.3). DynaSyms are also available in cut and paste and sticker formats, in both back-and-white and color books of 1,000 and 1,700 symbols each. Each symbol comes with the printed word above it. Aside from the study by Huer (2000) mentioned previously, no research has been conducted to compare DynaSyms with other types of communication symbols with regard to either learnability or transparency. However, because DynaSyms are quite similar to Picsyms, their predecessors, the research related to Picsyms is probably applicable. Several studies found that Picsyms were similar to or slightly more difficult to learn than PCS and rebus

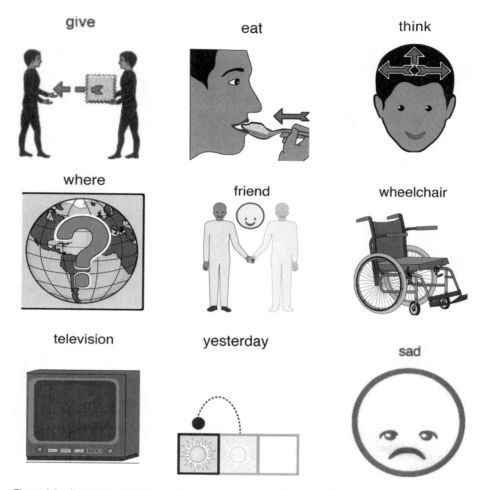

Figure 3.3. Examples of DynaSyms. (From Glennen, S., & DeCoste, D. [1997]. *Handbook of augmentative and alternative communication.* San Diego: Singular; reprinted by permission.)

symbols but easier to learn than Blissymbols (Bloomberg et al., 1990; Mirenda & Locke, 1989; Mizuko, 1987; Mizuko & Reichle, 1989; Musselwhite & Ruscello, 1984).

DynaSyms are available in dedicated communication devices available from DynaVox Systems LLC. Print versions in both black-and-white and color are available from Poppin and Company, along with communication bags, totes, posters, and yes/no symbol products.

Pictogram Symbols

Often confused in name with Picsyms and PCS, the Pictogram symbol set was developed in Canada and consists of almost 1,000 white-on-black symbols designed to reduce

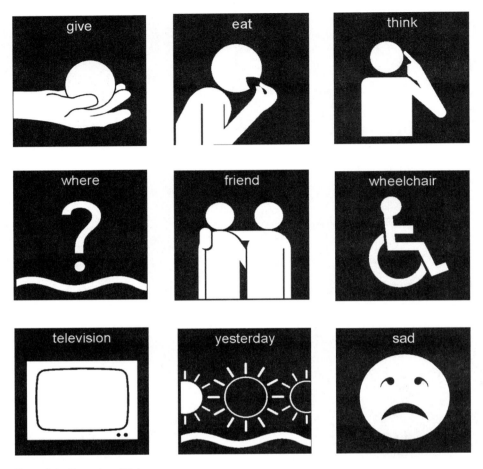

Figure 3.4. Examples of Pictograms.

figure–ground discrimination difficulties (Maharaj, 1980). Figure 3.4 illustrates some of these symbols.

Reichle and colleagues (1991) and Vanderheiden and Lloyd (1986) summarized a number of studies that indicate that white-on-black pictures are not necessarily more visually salient than standard black-on-white drawings. In a study with adults who did not have disabilities, Pictogram symbols (which at that time were called Pictogram Ideogram Symbols) were found to be less translucent than PCS and rebus symbols but more translucent than Blissymbols (Bloomberg et al., 1990). Leonhart and Maharaj (1979) reported that adults with severe to profound cognitive disabilities learned PIC symbols faster than Blissymbols. Pictogram symbols have also been used with people with other severe or profound disabilities (Leonhart & Maharaj, 1979; Reichle & Yoder, 1985) and with people with autism (Reichle & Brown, 1986), typically in conjunction with communication books or boards.

Pictogram symbols have been adapted for use in Sweden, Norway, Finland, Holland, Belgium, Iceland, Portugal, Italy, and Japan. In North America, Pictogram symbols are available from ZYGO Industries, Inc., in both print and CD-ROM (Windows) formats, with and without text captions.

Blissymbolics

The history of Blissymbolics is complex and fascinating (see the original work by Charles Bliss, 1965, as well as historical records of Blissymbolics development in Canada in the early 1970s [Kates & McNaughton, 1975] for an in-depth explanation of the history of Blissymbolics). Generally, the system was developed to function as an auxiliary language for international written communication. It consists of approximately 100 basic symbols that can be used singly or in combination to encode virtually any message (Silverman, 1995). The current system is composed of more than 3,000 symbols; new Blissymbols are added periodically by an international panel affiliated with Blissymbolics Communication International (BCI) (see Figure 3.5 for examples of several Blissymbols).

In addition, a collection of Blissymbols is available that has been enhanced by pink line-drawing cues (Blissymbolics Communication International, 1984). These enhanced Blissymbols are designed to remind both the new Bliss learners and novice instructors of the concepts that the symbols represent, and they appear to have positive effects on both acquisition and retention of Blissymbols (Raghavendra & Fristoe, 1990, 1995).

Blissymbolics is used in over 33 countries and has been translated into 17 languages. Blissymbolics dictionaries, software (e.g., AccessBliss), research reports, videotapes, teaching materials, and training workshops can be obtained through Blissymbolics Communication International (BCI, Canada). Enhanced Blissymbols books, stamps, flashcards, and a teaching manual are also available through BCI.

Numerous studies have indicated that of all the representational symbols in common use, Blissymbols are the least transparent, the most difficult to learn, and the hardest to retain (Bloomberg et al., 1990; Huer, 2000; Hurlbut, Iwata, & Green, 1982; Mirenda & Locke, 1989; Mizuko, 1987). Why, then, is this system so widely used in the AAC field? Vanderheiden and Lloyd (1986) noted some major strengths of Blissymbolics:

1. The principles and strategies for combining symbols enable expression of thoughts not on the communication board. The symbols are conceptually based and constructed using consistent, systematic rules.

2. The symbols can be introduced simply and later expanded.

3. The use of Blissymbolics is compatible with other techniques including reading and writing.

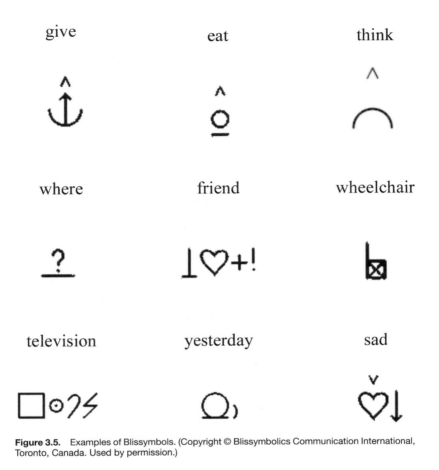

Figure 3.5.   Examples of Blissymbols. (Copyright © Blissymbolics Communication International, Toronto, Canada. Used by permission.)

Many computerized tools have been developed around the world to support Blissymbolics, including Blissvox from Hungary (Olaszi, Koutny, & Kálmán, 2002) and Bliss for Windows and other Bliss software products from the Netherlands (Handicom). In addition, BlissInternet and BlissWrite software can be used together to translate between text and Bliss in both directions, so that people who use Blissymbols can communicate via the Internet.

Other Pictorial Systems

Several additional representational symbol systems are also available, although they have not been studied in terms of relative guessability and learnability. Some of these merit brief mention.

The computerized COMPIC system from Australia contains over 1,700 pictographic symbols, most of which are available in both black and white and color formats (Bloomberg, 1990). COMPIC symbols, software, videotapes, and instructional materials are available from the Communication Resource Center in Victoria, Australia. In the province of Quebec, Commun.i.mage, a computer-based line-drawing symbol system of more than 1,000 symbols that is available with French, English, and Spanish labels, is available through the Centre Québécois de Communication Non Orale in Montreal (Flouriot & De Serres, 2000).

Pick 'n Stick   Pick 'n Stick symbols are color pictographs arranged categorically and available on peel-back pages as well as on CD-ROM for both Windows and Macintosh. The 2,500 symbols in the set are not accompanied by written labels, so each symbol can be used flexibly to represent one of many related concepts (e.g., a symbol of a person sunbathing may be used to mean *sunbathe, relax, weekend,* or *suntan*). There is no available research concerning the relative iconicity of these symbol sets.

Pick 'n Stick symbols and software are available from PRO-ED, Inc. (Austin, TX).

Talking Pictures   Talking Pictures are sets of black-and-white line drawings that are available on cards with printed labels in either ASL or in English, French, German, Italian, and Spanish on the reverse side of each card. They depict a range of functional, community living, and daily living vocabulary words. They also come in a sticker format, with a variety of support materials.

Talking Pictures I, II, and III can be ordered from Crestwood Communication Aids, Inc. (Milwaukee, WI).

Oakland Schools Picture Dictionary   The Oakland Schools Picture Dictionary consists of over 700 black-and-white line drawing symbols, more than 75% of which are nouns (Kirstein, 1981). The symbols have been translated into several languages, including French, Hebrew, and Spanish. Included are symbols for vocational concepts and adult vocabulary items not found in other similar sets of symbols. Oakland symbols compared favorably with PCS and rebus symbols on both transparency and translucency tasks with adults who had cognitive disabilities and those who did not in a study of symbols representing emotions (Francis, Nail, & Lloyd, 1990).

The Oakland Schools Picture Dictionary is available from Oakland Schools in Waterford, Michigan.

Pictographic Communication Resources   Pictographic Communication Resources (PCRs) were developed to assist health professionals and other conversation partners (e.g., family members) to communicate with adults who have aphasia and other acquired communication impairments. They include adult-oriented symbols designed to explain aphasia and to facilitate interactions between adults with disability and nurses, social workers, physical and occupational therapists, physicians, counselors, chaplains, and family members.

Pictographic Communication Resources are available through the Aphasia Institute in North York, Ontario (Canada).

Gus! Communication Symbols   Gus! Communication Symbols are the most recent North American addition to the symbol set family and they consist of 2,500+ color line-drawing symbols representing standard vocabulary words as well as words related to entertainment, sports, current events, politics, and other common topics of conversation. The set was designed to appeal to adolescents and adults as well as children, and free downloads of new symbols are available monthly. Another unique feature is the availability of custom-designed symbols based on photographs of specific people (e.g., family members, friends).

Gus! Communication Symbols are available from Gus Communications, Inc. (Bellingham, WA).

AIDED SYMBOLS: ABSTRACT SYMBOL SYSTEMS

Abstract symbol systems include symbols for which form does not suggest meaning. The most widely known and used abstract symbol set is Yerkish Lexigrams. Blissymbolics is not considered abstract because at least some symbols are pictographic.

Yerkish Lexigrams

The abstract Yerkish lexigram symbols resulted from a primate research project designed to develop a computer-based system for studying language acquisition in chimpanzees (Rumbaugh, 1977). The lexigrams are composed of nine geometric forms used singly or in combinations of two, three, or four to form symbols, and they usually appear as white element combinations on black backgrounds (Romski, Sevcik, & Pate, 1988). Because children and adults do not typically have experience with lexigrams, they have been used in research studies where it is important to control the amount of previous exposure to symbols (e.g., Brady & McLean, 2000). For example, lexigrams were originally used in studies investigating the symbol-learning abilities of institutionalized adolescents and young adults with mental retardation requiring extensive support (Romski et al., 1988; Romski, White, Millen, & Rumbaugh, 1984). Lexigrams have also been used successfully as symbols on SGDs with children with mental retardation requiring limited and extensive supports (Romski & Sevcik, 1996).

AIDED SYMBOLS: ORTHOGRAPHY AND ORTHOGRAPHIC SYMBOLS

Traditional orthography refers to the written characters used to transcribe a particular linguistic system (e.g., English letters, Chinese characters). Orthography has been used in AAC systems in the form of single letters, words, syllables (e.g., prefixes, suffixes), sequences of commonly combined letters (e.g., *ty*, *ck*, *th*), and phrases or sentences (Beukelman, Yorkston, & Dowden, 1985; Goodenough-Trepagnier, Tarry, & Prather, 1982).

The term *orthographic symbol* is used to refer to aided techniques that represent traditional orthography, such as braille and fingerspelling. These are differentiated from *orthographic codes*, which use letters as message abbreviations and are discussed later in this chapter.

Braille

Braille is a tactile symbol system for reading and writing that is used by people with visual or dual sensory impairments. Braille characters are formed by combinations of six embossed dots arranged within a cell of two vertical columns of three dots each (see Figure 3.6). From top to bottom, the dots are numbered 1–3 on the left column and 4–6 on the right. The characters represent letters, parts of words, or entire words. Each character is formed according to a standard pattern within the six-dot cell.

There are two methods of writing braille. One method uses one-to-one correspondence between each letter and braille cell; in this method, called "uncontracted braille," all

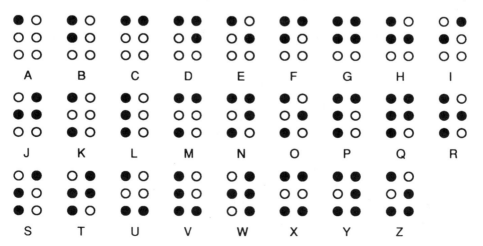

Figure 3.6. English braille alphabet. Darkened circles represent embossed dots.

words are spelled out. The second method uses special symbols (called contractions) that stand for entire words or combinations of letters (such as *-er, ch, -ation*); this method, called "contracted braille," is used to produce most textbooks and trade books. The official rules for braille transcription in both Canada and the United States can be found in *English Braille–American Edition* (1994, with a revision in 2002).

Anything that can be written in print can also be written in braille. The six-dot braille cell is used internationally, but different countries use specific contractions for different letter combinations in different languages. In addition to being the standard literacy code for reading and writing, the six-dot braille cell is also used to represent mathematics, scientific notation, music, and computer codes. In general, although there are hundreds of symbols in the various codes, all codes use the standard six-dot cell design but assign different meanings to the same symbol (Huebner, 1986). English-speaking countries (including Australia, Canada, New Zealand, South Africa, Nigeria, the United Kingdom, and the United States) are currently exploring the feasibility of adopting a single braille code for use with English texts.

The International Council on English Braille, which has representatives from Australia, Canada, New Zealand, South Africa, Nigeria, the United Kingdom, and the United States, is currently conducting the Unified Braille Code (UBC) Research Project. The goal of this project is to develop a single braille code providing notation for mathematics, computer science, and other scientific and engineering disciplines as well as general English literature.

Fingerspelling (Visual and Tactual)

Sign language systems such as ASL use fingerspelling to represent single letters of the alphabet that can be combined to spell words for which there are no conventional signs (i.e., proper names). Interest in literacy instruction for persons who rely on AAC has drawn attention to this feature of sign language because of its potential to assist beginning readers to learn the phonological code needed for reading and writing. Because many fingerspelled letters appear to be visually similar to their graphic counterparts, the learning of letter–sound relationships might be enhanced by pairing the two, at least during initial instruction (Koehler, Lloyd, & Swanson, 1994). There is some evidence of the efficacy of such an instructional strategy with individuals who can speak but have difficulty learning to read (Blackburn, Bonvillian, & Ashby, 1984; Wilson, Teague, & Teague, 1984).

In addition, the tactual reception of fingerspelling is a mode of communication that is commonly used by people with dual sensory impairments who are literate. Information is transmitted in fingerspelling by placing the hand of the information receiver over the hand of the individual formulating the letters (Jensema, 1982; Mathy-Laikko et al., 1987). Research has shown that, at communication rates of approximately two syllables per second (roughly half that of typical speaking rate), experienced deafblind individuals can receive key words in conversational sentences at roughly 80% accuracy using tactual reception of fingerspelling (Reed et al., 1990).

COMBINED SYMBOL SYSTEMS (AIDED AND UNAIDED)

Formal symbol systems that incorporate the use of at least manual signs with graphic symbols became popular in North America in the 1980s and have been used with people who do not speak. In general, use of such systems is based on the assumption that if a single augmentative communication technique works, then using more than one technique should work even better. These combined systems differ from individualized communication systems that incorporate multiple modes (e.g., Hooper, Connell, & Flett, 1987) in that symbols are combined in a standard intervention package. The combined symbol system that is currently used most widely in augmentative communication is the Makaton Vocabulary.

Makaton Vocabulary

Makaton is a language program offering a structured, multimodal approach for the teaching of communication, language, and literacy skills. Devised for children and adults with a variety of communication and learning disabilities, Makaton is used extensively throughout the United Kingdom. The approach combines speech, manual signs, and graphic symbols. The core vocabulary consists of approximately 470 concepts organized in a series of nine stages, plus an additional section, that correspond to the order in which the words are introduced. For example, Stage 1 consists of 39 concepts that meet immediate needs and can establish basic interactions, whereas Stage 5 consists of 50 words that can be used in the general community. In addition, there is a large resource vocabulary of approximately 7,000 concepts for which there are manual signs and symbols illustrated by the Makaton Vocabulary Development Project (MVDP). Makaton symbols are illustrated in Figure 3.7.

The MVDP requires that signs from the sign language of a country's Deaf community are matched to the Makaton Vocabularies, which are adapted to suit cultural needs in collaboration with the MVDP. Thus, in the United Kingdom, a combination of British Sign Language (BSL) and British Signed English signs are used, whereas in the United States, the signs are taken from American Sign Language (ASL). The MVDP has produced a specific collection of Makaton signs and symbols that are related to the main core subject areas of the British National Curriculum, including information on developing literacy skills through Makaton. These include Makaton symbols and signs (from British Signed English) for all the grammatical elements of English as well as for many European and Asian languages.

The Makaton Vocabulary program has been adapted for use in over 50 countries, including New Zealand, Australia, Canada, United States, France, Germany, Spain, Portugal, Switzerland, Norway, Malta, Greece, Turkey, Kuwait, Saudi Arabia, Bahrain, Egypt, Sri Lanka, Pakistan, India, Nepal, Hong Kong, Japan, Uganda, Namibia, and Zimbabwe. The Makaton Vocabulary Development Project distributes a variety of Makaton resource and training materials and organizes training courses in Great Britain and other countries.

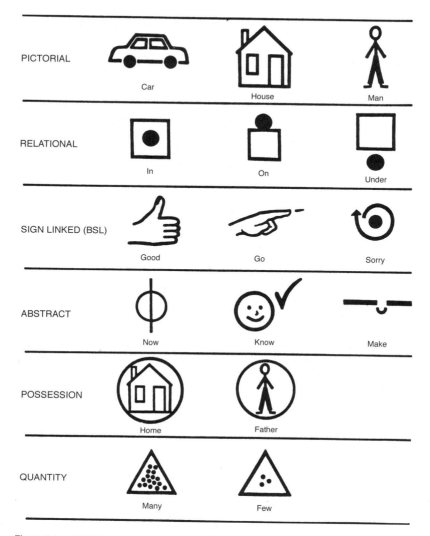

PICTORIAL

Car   House   Man

RELATIONAL

In   On   Under

SIGN LINKED (BSL)

Good   Go   Sorry

ABSTRACT

Now   Know   Make

POSSESSION

Home   Father

QUANTITY

Many   Few

Figure 3.7.   Examples of Makaton symbols. (From Grove, N., & Walker, M. [1990]. The Makaton Vocabulary: Using manual signs and graphic symbols to develop interpersonal communication. *Augmentative and Alternative Communication, 6,* 23; reprinted by permission of Taylor & Francis Ltd, http://www.tandf.co.uk/journals.)

With regard to instruction, Makaton can be used and taught either with a *key-word approach*, in which only the main information-carrying words are spoken, signed, and represented graphically, or with a grammatical translation approach, in which the complete word order of the language is used (much like SEE-2 is used with students in North America who are deaf). Makaton is taught through structured behavioral interventions and in natural contexts (Grove & Walker, 1990). Margaret Walker, the author of Makaton, emphasizes that, although the program is organized in stages and within a structure, practitioners are free to modify the system to meet individual student needs regarding the symbols used; the vocabulary introduced; and the procedures for assessment, instruction, goal setting, and data collection (Grove & Walker, 1990). The Makaton approach has been used successfully with children and adults with mental retardation, autism, specific language disorders, multiple sensory impairments, and acquired neurological problems affecting communication (Walker, 1987).

RATE ENHANCEMENT TECHNIQUES

The conversational speaking rates of natural speakers who do not have disabilities vary from 150 words per minute to 250 words per minute (Goldman-Eisler, 1986). These speaking rates allow for efficient communication of extensive messages, which are formulated and spoken virtually simultaneously. One has only to view the interaction patterns among a talkative, animated group of friends to realize the importance of efficiency in communication in order for all speakers to take their conversational turns and communicate their messages before someone else claims the floor.

In addition to communicating efficiently, natural speakers formulate spoken messages to meet the needs of the particular communicative situation. During spoken interaction, much of the meaning of a message can be derived from the context and the timing of the message. For example, we frequently mumble greetings to friends or colleagues as we pass them in the hallway at work. It is only because of the context that such poorly articulated messages can be understood. As we watch a sporting event with friends, someone may exclaim, "That's not fair!"—a message with no referent, which can be understood and appreciated only if it is produced in a timely fashion, not 3 minutes after someone has fumbled the ball.

Unfortunately, communication inefficiencies and message-timing limitations interfere with the communication interactions of many individuals who use AAC symbols to communicate. For example, the AAC rates of those who use aided symbols were reported to be less than 15 words per minute under most circumstances (Foulds, 1980, 1987). In many cases, the rates are much less—often two to eight words per minute. These rates are only a fraction of those achieved by natural speakers. Clearly, such drastic reductions in communication rate are likely to interfere significantly with communication interactions, especially in communicative situations with natural speakers who are accustomed to exchanging information at a much more rapid pace.

One factor contributing to the slowed communication rates of individuals who use aided AAC is that they usually compose messages by selecting the component parts (e.g., pictures or other symbols, letters of the alphabet, words) from their communication displays, one item at a time. Obviously, this requires considerable time and effort. A strategy that is often used to increase communication rates is to store complete words, phrases, or sentences in AAC systems and to assign a code of some type to the stored message. Then, rather than communicating messages incrementally, the individual is able to convey an entire message by using a single code.

Hoag, Bedrosian, McCoy, and Johnson (2004) examined the impact of both message informativeness and speed of message delivery on shopkeepers' attitudes toward adults who use SGDs. They found that messages that were delivered quickly but contained excessive information, and messages that were delivered slowly both with and without "floorholders" (e.g., "Please wait while I prepare my message") were rated similarly. However, quickly delivered messages with inadequate information were rated significantly lower. From this study, it appears that the accuracy of message content is more important than communication rate, when a trade-off between the two must be made.

AAC teams have developed and implemented a number of coding and retrieval strategies over the years. The term *encoding* identifies any technique in which the one gives multiple signals that together specify a desired message (Vanderheiden & Lloyd, 1986). How codes are represented—that is, the type of symbols used—is an individual decision that should be matched to a person's capabilities. Whether memory-based or chart-based codes are used is also an individual decision. Memory-based codes require that the person have excellent long-term memory skills while chart-based codes (i.e., codes that are presented on a chart or menu, or that are recited aloud so the person can choose) require either good visual skills or good auditory discrimination skills. A chart-based display that might be used for eye pointing is illustrated in Figure 3.8. In this figure, the AAC communicator looks at the numbers 5 and 2 sequentially. The partner decodes this message, which represents the letter *d*, using her chart. The person using AAC then continues to spell a message or send an alphabetic code by indicating additional letters. Obviously, the rate of communication depends on how efficiently the AAC communicator and the partner can visually locate the desired code or message on the chart.

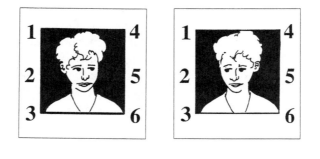

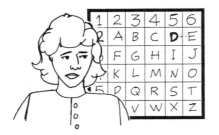

Figure 3.8.   Chart-based display used for eye pointing.

Word Codes

Several types of codes are used to represent single words. These include various letter, numeric, and alphanumeric techniques, as described in the sections that follow.

Alpha (Letter) Word Codes

Two types of letter codes are typically used for single words. Truncation codes abbreviate words according to the first few letters only (e.g., *HAMB = hamburger; COMM = communication*), whereas contraction codes include only the most salient letters (e.g., *HMBGR = hamburger; COMUNCTN = communication*). Truncation codes often have fewer letters and are thus easier to construct, but contraction codes may have the advantage of being more flexible. Both types of codes can be either memory-based or display-based.

Alphanumeric Word Codes

Alphanumeric codes use both letters and numbers for words. For example, *COMM 1* might mean *communicate; COMM 2 = communication; COMM 3 = community*, and so forth. As can be seen from these examples, the advantage of this approach is that the same letters can be used repeatedly across words that are differentiated by number.

Letter-Category Word Codes

When letter-category codes are used for words, the initial letter is usually the superordinate category and the second letter is the first letter of the specific word. For example, if *F = fruit* and *D = drinks, FA* might mean *apple, FB = banana, DC = coffee, DM = milk*, and so forth. Again, this encoding technique can be used in either memory- or display-based systems, depending on the ability of the person using it.

Numeric Encoding

Occasionally, numeric codes alone are used to represent words or messages. For example, numeric codes may be used when a communication display must be quite small, in order to accommodate a person's limited motor capabilities. In this case, it is advantageous if items in the small selection set can be combined in many ways to code words or messages. Usually, the relationship between the code and its corresponding word is completely arbitrary; thus, 13 might be the code for *Yesterday* and 24 might be the code for *Hello*. Most systems that use numeric encoding display the codes and the associated words or messages on a chart or a menu as part of the selection display so that neither the person communicating through AAC nor the communication partner must rely on their memory for recall or translation. Extensive learning and instruction is necessary to memorize the codes if this option is not available.

Morse Code

Morse code is an international system that uses a series of dots and dashes to represent letters, punctuation, and numbers (see Figure 3.9). When used in AAC applications, the dots and dashes are transmitted via microswitches through a device called an emulator that translates them into orthographic letters and numbers.

A	. _		V	... _
B	_ ...		W	. _ _
C	_ . _ .		X	_ .. _
D	_ ..		Y	_ . _ _
E	.		Z	_ _ ..
F	.. _ .		1	. _ _ _ _
G	_ _ .		2	.. _ _ _
H	....		3	... _ _
I	..		4	.... _
J	. _ _ _		5	.....
K	_ . _		6	_ ....
L	. _ ..		7	_ _ ...
M	_ _		8	_ _ _ ..
N	_ .		9	_ _ _ _ .
O	_ _ _		0	_ _ _ _ _
P	. _ _ .		period	. _ . _ . _
Q	_ _ . _		comma	_ _ .. _ _
R	. _ .		?	.. _ _ ..
S	...		error	....
T	_		wait	. _ ...
U	.. _		end	. _ . _ .

Figure 3.9. Morse code.

Morse Code emulators are available in a number of communication devices and communication software products, including EZ Keys (Words+, Inc.); HandiCODE (Microsystems Software, Inc.); and the Great Green Macaw and LightWRITER (ZYGO Industries, Inc.). In addition, computer access can be achieved through use of devices such as the Darci USB (WesTest Engineering Corporation).

Research on Learnability

In an early AAC study, the learning curves of typical adults for five encoding strategies used to represent single words were investigated (Beukelman & Yorkston, 1984). The five strategies were 1) arbitrary numeric codes, 2) alphabetically organized numeric codes in which consecutive numbers were assigned to words based on their alphabetic order, 3) memory-based alphanumeric codes, 4) chart-based alphanumeric codes, and 5) letter-category codes. Ten literate adults without disabilities served as participants (two per condition) and were introduced to 200 codes and their associated words during 10 sessions. The participants performed most accurately and retrieved the codes most quickly when using encoding approaches that grouped words according to a logical pattern—that is, the alphanumeric, alphabetically organized numeric, letter-category, and chart-based codes. The participants were least effective using arbitrary numeric codes. The learning curves for the arbitrary numeric codes and the memory-based alphanumeric codes did not show as much improvement over time as did learning curves for the other three encoding strategies.

Three single-word encoding techniques were also investigated (Angelo, 1987), including 1) truncation codes, 2) contraction codes, and 3) arbitrary letter codes. The 66 individuals without disabilities in this study attempted to learn 20 words during a series of 10 trials. The results indicated that the individuals recalled truncation codes most accurately, followed by contraction and arbitrary letter codes, respectively.

Studies investigating the learnability of Morse code by people who communicate through AAC are limited. One exception is a case study of a man with a spinal cord injury who wrote using Morse code at a rate of 25–30 words per minute. He learned to produce basic Morse code using a sip-and-puff switch within 2 weeks and became proficient in the use of the system within approximately 2 months (Beukelman, Yorkston, & Dowden, 1985). Hsieh and Luo (1999) also described the Morse code learning of a 14-year-old Taiwanese student with cerebral palsy who was able to read English at a grade 2 (Taiwanese) level. He earned to type English words at approximately 90% accuracy over a 4-week period. This is congruent with unpublished data suggesting that the threshold for learning Morse code is a second- or third-grade reading level (Marriner, Beukelman, Wilson, & Ross, 1989).

Message Codes

Many of the strategies used to encode words can also be used for messages. In the sections that follow, we discuss the various message encoding options and the research related to the learning demands they place on the people who use them.

Alpha (Letter) Encoding

Letters of the alphabet are used to encode messages in a wide range of AAC systems. These codes are usually memory based and incorporate different strategies to assist the person using them to remember each code and its referent.

Salient Letter Encoding   In salient letter encoding, the initial letters of salient content words in the message are used to construct the code. For example, the message *Please open the door for me* might be coded *OD*, because these are the initial letters of the primary words in the message *open door.* This technique attempts to establish a logical link between the code and how the message is spelled. Although the capability requirements for salient letter encoding have not been studied in detail, it seems that some familiarity with traditional orthography and the ability to spell at least the first letter of words are necessary. In addition, this technique is probably the most effective for those who are able to recall messages in their correct syntactic forms, as the codes are often determined by the usual word order of the most salient items.

Letter-Category Encoding   When letter-category message encoding is used, the initial letter of a code is determined by an organizational scheme that categorizes messages. For example, the messages *Hello, how are you? It's nice to see you, See you later,* and

Good-bye for now could be grouped in the category of greetings. The first letter of the code for each of these messages would then be the letter *G*, which represents the category. The second letter of the code would be the specifier within the category, which is based on the specific content of the message. Thus, the message *Hello, how are you?* might be coded *GH* (for *hello*), and the message *It's nice to see you today* might be coded *GN* (for *nice*).

Abbreviation expansion is a term that has also been applied to alpha encoding techniques. Vanderheiden and Lloyd (1986) defined abbreviation expansion as "a technique that can be used in conjunction with all techniques that include an alphabet in their selection vocabulary. . . . Words, phrases, or entire sentences can be coded and recalled by the user using a short abbreviation." (p. 135)

Alphanumeric Encoding

Alphanumeric message encoding utilizes both letters and numbers. Generally, the alphabetic part of the code refers to the category of messages, such as *G* for greetings, *T* for transportation, and *F* for food. The number is used arbitrarily to specify an individual message within the category. Thus, *G1* might refer to *Hello, how are you?* and *G2* might refer to *I haven't seen you in a long time!* and so forth. It is usually desirable to combine memory- and chart-based strategies when this type of code is used.

Numeric Encoding

As noted previously, numeric codes can be used to represent messages as well as words. When used for messages, some type of system is often applied to organize the codes into categories. For example, Chris is a man with multiple disabilities who uses a large repertoire of numeric codes, organized by the first number. Codes starting with 3 are about wants and needs, codes starting with 6 are about people, and codes starting with 8 are used sparingly because they are four-letter words or sarcastic comments! Using partner-assisted auditory scanning, Chris selects numbers up to three digits in length to communicate messages such as *Get me a cup of coffee* (326), *Can you phone my mom and tell her to get in touch with me?* (611), or *Eat my socks!* (825). Although Chris has memorized over 900 codes over the years, his communication partner looks them up in a code book in order to translate their meanings. Obviously, such a system requires a good memory on the part of the person who uses it unless they, too, have access to a code book for reference.

Iconic Encoding

Baker (1982, 1986) proposed an iconic encoding technique referred to as *semantic compaction*, or Minspeak. In this system, sequences of icons (i.e., pictorial symbols) are combined to store word, phrase, or sentence messages in one of the SGDs constructed to incorporate this technique. The icons used for this encoding are deliberately selected for their rich semantic associations.

Using iconic encoding, an apple icon might be associated with *food, fruit, snack, red,* and *round;* a sun icon might be used to refer to concepts such as *weather, yellow, hot, summer,* and *noon;* or a clock icon might represent *time, numbers,* and a *daily schedule.* Some of

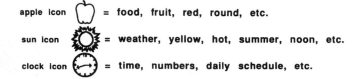

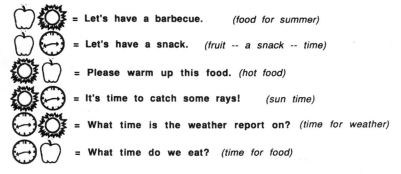

Figure 3.10. Examples of iconic codes. (Picture Communication Symbols copyright © 1981–2004 by Mayer-Johnson LLC. All Rights Reserved Worldwide. Used with permission. Some symbols have been adapted.)

the codes that might by constructed from these three icons are depicted in Figure 3.10. As illustrated in this figure, the message *Let's have a barbecue* might be encoded with an apple icon (food) and a sun icon (summer). Or, an apple icon might be combined with a clock icon to encode the message *It's time to have a snack.* Or a sun icon might be combined with a clock icon to signify *It's time to catch some rays!* These sequences and their corresponding messages are stored in an SGD that the person using AAC activates to produce synthetic speech for the message. Using iconic encoding, messages can be semantically organized by activities, topics, locations, or other categories to enhance retrieval. The semantic associations with icons assist with retrieval, as do the icon prediction lights available on some SGDs (Beck, Thompson, & Clay, 2000).

Unity software incorporates Minspeak and is available in most Prentke Romich communication devices. Minspeak applications have also been developed for use in Sweden (Ferm, Amberntson, & Thunberg, 2001) and Germany (Braun & Stuckenschneider-Braun, 1990).

Color Encoding

Color has also been utilized to encode messages, usually in conjunction with specifiers such as numbers or symbols. In particular, color encoding has been used to formulate messages for eye-pointing communication systems (Goossens' & Crain, 1986a, 1986b, 1987). Imagine an eye-gaze display with color squares in the eight common locations with letters of the alphabet assigned to each square. Such a display is depicted in Figure 3.11,

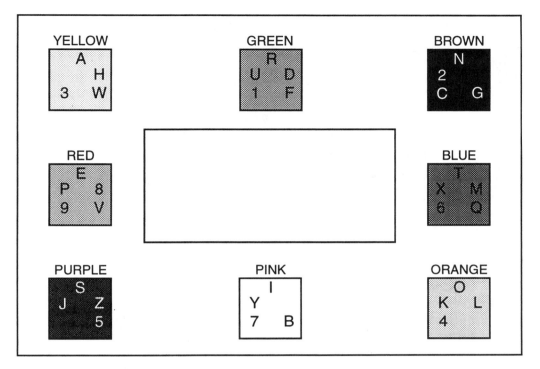

Figure 3.11. Color eye-gaze display.

using the standard ETRAN letter and number arrangement. A person might have a series of color and alpha codes to represent various messages that are cataloged in a decoding book for partners. For example, the message *Turn on the music* might be symbolized as *BLUE M* and the message *Can you scratch my foot?* might be *PURPLE F*. In order to select the first message, the person using AAC would first gaze at the blue square on the display and then shift his or her gaze to the letter *M*. The communication partner would then find the message that corresponds with *BLUE M* in the decoding book and follow with the requested action. Color coding can be used with other types of access techniques, such as communication books and electronic displays, to help individuals locate symbols more easily. For example, all of the people symbols might be colored with yellow backgrounds, all of the food symbols colored green, and all of the things-to-do symbols colored blue.

Research on Learnability

Several studies have investigated learning and instructional issues associated with various message encoding techniques. One study used undergraduate university students as participants (Egof, 1988), one involved typically developing 4- and 5-year-old children (Light, Drager, McCarthy, et al., 2004), and still others involved persons with cerebral palsy (Hochstein, McDaniel, & Nettleton, 2004; Light & Lindsay, 1992; Light, Lindsay, Siegel, & Parnes, 1990) or aphasia (Beck & Fritz, 1998).

In the Light and colleagues (1990) study, 30 salient letter, 30 letter-category, and 30 iconic codes were taught in three 15-minute sessions. In the Light and Lindsay (1992) study, 80 codes of each type were taught over an extended training period with multiple sessions. Hochstein and colleagues (2004) taught 30 nouns and 30 verbs over 12 practice sessions, using both a dynamic display device organized taxonomically (i.e., by semantic categories such as people and things) and static display iconic encoding. Light, Drager, McCarthy, and colleagues (2004) taught 12–15 concrete vocabulary items (i.e., nouns, verbs) and 12–15 abstract items (e.g., questions, relational items, greetings) over four learning and testing sessions. They compared iconic codes as well as various symbols or pictures in dynamic display devices organized either taxonomically, schematically (i.e., by event schemes such as eating cake and opening presents), or in visual-scene displays. The results of these four studies indicate that 1) letter-based codes were recalled most accurately, while iconic codes were associated with the least accurate performance (Light et al., 1990; Light & Lindsay, 1992); 2) three dynamic display conditions (taxonomic, schematic, and visual-scene display) resulted in more accurate and faster learning for typical children than the iconic encoding condition (Light, Drager, McCarthy, et al., 2004); 3) initially, children with cerebral palsy were more accurate with iconic codes than with taxonomic dynamic displays, but the reverse was true after eight practice sessions (Hochstein et al., 2004); 4) regardless of the study or the encoding/organizational technique used, concrete messages (e.g., nouns) were easier to learn than abstract ones (e.g., verbs); and 5) there was no apparent learning advantage of personalized codes—those selected by the person using AAC rather than by a researcher or a clinician—over nonpersonalized codes (Light & Lindsay, 1992).

Beck and Fritz (1998), in the only study to date examining iconic code learning in adults with aphasia, taught 24 messages over three learning sessions to five adults without disability and five individuals with each of Broca's and Wernicke's aphasia. They found that nondisabled adults learned more iconic codes than adults with aphasia, that adults both with and without disabilities learned more codes for concrete messages (e.g., "I want a drink") than for abstract messages (e.g., "I don't agree"), and that the performance of adults with aphasia deteriorated more than that of typical adults as the length of the iconic codes increased. They also found that adults with Wernicke's aphasia (i.e., poor language comprehension skills) had more difficulty learning codes longer than one icon for abstract messages than did those with Broca's aphasia (i.e., relatively good comprehension skills).

Clearly, the learning issues associated with iconic encoding in particular are extensive. Light, Drager, McCarthy, and colleagues (2004) noted that, at the observed rate of learning for iconic encoding found in their study, 4-year-olds would require close to 1,000 instructional sessions and 5-year-olds would require approximately 400–500 sessions to learn even a 1,000-word vocabulary. This is not to say that iconic encoding is not a useful technique; however, it requires significant learning time and places considerable cognitive demand on those who use it, especially in the early stages of acquisition. AAC teams need to be aware of and consider these issues carefully when making decisions about when and with whom specific encoding techniques should be used.

Message Prediction

In addition to word and message encoding, message prediction, a dynamic retrieval process in which options offered to the people who rely on AAC change based on the portion of the message that has already been formulated, can also be used to enhance communication rates. Message prediction algorithms generally occur at one of three levels: single letter, word, or phrase/sentence.

Single-Letter Prediction

In virtually all languages that can be represented orthographically (i.e., with letter symbols), individual letters of the alphabet do not occur with equal probability. Some letters occur more frequently than others; for example, in English, the letters *e, t, a, o, i, n, s, r,* and *h* occur most frequently, and *z, q, u, x, k,* and *c* occur least frequently (as any frequent watcher of the television show *Wheel of Fortune* is well aware!).

Orthographic languages are also organized so that the probability of the occurrence of a letter in a word is influenced by the previous letter. In English, the most obvious example of this is that the letter *q* is almost always followed by the letter *u*. Some letter combinations occur with more frequency than others. For example, *ch-, -ed, tr-, str-,* and *-tion* are frequent letter combinations in English, whereas combinations such as *sz, jq,* and *wv* occur rarely, if at all.

Some electronic AAC letter prediction systems rely on the probability of these letters and letter combination relationships so that when a letter is activated, a menu of the letters that are most likely to follow will be offered on a dynamic display. When this technology was first introduced, the entire display of a scanning system was electronically reorganized each time a new letter was selected. People who communicate with AAC complained, however, that this required extensive visual searching to find the letter they wanted to enter. In response to this problem, letter prediction systems were redesigned to keep the overall letter display intact and to include an additional, dynamic line of letter prediction at the top or the bottom of the display.

Another letter prediction technique involves the use of "ambiguous keyboards" such as those used on touch-key telephones, in which each key is associated with several letters (e.g., abc, def). A disambiguation algorithm is used so that a computer can predict which of the possible characters on each key was actually intended by the individual. Work in this area suggests that if the keyboard arrangement is optimized across a nine-key layout, keystroke efficiencies of up to 91% can be achieved (Lesher, Moulton, & Higginbotham, 1998a; see also Arnott & Javed, 1992, and Levine, Goodenough-Trepagnier, Getschow, & Minneman, 1987). For single-switch scanning, optimized layouts with character prediction can result in switch savings of approximately 37%, a 53% gain over a simple alphabetic matrix. This translates to substantial improvements in text production rates (Lesher, Mouton, & Higginbotham, 1998b). Work in this important area continues through the Rehabilitation Engineering Research Center-Augmentative and Alternative Communication (AAC-RERC) site at the State University of New York at Buffalo and Enkidu Research, Inc. (e.g., Lesher, Moulton, Higginbotham, & Alsofrom, 2002; Lesher & Rinkus, 2002).

Word-Level Prediction

There are three basic types of prediction strategies that can occur at the word level: word prediction, word-pattern prediction, and linguistic prediction. These are discussed in the following sections.

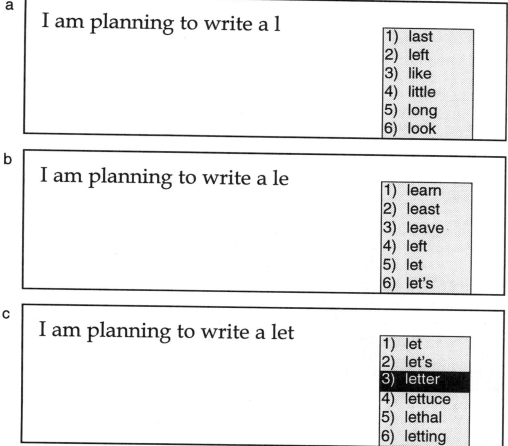

Figure 3.12. Dynamic menu display with word prediction (selecting the word *letter*). a) The screen displays the six most likely words that begin with *l* when that letter is typed; b) the screen changes to the six most likely words that begin with *le* when the letter *e* is added; c) screen changes to the six most likely words that begin with *let* when the letter *t* is added. The number 3 is typed to select the word *letter.*

Word Prediction   Electronic word prediction, in its simplest form, involves a computer program that provides a set of likely words (e.g., words weighted for frequency of use) in response to one's keystrokes. As an example, a typical word prediction system with a dynamic menu display is illustrated in Figure 3.12. Words are displayed in a menu or "window" at the upper right of the screen. The letters selected by the typist determine the specific words that the computer program presents in the menu. For example, if a person types the letter L, the six most frequently used words that begin with L will appear on the menu. If the word of choice is not included in the listing, then the person types the next letter (e.g., E) and six frequently used words that begin with LE will be presented in the menu. This process continues until the desired word is displayed in the menu. Once the person using the system sees the desired word, he or she can simply type its associated number code to insert the word in the text being formulated on the screen. Thus, this form of word prediction can also be thought of as a numeric encoding technique with dynamic displays.

The symbols or messages included in word prediction software can be selected in several ways. Some software contains preselected messages determined by the manufacturer. Other products allow the entry of specific words in the menus. Other programs monitor the communication performance of the person using the system and update the menu content based on frequency of word use. More than one of these options may be available in the same product.

Word-Pattern Prediction   Some AAC systems predict words based on the patterns of word combinations likely to occur in conversational interactions. For example, the probability is high that in the English language, an article such as *a, an,* or *the* will follow a preposition in a prepositional phrase (e.g., *on* the *bed, under* a *tree*). Designers of AAC systems have translated this word pattern information into prediction algorithms. These systems offer the typist a menu of words that are likely to follow each word that one selects. Thus, the words offered depend not on the letters typed (as with word prediction) but rather on the word *patterns* in the text. The person simply indicates in some way whether the predicted word is acceptable (e.g., by hitting the space bar) or unacceptable (e.g., by typing the next letter of the desired word).

Linguistic Prediction   In an effort to refine prediction strategies, some system designers have included algorithms that contain extensive information about the syntactic organization of the language. The predictions offered to persons who use these systems are based on grammatical rules of the language. For example, if an individual selects a first-person singular noun as the subject of a sentence (e.g., *Chris, mom*), only verbs that agree in subject and number will be presented as options (e.g., *is, likes, is going*). If the person selects an article (e.g., *a, an,* or *the*), the system will predict nouns rather than verbs as the next word, because it is unlikely that a verb will follow an article. Obviously, the algorithms that support linguistic prediction are complex. This type of message enhancement is becoming increasingly available, however, with decreasing costs of computer processing. Not only does this type of prediction enhance communication rate, but it may also enhance the grammatical performance of some people who have language or learning disabilities.

Letter and/or word prediction is available in many AAC products, such as Co:Writer 4000 (Don Johnston, Inc.); the WiViK 3 on-screen keyboard, Vanguard Plus, and Vantage Plus (Prentke Romich Co.); EZ Keys software (Words+, Inc.); Speaking Dynamically Pro and WordPower software (Mayer-Johnson, Inc.); Gus! Word Prediction software (Gus Communications, Inc.), and the LightWRITER (ZYGO Industries, Inc.).

Phrase/Sentence-Level Prediction

Two research teams have developed computer programs that incorporate sophisticated algorithms for predicting language units longer than single words. Research at the Universities of Abertay and Dundee in Scotland (File & Todman, 2002; Todman & Alm, 2003) resulted in development of TALK Boards (Mayer-Johnson, Inc.). This is a set of more than 700 phrase-based communication displays that can be individualized and used with the Speaking Dynamically Pro software program (Mayer-Johnson, Inc.) to assist literate individuals who use AAC to engage in social conversations. TALK studies involving individuals with amyotrophic lateral sclerosis (Todman & Lewins, 1996) and cerebral palsy (File & Todman, 2002; Todman, 2000; Todman, Rankin, & File, 1999) suggest that communication rates of between 42 and 64 words per minute may be attained with the TALK software—rates that are 3–6 times faster than those that rely on phrase construction during conversation. Meanwhile, researchers at the University at Buffalo and Enkidu Research (Higginbotham, Wilkins, Lesher, & Moulton, 1999) developed Frametalker, an utterance-based communication software program designed to support communication in structured situations such as doctors' offices and restaurants where interactions are highly sequential and more predictable. Preliminary data suggest that the keystroke savings achievable with Frametalker are far greater than that of other commercially available word-level prediction software programs (Higginbotham, Moulton, Lesher, Wilkins, & Cornish, 2000). These two research teams joined forces to develop a prototype hybrid communication system called Contact that incorporates features of both word- and phrase-level prediction for both social and structured conversation (Higginbotham, 2001; Lunn, Coles, File, & Todman, 2003).

Information about the TALK Boards, Frametalker, and Contact is available from Mayer-Johnson, Inc., the Division of Applied Computing at the University of Dundee (Scotland), and the Communication and Assistive Device Laboratory at the State University of New York at Buffalo. Another phrase-level system, ScripTalker (Dye, Alm, Arnott, Harper, & Morrison, 1998), was also developed at the University of Dundee and is available in The Netherlands and Germany.

Prediction Research

Because a number of human factors affect various rate enhancement strategies, the extent to which these strategies actually enhance communication rates may not be as great as implied by studies that have examined only one factor (Koester & Levine, 1998). As noted previously, the human factors associated with both encoding and predicting also vary depending on the interactions between visual monitoring and motor control. For example, Koester and Levine (1996) compared spelling with a letter-plus-word prediction technique in six men with cervical spinal cord injuries (SCI) and eight men who were able bodied (AB). All of the participants were given comparable sentences to transcribe with a standard keyboard and a mouthstick using either letter-only or letter-plus-word prediction, in which six numerically coded words at a time appeared on the screen based on the letters typed (see Figure 3.12). The authors analyzed the data along several dimensions and found that the benefits of any keystroke savings for the word prediction system were generally offset or even exceeded by the keystroke cost of making each selection. Thus, improvements in text generation rate with the prediction system relative to letters only were "much less than would be expected based on keystroke savings alone" (Koester & Levine, 1996, p. 164). The participants without disabilities selected items between 25% and 40% more slowly with the prediction system than with letters only, and the participants with SCI made selections from 50% to 70% more slowly. Much of the extra time was spent searching the menus; even by the end of the study (i.e., after several sessions of practice), the average search time was 0.47 seconds for the participants without disabilities and almost twice as long for those with SCI. Both groups of participants also rated the letter-plus-word prediction strategy as more difficult to use than the letter-only strategy, implying that the former placed higher cognitive demands on the participants than the latter.

Despite the complexity of this issue, there is no doubt that the rate and timing gains made possible by encoding and prediction strategies are potentially very important and can result in substantive interaction gains. In acknowledgment of the complexity of this issue, researchers have proposed several factors that should be considered when evaluating the efficacy of various rate enhancement strategies:

- Linguistic cost (i.e., the average number of selections needed to communicate a word) (Rosen & Goodenough-Trepagnier, 1981)

- Motor act index (i.e., the number of keystrokes necessary to produce a message) (Rosen & Goodenough-Trepagnier, 1981; Venkatagiri, 1993)

- Search time (i.e., the amount of time it takes to locate a letter, word, or phrase from a prediction menu) (Koester & Levine, 1998)

- Key press time (i.e., the amount of time it takes to activate a key or switch) (Koester & Levine, 1998; Venkatagiri, 1999)

- Time or duration of message production (i.e., how long it takes to produce a message) (Rosen & Goodenough-Trepagnier, 1981; Venkatagiri, 1993)

- Cognitive processing time needed to decide which selections or acts are necessary (Light & Lindsay, 1992)

- Productivity and clarity indices (i.e., measures of *which* meanings may be encoded and *how well* they are encoded) (Venkatagiri, 1993)

Currently, people who use AAC and their facilitators must weigh the relative benefits and costs of available strategies without much assistance from a research base. Research in message encoding and prediction continue to clarify the interactions among various human factors, while development efforts focus on innovative strategies that minimize costs to people who require AAC.

CHAPTER 4

ALTERNATIVE ACCESS

In the 1980s, in a junior high school in Edmonds, Washington, I received my first extensive lesson in alternative access. Kris, a middle school student with severe athetoid cerebral palsy, was "talking" with her mother at the end of a school day. As I observed from across the room, they faced each other. Her mother stared intently at Kris's face and talked quietly throughout the interaction. Kris did not speak at all; however, after watching for a while, it was clear to me that she was communicating a great deal. At the time, I was impressed with the magic of the interaction. Her mother was "reading" Kris's face, and they were discussing the schoolwork to be completed at home over the weekend. I was "listening" to a sincere interaction in which both individuals were contributing, adding their opinions, and arguing a bit.

My curiosity led me to move behind Kris's mother, where I observed a series of very rapid eye movements that were somehow being translated into letters, words, and eventually messages. As I came to know Kris and her mother better, they let me know the nature of their code. When Kris directed her eyes at her mother's feet, she was communicating the letter *F*. When she directed her eyes toward her mother's elbow, she signaled an *L*. When she looked at her mother's nose, she signaled the letter *N*. After they explained these codes to me, they seemed rather logical. Then, they told me that when Kris raised her eyes and looked slightly to the left, she was signaling the letter *Y*, referring to the "yellow curtains in the living room," the location where Kris and her father had developed this eye code.

At one point, I attempted to communicate with Kris using her system and quickly found that, although the system was technically inexpensive, it required extensive learning and ability on the part of a listener. I didn't have the training and practice to be an effective communication partner for Kris, so her mother and her speech-language pathologist patiently interpreted for me. Kris and I knew the same language, English. She communicated through spelling letter-by-letter, which was the same strategy that I used every day. I knew the words that she spelled, but I was not proficient with the form of alternative access (eye point) that she used so efficiently. Over the years, Kris learned other forms of alternative access so that she could control electronic communication and com-

puter technology; converse fluently; and complete high school, a university degree, and eventually a doctoral degree. (D. Beukelman, personal communication, February 2004)

Those of us who speak learned our verbal communication skills at an early age. These skills and processes are now so automatic that we have little awareness or understanding of them. Only when we begin to translate our spoken language into written form do we begin to realize that we code messages by combining and recombining a relatively small set of elements. In the English language, people who are literate are able to write nearly anything they wish by combining and recombining a set of 26 letters. A child's task in learning to write is to select the appropriate letters from the set of 26 and to formulate them so that they meet certain standards of accuracy, intelligibility, and aesthetics. Simi-larly, people who speak are able to say every word in spoken English by combining ap-proximately 45 sounds. Only those who have difficulty learning to speak need to know that words are made up of sounds and that certain sounds require special attention in order to be spoken correctly.

Communication is based on the selection of one or more types of symbols used alone or in combination to express messages. In natural speech, a person produces messages by combining specific sounds. In writing, a person forms orthographic symbols (i.e., letters) and places them in a systematic order. People who are unable to speak or write through traditional means need alternative strategies in order to communicate. The task of learn-ing alternative access methods is easier to understand when the organization of natural language is first considered. For a person with complex communication needs, learning alternative access methods involves the selection of messages or codes from a relatively small set of possibilities. The person then uses these elements alone or combines them in ways that allow for the communication of a variety of messages. Obviously, the person must present the message to the listener in a way that the listener can understand.

In the past, many people with complex communication needs operated standard communication devices such as typewriters by using headsticks and special keyguards. If they were unable to use these devices, interventionists considered these individuals to be inappropriate candidates for electronic communication options. However, beginning in the 1970s and continuing to the present time, alternative access options for people who were unable to use standard devices have expanded dramatically. In order to adequately cover the influx of new technology without making this book outdated before it pub-lished, we decided to offer readers only limited examples of communication devices that represent specific access techniques or features. This is in no way meant to imply that the products mentioned in this chapter are the only examples or even the "best" examples of the concepts they illustrate. It was not our intention to attempt to offer a comprehensive overview of the latest technology. The Resource List at the conclusion of this book con-tains the names and addresses of many of the major communication device manufactur-ers and distributors. In addition, the Barkley AAC Center's World Wide Web site (http://aac.unl.edu) contains links to most of the manufacturers associated with the aug-mentative and alternative communication (AAC) field.

THE SELECTION SET

The *selection set* of an AAC system includes the visual, auditory, and tactile presentation of all messages, symbols, and codes that are available at one time to a person who relies on AAC (see Chapter 3). Most AAC techniques utilize visual displays of items in the selection set. For example, electronic AAC technology is often used by people who have difficulty writing by hand. The displays of such computer devices contain a finite set of symbols that comprise the selection set. On standard computer keyboards, for example, these symbols include individual letters of the alphabet; punctuation characters; numbers; and control commands for the device, such as *enter, control, tab,* and *return.* Other individuals use visual displays that consist of pictorial symbols or codes. When visual displays are inappropriate because of an individual's visual impairments, the selection set may be displayed auditorily or tactually. Auditory displays usually involve presentation of the selection set through spoken words or messages. Tactile displays are composed of tactile representations of items in the selection set using real or partial objects, textures, shapes, or raised dots (braille).

The items in a selection set are determined in a number of ways. In the case of standard computer keyboards, the manufacturer assigns the symbols (numbers, letters, punctuation symbols, and commands) to specific locations. It is the task of the individual who relies on AAC to learn what the various symbols mean and how to use them. For many persons who use AAC systems, however, symbols and codes are selected on an individual basis so that relevant messages can be represented in a way that they are understood and used efficiently.

Messages in the Selection Set

At the time this book was written, we were providing support to a man with amyotrophic lateral sclerosis (ALS) who relied on AAC technology to communicate. The upcoming 2004 Olympics was of particular interest to him because he is a sports enthusiast and, more importantly, because he has a very close relationship with a woman who was one of the participants on the U.S. volleyball team. Months earlier, she had requested permission from the U.S. Olympic Committee to change the number on her jersey from 18 to 12 in honor of this man, because he had worn the number 12 throughout years of athletic performance.

As the Olympics approached, he and his wife invited friends to come to their home and join them to watch the coverage on television. In preparation for these evenings, he programmed his AAC device to support his communication. He selected specific messages for a number of different reasons. He needed to communicate some messages immediately, if they were to have meaning. For example, the message WHAT A GREAT PLAY! would only be meaningful if he could produce it at exactly the right moment during a fast-moving volleyball game. If he had to spell the message letter by letter, he would not meet this timing requirement, and the message—completed long after the play that elicited the comment—would lose its meaning. He chose to include other phrases (such as greetings, comments, and questions) because he anticipated that they would be used frequently, and because he needed to be able to retrieve them in a timely manner that also allowed him to conserve energy. Examples of some of these messages included HI, THANKS FOR COMING, WHAT DID YOU THINK OF THAT? I THINK THAT THEY WILL PLAY AGAIN ON _____; WOULD YOU LIKE SOMETHING TO EAT (OR DRINK)? and SEE YOU LATER. He also prepared several pages of jokes, news, and specific thoughts that he wanted to communicate to his friends. In addition, he programmed names of family members, friends, and athletes to enhance communication speed. Finally, alphabet and word prediction functions were available to him, so that he could prepare unique messages on a letter-by-letter basis. Obviously, choosing messages to be included in this selection set required cooperative effort by this individual and his facilitators. As is always the case, the symbolization and coding of the messages on his display depended on his unique linguistic and learning abilities, as well as on his personal preferences.

Types of Selection Set Displays

The display of a selection set depends on the technique and device employed in the AAC application. Displays are generally one of three main types—fixed, dynamic, and hybrid; a fourth type, called a visual scene display, was in development as this book was being written and is likely to be available relatively soon.

Fixed Displays

We use the term *fixed display* to refer to any display in which the symbols and items are "fixed" in a particular location. Fixed displays (also known as static displays; Hochstein, McDaniel, Nettleton, & Neufeld, 2003) are typically used in low-tech communication boards as well as in some speech-generating devices (SGDs). The number of symbols that a fixed display can include is limited, depending on a person's visual, tactile, cognitive, and motor capabilities. Often, individuals who rely on AAC use a number of fixed displays in order to accommodate all of their needed vocabulary items. For example, if a person wishes to change the topic of discussion from the Olympic Games to plans for an upcoming holiday, he or she might need to change from the display with sports symbols to one with travel and family vocabulary items.

Because of the obvious limitations imposed by the use of multiple fixed displays (e.g., difficulty with portability, inefficiency), interventionists have made extensive efforts to compensate for the limited symbols that a fixed display can contain. One compensatory technique is to organize a number of displays into levels. For example, a communication book in which symbols are arranged topically on pages is an example of a fixed display with several levels (in this case, each page is a different level). Many SGDs that contain visual or auditory selection sets also incorporate levels in their design and operation. Another compensatory technique involves various encoding strategies by which an individual can construct multiple messages by combining one, two, three, or more items (symbols) on a fixed display. Obviously, by coding messages this way, the number of messages a person can communicate can greatly exceed the number of items on the display (see Chapter 3).

Examples of SGDs with fixed displays include the TechTalk and TechSpeak (Mayer-Johnson, Inc.), Cheap Talk 8 (Enabling Devices), Parakeet 15 and Macaw (ZYGO Industries, Inc.), DigiCom 2000 (Great Talking Box Co.), Easy Talk (Saltillo Corp.), and Message Mate (Words+, Inc.).

Dynamic Displays

We use the term *dynamic display* to refer to computer screen displays with electronically produced visual symbols that, when activated, automatically change the selection set on the screen to a new set of programmed symbols. For example, if an individual has access to a dynamic display, he or she might first see a screen displaying symbols related to a number of different conversational topics, such as volleyball, jokes, personal care, news, or family. By touching the VOLLEYBALL symbol, he or she can activate the screen to display messages related to volleyball. When a break occurs during the volleyball game, he or she can return to the initial screen by touching an appropriate symbol, select a new topic (e.g., jokes, personal care), and have access to a new screen with related vocabulary. A wide variety of commercial AAC products offer dynamic displays. Figure 4.1 provides an example of how a dynamic screen display operates.

Hybrid Displays

We use the term *hybrid display* to refer to electronic fixed displays with a dynamic component, such as indicator lights that inform the individual which items in the selection set are available for activation. This technique is used in the Chatbox and the Pathfinder (Prentke Romich Co.), two AAC devices that use iconic codes to represent messages (see Chapter 3). When one activates the first icon in a sequence, indicators on the display screen light up next to each icon that could be chosen next. After a selection is made from one of these options, the lights change to indicate the icons that could come next in the sequence. AAC specialists designed this technique as a memory aid, particularly for individuals who use numerous icon sequences to communicate. In the only study that has examined this issue to date, college students without disabilities recalled significantly more codes when icon predictor lights were used compared to when they were not (Beck, Thompson, & Clay, 2000).

A few published studies have compared the learnability of electronic fixed and dynamic display devices when used by individuals with severe intellectual disability (Reichle, Dettling, Drager, & Leiter, 2000); cerebral palsy (Hochstein, McDaniel, & Nettleton, 2004; Hochstein, McDaniel, Nettleton, & Neufeld, 2003); and no disabilities (Hochstein et al., 2003). Initially, response time was faster and accuracy was greater for fixed displays, for all types of participants. However, Hochstein and colleagues (2004) and Reichle and colleagues (2000) both found that the fixed display advantage lessened or disappeared after eight or nine practice trials; Hochstein and colleagues (2003) did not address the impact of learning over time. Thus, it appears that if quickly achieving symbol recognition is more important than optimizing ease of recognition, initial training on a fixed display

a.

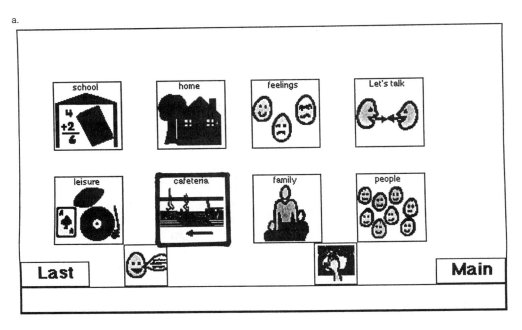

b.

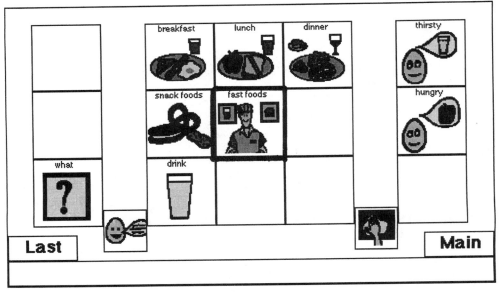

Figure 4.1. Example of a series of dynamic display screens using Speaking Dynamically. a) The main screen contains symbols depicting activity options; b) when the CAFETERIA symbol is selected, the screen changes to symbols for various food and drink categories; c) when FAST FOODS is activated, the screen changes to display food and drink items available in that type of environment; d) finally, when HOW MUCH? is activated, the screen changes again to display money, coin, and amount symbols. Note that the user can return to the previous screen at any time by activating LAST and can return to the main screen by selecting MAIN.

c.

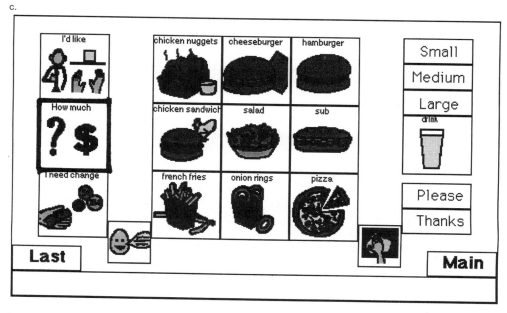

d.

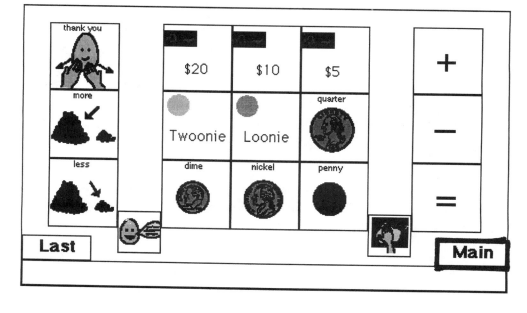

may be desirable. If the opposite is true, a dynamic display device can be introduced from the outset, providing that sufficient training time is available.

Examples of SGDs with dynamic displays include the Springboard, Vantage, and Vanguard (Prentke Romich Co.); DynaVox Series 4 and Impact Tablet (DynaVox Systems LLC); Chat PC (Mayer-Johnson, Inc.); Dialect (ZYGO Industries, Inc.); and TuffTalker (Words+, Inc.). Speaking Dynamically Pro is dynamic display software available from Mayer-Johnson, Inc./DynaVox LLC.

Visual Scene Displays

A visual scene display (VSD) is a picture, photograph, or virtual environment that depicts and represents a situation, place, or experience. Individual elements such as people, actions, and objects appear within the visual scene (Blackstone, 2004). For example, in a photograph of a birthday party, the people, food, and gifts all appear in a single picture. Messages such as the names of the guests or the food items that were served can then be accessed from the picture. Additional displays may also be accessed, such as those that contain more information about the person having the birthday and his or her family. While VSDs usually employ dynamic display technology, the concept can also be applied to fixed displays, at least in a limited way.

Figure 4.2 illustrates a VSD with a series of photographs of a vacation. An extended family is shown in a variety of settings, engaged in actual and implied activities. In addition to representing individuals and objects, these photographs provide topical information that can guide and support conversational interactions. Miniature photographs are located along the top, bottom, and right sides of the screen to allow navigation to content that represents other communication themes, such as food, shopping, personal care, maps, extended family, and so forth.

VSDs are quite different from the more typical grid displays that are widely used in AAC devices. The visual scene depicts a set of elements (people, actions, objects) within a coherent, integrated visual image, while a grid or matrix display arranges elements in separate boxes usually organized in rows and columns; the elements in the grids may or may not be related. Currently, visual scene display research and development work is ongoing with children with developmental disabilities, young adults with multiple disabilities, and adults with aphasia, and the preliminary results are very encouraging. It appears that visual scenes support conversational interactions for persons who find traditional grid displays challenging (Beukelman et al., 2003; Blackstone, 2004; Light & Drager, 2004).

Physical Characteristics of Selection Set Displays

Regardless of the type of display employed, several physical characteristics of the selection set display must be considered after the messages have been chosen (see Chapter 2) and the symbolization or encoding strategies for the various items have been identified (see Chapter 3). Intervention decisions should be based on a match among the cognitive,

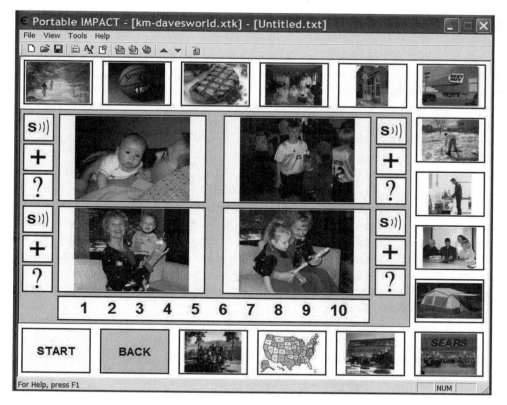

Figure 4.2.   Visual screen display of an extended family.

language, sensory, and motor capabilities of the individual who relies on AAC and the characteristics of the AAC technique.

Number of Items

Whether a display is visually, auditorily, or tactually based, the actual number of items in the selection set is a compromise involving many factors. The most important factor is the number of messages, symbols, codes, and commands that are required by the individual. When symbols other than those representing letters or codes are used exclusively, the size of the selection set increases with the number of messages because there is a one-to-one correspondence between messages and symbols. Thus, 500 symbols are typically required for 500 messages. When VSDs are used, more than one message may be integrated into a single photograph or picture, but multiple pictures will still be needed to represent various situations or topics. In contrast, the number of items in the selection set may be greatly reduced when encoding strategies are used, depending on the number of codes used. Thus, if a large number of codes are used, the display may contain fewer items than if a small number of codes are used. This is because each item can be used in multiple ways to make up numerous codes; for example, literally thousands of two-letter codes can be constructed by combining each of the 26 letters in the alphabet with the other 25.

Size

Intervention teams should consider two issues related to size when making selection set decisions: individual item size and overall display size. For visual displays, the actual size of the symbols or messages on the display is determined by an individual's visual capabilities, the motor access technique employed, the type of symbol, and the number of items to be displayed. For many individuals, visual capabilities determine individual item size; this factor is discussed in more detail in Chapters 6 and 7. For others, motor control is the critical variable because items need to be sufficiently large to allow accurate and efficient selection.

The overall size of the visual display also involves compromises among the number of items that must be displayed, the size of individual items, the spacing of items, mounting and portability factors, and the physical capabilities of the person using AAC. For example, if the system is to be carried around by the individual, its shape and weight must be manageable and nonfatiguing, and its exact dimensions will depend on the person's physical capabilities. If the individual uses a wheelchair, the AAC display must not be so large that it obscures vision. If the individual selects items using finger pointing or a headstick, the overall size of the display must accommodate the individual's range of movement or some items will be inaccessible.

With auditory displays, the size of the display is determined by the individual's memory and ability to retain the organizational scheme of the display. When large auditory displays are employed, individuals need to remember that a particular item will eventually be displayed (i.e., announced) if they wait long enough. When multilevel displays are available in electronic auditory scanners, the person must be able to remember the categorical scheme used for organization. For example, if messages are organized by main topic (e.g., food, drinks, places, people), the person must remember that COKE is a message under DRINK, whereas SHOPPING MALL is stored under PLACES. If the display contains more than two levels, this categorical scheme can become even more complex, and COKE might be a message under SODA POP, which is a subcategory of DRINKS.

For tactile displays, the size of the selection set depends on tactile recognition capabilities. Some individuals, such as those who use braille, require very little information to recognize options presented tactually, whereas others with less cognitive or tactile ability may require larger tactile symbols or actual objects.

Spacing and Arrangement of Items

Spacing and arrangement of items on a visual or tactile selection display is determined largely by the visual and motor control capabilities of the individual. For example, some individuals are more able to discriminate among items on the display if the items are widely separated and surrounded by a large empty area. For others, performance may be improved if the space surrounding the items is colored to contrast with the rest of the communication board. Still other individuals may have field cuts or blind spots that require irregular spacing arrangements to match their visual capabilities. Assessors need to make determinations such as these on an individual basis (see Chapters 6 and 7).

The motor control profile of each person also influences the spacing arrangement. Many people with physical disabilities who use AAC systems have better control of one hand than the other. The items on the display should be positioned accordingly to enhance access. For example, Figure 4.3 illustrates a communication board in which fre-

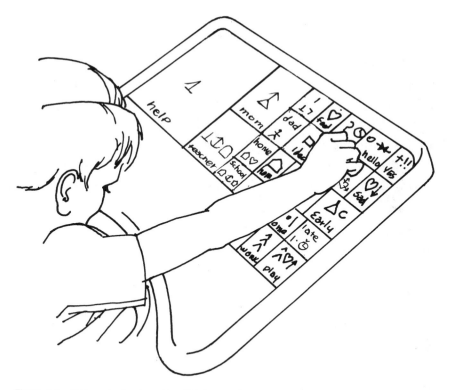

Figure 4.3. Communication board in which frequently used items are displayed to be most accessible to the individual's dominant hand.

quently used items are displayed to be most accessible to the individual's right hand, which has better motor control. In addition, the size of the items in the area where this person has the best motor control (i.e., the right side of the board) is smaller than in areas of reduced motor control (i.e., the left side of the board).

Another example of a communication board display, a curved array, is provided in Figure 4.4. This arrangement is designed to accommodate the motor control capabilities of a person using a headstick. By positioning the items in an arch, the forward and backward movements of the head and neck are minimized, compared with movements needed to reach items in a square or rectangular display.

Orientation of Display

Orientation refers to the position of the display relative to the floor. The orientation of a visual or tactile display is dependent on a person's postural, visual, and motor control capabilities. Visual and motor capabilities are the most critical in a direct selection display, where one needs to be able to point in some way to items on the display. If a scanning approach is used, visual and postural factors will probably determine the orientation decisions because these are critical skills for the switch activation required by this technique. These issues are detailed later in this chapter.

A visual/tactile display mounted on a table or wheelchair tray that is horizontal to the floor provides considerable arm and hand support, as well as stabilization, if weakness,

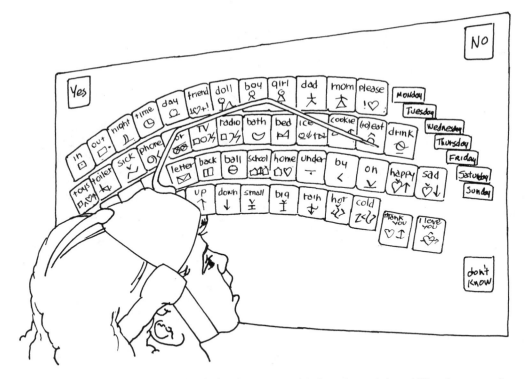

Figure 4.4.   Communication board display designed to accommodate the motor control capabilities of a person using a headstick.

tremor, or extraneous movements are present. This display orientation requires that the person maintain upright posture (either independently or with adaptive equipment) while viewing and using the display. Alternatively, a display positioned at a 30°–45° angle to the floor provides a compromise position for many people with physical disabilities. This orientation allows an individual to see the display clearly but avoids the neck flexion required by the horizontal display, while still providing some degree of hand and arm support and stability. Many people with very limited motor control due to weakness or extraneous movements may experience difficulty using a display that is oriented in this way. For these individuals, mobile arm supports may be used to elevate their arms and hands so that they can access a slanted display. Finally, displays that are used in combination with light or optical pointers are usually oriented at a 45°–90° angle to the floor, again depending on the individual's vision, motor control, and posture. When a display is positioned at a 45°–90° angle, care must be taken not to obstruct the person's vision for other persons or activities, such as operating a wheelchair or viewing instructional materials.

SELECTION TECHNIQUES

The term *selection technique* refers to the way an individual who relies on an AAC system selects or identifies items from the selection set. People who use AAC systems may choose from two principal approaches to item selection: direct selection and scanning.

Direct Selection

The person who relies on AAC indicates the desired item directly from the selection set with direct selection techniques. Most of us have experienced several types of direct selection. When typing, we are able to directly choose or activate any item on the typewriter or computer keyboard by depressing a key. Even those of us who are single-finger typists have the option to select any key that we wish. In addition, most of us have used natural speech and gestures, and many have either observed or used manual signing. These modes are direct selection techniques because we can directly select gestures or signs to communicate specific messages from a large set of options.

Direct Selection Options

Direct selection via finger pointing or touching is the most common selection method. Some individuals employ an optical pointer, light pointer, head mouse, or headstick to select items, point their gaze in order to indicate choices (see Kris's story at the beginning of this chapter), or use speech recognition. Options for direct selection are reviewed briefly in the following sections.

Physical Pressure or Depression   Individuals may activate many AAC devices by depressing a key or a touch-sensitive surface. A standard keyboard requires this activation mode, as does the touch pad (i.e., membrane switch) on many microwave ovens and AAC devices. If a device requires pressure for activation, an individual usually generates it with a body part, such as a finger or a toe, or with some device that is attached to the body, such as a headstick or a splint mounted on the hand or arm. The movement of the body part or body-part extension (e.g., a headstick) must be sufficiently controllable so that only a single item is activated with each depression. Facilitators can usually help individuals set pressure-sensitive keys and touch pads to a variety of pressure thresholds that enhance accurate activation.

Physical Contact   With many nonelectronic AAC options, individuals select items with physical contact rather than pressure or depression. For example, when a person uses a communication board, items are identified from the selection set by touching them. Because electronic activation is not involved, pressure is not required. Manual signs and gestures fall into this category because they are formed by hand and body movements rather than by making physical contact with a display.

Pointing (No Contact)   A person does not always need to make actual physical contact when selecting an AAC option. For example, in eye pointing (eye gazing), one looks at an item from the selection set long enough for the communication partner to identify the direction of the gaze and confirm the selected item. Many individuals who are unable to speak as a result of physical impairments employ eye pointing because these people often retain relatively accurate eye movements. In addition, eye pointing is often employed by young children who have not yet learned other communication techniques, as well as by those with poor positioning, chronic fatigue, or ongoing medical conditions that prevent them from utilizing more physically demanding options. Some nonelectronic eye-gaze communication techniques are quite advanced and incorporate complex encod-

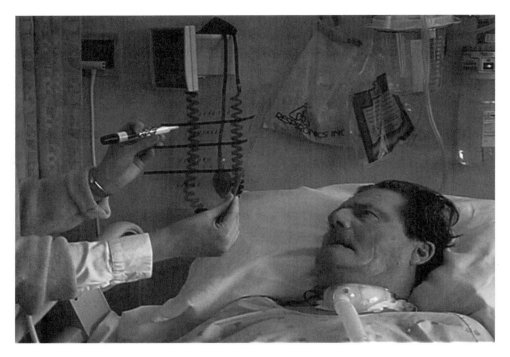

Figure 4.5. Eye-linking display. (From Goossens', C. [1989]. Aided communication intervention before assignments: a case study of a child with CP. *Augmentative and Alternative Communication, 5,* 20. Reprinted by permission of Taylor & Francis Ltd, http://www.tandf.co.uk/journals.)

ing strategies (Goossens' & Crain, 1987). Figures 4.5 and 4.6 illustrate an eye-linking display and an eye-gaze communication vest, respectively.

Those who use AAC strategies can also use pointing without contact with an optical or light (or laser)-generating device that is mounted on the head in some way (e.g., on a headband, attached to glasses; see Figure 4.7) or held in the hand. This technique can be used with both high- and low-tech AAC options. For example, an individual who uses a communication board can indicate his or her choice by directing a light beam toward the desired item. Individuals can also activate electronic AAC systems with optical or light pointing. Systems that incorporate this selection technique electronically monitor the position of the light beam or optical sensor and select an item if the beam or sensor remains in a specific location for a period of time. The two primary motor requirements for use of this technique are the ability to direct the light beam to a desired item and the ability to maintain the direction for a prescribed period of time. Because light pointers and optical sensors are usually mounted on the head, individuals must have head control without excessive tremor or extraneous movements for accurate and efficient use of these options.

Individuals can also make selections with sonar or infrared technology instead of direct physical contact. A receiving unit positioned near a computer screen display generates sound or infrared signals that are imperceptible to human senses. The person using AAC wears a sensor mounted on the forehead or eyeglasses (usually referred to as a "head mouse") that is directed to symbols on the screen through fine head movements. These

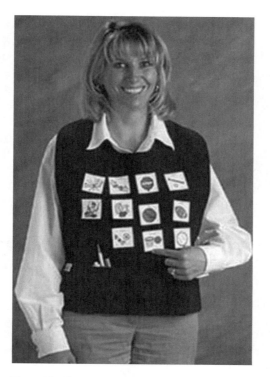

Figure 4.6.   Eye-gaze vest. (Used with permission, Mayer-Johnson LLC.)

movements control the cursor on the computer screen to indicate items from the selection set. The motor control requirements of sonar or infrared systems are similar to those for light pointing and optical systems.

The HeadMouse Extreme (Origin Instruments Corp.), Smart Nav (Natural Point), and HeadMouse (Words+, Inc.) are examples of sonar or infrared devices for direct selection.

Speech Recognition   In the past, individuals who were typical speakers but were unable to write or control a conventional computer keyboard (e.g., spinal cord injury) opted primarily for voice recognition strategies. AAC researchers and developers continue to focus on voice recognition as an alternative access selection mode for people who can produce consistent speech patterns even though their speech is mildly or moderately distorted. At the time this book was written, speech recognition strategies by persons with speech impairments have received considerable research attention but have not achieved routine acceptance to support those who rely on AAC technology; therefore, we have chosen not to discuss speech recognition strategies in this edition.

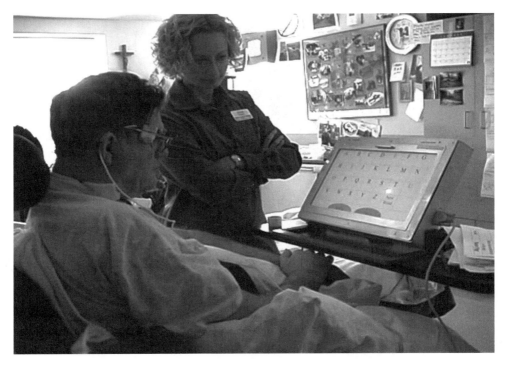

Figure 4.7.   Safe-laser head pointer (optical head pointer). (From *Handbook of Augmentative and Alternative Communication, 1st edition* by GLENNEN. © 1997. Reprinted with permission of Delmar Learning, a division of Thomson Learning. www.thomsonrights.com. Fax 800 730-2215.)

Direct Selection Activation Strategies

When an individual uses direct selection to choose an item from an electronic display, he or she must then activate the item so that the AAC system recognizes and translates it into usable output. Because many persons who rely on AAC have limited motor control capabilities, they must employ alternative activation strategies. For example, some individuals may be unable to isolate a pressure key on a selection display without dragging their fingers across the display, inadvertently activating other items. Several electronic options can compensate for these difficulties.

Timed Activation   Most electronic AAC devices that allow for direct selection offer the option of timed activation. This strategy requires one to identify an item on the display in some way (e.g., through physical contact or by shining a light or laser beam) and then sustain the contact (or dwell on a location) for a predetermined period of time in order for the selection to be recognized by the device. Timed activation allows persons to move their fingers, headsticks, or light beams across the display surface without activating each item that they encounter. The length of the "dwell time" can be adjusted to accommodate individual abilities and situations. The clear advantage of this strategy is that it reduces both inadvertent activations and motor control demands.

Release Activation   Release activation is another activation strategy available in electronic AAC devices. The individual can use release activation only with displays controlled by direct physical contact, either with a body part or with an extension of some type. The strategy requires the person to contact the display, for example, with a finger, and then retain contact until the desired item is located. The individual can move his or her finger anywhere on the display without making a selection as long as direct contact with the display is maintained. To select an item, the person releases contact from the display. Again, the contact time can be adjusted to accommodate individual abilities and needs. The advantages of this strategy are that it allows an individual to use the display for stability and that it minimizes errors for those who move too slowly or inefficiently to benefit from timed activation.

Filtered or Averaged Activation   Some persons who rely on AAC are able to select a general area on the display but have difficulty maintaining adequately steady contact with a specific item for selection. In other words, their selection ability is so limited that it is impossible to set a sufficiently low activation time to accommodate them. Often, these are individuals who are able to use head-mounted light or optical pointers but who do not have the precise and controlled head movements needed for accurate selection. Devices with filtered or averaged activation "forgive" (i.e., ignore) brief movements away from a specific item and sense the amount of time the pointer spends on each item in the general area of an item. The device averages this accumulated information over a short period of time and activates the item to which the light or optical device was pointed the longest. Facilitators can set the amount of time that elapses prior to activation to personalize the system.

Scanning

Some individuals who require AAC systems are unable to choose items directly from the selection set. Although this inability can occur for many reasons, the most common reason is lack of motor control. In such situations, the items in the selection set are displayed either by a facilitator (i.e., a trained communication partner) or by an electronic device in a predetermined configuration. The individual must wait while the facilitator or electronic device scans through undesired items before reaching the item of choice. At this point, the person who relies on AAC indicates in some way that the desired item has been presented. This type of item selection is called *scanning*. We discuss various aspects of scanning selection in the following sections.

Scanning Patterns

The configuration in which items in the selection set are presented is one important feature of scanning. It is important that items in the selection set be identified systematically and predictably so that the intention of the individual who uses AAC strategies and the actions of the facilitator or device are coordinated. Three primary selection set patterns are circular, linear, and group–item scanning techniques.

Circular Scanning   Circular scanning is the least complicated pattern that electronic devices use to present items in the selection set (see Figure 4.8). The device displays individual items in a circle and scans them electronically, one at a time, until the individual stops the scanner and selects an item. The scanner is usually a sweep hand like the big hand on a clock or takes the form of individual lights near each item in the selection set. Although circular scanning is visually demanding, it is relatively easy to master cognitively and for this reason is often introduced first to children or beginning AAC

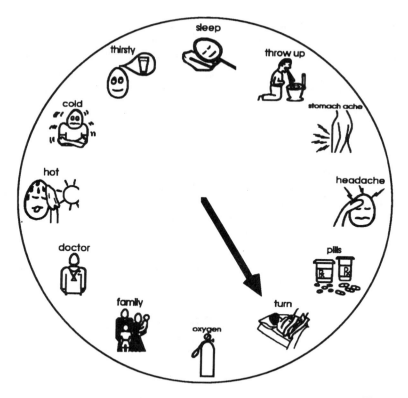

Figure 4.8. A circular scanning display for an individual in an intensive care unit. (Picture Communication Symbols copyright © 1981–2004 by Mayer-Johnson LLC. All Rights Reserved Worldwide. Used with permission.)

communicators. Horn and Jones (1996) provided a case report of a 4-year-old child involving circular scanning. They found that, for this child, scanning was more difficult than direct selection via headlight pointing, even though assessment information suggested that scanning would be the more appropriate option.

Linear Scanning   In visual linear scanning, a cursor light or an arrow moves across each item in the first row, each item in the second row, and each item in the subsequent row, until an item is selected. Figure 4.9 illustrates a visual display in which items in the selection set are arranged in three lines or rows. In auditory linear scanning, a synthetic voice or a human facilitator announces items one at a time until a section is made. For example, the facilitator might ask, "Which shirt do you want to wear today? The red one? The blue one? The striped one? The purple and green one?" until the individual answers YES. Linear scanning, although more demanding than circular scanning, is straightforward and easy to learn. Nevertheless, because items are presented one at a time in a particular order, it may be inefficient if the selection set contains many items.

Light (1993) reported a case study documenting a developmentally based instructional protocol to teach automatic linear scanning to a 5-year-old child with severe physical and communication disabilities. Previously, the child had failed to learn scanning from instruction focused primarily on the motor control process. Analyses of the per-

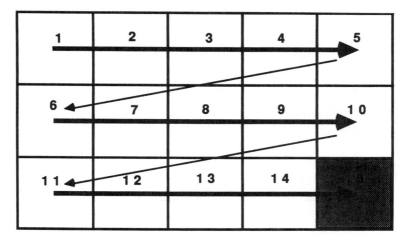

Figure 4.9. A linear scanning display with three rows of symbols.

formances of successful scanners suggested that the task of automatic linear scanning involves coordination of the relation of the cursor to the target symbol in the array and the relation of the switch to the selection process. Instruction was effective in providing the conceptual bridge that this child required to progress from her partial representation of the task (relation of the switch to the selection process) to the representation that allowed her to scan successfully.

Group–Item Scanning AAC device developers have developed a number of group–item scanning approaches in an effort to enhance scanning efficiency. Basically, group–item scanning involves identifying a group of items and then eliminating options gradually until a final selection is made. For example, in auditory group–item scanning, the device or facilitator might ask, "Do you want food items? Drink items? Personal care items?" and continue until the individual identifies the group or topic. Then, the device or facilitator recites a predetermined list of options within that group. For example, if the individual selects DRINK ITEMS, the facilitator might question, "Water? Pop? Tea? Beer?" until choice is made. Clearly, this would be more efficient than if the facilitator first went through a list of food items and then repeated the process for drink items before selection could be made.

One of the most common visual group–item strategies is row–column scanning (see Figure 4.10). Each row on the visual display is a group. The rows are each electronically highlighted in presentation until the target item is selected. Then, individual items in that row are highlighted one at a time until the scanning is stopped at the specific item desired.

There are also a number of row–column scanning variations. To increase efficiency, sophisticated AAC systems that contain many items in the selection set often employ group–row–column scanning, a common variation of row–column scanning. Group–row–column scanning requires one to make three selections. First, the entire display is highlighted in two or three groups. When the person identifies a group—for example, the group at the top of the screen—each row in that group is scanned. When the individual selects a specific row, the scanning pattern changes to highlight each item in that row. Finally, the person identifies the desired item within a row.

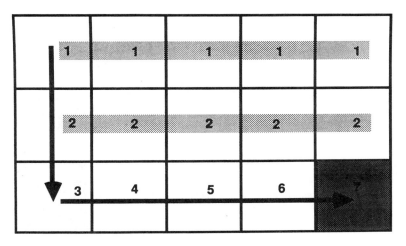

Figure 4.10. A row–column scanning display.

Scanning Timing and Speed

In addition to customizing the scanning pattern, the speed and timing of scanning must be personalized according to each individual's physical, visual, and cognitive capabilities. When nonelectronic scanning is used, a facilitator can announce the items audibly or point to them on a communication display (e.g., an alphabet or communication board) as quickly or as slowly as the individual requires. The facilitator can usually observe the individual's response patterns and adjust the speed of scanning accordingly. When electronic equipment is used, however, scanning speed must be individualized for or by the person because a facilitator is not involved in the scanning presentation. Most electronic AAC devices have sufficient scanning speed options to meet individual needs.

Selection Control Techniques

Persons who use auditory scanning or electronic visual scanning must be able to select an item while a device systematically scans items in a display. Generally, three selection control techniques are used: directed (inverse), automatic (regular or interrupted), and step scanning.

Directed (Inverse) Scanning   In directed scanning, the indicator or cursor begins to move when the person activates (i.e., holds down) a microswitch of some type. As long as the switch is activated, the indicator moves through the preset scanning pattern (e.g., circular, linear, row–column). The selection is made when the switch is released. Directed scanning is particularly useful for people who have difficulty activating switches but who can sustain activation once it occurs and can release the switch accurately.

Automatic (Regular or Interrupted) Scanning   In this type of scanning, the movement of the indicator or cursor is automatic and continuous, according to a preset pattern (e.g., circular, linear, row–column). The person activates a switch to stop the indicator at the group or item of choice in order to make a selection. This type of scanning is particularly useful for people who are able to activate a switch accurately but who have difficulty sustaining activation or releasing the switch. This is also the type of scanning that is employed when the display presentation is auditory. A facilitator might recite names of movies, for example, until the individual stops (or interrupts) the recitation at the one he or she wishes to see.

Step Scanning   In step scanning, the indicator or cursor moves through a preset selection pattern, one step (i.e., one group or item) at a time for each activation of the switch. In other words, there is a one-to-one correspondence between cursor movement and switch activation. In order to select a specific item, the individual simply stops activating the switch for an extended period of time or activates a second switch that indicates that the item displayed is the desired selection. Step scanning is often used by individuals who have severe motor control or cognitive restrictions or who are just beginning to learn to operate electronic scanners. Because step scanning requires repeated, frequent switch activations, it is often fatiguing for complex AAC applications.

FEEDBACK

The two primary purposes of feedback from a communication system are 1) to let the individual using AAC know that an item has been selected from the selection display (activation feedback) and 2) to provide the individual with information about the message that has been formulated or selected (message feedback). Some communication systems provide neither type of feedback, some provide one but not the other, and some provide both. Feedback can be visual, auditory, tactile, or proprioceptive.

Activation Feedback

Lee and Thomas defined activation feedback as "the information sent back to the person, upon activation of the input device" (1990, p. 255). Activation feedback differs from message feedback in that it informs the individual that activation has occurred but does not provide information about which symbol or message has been selected. It differs from output in that it provides information that is useful to the person operating the technology but not, generally, to the communication partner.

Activation feedback must occur in a sensory modality that is within the person's capabilities. Auditory activation feedback may be a beep, click, or other generic sound produced by an electronic communication device. Nonelectronic displays do not provide auditory activation feedback. Visual activation feedback on an electronic communication device may be provided via a light flash after a switch has been activated or via an area or symbol flash on a backlit display. Visual activation feedback on a nonelectronic display may consist of seeing one's body part contact the device. Contact with the textured surface of symbols on either electronic or nonelectronic devices provides tactile activation feedback. Finally, proprioceptive activation feedback is obtained when the individual applies pressure against a resistant surface (a switch or key) that moves when the pressure threshold is exceeded. Persons who produce manual signs and gestures also get proprioceptive and kinesthetic feedback from the position and movement of their hands in space.

Message Feedback

Message feedback provides information about the symbol or message itself after it has been formulated. Unlike activation feedback, message feedback may be useful to the communication partner as well, although this is of secondary importance. For example, when an individual interacts with a keyboard that echoes each letter as it is typed via synthetic speech, the echo provides message feedback. The echo may also serve as output for the communication partner, if he or she can hear the echo and chooses to listen, but this is not its primary purpose. Similarly, most dynamic display devices provide the person using AAC technology with message feedback in the form of a screen display of symbols as they are activated in a sequence.

Message feedback, like activation feedback, is available through auditory, visual, tactile, or proprioceptive modalities. Auditory message feedback may be provided on an electronic device as either a key echo (e.g., a speech synthesizer announces each alphabet letter as it is activated when using orthographic symbols) or a word/phrase echo (e.g., a speech synthesizer says individual words or phrases in a message as they are produced). With nonelectronic displays (both aided and unaided), the communication partner often provides auditory message feedback (sometimes referred to as "partner reauditorization"; Bedrosian, Hoag, Calculator, & Molineux, 1992) by echoing each letter, word, or phrase as it is produced or selected.

Visual message feedback may be provided on electronic devices as computer screen displays of letters, words, or phrases as they are selected. Many communication devices and software products are available that provide message feedback in screen displays of symbol sequences as each symbol is selected. Visual message feedback from aided and unaided nonelectronic devices is generally identical to activation feedback—the individual sees the symbol he or she produces. AAC applications do not provide tactile and proprioceptive message feedback, with the exception of writing aids used by people with visual impairments.

RESEARCH ON ALTERNATIVE ACCESS

The usefulness of a variety of alternative access options has been discussed in this chapter and is illustrated more comprehensively in Chapters 10–18. There has been considerable speculation but little systematic research regarding the effectiveness of various alternative access options.

> It has been speculated that scanning is more difficult than direct selection for several reasons. First, scanning is a slower selection technique than direct selection . . . . Using direct selection, the rate of production ranges from 6 to 25 words per minute (Yoder & Kraat, 1983); using scanning, it ranges from 5 to 10 words per minute (Foulds, 1985). The slow rate of scanning may place extra demands on . . . memory and attention. Others have speculated that scanning is cognitively more difficult than direct selection and have hypothesized that different forms of direct selection and scanning vary in their cognitive complexity . . . . However, there is limited empirical evidence to support any of these speculations about the cognitive differences between direct selection and scanning. (Mizuko & Esser, 1991, p. 44)

Research studies have addressed only some of these issues. Ratcliff compared direct selection and row–column scanning performance among typically developing children. The study reported that the children "made significantly more errors, and took longer to respond" (1994, p. xi) using scanning as opposed to direct selection. Ratcliff suggested that scanning requires more attention and short-term memory than direct selection. In contrast, the results of another study regarding the cognitive demands of direct selection and row–column scanning techniques appear to contradict those of Ratcliff. Mizuko and Esser (1991) found no significant differences among typically developing 4-year-old children on a visual sequential recall task performed with direct selection and circular scanning. The task in this study, however, was considerably less demanding than that used in the Ratcliff study. In a related report, Fried-Oken (1989) presented evidence suggesting that electronic auditory scanning places higher information-processing demands on adults without disabilities than does electronic visual scanning. Researchers have not confirmed these results either with children or adults who have disabilities. As is apparent from this brief discussion, research examining the requirements (sensory, motor, cognitive, and language) and the effects (rate, accuracy, and fatigue) of various access options is still limited.

Despite a lack of extensive research, persons of all ages and abilities have used and are using alternative access techniques successfully because AAC teams are able to match individual abilities and needs of individuals with the characteristics and capabilities of various techniques. Although one might think that there is a "best" or "ideal" alternative access method for each person, in reality most individuals utilize several different access options depending on the communication task, the time of day, and their fatigue level. The story of Kris, presented at the beginning of this chapter, illustrates this. Although Kris initially communicated using eye pointing, she eventually learned to control a Morse code–based AAC device with bilateral head switches in order to participate in school classes. Ten years later, she was communicating with eye pointing as well as with her Morse code device, depending on the situation. She used eye pointing when she "talked" with her family, when she was tired or ill, and when she was not in her wheelchair. She used Morse code when she was at the university to operate her computer, write papers, and talk with people who were not able to comprehend her eye-pointing system. In addition to her electronic communication device, Kris also controlled other assistive devices such as a powered wheelchair and a page-turner.

MESSAGE OUTPUT AND INPUT

The auditorium was nearly full as Michael Williams lectured, from his own experience, about AAC use in society. He illustrated his comments about how people who rely on AAC interact with the public by recounting a recent shopping trip to purchase a new suit. The story was funny and poignant. Looking around the room at the audience who were laughing, many with tears in their eyes, I realized how effectively Michael was communicating with more than 500 people. His message was not interpreted by a natural speaker or illustrated by text projection. He spoke independently using an AAC device with DECtalk (Perfect Paul) voice. When the "suit story" was finished, I imagined how completely proud Dennis Klatt would have been that day. Dennis was a noted speech acoustics researcher who had developed the DECtalk algorithms to simulate his own voice—rather, the voice that he had before the onset of throat cancer. Dennis died in 1987, so he had little opportunity to realize his impact on the AAC field; however, I suspect that he probably foresaw it. I also reflected on the fact that, while Michael Williams spoke that day in North America, people in many countries were speaking with synthetic voices (American English, British English, French, German, Italian, Norwegian, Spanish, and Swedish) that had been developed by Karoly Galyas and his colleagues at the Royal Institute of Technology in Stockholm, Sweden. Although Karoly also died of cancer, he had the opportunity to observe the impact of these voices before he died. (D. Beukelman, personal communication, August 1997)

Those who rely on AAC, like all of us, are both the senders and the receivers of messages during communicative interactions. In this section, the term *message output* refers to the information that they send to their communication partners. Examples of message output modes include synthetic speech, print, gestures, manual signs, and nonelectronic aided symbols. Conversely, the term *message input* refers to the information that they receive from others. Message input usually takes the form of natural speech, gestures, and vocalizations (assuming that most partners do not have disabilities), although input may also take the form of written or printed materials (e.g., letters, notes) or manual signs.

It is important to distinguish message input and output from *feedback*, which is primarily provided during rather than at the end of message construction and was discussed in the previous section. Feedback lets the individual know that an item has been selected and, in some cases, also provides them with information about the selected item.

For some, the input mode through which they receive messages may be as much of an intervention concern as the output mode by which they send messages. For example, Beukelman and Garrett noted that "the incidence of auditory reception problems among the adult population with aphasia is large" (1988, p. 119), and these individuals may need augmented input in the form of gestures, pictures, or writing in addition to natural speech. People with impairments that affect cognitive, sensory, and linguistic processing (e.g., mental retardation, traumatic brain injury [TBI]) may also require and benefit from augmented input techniques. The following sections review the major types of message output and input used in AAC applications in terms of general characteristics and the learning and performance abilities that they require.

Synthesized Speech

The advances in synthetic speech technology in the AAC field since the mid-1990s have been nothing short of remarkable! People who once had no choice but to use devices that produced robotic, barely intelligible English voices are now able to choose from an array of natural-sounding male, female, and childlike voices in dozens of languages! As we write this book, several new synthetic speech technologies are about to be introduced. At this time, we have minimal public information about the intelligibility or acceptability of these new voices. Readers are encouraged to follow research reports to learn about the characteristics of these new voices. The main types of synthesized speech are described in the following sections.

Speech technology research can be found in journals such as *Augmentative and Alternative Communication, Assistive Technology,* and the *International Journal of Speech Technology.*

Types of Synthesized Speech

Synthesized speech is produced from stored digital data. Discussions of the methods used to develop the digital data stores and to retrieve these data to produce synthesized speech follow.

Text-to-Speech   A common method used to generate synthetic speech in AAC devices is text-to-speech synthesis. According to Venkatagiri and Ramabadran (1995), this requires a three-step process. First, text (words or sentences) that has been entered into an AAC device or retrieved from its memory as codes is transformed into phonemes and allophones. Second, the device uses the stored speech data to generate digital speech signals that correspond to phonetic representations of the text. Finally, the device converts the digital signals to analog speech waveforms that listeners can interpret and understand.

Rule-generated speech involves a flexible mathematical algorithm representing the rules for pronunciation, pronunciation exceptions, voice inflections, and accents. In standard text-to-speech synthesis applications, the algorithms generate speech sounds that reflect the phonetic representation of the text. The device does not store speech itself in digitized form; rather, the device generates speech for each utterance by the rule-based algorithm. A complete discussion of the algorithms used for these applications is beyond the scope of this text (see Venkatagiri and Ramabadran, 1995, for additional information).

A second type of text-to-speech synthesis uses diphone-based strategies to produce speech. Because the diphones are extracted from carrier words recorded by natural speakers, the resulting speech is intended to be more natural sounding than conventional text-to-speech synthesis. New diphonic voices continue to be introduced regularly, but it is beyond the scope of this book to be current with these developments.

Digitized Speech   Digitized speech, also called waveform coding, is another type of electronic speech used in AAC systems. This method consists primarily of natural speech that has been recorded, stored, and reproduced. In digitized speech, natural speech is recorded with a microphone and passed through a series of filters and a digital-to-analog converter (Cohen & Palin, 1986). When reproduced, the speech is a close replica of the original speech entry.

Combination Speech   Some individuals use a combination of text-to-speech and digitized speech techniques. The AAC device converts text entered via a keyboard to a pronunciation code using a dictionary and a set of rules in an algorithm. The device converts this code again to produce intonation, duration, and proper stress. Finally, the device creates speech from the code with a digital-to-analog converter (Cohen & Palin, 1986). The process requires a moderate amount of computer memory, involves no more time than the standard text-to-speech method requires, and results in very natural sounding speech.

For those with a particular interest in the role of speech output in AAC, the March 2003 issue of the journal *Augmentative and Alternative Communication* contains some excellent summary articles by Schlosser (2003e); Blischak, Lombardino, and Dyson (2003); Koul (2003); and Schepis and Reid (2003).

Only a few studies have been conducted regarding the intelligibility of digitized speech. Because it is a digital recording of natural speech, the assumption has been that the intelligibility of digital voices rivals those of natural speech. However, in practice, researchers and clinicians are realizing that that is not always true. Differences may occur in the quality of the digital-to-analog converters, playback mechanisms, or other components that produce better speech in some systems than in others. This evaluation awaits future comparative research.

Advantages and Disadvantages of Synthesized Speech

The major advantages of reasonably intelligible synthesized speech are that it 1) may significantly reduce the communication partner's burden in the interaction because interpretation of the output requires only the ability to understand spoken language, 2) provides information in a mode that is relatively familiar and nonthreatening to communication partners, 3) allows communication even with communication partners who are not literate (as long as they understand spoken language) and with those who have visual impairments, 4) allows the person using AAC to send messages without first obtaining his or her partner's attention through some other mode, and 5) allows communication to occur at a distance. Telephone interactions can also be enhanced by the use of synthetic speech. For example, Drager, Hustad, and Gable (2004) reported that synthetic voices were more understandable over typical audio speakers and over the telephone than the natural speech (which was 85% intelligible) of a 45-year-old woman with cerebral palsy.

To illustrate these advantages, consider Ahmad, a boy with severe disabilities who is included in a general kindergarten classroom of 30 children, has limited receptive language skills, and does not speak. If he uses an unaided AAC technique such as manual signing or a low-tech aided system such as a communication board, his teacher and his classmates must also learn to use and understand the symbols in that system. In fact, if Ahmad uses a communication board, his communication partners must be near him when he communicates so that they can see the symbols on the display. Now, imagine Ahmad using an AAC device that produces high-quality synthetic speech output when he touches a symbol on the display. His teacher and classmates now face fewer learning demands regarding reception and comprehension of the output, and Ahmad can communicate from anywhere in the classroom assuming that he can adjust the volume on the device sufficiently.

Speech output has several disadvantages as well. Even when synthetic or digitized speech is fairly intelligible, it may be difficult to hear and understand in noisy environments by people with hearing impairments, non-native language speakers, or those with reduced receptive language ability (e.g., aphasia, congenital learning disabilities, cognitive disabilities). AAC teams must consider such limitations individually before deciding whether speech output is appropriate for a particular individual.

Visual Output

As the quality of synthetic speech has improved over the years, visual output has changed from being a primary output method in AAC to being a supportive one. Generally speaking, visual output serves to clarify messages when the listener does not understand synthetic or natural speech. When an AAC device has a computer output screen, the listener may request clarification or message reformulation less frequently (Higginbotham, 1989). Visual output is particularly important for communication partners who have hearing impairments, who are unfamiliar with the person using AAC and his or her system, or who communicate in noisy environments where synthetic speech may not be intelligible. In addition to employing visual output to supplement synthetic speech output, many individuals utilize printed output in similar ways as do the rest of us—to write letters, complete assignments, leave notes, make lists, and keep personal journals.

AAC teams have often considered the type of visual display that electronic devices provide to be secondary to selection of the symbol set, access mode, and encoding technique. Nevertheless, as an increasing number of options have become available, and as stationary AAC computer displays have become increasingly common in schools and vocational settings, information concerning visual display options has become more relevant to device selection. A detailed discussion of the visual technology used in AAC devices, however, is well beyond the scope of this book (see Cook & Hussey, 2002, for a discussion of visual screens).

Hard Copy Print

A printer that may be part of a communication device or an adjunct to it produces permanent, "hard copy" output on paper. Many communication devices can be connected to standard peripheral printers or interfaced with small, portable printers. The printer may produce full-page, wide-column, or strip output in many paper and font sizes. Some software/hardware combinations can also print messages with nonorthographic symbols. For example, Macintosh computers can display and print PCS symbols using software programs such as Boardmaker and Speaking Dynamically Pro (Mayer-Johnson, Inc.) and Blissymbols can be printed using programs such as StoryBliss and AccessBliss (McNaughton, 1990a, 1990b).

Computer Screen Messages

Computer-generated messages are widely used in AAC devices as feedback and output. This technology can manage both orthographic and specialized symbols. A variety of technologies help display computer-generated symbols on screens (see Cook & Hussey, 2002, for detailed information).

Unaided Symbols

Nonelectronic forms of output such as gestures or manual signs impose memory requirements on both of the participants in the communicative exchange. Because no permanent display is available, all of the gestures or manual signs must be produced from memory by the sender and processed in memory by the receiver. These may be very difficult tasks for people who have memory impairments (e.g., people with TBI) or who have difficulty processing transitory information (e.g., people with autism; see Mirenda, 2003b). Many researchers and clinicians have encouraged the use of aided systems with permanent displays as a solution for people with memory impairments.

Another major concern regarding unaided symbol output is that relatively few people without disabilities are likely to understand it. For example, it appears that only 10%–30% of American Sign Language (ASL) signs and 50%–60% of Amer-Ind gestures are guessable by typical adults (Daniloff, Lloyd, & Fristoe, 1983; Doherty, Daniloff, & Lloyd, 1985). Thus, if an individual produces unaided symbols as the sole output to unfamiliar partners, he or she will almost always require a translator. Again, multimodal systems that incorporate both aided and unaided symbols often serve to resolve this dilemma.

Aided Symbol Displays

In nonelectronic applications that use aided symbols, communication partners interact directly with the symbol set itself. As the person who uses AAC identifies the symbols of choice, the partner formulates the message, often speaking it aloud as feedback. Whenever unfamiliar (i.e., translucent or opaque) symbols are used to form messages in communication systems, constraints may be placed on the range of communication partners who will comprehend the message. Potentially problematic aided symbols include textured symbols with arbitrarily assigned meanings, selected symbols from all the pictorial line-drawing sets discussed in Chapter 2, Blissymbols, orthographic symbols, abstract lexigrams, and other symbols such as braille and Morse code. To maximize aided output intelligibility in such situations, AAC teams often choose systems that provide simultaneous written translations of aided messages for literate communication partners. To facilitate interactions with nonliterate partners, AAC teams may opt for a multimodal AAC system with at least one component that provides synthetic speech output for the communication partner(s).

Another difficulty with the output provided by nonelectronic AAC options has to do with partner attention to the display. When people communicate with books, boards, or other low-tech displays, they must first get their partners' attention. Then, the partner must be able to turn or move toward the individual using AAC in order to see the board, book, or device that displays their message symbols. Finally, the communication partner must possess sufficient sensory acuity to see the output. There are many situations in which one or more of these requirements is difficult or impossible to fulfill. Such situations include communicative interactions in which a partner has a visual impairment and interactions in busy, crowded, or dimly lit environments or places that allow limited mobility (e.g., classrooms, factories, movie theaters, football games). The best solution in these situations may be for AAC teams to introduce one or more forms of speech or print output as part of a multimodal, individualized communication system.

> The role and potential impact of communicative [input] . . . has been underutilized in intervention approaches to date . . . . Research focus should be directed to the influence of the partner's communication [input] in [AAC] system exchanges. (Romski & Sevcik, 1988b, p. 89)

Visual Input

The availability of visual input appears to facilitate receptive language comprehension for some individuals. People with autism spectrum disorders, for instance, have been found to process concrete visuospatial information more readily than temporal or visuotemporal information such as speech or manual signs (Biklen, 1990; Mirenda & Schuler, 1989). Providing visual input models also appears to enhance their communication and language abilities or literacy skills, as exemplified by the work of Romski and Sevcik (1996; see Chapter 12 for additional information). Some individuals with aphasia may also benefit from augmented input, as discussed in Chapter 16.

Unaided Symbols

Gestures and signs are convenient types of input because they require no additional paraphernalia (e.g., books, boards, computers) and are always available for use because they do not have to be switched on as do electronic devices. Teachers and family members of persons with developmental disabilities often use manually signed input within a total (or simultaneous) communication paradigm, in which the communication partner accompanies spoken words with their corresponding signs (Carr, 1982). Some evidence suggests that communication partners who use total communication slow their rates of both speaking and signing and insert more pauses than when they use speech alone (Wilbur & Peterson, 1998; Windsor & Fristoe, 1989, 1991). This may account, at least in part, for the expressive and receptive language gains that some people with autism and other developmental delays display when using this approach (Kiernan, 1983). The type and amount of input that partners should provide to the child or adult are, however, major considerations. Should manually signed input accompany all or most spoken words, or should communication partners opt for a telegraphic or key-word approach instead? Should the individual employ a total communication approach throughout the day or only during designated instructional periods? Unfortunately, existing research does not supply the answers to these important questions, so clinicians must use their best judgment to make individualized decisions in these areas.

Aided Symbols

Communication partners can also provide input to people who rely on AAC, using aided symbols of many types. For example, a facilitator may draw simple pictures or write letters and words while speaking to a person with receptive aphasia to help him or her to comprehend messages (see Chapter 16). The two most prevalent input methods that utilize aided symbols are *aided language stimulation* (Elder & Goossens', 1994; Goossens', Crain, & Elder, 1992) and the *System for Augmented Language* (Romski & Sevcik, 1996). In both methods, a facilitator points to key symbols while speaking, in a manner parallel to that used in total communication. In order to accomplish this, facilitators must have the necessary symbols available for transmission and must organize the environment in order to apply the symbols appropriately. For aided language stimulation, facilitators must prepare activity boards with the necessary symbols in advance and have them available when needed (Goossens', 1989). Unfortunately, the logistical demands of aided symbol input often prevent facilitators from using the technique extensively, despite research evidence that it can have positive effects on both speech and language development over time (Romski & Sevcik, 1996; see Chapter 12 for additional information about these techniques).

CHAPTER 5

Team Building for AAC Assessment and Intervention

The office of the International Society of Augmentative and Alternative Communication (ISAAC), located in Toronto, Ontario, Canada, is an excellent source of information about AAC activities, policies, and services around the world. Information about the journal *Augmentative and Alternative Communication*, the *ISAAC Bulletin*, and other AAC publications such as *Communication Outlook*, *Communicating Together*, *Augmentative Communication News*, and *Alternatively Speaking* can be obtained from ISAAC.

The AAC field has developed and continues to develop in the context of a broad-based international community of persons who rely on AAC, family members, professionals, researchers, developers, and manufacturers. (See Zangari, Lloyd, & Vicker, 1994, for a detailed chronology of the development of the AAC field.) Although the models used to deliver AAC services vary widely from country to country, one common goal unites these efforts: to enable people to communicate to the best of their abilities. And, although the policies, legislation, and organizations that affect AAC continue to change, the efforts of teams of people, including the individual with complex communication needs and his or her family, are essential during the assessment and intervention process. Because a team approach is so important to the success of any AAC intervention, this chapter focuses on the skills needed for effective collaboration within a team.

TEAM DEVELOPMENT

Why work within a team structure anyway? Wouldn't it be easier for professionals to "do their own thing" in each specialty area and have occasional meetings to share information? The answer is yes, it would be easier for professionals, but it would not be better for those who rely on AAC and their families! It is essential to involve them as well as other significant individuals as members of the team from the outset of intervention. Furthermore, AAC teams should base intervention decisions on a broad range of information. For example, teams need information regarding the cognitive, language, sensory, and motor capabilities of the individual, as well as information regarding the operational, linguistic, social, and strategic competence of the individual's current communication strategy. Teams also need to know about current and future communicative contexts and about the support system available to the individual. Intervention teams must also identify and respect the preferences of those with complex communication needs, their families or guardians, and their personal advisers. Few individual AAC specialists are capable of assessing and intervening in all these areas; therefore, it is nearly always necessary to involve a team of individuals to provide appropriate AAC services. When it comes to AAC, the old adage that "two heads are better than one" holds true—collaborative efforts are integral to the success of most interventions (Utley & Rapport, 2002).

Early efforts to build inclusionary, cooperative teams may prevent problems and discord later on. "Consensus today keeps dissension away."

Two kinds of issues affect the ability of a team to function harmoniously and efficiently: structural issues and relational issues. Structural issues include concerns such as

- The model of service delivery that guides the functioning of the team

- The goals and purposes of the team

- Membership on the team

- Who can be referred to the team and how the referral process is organized

- How services are organized and delivered

- How resources are managed

- How and by whom team meetings are run

Blackstone (1990) identified several structural factors deemed critical by AAC interventionists. These include conducting interventions in natural contexts, involving families throughout the assessment and intervention, and using a team approach. She also noted several structural factors that clinicians believe impede service delivery, such as insufficient funding, center-based evaluations, lack of a team approach, lack of follow-up, and pull-out therapy services. Structural problems often appear in the form of confusion about the purposes of the team or how it operates; a perception that services are delivered inequitably; long lag times between referral and service delivery because of inefficient team operation; team meetings that are disorganized and consume inordinate amounts of time; and, ultimately, less-than-adequate outcomes for the consumer.

Similar problems can also be the result of relational problems on the team, including

- Frequent violation of the implicit and/or explicit social norms established by the group for interaction

- A feeling that it is not safe for team members to express their feelings and opinions
- Inequitable or dysfunctional interactions among team members
- An inability to give and receive criticism, resolve conflicts, and take others' perspectives
- Decision-making processes that leave some members feeling devalued or marginalized
- Team members who regularly dominate meetings and interactions
- A lack of creative problem-solving skills among team members
- Freeloading, perpetual lateness, or work avoidance by some team members
- A lack of positive interdependence ("all for one, one for all")

Initially, relational problems affect how team members interact and cooperate, but over time they also affect team functioning and productiveness. Team members often ignore relational issues until the problem is like a "whale in the living room"—so big that it can't be ignored any longer! Unfortunately, by this time team members are often so angry and demoralized that it is difficult for them to deal openly and honestly with the concerns. The trick, of course, is to avoid such problems by setting up the team in ways that are likely to prevent it from becoming dysfunctional. The sections that follow focus on strategies for building functional, effective teams.

STRUCTURAL ISSUES

Teams can be organized in a variety of ways. On a *multidisciplinary* team, each specialist independently completes his or her portion of an AAC assessment and makes discipline-specific intervention decisions. The team members then share the assessment results and intervention plans at a team meeting, after which each team member provides direct services to the individual. Within an *interdisciplinary* team model, specialists also assess students individually but then meet to discuss their individual findings and make collaborative recommendations regarding an intervention plan. Team members may meet regularly to discuss progress and make revisions in the intervention, which is usually overseen by one team member (often called the "case manager"). Alternatively, all of the interdisciplinary team members may meet regularly to discuss progress and make revisions in the intervention. Finally, on a *transdisciplinary* team, information is shared among professionals so that direct services providers become proficient in areas other than their primary specialties (Locke & Mirenda, 1992). Assessment is often completed through the collaborative efforts of all team members and is followed by a team meeting to establish the goals and objectives for intervention. According to Hart (1977), once decisions are made, each team member is responsible for the care of the whole individual, rather than only one facet of his or her life.

What is the "best" structure for an AAC team? This question cannot be answered without first considering the goals and purposes of each team and whom it is meant to serve. Thus, successful AAC teams may work within any of these models, although Yorkston and Karlan (1986) suggested that the interdisciplinary model is perhaps the most common. There is certainly a growing trend toward and a need for service-delivery structures in which center-based and community-based programs work together in one system. Alm and Parnes recommended models that combine community-based rehabilitation with "Centers for Excellence" (1995, p. 183) that focus on specialty areas of AAC, research and development, and high-tech assistive technology approaches. The trend toward such models is becoming increasingly prevalent around the world in such places as Sweden, South Africa (Alant, 1993; Alant & Emmett, 1995), the United Kingdom (Leese et al., 1993), and the United States. Alm and Parnes noted that systems that operate as a "dynamic continuum" (1995, p. 183) are more likely to encourage accessible and flexible programs that are effective and cost-efficient while also providing for a concentration of expertise as needed for technological and training supports. Alant suggested that, especially in less developed countries, community-based service delivery requires a "dialogical strategy" (1996, p. 3), which accommodates both an intellectualized level of knowledge (from professionals) and an experiential level of attitudes and social structures (from the community).

> One factor that hampers intervention in less developed countries can be identified as the separation of the technical AAC strategy skill of professionals and their ability to understand the contextual demands for implementation . . . . This . . . often contributes to a superficial understanding of the reality within which service provision occurs within these contexts, leading to inappropriate recommendations of "what is needed." . . . It is clear that, when dealing with different communities, one of the most important issues remains the redefinition of AAC strategies within the infrastructure of that community. (Alant, 1996, p. 2)

Team membership often needs to be quite broad and must include the person who relies on AAC and family members as integral—not just "token"—members. Several negative outcomes can result if these individuals are not incorporated into the team before the assessment and intervention-planning processes. First, the team will lack information that pertains to subsequent intervention efforts. Second, the individual who relies on AAC and his or her family may not be able to assume "ownership" of interventions that are formulated by others on the team without their input and agreement. Third, distrust of the agency delivering AAC services may develop if the family is not permitted to participate, regardless of the quality of the evaluation or interventions. Fourth, they may not learn to participate as team members if they have been excluded when team dynamics and interaction styles are established.

These consequences are also likely to result if key professionals, especially those who manage the natural environments in which the persons with complex communication needs participate, are excluded or ignored as team members. For example, general and special education teachers usually manage a child's educational environment, speech-language pathologists often manage the communication-conversation environment, employers manage the work environment, and family members or residential staff may manage the living environment. One or more of these individuals is likely to be affected by any of the team's decisions. Therefore, their involvement is absolutely critical in order to avoid later problems that are related to a lack of collaboration or a failure to follow through with team decisions.

Galvin and Donnell (2002) noted that what they call "technology lust" can "cause one to forget that there is a process for selecting a device, a process that involves the consumer in identifying his or her goals, the tasks to be accomplished, and his or her attitude toward technology. The result, if the assessment is conducted appropriately, may be an item of high technology or one of low technology . . . " (pp. 156–157)

Another important structural issue involves the creation of systems for managing resources. In particular, it is important to have ready access to rental or loan equipment that can be used for trial periods during an AAC evaluation. Rental equipment can be housed in centralized loan banks or can be located in community settings such as health units or school districts (Blackstone, 1990, 1994b). In fact, loan banks or similar systems may help to reduce the prevalence of technology abandonment, which occurs worldwide. The phenomenon of technology abandonment, which is all too familiar to most AAC professionals, occurs when communication technology is discarded by the person whom it was meant to benefit. As Turner and colleagues noted, "At first glance, technology abandonment seems somewhat understandable because people with disabilities are the ones sticking technology in their closets, attics, and basements. Yet the responsibility for this phenomenon does not rest solely with the disability community" (1995, p. 288). Technology abandonment appears to be the result of a number of interrelated factors, including the following:

- Recommendations for electronic AAC devices that produce inadequate synthetic speech; that demand message programming or retrieval skills that are too complex for the individual who relies on AAC; and/or that are not cosmetically pleasing to the person using the device (Galvin & Donnell, 2002; Jinks & Sinteff, 1994; Riemer-Reiss & Wacker, 2000)

- The use of professional-centered rather than consumer- and family-centered decision-making processes (Riemer-Reiss & Wacker, 2000; Turner et al., 1995)

- Inadequate availability of AAC systems in relevant environments, a lack of responsive communication partners, inadequate training of communication partners, insufficient time for consumer training and support (i.e., follow-up), inadequate selection of vocabulary for systems, and lack of acknowledgment of the multimodal nature of communication (Galvin & Donnell, 2002; Murphy, Marková, Collins, & Moodie, 1996)

- Poor or inadequate services related to the mounting and portability of AAC systems (Jinks & Sinteff, 1994; Murphy et al., 1996)

Table 5.1.   Symptoms of structural difficulties in AAC service delivery programs

1. Because the AAC program includes people from many professional disciplines, there is no administrator who assumes overall responsibility for the program.
2. The agency has no policies regarding the use of AAC equipment or materials.
3. There is no staff development plan for the AAC team members.
4. A person who relies on AAC is placed at the beginning of the school year in a classroom in which the "new" teacher has had no preparation regarding AAC.
5. The AAC efforts of the agency are inefficient or haphazard because there is no designated team leader.
6. AAC interventions are often "stalled" because it is not clear who is responsible for obtaining funds to purchase AAC systems.
7. Funds for purchasing the AAC equipment and materials that are needed for assessment must be "squeezed out" of the budgets of the speech-language pathology and occupational therapy departments because the AAC program has no independent budget.
8. People with AAC systems receive as much (or less) intervention time from the speech-language pathologist as people with mild communication impairments (e.g., mild articulation disorders).
9. Although one or two schools in a school district have well-developed AAC programs, there is no systematic plan for establishing such programs in other schools that serve students with complex communication needs.
10. Although a person with complex communication needs and his or her family desire AAC services, they cannot figure out how to obtain them or who is responsible for delivering services

Clearly, these are all issues related to the adequacy of assessment and implementation (i.e., issues related to the quality and quantity of available services), not simply issues that stem from simple consumer or family "noncompliance." Service delivery systems that are structurally sound and that have efficient systems for managing resources are more likely to experience fewer problems in this area. Table 5.1 lists symptoms of structural difficulties that may be found in agencies that deliver AAC services.

> Having a collection of people is not the same as having a team. (Giangreco, 1996a, p. 21)

RELATIONAL ISSUES

How do a "collection of people" come together to form a team? If you are lucky enough to be a member of a team that functions like a well-oiled machine, you may not have had the need to stop and ask yourself how it came to be that way. But if you (like most of us) are now or have ever been on a team whose gears are sometimes out of alignment, this is more than an academic question. When conflicts occur, the roots frequently can be traced to early failure to develop productive consensus patterns among team members. Table 5.2 lists 10 symptoms commonly seen among AAC teams that do not practice consensus-building strategies during assessment and decision making.

Fortunately, we know a lot about what helps and what hinders the ability of a collection of people to collaborate efficiently and effectively as a team. According to Thousand and Villa (2000), all members of truly collaborative teams employ a process that involves 1) frequent face-to-face interactions in which each member's input is equally valued;

Table 5.2.   Ten symptoms of AAC teams that do not practice consensus building

1. Parents or guardians who have not been included in the assessment or decision-making processes are asked to sign individualized education programs (IEPs) that delineate AAC interventions.
2. People with complex communication needs are not asked for input during assessment or intervention planning.
3. A person's new AAC system is a surprise to his or her classroom teacher, parents, or employer.
4. Although many team members attend a meeting, only a few give reports. These few team members also control the discussion so that other members are neither required nor expected to contribute their opinions or preferences.
5. A parent or guardian refers to an AAC intervention as something "they" said to do.
6. Paraprofessionals, educational aides, or direct care staff are not invited to attend team meetings.
7. A school administrator rejects an intervention plan without having attended the team meeting at which it was formulated.
8. Parents or guardians are not provided with opportunities early in the assessment process to express their opinions and preferences.
9. When parents speak at a team meeting, team members do not take notes as they do when other team members speak.
10. The members of the AAC team have never met the staff who manage the individuals' residence or employment site.

2) positive interdependence; 3) practicing, monitoring, and processing interpersonal skills; and 4) individual accountability. We examine each of these in detail.

Frequent Face-to-Face Interactions

It might seem obvious that team members need to meet regularly in order to function as a team, but there are many ways in which teams can compromise this most basic requirement. Groups can be so large that there is little opportunity for each member to express his or her ideas or feelings. Scheduling a common meeting time for people who are very busy can be difficult. Then there are the latecomers, the early leavers, and the sporadic attenders; teams thus have the challenge of efficiently communicating decisions and assignments to members who are absent. There may also be power imbalances or learning style differences among team members that can create challenging interpersonal dynamics. Even physical arrangements can make it difficult to interact and plan effectively. It's no wonder that the simple requirement for face-to-face interaction is often problematic!

Haaf, Millin, and Verberg described the ideal relationship between a consumer and a team of AAC professionals in a story about Sheila, a fictitious 16-year-old girl with cerebral palsy:

When decisions are being made regarding assistive technology, Sheila's opinions and ideas are listened to, and her needs (not the preferences of the professional team or convenience of family member[s] or school staff) are paramount . . . . Recently, Sheila expressed a desire to try a standard keyboard with a keyguard on her computer at school. Although clinicians on her team expressed their opinion that this was not as functional for her as using her Touch Talker (SGD), the clinicians recognized that Sheila needed to try it for herself and make her own decision. The consequence of this level of responsibility is that although the decision is ultimately Sheila's, she needs to assume responsibility for the decisions that are made, even if they turn out to be wrong. (1994, pp. 4–6)

Team Membership and Participation

It is important to make thoughtful decisions about who should be on a team. The following three questions should be asked when formulating any team:

1. Who has the expertise needed by the team to make the best decisions? The days when "the more, the merrier" was the predominant approach to team membership are long past. Funding, time, and other constraints often make it necessary to economize for the sake of efficiency, but smaller teams can also be more effective. The literature on this issue suggests that a team of four to six members is ideal to ensure diversity of viewpoints while supporting effective communication (Johnson & Johnson, 1987b). However, at any given time, team membership might change as the consumer's needs dictate. For example, during the initial assessment for an AAC system or device, the involvement of one or two team members might be sufficient if the issues are quite clear. Later on, teams might invite additional members to consult about specific motor, sensory, or other concerns that arise. This concept of utilizing a small "core team" of people who are most immediately and directly involved with a specific individual with complex communication needs plus an "expanded team" of people with additional expertise as needed is likely to enhance both team effectiveness and team efficiency (Swengel & Marquette, 1997; Thousand & Villa, 2000).

2. Who is affected by the decisions? In almost all cases, the answer to this question is simple: the person who relies on AAC and his or her family. Ironically, these are often the individuals who are least involved and least consulted in the AAC assessment and intervention process! As a result, the outcomes desired by the consumer may take a "backseat" to the goals identified as important by the professionals on the team. For example, one of us was told about the experience of an older man with cerebral palsy who lives in a group home and whose speech is insufficient for talking on the telephone (but is sufficient for most day-to-day interactions). During the initial meeting with the AAC team, he made it quite clear that all he wanted was to be able to use the telephone to talk to his family and order pizza or do other tasks. Six months later, after many hours of assessment and experimentation, he ended up with a very sophisticated SGD that can do just about everything, including help him talk on the telephone—and that's exactly what he uses it for! The rest of the time, this expensive piece of equipment sits by the telephone waiting for the next time he has a taste for pizza! When members of the AAC team that provided the device were told about this outcome, they shook their heads and bemoaned his lack of vision for himself and his reluctance to use the technology provided to him. This example illustrates the kind of problem that can arise when the consumer and family members are "token" but not "real" members of the team and when goals and outcomes are professionally defined rather than consumer defined. As Michael Williams asked, "Whose outcome is it anyway?" (1995, p. 1).

3. Who has an interest in participating? This question is meant to encourage the team to think beyond the obvious. In every community, there are people who might be interested in helping to solve particular problems or in lending their expertise. For example, we know a high school computer science teacher, Mr. Reilley, who acts as an informal "technology consultant" to his daughter's elementary school. In this capacity, he has made numerous suggestions for simple adaptations that have resulted in better computer access for students with physical disabilities. Although unusual, Mr. Reilley's membership on the team has been a critical factor in those students' successful use of technology. Thinking broadly about team membership will often reveal such opportunities to "build bridges" into the larger community.

> The speech teacher did ask me if I liked it [a Canon Communicator] and I said "no" but she said, "Hang in there; it's not going to be overnight." Most of the time nobody asked. And, if they did, it didn't seem to make them change anything. I felt like they were the experts; listen to them . . . . My doctor told my speech teacher what to put on my board so I could tell him what my problem is . . . . Nobody asked me if the pictures were okay. The doctor said it and the speech teacher did it . . . . They made me feel like I'm not the one who has to carry it and use it; but I am. Does it matter if they are wrong? No. Just do what they say and don't make waves! (Dawn, a young woman with cerebral palsy, describing the "flip side" of the consumer–professional relationship, in Smith-Lewis & Ford, 1987, p. 16)

More challenging than decisions about who should be on a team are decisions about how to create an environment in which team members can function most efficiently and effectively. This goes beyond arranging the physical environment and encompasses such nitty-gritty issues as organizing meetings for maximal effectiveness, establishing guidelines for communication and attendance, and dealing with time constraints. We discuss these issues in more detail later in this chapter.

> Positive interdependence is the perception that one is linked with others in a way so that one cannot succeed unless they do (and vice versa), and that their work benefits you and your work benefits them. It is the belief that "you sink or swim together." (Johnson & Johnson, 1987a, p. 399)

Positive Interdependence

Perhaps the most important aspects of team functioning are the relationships and interactions among team members. Often, the mutual respect and ability to work in an "all for one and one for all" atmosphere will determine the success of a team effort (Giangreco, 2000). Four processes are particularly relevant to interdependence, especially when new teams are being formed or when new members join an existing team.

Discussing Individual Philosophies, Goals, Roles, and Needs

Having team members discuss individual philosophies, goals, roles, and needs is an important yet often overlooked step in forming a collaborative team. It is natural for each member of the team to have his or her own experiences, goals, perception of his or her roles, and needs. However, it is generally assumed that individuals will put all of these preconceptions aside "for the greater good," even during team conflict. When teams first come together, it is important for members to discuss individual goals and needs publicly. This is particularly important in order to involve consumer and family members productively because their perceptions of their needs and the perceptions of the rest of the team may differ. In addition, the needs and priorities of parents may change over time, as reflected in two related studies that examined this issue in families with young children (Angelo, Jones, & Kokoska, 1995) and with adolescents or young adults who use AAC (Angelo, Kokoska, & Jones, 1996). Table 5.3 summarizes the top needs and priorities identified by both mothers and fathers across these two studies, which may differ quite dramatically over the years as mothers and fathers assume different roles on the AAC team.

Similarly, professional members of the team, especially those who join the team on a case-by-case basis (e.g., a vision specialist who participates on behalf of specific indi-

Table 5.3.   Needs of mothers and fathers of people who rely on AAC in two age groups

	Families with young children		Families with adolescents and young adults	
	% Mothers (*n* = 56)	% Fathers (*n* = 35)	% Mothers (*n* = 85)	% Fathers (*n* = 47)
Increasing knowledge of assistive devices	44.4	48.5	46.4	44.7
Planning for future communication needs	42.8	45.7	44.6	50.0
Integrating assistive devices in community settings	49.0		48.8	
Integrating assistive devices at home		41.1		44.7
Getting computer access	44.4			43.2
Developing community awareness and support for assistive device use	47.2			
Finding advocacy groups for parents of children using assistive devices	41.0			
Finding trained professionals to work with my child	41.0			
Finding volunteers to work with my child		44.1		
Getting funding for an assistive device		42.8		
Knowing how to teach my child using an assistive device		41.1		
Having social opportunities with peers without disabilities			54.1	
Having social opportunities with others who use assistive devices			47.6	
Knowing how to maintain or repair an assistive device				48.9
Integrating assistive devices in educational settings				43.5
Knowing how to program an assistive device				43.5

viduals but is not a consistent member), should be included in a discussion related to their needs and roles from the beginning of their involvement. For example, Locke and Mirenda (1992) reported that teachers on AAC teams often assume a wide variety of responsibilities, ranging from traditional "teacher roles," such as writing goals and objectives (82%) and assessing cognitive abilities (81%), to those that might be within the traditional domain of other team members, such as designing and constructing adaptive devices (35%) or assessing symbolic representation (34%). Thus, these individuals join each new team with expectations colored by their past experiences (positive and negative) that may not represent the expectations of the rest of the team. It is important to achieve clarity and negotiate agreement on such issues early in the collaborative process.

A major reason for having team members clearly articulate their needs, role perceptions, and priorities is to avoid some of the negative effects of not doing so! Such effects may include the sabotage of team efforts by individual members, passive-aggressive behaviors such as "forgetting" to come to meetings or "not having time" to complete essential tasks, or even expressions of outright hostility in some cases. If everyone declares their personal agendas "up front," these agendas are more likely to be met or accommodated. Most important, declaring one's own goals and needs publicly is the first step in establishing a standard of honest, trusting, and trustworthy behavior among all team members (Locke & Mirenda, 1992).

Ada Huston is a speech-language pathologist who worked for the past 6 years in a school district where she had a caseload of 52 students, 6 of whom relied on AAC technology (see Blackstone, 1997, for information about "typical" speech-language pathologist caseloads in schools and other settings). She is most familiar with a two-tiered AAC service delivery model in which school district personnel assess and serve students with less complex communication needs and specialists help those with more complex needs at a regional assessment center. Recently, she moved to a new city and is now part of a team that supports children and adults with acquired disabilities. When she meets the other members of her team for the first time and they each talk about their personal goals, she says that she wants to learn more about AAC technology for children and adults. She also says that her long-term goal, maybe 5 years down the road, is to start a private practice specializing in communication supports for children and adults with traumatic brain injury.

Identifying Learning and Work-Style Needs

One area in which goal and need identification is particularly important for AAC professionals has to do with learning and work style issues, especially as they relate to technology learning. From our clinical, research, and classroom experiences, we have come to think about professionals in three groups: mastery learners, performance learners, and social learners (Beukelman, Burke, Ball, & Horn, 2002; Beukelman, Hanson, Hiatt, Fager, & Bilyeu, 2004; Burke, Beukelman, Ball, & Horn, 2002). *Mastery learners* are individuals who prefer to learn alone and will strive to master completely new pieces of software or equipment. They tend to be very systematic in their learning; they will often read instruction manuals thoroughly, explore all of the options and features of each new product, and so forth. These individuals are often solitary learners who prefer to be self-directed rather than work in groups. In addition, they often have considerable self-efficacy—that is, the confidence that they can learn if they apply themselves. In contrast, *performance learners* work well in a team structure and usually learn new technologies in order to provide good service. Their goal is to learn what they need to enhance client performance rather than to completely master the technology; they learn best when they are faced with actual clinical problems that they can resolve as part of the learning process. Because performance learners are more "practically oriented" than "thoroughness oriented," they may appear (at least to mastery learners) to be rather haphazard in their approach, when, in fact, they are simply more focused on technology as a means to an end rather than as an end in itself. Performance learners with high self-efficacy may enjoy learning alone or in small groups, whereas those with low self-efficacy often prefer direct instruction from an expert.

Finally, *social learners* enjoy the social aspects of team participation. They tend to be motivated to learn so that they are included in (or at least not excluded from) the group. If they have high or moderate self-efficacy in an area, they often prefer to work in interactive groups so that their social needs can be met while they are learning. If they have low self-efficacy in an area, they may prefer direct instruction from an expert. Social learners tend to provide the relational "glue" for an AAC team.

Previous exposure to and experience with computers in general and AAC in particular appears to be one of the factors that determines technology learning style. For example, many AAC specialists tend to be mastery learners (Burke et al., 2002), while students and professionals with less experience tend to be performance learners (Beukelman, Burke, et al., 2002). Clearly, it is important for each team member to think about and articulate his or her technology learning style needs early in the formation of the team. In that way, accommodations can be made for the different (and sometimes conflicting!) styles. For example, performance and social learners are often intimidated by mastery learners who, in turn, may be quite impatient and frustrated with their extremely people-oriented colleagues. Putting these three types of learners together to learn a new product is often a recipe for stress and conflict. Yet, mastery learners are invaluable on a team because they are the ones to whom everyone turns when there is a technological problem or unusual challenge. By the same token, social learners have the "people skills" that make them good group instructors for other social learners (once they have learned the technology themselves). Similarly, performance learners often make good technology instructors because they can appreciate and explain both the clinical implications and the technical aspects of a product. We find that effective teams often have a good "mix" of each type of learner and assign responsibilities within the team to take advantage of each person's learning and work-style strengths.

Ms. Huston and her colleagues talk at their first meeting about learning and work styles. She admits (somewhat sheepishly) that she has not had a lot of experience with high-tech AAC devices and computer software and that she is a bit worried about her ability to contribute to the team efforts in this area. She says that she is used to being socially active throughout her day and, although she is quite able to be independent, she prefers collaborating with others to learn and to solve problems. Her colleagues laugh and tell her to "stay away from Jake," the physical therapist on the team who they fondly call a "tech-head" because his style is exactly the opposite! Two team members suggest that she participate in a series of hands-on workshops they are running for parents and teachers over a 6-week period to learn the basic operations of several pieces of equipment, and she quickly agrees. They also reassure her that they all learn differently and that she'll do just fine (as long as she steers clear of Jake!).

Agreeing on Mutual Team Goals

Once individual goals have been identified, the team can move on to identifying mutual goals that are needed for effective functioning. Some of these may be congruent with individual goals, and some may conflict. When conflicts occur, it is important for members to examine the conflict within a "win-win" framework (Fisher, Ury, & Patton, 1991) and attempt to discover together how the goals of all conflicting parties can be accommodated. This may take some time but is surely worth the effort in the long run because the process of arriving at solutions together can help the team to develop some of the negotiation and listening skills that are critical for long-term success. The process of identifying mutual goals is really a process of "vision planning" and should be repeated periodically in teams that are longstanding.

At the rehab team's first meeting, members also did some "vision planning" for 1-year and 3-year markers. They decided that their 1-year goal was to explore ways to improve the efficiency of their service delivery model in light of the funding restrictions imposed by managed care. Specifically, they decided to modify the transdisciplinary, or "arena assessment," model they've used in the past. Within this model, all team members meet to complete the assessment and then establish collaborative goals and objectives for intervention. They decided to try a modified approach in which the team will first meet to decide who should be involved in the assessment for each client (Glennen, 1997). The selected members will then work collaboratively as a "mini-team." They also decided that over the next 3 years they want to improve their ability to do field-based research to document the outcomes of their interventions. A subgroup volunteered to discuss some strategies for accomplishing this and report back with suggestions in 1 month.

Creating Positive Resource, Role, Task, and Reward Interdependence

Positive interdependence means that team members share resources and take different roles as needed, create an equitable division of labor, and create common rewards for group members' work. It also means that the team shares the knowledge, skills, and material resources of each member to complete the job at hand and that team roles may be explicitly distributed and shared among members during team meetings on a rotating basis. Some of the most common of these roles are summarized in Table 5.4. Finally, interdependence requires that all members participate equally in completing the necessary tasks, even if this means crossing "disciplinary boundaries" at times (Soto, Müller, Hunt, & Goetz, 2001b). For example, the motor specialist on a team might offer to assist her "temporarily swamped" speech-language pathologist colleague to create communication displays. Her colleague might then reciprocate later by helping to create a specialized switch mount for a wheelchair. When task interdependence is held as the norm, work assignments should be reviewed periodically by the team to ensure that no one is either "freeloading" by taking on fewer tasks or having trouble "letting go" of tasks that could be shared with others. Finally, when successes are celebrated collectively so that no one person gets special recognition, all team members can share in the gratification of having contributed to the achievement. By the same token, teams that swim together may sometimes sink together—so when things don't go the way they were planned, the collective "we" rather than a single person takes responsibility for setbacks.

It is now 4 months after the team's first meeting, and Ms. Huston has been busy! She's had to get used to working in a setting where resources and job responsibilities are shared. At first, she felt a bit threatened and was concerned that her skills were not respected or utilized, because everyone on the team seemed to know a lot about everything! Over time, though, she has realized that her expertise is valued and that she can be an active contributor to the AAC assessment and intervention process. Plus, she's learned a lot of things that she never imagined she would learn—from the operation of several new devices to how to recognize primitive reflex patterns that might interfere with their use. She's also learned about how *not* to conduct team meetings—it seems to her that her colleagues waste a lot of time each week complaining about their workloads! Ms. Huston, however, does enjoy the 10 minutes at the end of each meeting when the outreach team reports about the status of individuals who have been discharged, because most of them are doing well in the community. Overall, she's a bit overwhelmed but proud to be part of a team that works and celebrates their successes together!

Practicing, Monitoring, and Processing Interpersonal Skills

People are born into the world one at a time, not in groups—perhaps that's why most of us don't automatically have the skills needed to collaborate in group situations! Although such skills go far beyond those required in one-to-one interactions or most other social situations, it is not unusual for teams to assume that all members will just "have" the interpersonal skills that are needed to work together effectively. Of course, that's not always the case—and problems with interpersonal communication among the members of a team are both common and stressful for all involved. In this section, we examine some of the strategies that might be useful to teams who are dissatisfied with the ways in which members interact with one another.

Table 5.4.   Areas of expertise for an AAC team

Speech-language pathology

  Communication sciences

  Normal and disordered communication

  Receptive and expressive language

  Development and disorders

  Alternative and augmentative aids, symbols, techniques, and strategies

  Management of communication interventions

Medicine

  Management of therapeutic program

  Natural course of the disorder

  Medical intervention

  Management of medication regimes

Physical therapy

  Mobility aids

  Motor control and motor learning

  Positioning to maximize functional communication in all environments

  Maintenance of strength and range of motion

  Physical conditioning to increase flexibility, balance, and coordination

Occupational therapy

  Activities of daily living

  Positioning to maximize functional communication in all contexts

  Adaptive equipment

  Mobility aids

  Access to aids, computers, and splints

Engineering

  Application and modification of existing electronic or mechanical aids and devices

Education

  Planning for appropriate social and academic experiences

  Development of cognitive/conceptual objectives

  Assessment of sociocommunicative components in the classroom

  Integration of augmentative components in the classroom

  Development of an appropriate vocational curriculum

Psychology

  Documentation of level of cognitive functioning

  Selection of appropriate learning styles

  Estimation of learning potential

Social services

  Evaluation of total living situation

  Identification of family and community resources

  Provision of information about funding options

Vocational counseling

  Assessment of vocational potential

  Identification of vocational goals

  Education of co-workers

  Identification of augmentative components in vocational settings

Computer technology

  Evaluation of software programs for potential use by clients

  Modification of existing software programs

  Developing programs to meet existing communication needs

Establishing Group Norms

All groups have norms (i.e., expectations about standard practices and operations), but they are usually informal (i.e., unstated) rather than explicit. Norms are important because they help to equalize the influence between outspoken and more timid group members and because they establish a set of expectations that are understood by all. For some teams, it is important to discuss and determine group norms quite explicitly, especially if there is frequent team member turnover or if some members tend to function more autonomously than others. It might even be useful to post the agreed-on norms or include them as part of a new team orientation handbook. Some of the social norms that might be stated explicitly include, for example, not using foul language or sarcasm, treating each other with respect and dignity at all times, understanding that the process is just as important as the product, and so forth. The team may also decide to be explicit about one or more task-related norms such as, "We will get all reports done by the third Thursday of the month" or, "We will start and end all meetings on time."

> Over time, Ms. Huston learned that a social norm on her new team is that everyone uses first names when addressing each other, so she had to get used to being called Lavinia by her colleagues. She also learned that there is a very strong ethic that everyone participate actively at team meetings, which she knows will be a challenge for her because she is quite shy by nature. But it's all part of the growth process!

Practicing Interpersonal Skills for Collaboration

Johnson and colleagues (Johnson, Johnson, & Holubec, 1993; Johnson, Johnson, Holubec, & Roy, 1994) identified four sets of skills needed for effective collaboration:

1. Forming skills: Forming skills are the initial trust-building skills needed to establish a team. Forming skills are necessary to establish trust as well as to ensure that everyone is focused on the task at hand.

2. Functioning skills: Functioning skills are the communication and leadership skills needed for management and organizational purposes. They are also needed to ensure that tasks are completed and relationships are maintained. When functioning skills are present on a team, they are often taken for granted, but when they are not present, they are sorely missed! It is important that all team members value the same functioning skills; otherwise, mixed messages are likely to abound, with the associated stresses that accompany them. For example, if some team members are "solo players" and others are "team players," there is likely to be a conflict each time one of the latter members asks one of the former for assistance, unless it is clear that such co-teaching is expected and valued as part of the job.

3. Formulating skills: Formulating skills are those skills needed for learning, creative problem solving, and decision making, such as asking why or how a particular solution was chosen or asking for feedback, rationales, or elaboration. Formulating skills also include diagnosing and talking about group difficulties regarding both tasks and interpersonal problems and generating multiple solutions through creative problem-solving strategies. Many teams exert insufficient effort in this area in terms of both in-service education and actual practice.

4. Fermenting skills: Fermenting skills are needed to manage controversy and conflicting opinions, search for more information, and stimulate revision and refinement of solutions. The better the fermenting skills of a team, the more likely it is that members will see diversity as an asset rather than as a problem. It is important to note that although fermenting skills often do not come naturally, they can be learned. Some useful resources include game theory (Zagare, 1984) and the "win-win" techniques developed by Fisher et al. (1991).

It should be clear from this description that the interpersonal skills needed for collaborative teaming are multiple and complex! You might want to examine the forming, functioning, formulating, and fermenting skills evident in your own team by using the assessment form in Figure 5.1. You can use it to reflect on your own behavior as well as that of your team as a whole. Without a good balance of skills in each of these four areas, it is likely that decisions will be made autocratically (i.e., by one person) rather than after consultation with all members. The problem is that autocratic decision making is likely to perpetuate disjointed and fragmented service delivery as well as create conflicts among team members. An often-used alternative is to take a democratic approach to decision making in which the "majority rules"—but this, too, may be problematic in that it tends to polarize factions within teams and discount the potential value of dissenting opinions. A democratic approach is particularly problematic when the dissenting opinion is held by the person with complex communication needs and/or family members who, after all, will ultimately be the most affected by decisions. Arriving at decisions through consensus may take more time in the short run but can save time by avoiding the aftermath of more "efficient" processes over the long run. Regardless, as each team decides on its own decision-making process and style, the skills needed for cooperation and collaboration must be part of the members' learning agenda.

Ms. Huston and her team have decided to tackle the complaints about workload that seem to be growing in both frequency and magnitude. At a team meeting, they each take 5 minutes to share their experiences and their perceptions of the causes of the problem. They identify several issues: a perception that some members are overworked whereas others are not very busy, differences in individual work styles that make some appear to be more efficient than others, and the belief that there are just too few professionals for the number of individuals referred to the team. They spend some time brainstorming potential solutions without making any judgments about their potential efficacy and then talk about each idea in turn. By the end of the meeting, they have made two decisions: 1) to institute an absolute moratorium on complaining about the workload for 2 weeks and 2) to devise a system for collecting data that will allow them to identify how much time the various tasks assigned to each member currently take. They hope that, with such data, they will be able to determine whether they are actu-

Name: _____   Team name: _____

Directions for Individual Assessment

Reflect on your behavior while working as a member of your team. On a five-point scale (1 = *I never do;* 5 = *I always do*), rate yourself on the following skills. Select and place a star next to the two to four skills that you wish to improve.

Directions for Group Assessment

Reflect on your team's functioning. On a five-point scale (1 = *We never do;* 5 = *We always do*), rate your entire team on the following skills. Compare your ratings with those of your teammates and jointly select two to four skills to improve. Place an arrow next to the skills that your team has selected.

Forming Skills
(Trust building)

Self		Group
_____	I/We arrive at meetings on time.	_____
_____	I/We stay for the duration of the meeting.	_____
_____	I/We participate(d) in the establishment of the group's goal.	_____
_____	I/We share individual personal goals.	_____
_____	I/We encourage everyone to participate.	_____
_____	I/We use members' names.	_____
_____	I/We look at the speaker.	_____
_____	I/We do not use put-downs.	_____
_____	I/We use an appropriate voice volume and tone.	_____

Functioning Skills
(Communication and distributed leadership)

Self		Group
_____	I/We share ideas.	_____
_____	I/We share feelings when appropriate.	_____
_____	I/We share materials or resources.	_____
_____	I/We volunteer for roles that help the group accomplish the task (e.g., timekeeper).	_____
_____	I/We volunteer for roles that help to maintain a harmonious working group (e.g., encourage everyone to participate).	_____
_____	I/We clarify the purpose of the meeting.	_____
_____	I/We set or call attention to time limits.	_____
_____	I/We offer suggestions on how to accomplish the task effectively.	_____
_____	I/We ask for help, clarification, or technical assistance when needed.	_____
_____	I/We praise team members' contributions.	_____
_____	I/We ask team members' opinions.	_____
_____	I/We use head nods, smiles, and other facial expressions to show interest and/or approval.	_____
_____	I/We offer to explain or to clarify.	_____
_____	I/We paraphrase other team members' contributions.	_____
_____	I/We energize the group with humor, ideas, or enthusiasm when motivation is low.	_____
_____	I/We relieve tension with humor.	_____
_____	I/We check for others' understanding of the concepts discussed.	_____
_____	I/We summarize outcomes before moving to the next agenda item.	_____

Figure 5.1.   Individual and group assessment of collaboration skills. (From Thousand, J.S., & Villa, R.A. [2000]. Collaborative teams: A powerful tool in school restructuring. In R.A. Villa & J.S. Thousand [Eds.], *Restructuring for caring and effective education: Piecing the puzzle together* [pp. 254–292]. Baltimore: Paul H. Brookes Publishing Co.; adapted by permission.)

Formatting Skills

(Decision making and creative problem solving)

Self   Group

_____ I/We seek accuracy of information by adding to or questioning summaries.   _____

_____ I/We seek elaboration by relating to familiar events or by asking how material is understood by others.   _____

_____ I/We ask for additional information or the underlying rationale.   _____

_____ I/We seek clever ways of remembering ideas and facts (e.g., posters, visual aids, notes, mnemonics, public agendas).   _____

_____ I/We ask other members why and how they are reasoning.   _____

_____ I/We encourage the assigning of specific roles to facilitate better group functioning (e.g., process observer).   _____

_____ I/We ask for feedback in a nonconfrontational way.   _____

_____ I/We help to decide the next steps for the group.   _____

_____ I/We diagnose group difficulties regarding tasks.   _____

_____ I/We diagnose group difficulties regarding interpersonal problems.   _____

_____ I/We encourage the generation and exploration of multiple solutions to problems through the use of creative problem-solving strategies.   _____

_____ I/We communicate the rationale for ideas or conclusions.   _____

_____ I/We ask for justification of others' conclusions or ideas.   _____

_____ I/We extend or build on other members' ideas or conclusions.   _____

_____ I/We generate additional solutions or strategies.   _____

_____ I/We test the "reality" of solutions by planning and by assessing the feasibility of their implementation.   _____

_____ I/We see ideas from other people's perspectives.   _____

_____ I/We criticize ideas without criticizing people.   _____

_____ I/We distinguish differences of opinion when there is a disagreement.   _____

Augmentative and Alternative Communication: Supporting Children and Adults with Complex Communication Needs, Third Edition, by David R. Beukelman and Pat Mirenda. Copyright © 2005 Paul H. Brookes Publishing Co., Inc. All rights reserved.

---

ally short-staffed or whether they need to work on improving efficiency. They all agree that they are "sick and tired" of listening to each other complain and that they feel better now that they have an action plan that might help to institute change. They decide to meet again in 2 weeks to review the workload study proposal (see Blackstone, 1997, for three examples of how this might be done).

Monitoring and Processing Group Functioning

There's not much point to having norms and identifying interpersonal skills that need refinement without having some way to monitor and process the outcomes. Are team members honoring the agreed-on norms? Are certain interpersonal problems occurring regularly among team members? Are problems solved collaboratively and efficiently? If there are difficulties, what solutions can be created and implemented? Finally, how well do the solutions work? Teams can employ many strategies to monitor and process the answers to such questions. For example, Thousand and Villa (2000) suggested that a different team member be assigned the role of observer from week to week or meeting to meeting to observe and record the frequency of use of specific interpersonal skills of concern (e.g., the fermenting skill of "criticizing ideas without criticizing people"). Alternatively, the team could ask an outside observer to provide such input; or both types of individuals could assist. Another strategy is to take time regularly (e.g., during the last 10 minutes of each team meeting, once a month) to discuss team dynamics openly, using a comfortable format. This might include a "group sharing" process, in which team members discuss what they think is going well and not so well with regard to collaboration, or periodic use of the assessment tool presented in Figure 5.1. The point is to have some way of monitoring the use (or lack of use) of interpersonal skills that team members themselves have identified as needing work and then to share and process this information with the group as a whole. This helps to foster the "all for one and one for all" attitude that is central to the collaborative team process.

Individual Accountability

The final element necessary for effective teamwork is individual accountability. This exists when team members believe that their work is both identifiable and valued and that they must fulfill their responsibilities in order for the group (and themselves) to be successful. There are two sides to this issue, both of which are important. One side is the question of how the team can provide incentives and rewards for performance that meets or exceeds expectations; the other side is the question of what to do when a team member is not fulfilling his or her responsibilities. With regard to the first issue, the principles of teaming suggest that any extrinsic rewards be distributed to the team as a whole rather than to individuals because public recognition of one individual over another is likely to promote competition rather than collaboration (Villa & Thousand, 2000). Even more desirable is the fostering of intrinsic rewards such as feelings of personal satisfaction and pride in one's accomplishments. Traditional management theory is based on the principle that "What gets rewarded gets done" (Sergiovanni, 1990, p. 22). A better strategy on which to base team efforts is "What is rewarding gets done. When something is rewarding, it gets done even when no one is looking."

This is not to say that teams should avoid giving extrinsic rewards, particularly those that are ongoing and social in nature. No one likes to go to work day after day when the atmosphere is one in which productivity and excellence are taken for granted or ignored altogether! In fact, productive teams are characterized by the offering of frequent and mutual praise (by team members, not just by administrators), complimenting, and other forms of positive acknowledgment for efficient, high-quality work. These are the elements that make team efforts seem both rewarded and rewarding.

And what about the other side of the issue—the team member who is not doing his or her part? If dysfunctional behaviors occur infrequently or in isolated situations, the best strategy is to ignore them—after all, no one is a perfect team player all of the time. But if behaviors such as freeloading, rudeness, sloppy or late work, or other problems persist, direct confrontation is the best strategy. Of course, this should always be done on an individual basis and in private so that the person doesn't feel that the team is "ganging up" on him or her. Any team member can initiate the process if it is likely that the person will respond positively; otherwise, either a supervisor or one of the team members with whom the person has a positive relationship should offer the feedback. Although this kind of interaction is always uncomfortable for both the giver and the receiver, it is important to deal with such situations as soon as they are identified. Otherwise, team unity and morale is likely to be negatively affected as team members begin to complain to each other behind closed doors about the problem member.

After Ms. Huston has been on the job for about 6 months, one of her colleagues asks to meet with her for coffee. At that time, he tells Ms. Huston that he has some concerns about the fact that she was late the last few times they were scheduled to do an AAC evaluation together and asks if they could talk about it. Ms. Huston is initially quite defensive, saying that he should "cut her some slack" and implying that he is making a big deal about nothing. But her colleague persists, reminding her that last week he and a client had to wait 15 minutes before she appeared. She acknowledges that he is correct and that punctuality has never been her strong point. Together, they discuss some strategies for improving her time management skills, and she decides to invest in a digital watch with an alarm that can be set for 10 minutes before each appointment of the day. Although Ms. Huston feels embarrassed about being confronted, she is also grateful that her colleague brought it to her attention rather than just grumbling to himself about her lateness. She resolves to conquer her "time gremlins," and they part on a positive note.

The process of team development requires commitment, energy, patience, and practice from all concerned. Effective teams are not built in a day, and ineffective teams are often the result of inattentiveness to the "little things" that eventually grow to be "big things." Effective teams are structured in ways that allow team members to deal with internal business regularly and openly in order to both solve and prevent problems.

CHAPTER 6

Principles of Assessment

In the broadest sense, the goals of augmentative and alternative communication (AAC) interventions are 1) to assist individuals who rely on AAC to meet their *current* communication needs and 2) to prepare them to meet their *future* communication needs. AAC assessment involves gathering and analyzing information so that people who communicate through AAC and those who assist them can make informed decisions about 1) the adequacy of current communication, 2) the individual's current and future communication needs, 3) the AAC techniques that appear to be most appropriate, 4) how to provide instruction regarding use of these techniques, and 5) how to evaluate the outcomes. This chapter presents some of the general principles and procedures of AAC assessment. (See Chapter 7 for information about assessment of specific capabilities related to selection of an AAC system.)

AAC ASSESSMENT MODELS

Many models have been developed over the years to guide the AAC assessment process. These include candidacy models (which are no longer considered best practice and should not be used, but are included here because of their historical significance), communication needs models, and the Participation Model on which this book is based. We describe each of these briefly in the following sections.

Candidacy Models

A primary goal of an AAC assessment is to determine whether an individual requires or continues to require AAC assistance. This might appear to be an easy task, because it seems obvious that *all* people who are unable to meet their daily communication needs through natural speech require AAC interventions. Nevertheless, in the 1970s and 1980s in particular, considerable controversy was generated about "candidacy" or "eligibility" criteria for AAC services. In some cases, individuals were considered to be "too something" to qualify for AAC services—for example, too young, too old, or too cognitively (or motorically or linguistically) impaired. Ironically, some individuals were also excluded from AAC services because they were perceived as having "too many" skills, especially with regard to natural speech. For example, AAC supports were often withheld from children with developmental apraxia of speech in the hopes that their speech abilities might improve and/or out of concern that if they received AAC systems they might not exert the effort required to become natural speakers. Similarly, adults with aphasia and individuals with traumatic brain injury were often considered to be inappropriate candidates for AAC interventions until it became clear—sometimes months or even years after their injuries—that speech recovery had failed to occur. Consequently, these individuals were deprived of the ability to communicate their wants, needs, preferences, and feelings, often during the very period of time when they were attempting to restructure their lives in order to live with their severe communication limitations and other disabilities.

In other cases, "not ready for" criteria were used as a result of misguided interpretations of research examining communication and language development in typical children (see Kangas & Lloyd, 1988; Reichle & Karlan, 1985; and Romski & Sevcik, 1988a, for refutations of this practice). In particular, people with severe expressive communication problems secondary to intellectual impairments, autism spectrum disorders, congenital deafblindness, or multiple disabilities were frequently viewed as "not ready for" AAC. This thinking predominated so much that the service delivery guidelines of educational agencies often imposed specific requirements of cognitive or linguistic performance before interventionists would consider an individual to be an appropriate AAC candidate. In order to "become ready," these individuals were often expected to work on a variety of activities that were hypothetically designed to teach them the "prerequisite" skills that they lacked. Most of these activities, such as learning about object permanence by finding toys hidden under towels or learning about visual tracking by following stuffed animals moved across the line of visual regard, were nonfunctional and often age inappropriate, and usually failed to lead to the "readiness" they were intended to promote.

Finally, many individuals were excluded from AAC services because there was an "insufficient" amount of discrepancy between their cognitive and language/communication functioning on formal tests, because they had a specific medical condition or diagnosis that was thought not to be amenable to AAC supports (e.g., a degenerative disorder such as Alzheimer dementia, Huntington disease, or Rett syndrome), or because they had not benefited from previous communication services. External factors such as restrictive interpretations of educational, vocational, and/or medical necessity with regard to insurance regulations; lack of appropriately trained personnel; and lack of adequate funds or other resources have also been used—alone or in combination—to restrict access to AAC services. The fact is that *none* of these eligibility criteria is supported by research, and none is appropriate to apply for access to AAC services.

In 2003, the U.S. National Joint Committee (NJC) for the Communication Needs of Persons with Severe Disabilities issued a position statement on eligibility for communication services and support. The statement emphasized that "decisions regarding . . . types, amounts, and duration of services provided, intervention setting, and service delivery models should be based on the individual's communication needs and preferences. Eligibility determinations based on a priori criteria violate recommended practice principles by precluding consideration of individual needs. These a priori criteria include, but are not limited to: (a) discrepancies between cognitive and communication functioning; (b) chronological age; (c) diagnosis; (d) absence of cognitive or other skills purported to be prerequisites; (e) failure to benefit from previous communication services and supports; (f) restrictive interpretations of educational, vocational, and/or medical necessity; (g) lack of appropriately trained personnel; and (h) lack of adequate funds or other resources." (National Joint Committee, 2003a, 2003b; the complete position statement and supporting materials are posted on the NJC Web site at http://www.asha.org/NJC/eligibility.htm)

Communication Needs Model

Since the mid-1980s, "candidacy" guidelines for AAC intervention have been gradually replaced by guidelines based on communication needs, as a result of several influential factors. First, the definition of AAC services was expanded to include communication strategies and technologies that could be used by individuals who were not literate (i.e., those who could not type messages letter by letter). Initially, this expanded view of AAC allowed teams to provide communication options to individuals who were preliterate, such as preschoolers. In time, AAC teams also extended these options to people who were nonliterate.

Second, it became increasingly clear that when people were excluded from AAC services because of their "inadequate" capabilities, they were also usually excluded from the experiences, instruction, and practice necessary to improve those capabilities. In time, the concept of prerequisite skills was (for the most part) abandoned, and interventions were organized to match the individual's needs and capabilities for today while building future capabilities for tomorrow (see Chapter 7 for a more complete discussion). As a result of these changes, AAC teams now determine—or *should* determine—candidacy for communication interventions based on an individual's unmet communication needs rather than on some arbitrarily constructed profile of his or her impairments. Beukelman, Yorkston, and Dowden (1985) described the goals of the Communication Needs Model that was developed in this regard as follows:

- To document the communication needs of an individual

- To determine how many of these needs are met through current communication techniques

- To reduce the number of unmet communication needs through systematic AAC interventions

The Communication Needs Model works well for assessment and intervention when the communication needs of an individual are easy to define. For example, some adults with severe communication limitations have well-established lifestyles with consistent support systems. They are often successful in reaching consensus with their families and attendants about their communication needs; as a result, intervention plans can be quite straightforward. Determining the communication needs of individuals with less clearly defined or changing lifestyles is, however, more difficult. For these individuals, the Communication Needs Model has limitations because it is not sufficiently comprehensive and does not facilitate planning for the future.

In a 2004 technical report, the American Speech-Language-Hearing Association (2004) endorsed the Participation Model as a framework for carrying out AAC assessment and interventions.

Participation Model

In an effort to broaden the Communication Needs Model, Beukelman and Mirenda (1988) expanded on concepts that were initially described by Rosenberg and Beukelman (1987) and developed what they termed the "Participation Model" to guide AAC decision making and intervention. Over the past 5 years, minor modifications to the model were suggested by several authors based on research in which the model was implemented (Light, Roberts, Demarco, & Greiner, 1998; Schlosser et al., 2000). The revised Participation Model, shown in Figure 6.1, provides a systematic process for conducting AAC assessments and designing interventions based on the functional participation requirements of peers without disabilities of the same chronological age as the person who may communicate through AAC. This is similar to the Human Activity Assistive Technology (HAAT) model proposed by Cook and Hussey (2002), in which interventionists consider the interactions among the individual who relies on assistive technology, the activity to be completed, and the context in which the activity is performed.

Throughout this text, we use the Participation Model to discuss assessment and intervention strategies in AAC. First, however, we define and examine basic principles that underlie the Participation Model. These include the need for multiphase assessment and the importance of consensus building.

Some researchers have explored the usefulness of communication participation as a "unit of analysis for gaining information about children's communication in everyday contexts" (Kovarsky, Culatta, Franklin, & Theodore, 2001, p. 1). They conceptualize communication participation as consisting of five overlapping layers, four of which are roughly equivalent to the components of communicative competence described by Light (1989b): 1) lifeworld participation, 2) participant structures (e.g., knowing how and when to communicate in specific ways, similar to Light's social competence), 3) participant stances (i.e., the roles of speaker, author, and principal that can be assumed during a communicative interaction; the author role is similar to Light's operational competence), 4) participant accommodations (i.e., how individuals modify their messages to the needs of their communication partners, similar to Light's strategic competence), and 5) participant resources (i.e., the verbal and nonverbal resources that each person contributes to an interaction, similar to Light's linguistic competence).

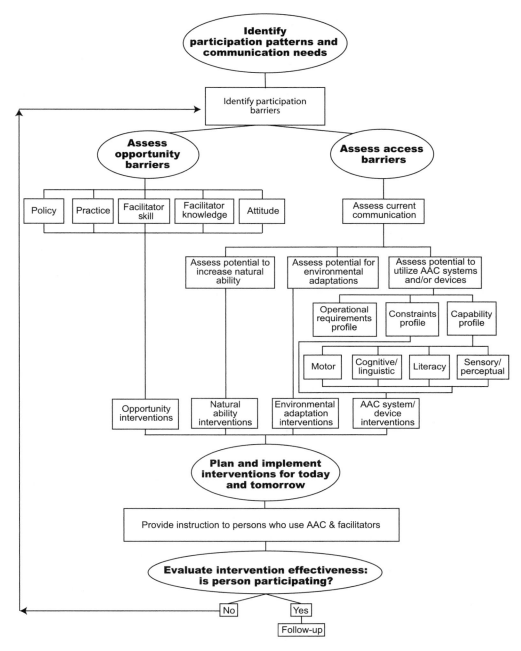

Figure 6.1. The Participation Model.

PHASES OF AAC ASSESSMENT

AAC interventions are usually ongoing, long-term processes, because the individuals who require them usually are unable to speak or write due to chronic rather than temporary disabilities. The communication problems of these individuals usually persist because of severe physical, cognitive, language, and sensory impairments. Nevertheless, as people who use AAC mature and age, their communication needs and capabilities often change. Some people experience an expanding world with increased opportunities, whereas others become less able to participate as they age or as their impairments become more severe. Thus, AAC assessment and intervention is a dynamic process and usually consists of three general phases.

Phase I: Initial Assessment for Today

During this phase, the AAC team assesses the individual's current communication interaction needs and physical, cognitive, language, and sensory capabilities so that efforts to support immediate communication interaction and communication can begin. Thus, the goal of initial assessment is to gather information to design an initial intervention to match today's needs and capabilities. These initial AAC interventions usually undergo continuous, subtle refinements as individuals learn about the operational requirements of their AAC techniques. Gradually, the AAC team develops a basic communication system to facilitate interactions with family members, friends, and other individuals familiar with the person who communicates through AAC.

Phase II: Detailed Assessment for Tomorrow

The goal of assessing for tomorrow is to develop a communication system that will support individuals who use AAC in a variety of specialized environments, beyond the familiar ones. These environments reflect the individual's lifestyle and may include school, employment, living (independent, assisted, retirement), and recreational and leisure environments. Such settings require basic conversational communication as well as specialized communication that matches the participation requirements of each setting. For example, a child in a classroom must have access to a system that allows academic and educational participation as well as social participation. Similarly, an adult at work might need to write and talk on the telephone as well as to converse with co-workers during break times. Or, an older adult may anticipate transitioning into a retirement or supported care facility after living in a family home for years. Thus, this phase requires careful assessment of the individual's expected participation patterns, as well as assessments to refine the basic communication system to accommodate future participation.

Phase III: Follow-Up Assessment

Follow-up, in general, involves maintaining a comprehensive AAC system that meets the changing capabilities and lifestyle of the individual. Assessment in this phase may involve periodically examining communication equipment to detect replacement and repair needs, assessing the needs and abilities of communication partners and facilitators, and re-assessing an individual's capabilities if they change. For individuals whose lifestyles and capabilities are relatively stable, follow-up assessment may occur irregularly and infrequently; for others, such as those with degenerative illnesses, follow-up assessments may be a major part of intervention planning.

IDENTIFY PARTICIPATION PATTERNS AND NEEDS

The remainder of this chapter follows the Participation Model flowchart depicted in Figure 6.1. The top part of the model depicts the process for describing the participation patterns and communication needs of the individual, referenced against the participation requirements made of same-age peers without disabilities. The sections that follow describe this process.

Conduct a Participation Inventory

The assessment of participation patterns begins with a Participation Inventory (see Figure 6.2), which can be completed for each of the regularly occurring activities in which the individual who uses AAC participates at home, school, work, or other settings. In addition to an inventory of activities, it is also helpful to identify those individuals who are active in the social networks of persons who rely on AAC. Blackstone and Hunt Berg (2003a, 2003b) provided an assessment tool to document and describe five categories of individuals who might constitute a social network: family members/life partners, friends, acquaintances, paid professionals, and unfamiliar persons.

Obviously, an individual's specific activities and communication partners will depend on numerous social, vocational, and educational factors. In any case, it is important at this stage of assessment for team members to reach a consensus regarding the activities to be assessed with the Participation Inventory, because this list will influence the subsequent assessment process and intervention program. Furthermore, if the team cannot reach a consensus about the key activities in a person's life, it will be very difficult to determine whether or not the AAC intervention has been effective and has achieved the desired outcomes.

Identify Participation Patterns of Peers

The first step in completing a Participation Inventory for a specific activity is to determine how peers participate in it, by recording the critical steps required for successful completion. The team should select as a model a peer of the same gender and approximately the same age as the individual, whose participation is representative of the desired performance in a given situation. This may necessitate selecting several peers, depending on the activities involved in the analysis. As team members observe and document participation patterns in each delineated activity, they base peer performance standards on the following criteria and record them in Figure 6.2 in the section entitled "Level of Independence—(P)eer–(T)arget":

- **Independent:** The peer is able to participate in the activity without human assistance.

Person's name: _____ Date: _____ Completed by: _____

Activity: _____ Goal of activity: _____

Critical steps to meeting the activity goal	Level of independence (P)eer–(T)arget					Opportunity barriers				Person barriers			
	Independent	Independent with setup	Requires verbal assistance	Requires physical assistance	Does not participate	Policy	Practice	Knowledge/ skill	Physical/ motor	Cognitive	Expressive communi- cation	Literacy	Visual/ auditory
1.													
2.													
3.													
4.													
5.													
6.													

In *Augmentative and Alternative Communication: Supporting Children and Adults with Complex Communication Needs, Third Edition*, by David R. Beukelman and Pat Mirenda. Copyright © 2005 Paul H. Brookes Publishing Co., Inc. All rights reserved.

Figure 6.2. Participation inventory. (From Blackstien-Adler, 2003.)

- **Independent with setup:** The peer is able to participate independently once human assistance has been provided to set up the activity (e.g., art materials are laid out for a student in school, the raw data for an engineering report are compiled for an employee).

- **Requires verbal or physical assistance:** The peer is able to complete an activity if provided with verbal or physical prompts or instruction (e.g., a trainer prompts an employee verbally as he or she learns to operate a new piece of equipment, a parent or a teacher provides physical guidance while a student completes an activity).

- **Does not participate:** The peer does not participate actively in the activity at all.

Accurately determining the critical steps required to complete an activity is an important step in the AAC assessment process. People who use AAC, their teachers, co-workers, caregivers, or family members may at times set unrealistic goals for an activity. For example, a junior high school social studies teacher once indicated to us that a student in her class who had severe cerebral palsy should be prepared to attend class and to discuss the assigned readings during every class. An assessment of the peer participation patterns in the classrooms revealed that few, if any, of the peer students were prepared to discuss the readings daily, and, in fact, some of them were almost never prepared to do so. If the AAC team had accepted the teacher's standard as its goal, they would have placed excessively high expectations on the student with the AAC system. Instead, the teacher, who was a member of the team, agreed to alter her expectations of the target student once she received the results of the peer participation analysis.

Assess Participation Effectiveness of the Target Individual

When team members have identified the critical steps required of peers to complete an activity, they can assess and document the actual participation pattern of the target individual against the same criteria they used to establish peer participation standards. The individual may be able to participate in some steps at a level similar to the peer, and in such situations, no participation gap exists. For other steps, however, discrepancies will be evident between the participation level of the peer and that of the individual. These can be indicated on Figure 6.2 in the section entitled "Level of Independence—(P)eer–(T)arget."

Identify Participation Barriers

According to the Participation Model, two types of barriers may result in a failure to participate—those related to opportunity and those related to access. *Opportunity barriers* refer to barriers that are imposed by people other than the individual with the severe communication disorder and that cannot be eliminated simply by providing an AAC system or intervention. For example, an individual may be unable to participate at the desired level because of the attitudes of those around him or her, even though an appropriate AAC system has been provided. *Access barriers* are present primarily because of limitations in the current capabilities of the individual or his or her current communication system. For example, an access barrier might occur because an individual's AAC device does not have sufficient memory for the specialized vocabulary needed for specific activities. Assessments aimed at identifying the source of barriers to participation are needed in order to formulate effective assessment and intervention strategies for each barrier.

Figure 6.2 provides the AAC team with an area for indicating what they believe the primary opportunity and access barriers to be, but additional assessment is almost always needed to identify specific concerns for remediation. In the sections that follow, we describe the specific issues related to opportunity and access assessment in more detail.

OPPORTUNITY BARRIERS

Figure 6.2 contains a section in which the AAC team can record four types of opportunity barriers that may exist: policy, practice, knowledge, and skill barriers. We discuss each of these briefly in the sections that follow.

Policy Barriers

Policy barriers are the result of legislative or regulatory decisions that govern the situations in which many individuals who use AAC find themselves. In schools, vocational environments, residential centers, hospitals, rehabilitation centers, and nursing homes, policies are usually outlined in the written documents that govern the agency. In less formal situations, such as a family home, policies may not be written but are nonetheless set by the decision makers (e.g., parents, guardians) in the environment.

A wide variety of policies can act as barriers to participation. For example, many educational agencies and school districts still have policies that segregate students with disabilities into classrooms or facilities that separate them from their peers without disabilities. In such situations, by policy, students with disabilities cannot be included in general education classrooms, participate in the school district's general education curriculum, or communicate regularly with peers who do not have disabilities. Furthermore, because many school districts with segregation policies offer such educational programs only in "cluster sites" or special schools, students may be bused to facilities far away from their neighborhoods. This not only limits these students' access to peers without disabilities during the school day, but it also greatly reduces these students' opportunities to make friends in their neighborhoods. The combination of these restrictions severely limits the communication opportunities afforded to students with disabilities. Similar situations can occur in sheltered workshops, segregated group homes or institutions, and in other "disabled-only" settings.

Another example is the "limited-use" policy that exists in many acute medical settings and intensive care units (ICUs) that contain complicated and expensive equipment. To prevent mechanical or electronic interference with this equipment, some hospitals have stringent policies regarding other types of equipment that patients can bring with them. People with electronic AAC devices may face opportunity barriers in such medical settings due to such policies. This situation may also exist in agencies or nursing homes that serve adults who use AAC.

Practice Barriers

Whereas policy barriers are legislated or regulated procedures, *practice barriers* refer to procedures or conventions that have become common in a family, school, or workplace but are not actual policies. The staff of an agency may think that long-standing practices are legislated policies, but a review of actual agency policies usually reveals that this is not the case. For example, it is a matter of practice in many school districts to restrict the use of district-funded AAC equipment outside the school, although this is not part of "official" district policy. We know of several cases in which school district representatives have told families and staff that such practices are state education department policies, although no such policies existed. The same may be true of the segregation practices of many schools or businesses. In fact, it is illegal in many countries, including the United States, to institute *policies* that prevent students with disabilities from attending general education classes or that prevent workers with disabilities from obtaining competitive employment. Nevertheless, there are often very strong *practices* in place that do not encourage or permit such participation.

Professional practices may also limit participation opportunities for individuals with AAC needs. Early in AAC history, for example, some speech-language pathologists made it their practice not to work with individuals who were unable to speak, believing that this would be inappropriate because they were trained to assist people with speech problems. Since then, speech-language pathologists have largely abandoned this practice, although it may still exist within some agencies.

Knowledge Barriers

A knowledge barrier refers to a lack of information on the part of someone other than the person who uses AAC that results in limited opportunities for participation. Lack of knowledge about AAC intervention options, technology, and instructional strategies often presents tremendous barriers to effective participation by individuals with disabilities. Knowledge barriers on the part of some members of the intervention team are likely to exist at some point during nearly every AAC intervention. One purpose of assessment is to identify these barriers in advance, so that information can be provided in order to eliminate or minimize them.

Skill Barriers

Skill barriers occur when, despite even extensive knowledge, supporters have difficulty with the actual implementation of an AAC technique or strategy. For example, we have all had the experience of attending a class, conference, or workshop that was full of good ideas and information and then encountering difficulty putting our newly acquired knowledge into practice at work on Monday morning! Numerous technical and interaction skills are often necessary to assist someone to become a competent communicator. It is important to assess the skill level of individuals who will be responsible for various aspects of the AAC intervention plan in order to identify skill impairments and to design interventions to reduce these barriers to communicative competence.

Not too long ago, we were involved in a situation in which a university professor did not want to permit a student with a disability who used AAC to enroll in his course. The *policy* of the university was clear: People with disabilities who had been admitted to the university were entitled to enroll in all courses. It was also the *practice* of the university to comply with this policy, even if this meant moving classes to more accessible locations. In addition, the university's Disability Resource center had staff with the *knowledge* and the *skills* that were needed to support both the student and the faculty members who taught the courses in which she was enrolled. Nevertheless, an individual professor, because of his *attitude* about students with disabilities, attempted to set up a barrier. Of course, he was not permitted to maintain this barrier in the face of the policies and practices of the institution, and the student was granted access to (and support within) his course.

Attitude Barriers

A fifth type of barrier, in which the attitudes and beliefs held by an individual present a barrier to participation, can also exist. We did not include the barrier related to attitude in Figure 6.2 because, if it is present within one or more members of the AAC team, it is probably not helpful to identify it publicly as such. Telling someone "You have an attitude problem!"—either implicitly or explicitly—is unlikely to solve the problem! Nonetheless, it is important to be aware of the potential for attitude barriers that may occur for a variety of reasons and may be manifested in a number of ways. Parents, relatives, coworkers, supervisors, professionals, peers, and the general public all may hold negative or restrictive attitudes. At times, attitude barriers are quite blatant, but more often they are subtle and insidious because most people realize the social unacceptability of such views. The result of most attitude barriers is that one or more members of the team have reduced expectations of individuals with disabilities, which in turn results in limited participation opportunities. It is outside the scope of this book to discuss the wide range of attitude barriers that exist. However, assessors should be sensitive to restrictive attitudes that may prevent an individual with a severe communication disorder from participating in activities with their same-age peers who do not have disabilities.

Even though persons who rely on AAC are receiving increasingly better elementary, secondary, and post-secondary educational opportunities, opportunities for employment remain severely restricted. For example, the Americans with Disabilities Act was passed in the United States in 1990, yet persons who rely on AAC are still routinely screened out at the initial interview stage when they seek employment. As two men with cerebral palsy who rely on AAC noted: "The REAL barrier . . . [is] people's stagnant and outdated attitudes toward . . . people with speech disabilities . . . . When people see me, they do not see me. They just see a person in a wheelchair." (McNaughton, Light, & Arnold, 2002, p. 66)

ACCESS BARRIERS

In the Participation Model (see Figure 6.1), *access barriers* pertain to the capabilities, attitudes, and resource limitations of individuals who communicate through AAC, rather than to limitations of their societies or support systems. Many types of access barriers can interfere with an individual's participation. Although access barriers related to communication are of primary importance in this book, it is important to remember that access barriers might also be related to lack of mobility or difficulty with manipulation and management of objects, problems with cognitive functions and decision making, literacy deficits, and/or sensory-perceptual impairments (i.e., vision or hearing impairments). Figure 6.2 contains a section in which the AAC team can record their general impressions about the types of access barriers that appear to affect participation. However, it is important to identify the nature and extent of an individual's capabilities as they relate to communication in particular. An individual's current communication, potential to use and/or increase the ability to use natural speech, and potential to use environmental adaptations should all be assessed.

Assess Current Communication

It is important to remember that everyone communicates in some fashion. Thus, the initial step in assessing communication access is to determine the effectiveness and the nature of the individual's current communication system. In general, the assessment of current communication focuses on two aspects of communicative competence: operational and social. Some individuals have a very difficult time using a particular communication technique. For example, a child may be unable to use eye gaze consistently, or an adult with aphasia may be unable to write messages with a standard pen or pencil. Some individuals, however, may be operationally competent but not socially competent with a specific technique. For example, an individual might be able to operate an electronic communication device but might never use it to initiate interactions. Therefore, when assessing the current communication system, it is necessary to rate both the individual's operational and social competence for each technique currently used. Figure 6.3 can be used in this regard. In addition, a number of excellent observation and/or interview instruments are available to assist the AAC team to identify both the forms and functions of a person's current communication. Table 6.1 summarizes some of the instruments that can be used in a variety of environments and with a variety of individuals.

The *Communication Matrix* (Rowland, 1996, 2004) is an assessment tool "designed to pinpoint exactly how a child is currently communicating and to provide a framework for determining logical communication goals." The complete *Matrix* and supporting information can be purchased from Design to Learn, Inc. In addition, an on-line version designed specifically for parents is accessible at no cost at http://www.communicationmatrix.com.

Table 6.1.   Selected instruments for documenting current communication behaviors and/or functions

Instrument	Use to assess . . .	Population	Source
Achieving Communication Independence (ACI): A Comprehensive Guide to Assessment and Intervention (Gillette, 2003)	Communication opportunities, behaviors, and functions in community, work, leisure, school, and home activities and environments	Children and adults who use AAC	Thinking Publications
Chalk Talk (Culp & Effinger, 1996)	Classroom communication behaviors and functions	Individuals who use AAC in general education classrooms	http://www.callier .utdallas.edu/ ACT/ChalkTalk.html
Communication Matrix (Rowland, 1996, 2004)	Communication behaviors and functions	Individuals who use any form of communication, including presymbolic communication or AAC	Design to Learn, Inc.
Home Talk: A Family Assessment of Children Who are Deafblind (Harris et al., n.d.)	Communication behaviors and functions in the home	School-aged children who are deafblind and have other disabilities	http://www.tr.wou.edu/ dblink/newresources 2.htm
Interaction Checklist for Augmentative Communication, Revised Edition (Bolton & Dashiell, 1991)	Communication behaviors and functions	Individuals who use any form of communication, including presymbolic communication or AAC	PRO-ED, Inc.
Inventory of Potential Communicative Acts (IPCA) (Sigafoos et al., 1998)	Prelinguistic communication behaviors and functions	Presymbolic communicators with developmental and/or physical disabilities	Contact Dr. Jeff Sigafoos at j.sigafoos@mail .utexas.edu
Social Networks: A Communication Inventory for Individuals with Complex Communication Needs and their Communication Partners (Blackstone & Hunt Berg, 2003a, 2003b)	Communication skills and abilities, communication partners, modes of expression, representational strategies, selection techniques, strategies that support interaction, topics of conversation, and types of communication	Individuals who use AAC across the range of age and ability	Augmentative Communication, Inc.

Once the AAC team has assessed a person's current communication system and how it is used, they can then begin to examine the potential of various solutions to existing communication barriers. One solution might be to help increase the person's natural communication abilities, as discussed briefly in the next section.

Assess Potential to Use and/or Increase Natural Speech

One of the most contentious issues in AAC assessment, especially with children, is whether AAC is necessary to augment existing but insufficient speech or (much less commonly) to serve as a replacement for speech altogether. Understandably, parents often worry that the use of AAC will discourage speech development, reasoning that children might be less

Directions:
1. List all of the various *techniques* the target individual currently uses to communicate. Examples: natural speech, vocalizations, gestures, body language, manual signs, pointing to a communication board with pictures, eye gaze to photographs, scanning with _____ device, typing on a typewriter, headlight pointing to device.
2. Describe the *body part* used for each technique listed (e.g., both eyes, right hand, left thumb, right side of head).
3. Describe any *unique adaptations* needed for each technique (e.g., must sit on Mom's lap, uses keyguard, needs to have eye-gaze chart held 6 inches from face).
4. After observing use of the technique, rate the person's *operational competence* (1 = poor; 5 = excellent). (Operational competence is the person's ability to use the technique *accurately and efficiently* over time without becoming fatigued.)
5. After observing and interacting with the person, rate his or her *social competence* (1 = poor; 5 = excellent). (Social competence is the person's ability to use the technique in an interactive, socially appropriate manner.)

Technique	Body part	Adaptations	Operational competence Poor 1	2	3	4	Excellent 5	Social competence Poor 1	2	3	4	Excellent 5
1.												
2.												
3.												
4.												
5.												
6.												

Augmentative and Alternative Communication: Supporting Children and Adults with Complex Communication Needs, Third Edition, by David R. Beukelman and Pat Mirenda. Copyright © 2005 Paul H. Brookes Publishing Co., Inc. All rights reserved.

Figure 6.3. Current communication techniques.

inclined to speak if they have access to an "easier" alternative like using a manual sign, pointing to a picture, or activating a speech-generating device (SGD). Family members of adults affected by an acquired brain injury as a result of trauma or stroke are often concerned about this issue as well, reasoning that their loved one may be less motivated to participate in the (often arduous) therapy needed for speech recovery if an alternative is provided.

These legitimate concerns must be addressed with sensitivity and objectivity as part of an AAC assessment. Fortunately, a growing number of research studies focused on children have provided evidence that the use of AAC techniques does not inhibit speech production and may facilitate it. For example, increased speech production has been documented in some participants following the introduction of manual signing (DiCarlo, Stricklin, Banajee, & Reid, 2001), communication boards with pictures and words (Garrison-Harrell, Kamps, & Kravits, 1997), tangible symbols (Rowland & Schweigert, 2000a), the Picture Exchange Communication System (Charlop-Christy, Carpenter, Le, LeBlanc, & Kellet, 2002; Kravits, Kamps, Kemmerer, & Potucek, 2002; Schwartz, Garfinkle, & Bauer, 1998), and SGDs (Mirenda, Wilk, & Carson, 2000; Romski & Sevcik, 1996; Sigafoos, Didden, & O'Reilly, 2003).

Cress and Marvin (2003) provided an excellent resource for parents of young children considering AAC and the teams that support them. The authors summarized much of the research to date related to nine common questions often asked by parents, including "Will the use of AAC interfere with my child's vocal development?" and "Will my child talk?" A summary of this article is available at http://www.unl.edu/barkley/present/cress/questions.shtml.

Most individuals with severe communication disorders demonstrate at least some ability to communicate using natural speech—that is, they are not 100% unable to vocalize or speak. Functionally, the effectiveness of natural speech for communicative interaction can be divided into 10 levels, according to the Meaningful Use of Speech Scale (MUSS; Robbins & Osberger, 1992):

1. Vocalizes during communicative interactions

2. Uses speech to attract others' attention

3. Varies vocalizations with content and intent of messages

4. Is willing to use speech primarily to communicate with familiar people on known topics

5. Is willing to use speech to communicate with unfamiliar people on known topics

6. Is willing to use speech primarily to communicate with familiar people on novel topics or with reduced contextual information

7. Is willing to use speech primarily to communicate with unfamiliar people on novel topics or with reduced contextual information

8. Produces messages understood by people familiar with his or her speech

9. Produces messages understood by people unfamiliar with his or her speech

10. Uses appropriate repair and clarification strategies

The AAC team can assess natural speech by interviewing family members using the MUSS to get an estimate of typical speech usage. Each item is scored on a scale of 0–4, with 0 indicating that the behavior never occurs and 4 indicating that it always occurs. Although the MUSS was designed for use with children with severe hearing impairments, Kent, Miolo, and Bloedel (1994) suggested that it can also be used appropriately with children who produce speech with reduced intelligibility of any kind. More specific information related to speech intelligibility in children can be obtained through the use of standardized measures such as the Assessment of Phonological Processes–Revised (Hodson, 1986), Bankson-Bernthal Test of Phonology (Bankson & Bernthal, 1990), Children's Speech Intelligibility Measure (Wilcox & Sherrill, 1999), and the Goldman-Fristoe Test of Articulation–Second Edition (Goldman & Fristoe, 2000). Cress, Sterup, and Hould (2003) successfully adapted the Bankson-Bernthal Test of Phonology for use with typically developing children as young as 18 months of age as well as children with severe expressive communication impairments. Adult intelligibility can be assessed with measures such as the Sentence Intelligibility Test (Yorkston, Beukelman, & Tice, 1996).

It is important to note that *intelligibility*, which refers to the adequacy of the acoustic signal to convey information, is affected by many intrinsic factors such as articulation, respiration, phonation, rate of speech, positioning, utterance length, and so forth (Kent et al., 1994; Yorkston, Strand, & Kennedy, 1996). Typically, intelligibility scores for someone who communicates through AAC will be either extremely low or fluctuate widely because of the combined influence of these factors.

A second measure, *supplemented intelligibility*, refers to the extent to which a listener can understand an individual's speech when he or she is provided with contextual information, such as the topic, first letters of words, and gestures. Hanson, Yorkston, and Beukelman (2004) completed a meta-analysis and developed practice guidelines for the use of supplemented speech techniques. In response to the need to assess supplemented intelligibility, specialists have begun to develop assessment tools for clinical use. For example, The Index of Augmented Speech Comprehensibility in Children (I-ASCC) was developed for use with children as young as 30 months of age (Dowden, 1997). Target words from common categories such as "something children eat at snacktime," "things children play with in the bathtub," and "a number less than 11" are identified. The target words are then elicited via speech in the following order: 1) picture cue only (e.g., "What is this?"); 2) picture plus context cue (e.g., "It's a place you might go with your family. What is it?"); and 3) picture plus embedded model ("It's a shirt. Now you say it."). Assessors tape-record the speech productions of the individual being assessed and then familiar and unfamiliar listeners review the recordings with and without supporting contexts. In the no-context listening task, assessors ask listeners to play the recording of each word twice and then write down what they hear. In the context condition, listeners receive a context cue phrase (e.g., "Something a person might eat for dinner") related to each word and are asked to listen and then write down the word they hear that best fits the context. This assessment is designed specifically to evaluate the extent to which speech is comprehensible under different conditions rather than the degree to which speech is simply intelligible without context. Dowden (1997) provided several illustrative clinical examples of the applicability of such assessment and suggested that it be used primarily to determine the effects of speech supplementation strategies on an individual's functional speech, resolve disagreements about the need for alternative communication strategies, assist in guiding a team that sees an SGD as a quick solution when it might not be, and clarify the role of speech and alternative strategies with unfamiliar partners in particular.

Assess Potential for Environmental Adaptations

Environmental adaptations may be successful and relatively simple solutions to communication access barriers. Such adaptations may include altering physical spaces or locations or altering physical structures themselves. For example, in the classroom, teachers can lower a blackboard or create a storage area that a student in a wheelchair can reach. School staff can raise or lower desks and tables, create a vertical work surface with a slanted board, or cut out countertops to accommodate wheelchairs or standing frames. Assessment of the need for such adaptations is a common-sense process and teams can almost always conduct such assessments by observation of problematic situations.

Assess Potential to Utilize AAC Systems or Devices

In the Participation Model (see Figure 6.1), four assessments determine an individual's ability to use AAC systems or devices in order to reduce access barriers. These include an operational requirements profile, a constraints profile, a facilitator skills profile, and a capability profile. We discuss the first three of these profiles in the following section, and the capability profile is discussed in Chapter 7.

Operational Requirements Profile

Often, AAC teams will need to institute either low-tech (nonelectronic) or high-tech (electronic) techniques to reduce existing access barriers to communication. Thus, it is necessary to identify which of the many AAC device options may be appropriate. The first step is for the assessment team to become familiar with the operational requirements of the various AAC techniques. For example, there may be display requirements regarding the number of total items in the selection set as well as the size and layout of the array. There are always alternative access system requirements regarding the motor and sensory interface between the individual and the device, so that the individual can operate the device accurately and efficiently. In addition, the output provided by the device may require the individual to have certain skills or abilities. (See Chapters 3 and 4 for descriptions of the operational and learning requirements of many AAC options.)

In order to obtain accurate [information], the *right person* must ask the *right questions* of the *right people* in the *right way* at the *right place* and *time* (the six R's). (Bevan-Brown, 2001, p. 139)

Constraints Profile

Practical issues, aside from those directly related to individuals and AAC techniques, may influence the selection of an AAC system and the strategies for instruction. The AAC team should identify such constraints early in the assessment process so that subsequent decisions do not conflict with the constraints and so that team members can make efforts to reduce them whenever possible. The most common constraints are those related to individual and family preferences, the preferences and attitudes of other communication partners, communication partner and facilitator skills and abilities, and funding.

Preferences and Attitudes of People Who Use AAC and Their Families

Undoubtedly, the most important constraints that AAC teams must assess are those related to the preferences of the person communicating through AAC and his or her family. These may include concerns about 1) system portability, durability, and appearance (i.e., cosmetic appeal); 2) the time and skills required to learn the system (this may be particularly relevant for manual sign and technology-based approaches); 3) the quality and intelligibility of speech output in SGDs; and 4) the "naturalness" of the communication exchange achieved through the system.

In an interesting Canadian study, O'Keefe, Brown, and Schuller (1998) asked 94 people who communicated using AAC, their familiar communication partners, AAC service providers, AAC device manufacturers, and people unfamiliar with AAC to rate the importance of 186 possible features of AAC devices. People who used AAC rated items related to situational flexibility, reliability, learning ease, and intelligibility of speech output significantly higher than did people in the other four groups. In addition, people who used AAC made several suggestions about a number of desirable features *not* included in the survey, including the need for devices that "speak" languages other than English, that enable private conversations when necessary, that can be used in bed, and that are easy for partners to program. What is clear from this study is that people who use AAC and their familiar partners may be considerably "more demanding than those who work with them clinically or who are responsible for the design, manufacture, and distribution of AAC communication aids" (p. 47), and that the preferences of the former two groups are of paramount importance when making AAC device decisions.

A number of factors can account for the wide variability in individual and family preferences related to AAC. One of the most salient has to do with the impact of ethnicity and culture on peoples' perceptions of disability in general and communication or AAC in particular. In both North America and elsewhere, AAC assessment and intervention approaches based on Anglo-European ideals and values tend to predominate, even though they may conflict with the values embraced by families from other cultural groups (Hetzroni, 2002; Judge & Parette, 1998). For example, in the dominant Anglo-European culture in North America, there tends to be an emphasis on individualism and privacy, equality, informality, planning for the future, efficient use of time, work and achievement, directness, and assertiveness (Judge & Parette, 1998). Children in Anglo-European cultures are often encouraged to be independent, self-reliant, hard-working, and competitive. Disability is often viewed as having multiple causes; disability "labeling" is widely accepted as a necessary step to obtaining services; and technology in the form of drugs, surgeries, adaptive equipment, and so forth is generally valued as a potential solution to disability-related obstacles.

These values may be in sharp contrast to the values of many other cultural groups that place a high value on attributes such as collectivism and cooperation, interdependence, hierarchical family structures, politeness, living in the here and now, a fluid understanding of time, indirect communication, and/or respect and agreement of elders and authority figures. Although children from other cultures are often raised to value education and hard work, they may also be taught to assume a relatively passive role in social interactions and encouraged to place family loyalty above all other alliances. Views of disability may also vary widely and may emphasize both natural and supernatural causes; a view that "labeling" is both stigmatizing and unnecessary; and a reluctance to employ modern technologies to the exclusion of folk, spiritual, and/or natural remedies.

To help fill the "culture-to-practice" gap, a team of U.S. researchers produced a very useful interactive, multimedia education tool entitled "Families, Cultures, and AAC" (VanBiervliet & Parette, 1999; see also Parette, VanBiervliet, & Hourcade, 2000). It features video segments of family members from diverse cultural backgrounds whose children use AAC, along with interactive learning games, Web site links, a glossary, and numerous printable documents. It can be used on both Windows and Macintosh platforms and has both English and Spanish text narration and controls. It is available from Program Development Associates.

Of course, these generalizations do not apply "across the board" to families from diverse backgrounds. Fortunately, since the late 1990s, a number of researchers have examined these issues as they relate to specific ethnic/cultural groups that are prevalent in North America. For example, Parette, Huer, and their colleagues have written extensively about the attitudes and preferences of African American (Huer & Wyatt, 1999; Parette, Huer, & Wyatt, 2002), Mexican American (Huer, Parette, & Saenz, 2001), Asian American (Parette & Huer, 2002), Vietnamese American (Huer, Saenz, & Doan, 2001), and Chinese American families (Parette, Chuang, & Huer, 2004) with regard to educational and AAC assessment practices, devices, and interventions. Other authors have summarized research related to the communication styles, practices, and/or preferences of American Indian (Bridges, 2000), Hispanic American and Mexican American (Harrison-Harris, 2002; McCord & Soto, in 2004), Filipino American (Roseberry-McKinnon, 2000), Southeast Asian (Hwa-Froelich & Westby, 2003), Chinese Canadian (Johnston & Wong, 2002), and Indo-Canadian families (Simmons & Johnston, 2004), among others. From studies such as these, AAC teams can learn much about the importance of truly understanding the values, expectations, historical contexts, child-rearing and communication styles, and perceptions of families from diverse backgrounds. Team members can also appreciate the importance of self-evaluating their own knowledge, awareness, attitudes, and skills both prior to and during the AAC assessment and intervention processes. Huer (1997) provided a Protocol for Culturally Inclusive Assessment of AAC, including the self-evaluation component presented in Figure 6.4 (see Table 6.2 for a description of the complete protocol).

The Protocol for Culturally Inclusive Assessment of AAC
Self-Assessment: Extent of Multicultural Competencies
©Mary Blake Huer, Ph.D.

Criteria: During self assessment, read the 20 statements below. Next to each statement place a "yes" if you feel you possess the competence and a "no" if you feel you do not. Participate in AAC service delivery when you have acquired at least 70% (14 of 20) of the competencies.

Knowledge base

———— I have extensive knowledge regarding AAC components, techniques, strategies, symbols, and assistive technology.

———— I have studied the characteristics of several different disabling conditions.

———— I have knowledge regarding the history of and attitudes toward multiculturalism.

———— I can identify cross-cultural similarities and differences in the communicative behaviors of my own culture as well as among culturally/linguistically diverse populations.

———— I have knowledge regarding policy and laws impacting AAC and multiculturalism.

———— I have knowledge of community and professional resources for all clients.

———— I can define terms such as ethnicity, world view, and acculturation.

Awareness of own cultural biases and beliefs

———— I enjoy interacting with persons from other cultures as much as when interacting with persons from my own culture.

———— I feel comfortable interacting with families from cultural backgrounds different from my own.

———— I am sure of what to expect from families.

Awareness of culturally appropriate assessment strategies

———— I am confident in my ability to evaluate linguistically diverse persons needing AAC services.

———— I use all family members, as appropriate, during the collection of information, e.g., parent(s), grandparents(s), aunt(s)/uncle(s), cousins(s), friends, elders, and folk healers.

———— I am confident in my ability to utilize comprehensive evaluation instruments.

———— I have experience conducting a culturally sensitive interview and a nonbiased assessment.

———— I use different methods for collecting information, i.e., observations, interviews, open-ended questions, and secondary sources.

———— I can conduct an effective interview with a family from a cultural background different from my own.

———— I monitor and correct my own errors, defensiveness, anxiety, and misunderstandings when communicating with persons form cultures other than my own.

Relationships with culturally/linguistically diverse families

———— I believe that I am perceived by most families to have the quality of trustworthiness.

———— I believe that families feel comfortable when interacting with me over time.

———— I believe that most persons do not perceive me as having biases or using stereotypes.

Total self score: ————————————   Date: ——————   Action: ——————————————

In *Augmentative and Alternative Communication: Supporting Children and Adults with Complex Communication Needs, Third Edition,* by David R. Beukelman and Pat Mirenda. Copyright © Mary Blake Huer, Ph.D. All rights reserved.

Figure 6.4. Self assessment: Extent of multicultural competence. (From Huer, M.B. [1997]. Culturally inclusive assessments for children using augmentative and alternative communication [AAC]. *Journal of Children's Communication Development, 19,* 27.)

In addition, team members must appreciate the complexities of conducting AAC assessments with individuals who are bilingual and who represent an increasingly large proportion of the population. For example, it is estimated that by the year 2050, 40% of school-age children in the United States will come from homes in which English is not the first language (Harrison-Harris, 2002). Because very little research exists to guide AAC

Table 6.2. The protocol for culturally inclusive assessment of AAC

Section	Description	Format
Self-assessment for practitioners	Assesses clinician's knowledge base, awareness of cultural values and biases, ability to use culturally appropriate assessment strategies, and ability to form relationships with families	Self-assessment (yes/no) form with 20 questions (form provided; see Figure 6.4)
Communication partner inventory	List of family members and others who regularly interact with the person using AAC; descriptions of family communication style, priorities, perceptions of disability, and expectations	Interview (form provided) and observation
Communication needs assessment	Description of communication patterns and needs of the child and family across languages and interaction styles	Interview (form provided)
Capability and technology assessment	Assessment of the abilities of the person using AAC (e.g., cognitive, motor, language, literacy, social skills, sensory skills, ability to use technology)	Direct assessment, observation, record review, interview (forms provided)

practices for individuals who are bilingual, team members must work closely with families to accommodate individual situations and needs. Fortunately, an increasing number of assessment tools are available in languages other than English and can be accessed by searching the Web sites of the major test distributors (see the Resources section).

Factors other than culture also influence people's attitudes and preferences with regard to disability and intervention in general and AAC in particular. One such factor has to do with people's experiences with and attitudes toward technology. Angelo (1998) reported that the majority of two-parent, Caucasian, middle-income families she surveyed did not believe that the amount of time required to program electronic AAC devices was burdensome for them and did not find the frequency with which such devices required repair to be excessive. However, these opinions certainly do not represent those of all families or even of all members within a family. For example, one parent of a child with a communication disorder may be very interested in an electronic AAC option, whereas the other parent may strongly prefer a low-tech approach. The basis for such disagreements may come from a variety of sources. One individual may have had more positive experiences with technology than the other, or one of the parties involved may be lured by the magic of technology, regardless of its appropriateness in a given situation.

Communities and countries that are economically and socially disadvantaged present unique circumstances that must be taken into account when planning and implementing AAC interventions. An edited book entitled *Augmentative and Alternative Communication: Beyond Poverty* (Alant & Lloyd, 2005) explores both the challenges faced by AAC providers who support individuals from around the world who live in poverty, as well as a wide range of potential solutions. It is available from Whurr Publishers.

There may also be a general consensus against the use of *any* type of AAC—either low tech or high tech—in some situations. As noted previously, it is not uncommon for the parents of young children to be biased against AAC because they are worried that natural speech will not develop if an alternative option is available. Family members of an individual who has experienced an acquired brain injury may also reject AAC options either because they have a strong desire that their child, spouse, or parent regain the use of natural speech or because they just cannot imagine their relative operating a system that produces artificial speech. Individuals may also reject AAC options when they are overwhelmed with a medical situation. For example, some individuals do not wish to attempt alternative forms of communication in an ICU, even if they cannot communicate important information because of a temporary absence of speech. It often seems that such individuals simply do not have the cognitive or emotional resources that are needed to acquire basic operational skills in the midst of high levels of existing stress.

In an assessment of constraints, it is important to help individuals who are considering the use of AAC and their families identify their preferences and attitudes so that AAC teams can consider these during subsequent decision making. Sensitivity and attention through consensus building are critical in an assessment of constraints, even if this means that the final assistive device decision is "less than perfect" from the perspective of the AAC professionals on the team. After all, it is the person who will use the AAC system and his or her family who will have to live with whatever decision is made. Failure to consider individual and family preferences will almost certainly result in a widespread lament: "The individual has this great system/device but hardly ever uses it!" (Creech, Kissick, Koski, & Musselwhite, 1988).

Preferences and Attitudes of Other Communication Partners   Less important than preferences of those who rely on AAC and their family members, but still of concern, are the technology-related preferences and attitudes of other individuals with whom an individual who uses AAC interacts, either regularly or occasionally. A number of studies have sought to empirically measure the influence of various communication techniques on the perceptions of unfamiliar communication partners. Individuals without disabilities in these studies typically have watched videotapes of interactions between a person using AAC and a natural speaker and have rated their perceptions or attitudes along a number of dimensions.

In studies involving school-age children, it appears that those who are already familiar with peers with disabilities have more positive attitudes toward AAC than those who are not familiar (Beck & Dennis, 1996; Beck, Kingsbury, Neff, & Dennis, 2000; Blockberger, Armstrong, & O'Connor, 1993). In most studies, girls have been found to have more positive attitudes toward AAC than boys (e.g., Beck, Bock, Thompson, & Kosuwan, 2002; Beck, Kingsbury, et al., 2000; Blockberger et al., 1993; Lilienfeld & Alant, 2002), although this may change as children get older (Beck, Fritz, Keller, & Dennis, 2000). With regard to specific AAC techniques, several studies have found no differences with regard to children's attitudes after they viewed videotapes of peers using electronic, aided nonelectronic (e.g., alphabet board), and/or unaided (i.e., manual sign) systems (Beck et al., 2002; Beck & Dennis, 1996; Beck, Fritz, et al., 2000; Blockberger et al., 1993). However, Lilienfeld and Alant (2002), in the only study to date involving adolescents as both the person using AAC and as raters, found more favorable attitudes when an SGD was employed rather than a low-tech alphabet display. This is similar to two studies involving adult raters, in which SGDs were also related to more positive attitudes than low-tech devices when used by adults with cerebral palsy (Gorenflo & Gorenflo, 1991) and aphasia (Lasker & Beukelman, 1999). Finally, there is some evidence that, regardless of the type of AAC device (i.e., low-tech vs. electronic) or the age of the individual using the device, more positive attitudes are associated with communication displays that employ phrase- or sentence-length messages rather than just single word messages (Beck, Kingsbury, et al., 2000; Raney & Silverman, 1992; Richter, Ball, Beukelman, Lasker, & Ullman, 2003).

Given that AAC devices are selected primarily to meet the communication needs of the people who will use them rather than unfamiliar communication partners, what can we make of these results? First, it appears that children are less influenced by the type of AAC system than by past, positive experiences with children with disabilities in general. This suggests that children in schools that include students with disabilities in regular classrooms may be relatively open to AAC techniques in general and may require only basic orientation when encountering classmates who use AAC for the first time. Males may require somewhat more support than females, but this will vary, depending on age. Supports that may result in more positive attitudes include providing information about AAC to adults (Gorenflo & Gorenflo, 1991) and providing opportunities to role play using AAC techniques to children (Beck & Fritz-Verticchio, 2003).

Second, although there is some evidence that electronic devices are perceived more positively than low-tech displays by adolescents and adults, there is also evidence to suggest that *either* AAC option is strongly preferred over poorly intelligible speech (Richter et al., 2003). Finally, we are reminded by this research that efficiency with regard to the rate of communication is an important consideration for unfamiliar communication partners regardless of age, and that strategies in this regard are critical, regardless of the type of AAC device that is used. Unfortunately, information about the attitudes of communication partners from various cultural, ethnic, and socioeconomic backgrounds is sorely lacking, and research is needed in this area.

Skills and Abilities of Communication Partners and Facilitators   Beyond the complex issues related to attitudes and preferences are those related to the skills and abilities of potential communication partners, since it is imperative that they are able to understand the messages conveyed through a communication system and/or provide the necessary supports to optimize its use. For example, if unfamiliar listeners cannot readily understand the AAC system output, as may be the case with manual signs or low-quality synthetic speech, frequent communication breakdowns will occur (see Chapter 4). If communication partners do not know how to interact appropriately with the person using AAC—for example, if they dominate interactions by asking many directive questions and failing to provide sufficient time for message construction—the quality of communication interactions will suffer as a result (Müller & Soto, 2002). Other constraints that may influence the selection of one system over another are the ages and literacy skills of potential partners and other display-related issues. At present, common-sense considerations such as these guide the assessment of partner abilities, because the field has accumulated little empirical research investigating the impact of such issues on AAC system use.

Facilitator skills also affect communication system use in a number of ways. Here, we use the term *facilitator* to refer to family members, professionals, and frequent communication partners who, in one way or another, assume some responsibility for keeping the AAC system current and operational and/or for teaching the person using it to do so effectively. If these individuals do not have the skills or the commitment to providing the supports needed for AAC system use, abandonment of the system is likely (Galvin & Donnell, 2002). The knowledge and skills of these individuals frequently must exceed those needed to interact with natural speakers. For example, facilitators typically need to be operationally competent in the programming, use, and maintenance of electronic AAC devices. They may need to know how to operate various technologies (e.g., software programs, digital cameras) that are used to create communication displays on an ongoing basis. They may need to provide extensive instruction to individuals who are learning to use iconic encoding or other learning-intensive communication techniques, or who are working to improve their grammar, social interaction, or other skills (e.g., Light & Binger, 1998; Lund & Light, 2003). They must also demonstrate social and strategic competence with AAC techniques in order to provide good models and instruction to the individuals they support. A lack of adequate facilitator skills may place constraints on the intervention selected, simply because the necessary, ongoing expertise is unavailable. Failure to specifically consider adequate facilitator skills in the assessment process will almost always result in implementation failure later on; this is especially true for more demanding high-tech devices.

Unfortunately, few assessment tools for evaluating the capabilities of potential facilitators are currently available. One exception is a Partner Rating Scale designed by Culp and Carlisle (1988) that assessors can use to evaluate facilitator attitudes and knowledge concerning AAC techniques used by children. Another, designed for use with the facilitators of adults with intellectual disabilities, can be found in a manual by Light, McNaughton, and Parnes (1986) which, while several years old, is still commercially available. Finally, Garrett and Beukelman (1992) provided a Partner Skill Screening Form and Partner Attitudinal Survey for use with partners and facilitators of adults with aphasia. In the absence of additional assessment instruments, the AAC team must rely on informal methods for evaluating partner and facilitator expertise.

Funding   The funding of AAC technology and services varies considerably from country to country. Even within countries, funding patterns often change from region to region as well as over time. Thus, a detailed discussion of AAC funding will not be provided here. Readers in the United States are referred to the Rehabilitation Engineering and Research Center for Communication Enhancement (AAC-RERC) Web site, which contains current information about funding patterns and procedures. Readers in other countries should consult a local AAC Center for funding information.

CHAPTER 7

ASSESSMENT OF SPECIFIC CAPABILITIES

Capability assessment is the process of gathering information about an individual's capabilities in a variety of areas in order to determine appropriate augmentative and alternative communication (AAC) options. In this chapter, we present some general principles and procedures for constructing a capability profile. In Chapters 9–19, we review additional capability assessment considerations for people with specific disabilities. First, however, we discuss some of the approaches that can be used for capability assessment in general.

OVERVIEW OF APPROACHES TO CAPABILITY ASSESSMENT

According to Yorkston and Karlan (1986), capability assessment involves identifying an individual's level of performance in critical areas that pertain to AAC intervention, such as cognition, language, literacy, and fine motor control. An assessment should result in a profile of the individual's capabilities that can be matched to the operational requirements of particular AAC options. One of the characteristics of a capability profile is that it emphasizes an individual's strengths and unique skills rather than his or her impairments. A strengths-based approach is critical to the endeavor because the assessor will match these strengths to one or more AAC techniques.

Several assessment approaches can be used to assess a person's skills with regard to AAC use. Two of these, criterion-referenced assessment and predictive assessment, predominate in current practice; while the third, norm-referenced assessment, must be used with considerable caution. We begin by discussing the limitations of norm-referenced assessment.

Limitations of Norm-Referenced Assessment

Many professionals in fields such as psychology, education, and speech-language pathology have been trained to use a norm-referenced approach to assessment. In this approach, formal or standardized tests are administered to compare an individual's abilities with those of same-age peers. Professionals are often frustrated when they attempt to use norm-referenced assessment tools to evaluate people who require AAC systems because the professionals cannot administer the tests in a standardized manner. For example, an assessor cannot use a test that requires verbal responses if the individual is unable to speak. A test that requires object manipulation may be useless for assessing an individual with upper-extremity impairments. Even instruments that incorporate multiple-choice formats can present difficulties because individuals may not be able to complete the tests within standard time limitations.

Fortunately, AAC assessment almost never requires that professionals administer norm-referenced tests in a standardized manner, because the purpose of such an assessment is not to compare the individual with peers of the same age. Thus, many professionals use norm-referenced tests that contain appropriate content during an AAC assessment, with test modifications as needed. For example, some individuals may require response options to be presented in a yes/no format instead of an open-ended format or multiple-choice array. Many formal language assessment instruments can be adapted for use with people who have upper-extremity impairments and need to use eye gaze or alternative techniques to respond. When these tests are administered with modifications, they can be useful for obtaining general information related to the person's capabilities rather than for obtaining scores that categorize people according to a developmental or mental age.

Admittedly, there may be situations in which educational or similar agencies require the administration of standardized tests to verify an individual's "eligibility" for services. Indeed, verification testing is one of the most frustrating aspects of agency policy and practice for those who serve people with severe communication disorders. The AAC team may need to address the problem of verification testing, which is an excellent example of a policy and practice issue that can become a barrier to communication opportunities. Professionals, people who use AAC, their families, and involved individuals may need to advocate to change such policies or practices so that service availability is not limited by such a barrier (Snell et al., 2003).

Criterion-Based Assessment

AAC specialists often use criterion-based assessment to determine whether an individual meets the performance thresholds necessary for successful implementation of specific communication techniques or devices. Yorkston and Karlan (1986) described this approach in detail:

> The team frequently has at its disposal some basic information regarding the individual. This information is usually obtained through a screening procedure that may involve a survey of the broad areas of cognitive and language function, hearing, and speech as well as environmental factors. Based on this screening, a decision is generally made not to conduct a comprehensive assessment. For example, when the goal of assessment is to select a portable writing/text editing system for an individual who has successfully attended a community college, in-depth assessment to identify the specific grade level in spelling or grammatical composition may not be necessary.
>
> The criteria-based assessment approach is used to expedite assessment because it is based on a series of branching decisions that allow the team to exclude a large number of possible questions and proceed to critical decisions. For example, when selecting the most appropriate interface by which an individual can access an AAC device, one of

the first questions asked is, "Can this individual access the aid in a direct selection mode?" If the answer is no, then a number of scanning options are explored in more detail. However, if the answer is yes, then a large number of scanning options are eliminated from consideration, and attention is focused on selecting the most appropriate direct selection option (pp. 175–176).

From this description, it should be clear that criterion-based assessment requires the professionals involved in the process to work together when gathering information and making decisions.

Predictive Assessment or Feature Matching

Several authors have suggested predictive profiling or *feature matching* as an extension of the criterion-based approach (Costello & Shane, 1994; Glennen, 1997; Yorkston & Karlan, 1986). In the predictive assessment approach, the team first assesses the capabilities of the individual using a number of carefully selected, criterion-referenced tasks. Based on the results of this assessment, the AAC team then predicts the efficiency with which the individual might utilize one or more devices or techniques. The team then uses its predictions to set up a "trial" of the selected AAC system for a designated period of time (e.g., from a few weeks to several months, depending on the technique involved). Feature matching requires that AAC team members be knowledgeable about the operational and learning requirements of a wide variety of AAC options. If the team does not use a feature-matching approach, it is often necessary to have many AAC options available at the time of the assessment or later so that members can complete successive trials with each device. In many settings, such equipment availability is simply impossible.

Assistivetech.net is an on-line resource for assistive technology (AT) and a link to a wide variety of AT and disability-related information. The searchable database of AT is designed to help people with disabilities, families, professionals, and others to target solutions, determine costs, and link to vendors that sell products. It has replaced the Trace Research and Development Center's CoNet and HyperABLEDATA resources.

In the United States, in response to the requirements of the Assistive Technology Act Amendments of 2004 (PL 105-394), all 50 states and U.S. territories have established assistive technology (AT) centers whose mandate is to increase the availability and utilization of AT devices and services for individuals with disabilities. Through these centers, a variety of AT assessment protocols and information-gathering tools have been developed, many of which are relevant to AAC assessment. In addition, a variety of AAC assessment software products are available to facilitate the capability assessment process, provide guidance to clinicians with regard to feature matching after assessment, or both. Table 7.1 provides information about some of the most widely available tools and software products that pertain to AAC assessment.

Table 7.1. Assistive technology (AT)/AAC assessment tools

Assessment tool/protocol	Purpose	Features	Target population	Availability
Assistive Technology Assessment Questionnaire (2002)	To help AT teams gather information about client needs and capabilities	Printed forms with sections for gathering client information in areas such as functional vision, hearing, mobility (upper and lower limbs), cognitive functioning (i.e., memory and information processing), and current communication use	Adult	Tech Connections, Atlanta, GA
Assistive Technology Predisposition Assessment (Scherer, 1994)	To facilitate the selection and evaluation of AT use in educational, workplace, and health care settings	An assessment battery for both technology providers and potential consumers: *Survey of Technology Use*, to measure consumers' current experiences and attitudes toward AT; *Assistive Technology Predisposition Assessment*, to help select appropriate AT; *Educational Technology Predisposition Assessment*, to identify educational goals and psychosocial issues related to AT use at school; *Workplace Technology Predisposition Assessment*, to identify workplace factors that might inhibit AT use; and *Health Care Technology Predisposition Assessment*, to identify factors that might inhibit use of health care technologies	Adolescent and adult	Institute for Matching Person and Technology, Inc.
Assistive Technology Screener© (Judd-Wall, 1995)	To assist professionals to determine the AT needs of students	Printed forms with sections for documenting past and current AT/AAC use and degree of success; and for considering the need for additional supports in nine areas, including AAC	School age	Technology and Inclusion, Austin, TX
Augmentative Communication Assessment Profile (Goldman, 2002)	To determine an appropriate low-tech AAC technique	Printed profile to identify skills that are related to manual signing (Makaton), low-tech communication displays that require pointing, and low-tech communication displays that require picture exchange	Children ages 3–11 with autism spectrum disorders	Speechmark Publishing
Matching Assistive Technology & Child (MATCH) (Scherer, 1997)	To determine which technologies are appropriate	Printed forms to help parents and team members determine a child's functional limitations and related goals, family considerations that may impact technology use, and appropriate technologies and training strategies	Infants and young children	Institute for Matching Person and Technology, Inc.

Name	Purpose	Description	Population	Source
Medicare Funding of AAC Technology Assessment/Application Protocol (2001)	To document the need for a speech-generating device (SGD) for AAC	Protocol includes directions for documenting the nature of the communication impairment, assessment results (hearing, vision, physical, language, and cognitive skills), daily communication needs, functional communication goals, and features of the recommended SGD and accessories. Protocol is required for Medicare funding of SGDs in the United States.	Adults with acquired communication disorders	Posted on the RERC on Communication Enhancement Web site
Protocol for Culturally Inclusive Assessment of AAC (Huer, 1997)	To document AAC-related assessment information	Protocol includes a cultural self-assessment for professionals as well as an assessment of communication partners, communication needs, capabilities related to AAC use, and technology use.	Children from diverse cultural/linguistic backgrounds	Huer, 1997
UKAT Toolkit (University of Kentucky, 2002)	To guide professionals through the AT service delivery process	Includes printed forms for information gathering, observational assessment and data collection, summarizing assessment data, documenting the results of equipment/device trials, planning implementation, monitoring student progress, and professional self-assessment of AT knowledge and skills.	School age	University of Kentucky Assistive Technology Project
W.A.T.I. Assistive Technology Assessment (2004)	To evaluate a student's need for AT in his or her customary environment	Printed forms to guide the assessment team in gathering information related to a student's abilities/difficulties, identifying relevant environments and tasks, setting priorities, generating potential solutions, making decisions, implementing equipment/device trials, and monitoring trial results and long-term outcomes.	School age	Wisconsin Assistive Technology Initiative
AAC Feature Match (1996)	To assist AAC teams to match client needs to the relevant features of AAC devices	Software (CD-ROM) presents a series of screens requesting information about a client's needs with regard to symbols, encoding technique, selection technique, microswitch type(s), feedback, display characteristics, output, mounting, and other features. Requires that an AAC assessment has already been completed. Results in recommendations of potential AAC devices that match the identified features, along with a report and vendor request letters. Annual software update available on-line at no cost.	School age and adult	Doug Dodgen and Associates

continued

Table 7.1. (continued)

Assessment tool/protocol	Purpose	Features	Target population	Availability
AAT Assessment Tool (1998)	To guide the adaptive/assistive technology assessment process	Software (CD-ROM) presents a series of screens that request information about the client in areas such as communication goals and needs; vision, hearing, fine motor, and gross motor abilities (upper and lower limbs); and cognitive, expressive language, literacy, and oral-motor skills. Results in a printed report of the assessment results.	School age and adult	Doug Dodgen and Associates
EvaluWare™ (Assistive Technology, Inc., 1999)	To help AT professionals identify the best computer access and AAC setups	Software (CD-ROM) presents fun, interactive tasks designed to assess motor access skills (e.g., input method and settings), looking skills (e.g., symbol type and size of visual arrays and targets), and listening skills (e.g., preferred feedback and type of voice output) as well as ability to use an on-screen keyboard and word prediction software. Results in report of assessment outcomes.	School age	Assistive Technology, Inc.
Lifespace Access Profile (Williams, Stemach, Wolfe, & Stanger, 1998)	To assist team to assess AT/AAC needs	Printed forms and software include rating scales to gather information on client strengths and weaknesses with regard to physical, cognitive, emotional, and technology support resources, as well as the extent of participation in school, home, community, work, and recreation/leisure activities and environments. Results in AT/AAC recommendations.	School-age and adult individuals with severe physical and/or cognitive impairments	Don Johnston, Inc.
Needs First (1996)	To assist AAC teams to match client needs to the relevant features of AAC devices	Software (CD-ROM) presents yes/no questions designed to help identify client needs related to AAC. Requires that an AAC assessment has already been completed. Results in a printable list of AAC devices whose features match the identified needs. Also available as on-line resource by subscription.	School age	Computer Options for the Exceptional, Inc.

ASSESSMENT DOMAINS

Several domains usually require investigation as part of an AAC assessment. These include assessment of positioning and seating; motor capabilities for direction selection and/or scanning; cognitive/linguistic capabilities; literacy skills; and sensory/perceptual skills.

Assess Positioning and Seating

Assessment of positioning and seating is critical for individuals with a range of motor impairments. People who have disabilities that severely restrict movement (e.g., cerebral palsy, spinal cord injury, amyotrophic lateral sclerosis [ALS]) may spend the majority of the day in a seated position; therefore, they need to be able to do so safely and without sacrificing functional communicative effectiveness. Other individuals may have more subtle motor impairments that affect their concentration, range of movement, and ability to use AAC functionally in a variety of positions. Consequently, it is important to consult with clinicians such as occupational and physical therapists, who specialize in motor control and can aid in assessing seating and positioning, as an initial step toward capability assessment in general. In that spirit, we welcome the contributions of Donna Drynan, an occupational therapist at the University of British Columbia and the Sunny Hill Health Centre for Children in Vancouver, British Columbia, Canada, who assisted us with developing this section on seating and positioning.

Neuromotor Impairments

Several types of neurological and motor impairments can affect positioning and movement. Some individuals have increased or decreased *muscle tone*, which refers to the "degree of vigor or tension in skeletal muscles" (Fraser, Hensinger, & Phelps, 1990, p. 279). Too much tone makes voluntary movement difficult, whereas too little tone creates problems with maintaining posture, balance, and strength. Many individuals have high tone or spasticity in their extremities and low tone in their trunk area and, therefore, may experience all of the above problems, depending on the task at hand. Efficient use of AAC devices necessitates providing external support or adapting the environment to compensate for these difficulties.

Other problems can result from the presence of *primitive reflexes*, involuntary muscle responses that are present in typically developing infants but disappear as they grow and mature. For example, you may have noticed that, if you stroke an infant's cheek, the child will turn his or her head and open his or her mouth to that side. This response is the *rooting reflex*, which usually disappears within the first few months of life. If the reflex persists it can interfere with voluntary head control (Orelove & Sobsey, 1996). Care must be taken not to position an access switch such that this reflex is elicited.

Other reflex patterns, such as the asymmetrical tonic neck reflex (ATNR), can affect the motor control needed for the use of switches or other adaptive devices. ATNR usually disappears by the time the infant is 6 months of age. It is activated when the infant's head is turned to the side, causing the child to extend the arm and leg on the same side to which his or her face is turned and also prompting the flexion of the infant's arm and leg on the opposite side (see Figure 7.1a). Once the reflex has been activated, many individuals become "stuck" in the abnormal motor pattern and are unable to resume a midline position without assistance. Therefore, AAC systems for individuals who exhibit ATNR should be designed to prevent the need for head rotation to scan a display, because once the person's head is turned, he or she will be unable to use the arm on that side for direct selection (see Figure 7.1b, c). The AAC team should conduct a thorough motor assessment to ensure appropriate switch placement for each individual (see Figure 7.1d, e).

Another common reflex pattern is the symmetrical tonic neck reflex (STNR), which occurs in response to either extension or flexion of the neck. When the individual's neck flexes (i.e., bends forward), STNR prompts flexion of the arms at the elbows and extension of the hips (see Figure 7.2a). The opposite occurs when his or her neck extends (i.e., moves backward): The individual's arms extend outward and his or her hips flex (see Figure 7.2b). Again, the individual often becomes "stuck" in the reflex position and requires assistance to resume a functional position. Because STNR interferes with the individual's functional use of his or her arms, its presence affects AAC motor access. One technique to avoid triggering the STNR reflex is to position displays or switches that are oriented vertically rather than horizontally (e.g., on a desk); (see Figure 7.2c, d). Similarly, people interacting with the individuals should not approach them from above (see Figure 7.2e) but should approach them at eye level (see Figure 7.2f).

Some individuals also have *skeletal deformities* that affect various aspects of positioning. Two common examples include scoliosis (lateral curvature of the spine), which can affect upright posture as well as comfort, and the windswept position of the hip (i.e., hip dislocation, pelvic rotation, and scoliosis), which affects sitting balance and posture. Prevention of such conditions is of primary importance, but if they have already developed in the individual and are fixed, the motor experts on the AAC team will need to compensate for the resulting difficulties.

Finally, *movement disorders* such as athetosis, which is characterized by involuntary movements of the face and limbs during muscle activation, are common in people with certain types of brain lesions. These individuals may not have sufficient control of their upper extremities to be able to write or point to symbols on a display, and as a result they may need to use switches to activate AAC devices.

Principles and Techniques

Most individuals with neuromotor impairments are likely to use their AAC devices while in a seated position—in a wheelchair, at a school or work desk, or at home. It is possible to grossly underestimate an individual's capabilities if he or she is not properly positioned and supported in a seated position. Improper positioning and inadequate physical support can affect a person's fatigue and comfort levels, emotional state, and ability to move and attend to a task. Therefore, the first step in an assessment should involve optimizing the individual's positioning so that the AAC team can accurately assess cognitive, language, and motor capabilities. This does not mean that the team should delay all other AAC assessment until the optimum wheelchair or seating insert has been developed to improve an individual's posture. Rather, it means that the team members who are experts at evaluating physical posture and control should be prepared to at least temporarily po-

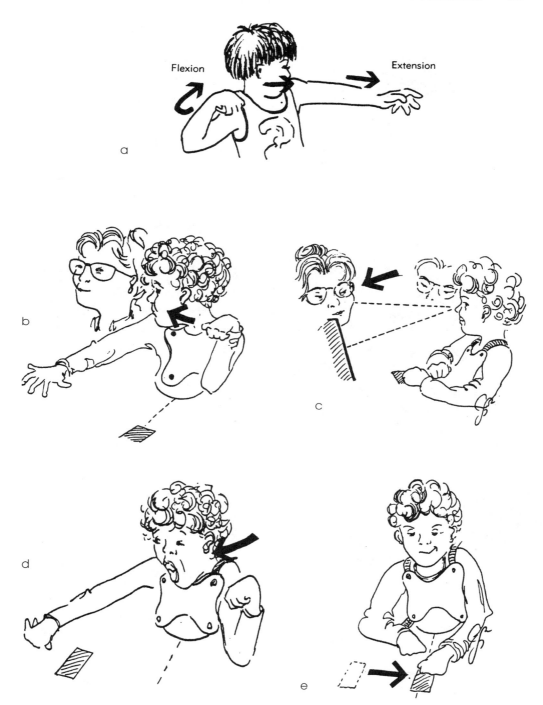

Figure 7.1. a) Asymmetrical tonic neck reflex (ATNR); b) facilitator and/or AAC display should not be placed to the side; c) midline placement of facilitator and/or AAC display is preferred; d) switches should not be placed to the side; e) midline placement of switches is preferred. (From Goossens', C., & Crain, S. [1992]. *Utilizing switch interfaces with children who are severely physically challenged* [p. 40]. Austin, TX: PRO-ED; copyright © Carol Goossens'.)

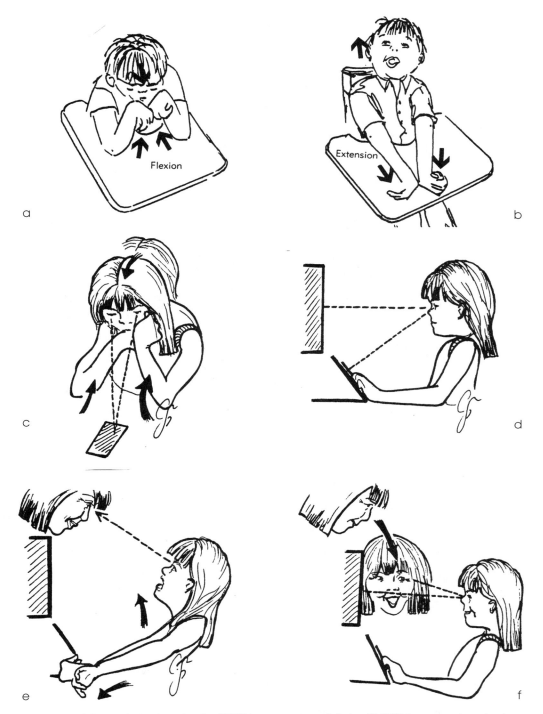

Figure 7.2.   a) Symmetrical tonic neck reflex (STNR) in response to neck flexion; b) STNR in response to neck extension; c) horizontal placement of AAC display and/or switches may activate STNR; d) AAC display should be placed at eye level and switches should be aligned vertically; e) approaching from above may activate STNR; f) facilitator should approach at eye level. (From Goossens', C., & Crain, S. [1992]. *Utilizing switch interfaces with children who are severely physically challenged* [p. 43]. Austin, TX: PRO-ED; copyright © Carol Goossens'.)

sition the individual so that they can complete an appropriate assessment. Over time, a comprehensive assessment of the individual's seating and positioning needs should be completed so that solutions for the individual's postural and movement difficulties can be implemented as part of the AAC intervention.

Ideally, a symmetrical seated position should be the goal; however, this will not be possible for many individuals with severe neuromotor impairments, especially those with fixed deformities. A number of principles should guide the assessment of (and the later design of supports for) positioning and seating. These principles, adapted from Radell (1997) and York and Weimann (1991), include the following.

1. Use yourself as a reference. Almost automatically, people without disabilities position themselves for comfort, stability, and functional movement during tasks. Therefore, in evaluating the position of a person with motor impairments, using yourself as a reference is usually a good idea. The process of using yourself as a reference involves engaging in a task (e.g., activating a switch, using a keyboard) and asking yourself questions such as "How would I position myself for this task?" "How would I align my trunk?" and "How would I position my head, arms, and legs?" The answers can then be used as guidelines to optimize positioning for the individual who is being assessed.

2. Ensure a stable base of support. It is impossible for a person to move in functional ways if his or her trunk and extremities are not sufficiently stable. For instance, if you place a piece of paper on a table and try writing without resting your forearms on the table surface, you will probably find the task fairly difficult. This is because the forearms stabilize the arms, shoulders, upper trunk, and wrists; so, in order to use any of these, the forearms must be supported. Similarly, the feet stabilize the lower part of the body and the trunk, which is why it is difficult to sit for long periods of time without resting your feet on the floor. For the individual undergoing AAC assessment, this stability can be achieved through the use of seat belts, bars, harnesses, lap trays, and other adaptive devices designed for static positioning (see Figures 7.3–7.5).

3. Decrease the influence of atypical muscle tone. An individual with low muscle tone often requires external supports to achieve a proper seated position for AAC assessment. For example, a person who cannot keep his or her head in an upright position may need a headrest or neckrest, either temporarily or permanently. Individuals with high muscle tone (i.e., spasticity) require the careful positioning of AAC displays, switches, and other assistive devices to avoid triggering reflex patterns and to maximize their ease of movement. Often, professionals use a trial-and-error approach to identify the position(s) that allows the individual to have the most functional movement.

4. Accommodate fixed deformities and correct flexible deformities. As noted previously, the ideal seated position is one that is symmetrical and stable. By applying the first principle ("use yourself as a reference"), AAC team members can correct most flexible deformities through the appropriate use of positioning devices. In many cases, fixed deformities may prevent the attainment of symmetry, and the individual may require accommodations to maintain residual movement, maximize comfort, decrease fatigue, and minimize the effort required for movement. For example, an individual with severe scoliosis or other deformities may be unable to sit in an upright position and the team will need to utilize ei-

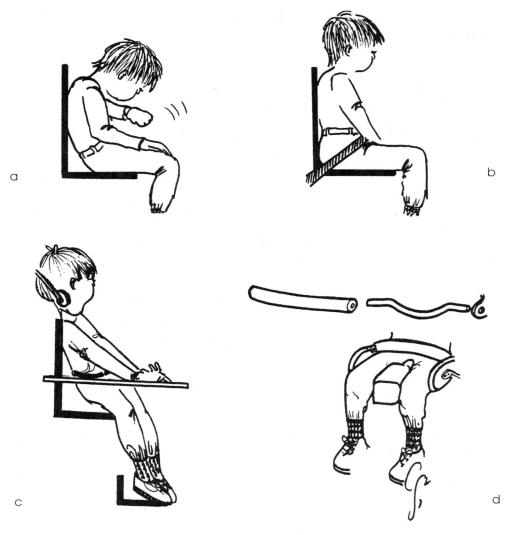

Figure 7.3.   a) Poor positioning in a chair; b) good positioning with pelvis back in the chair and stabilized with a seatbelt at a 45° angle across the hips; c) extensor thrust with hips extended and buttocks raised off the seat; d) subasis bar (rigid pelvic restraint used to stabilize the pelvis and prevent extensor thrust) in place, with two variations shown. (From Goossens', C., & Crain, S. [1992]. *Utilizing switch interfaces with children who are severely physically challenged* [p. 26]. Austin, TX: PRO-ED; copyright © Carol Goossens'.)

ther temporary or permanent supports to achieve alignment in as functional a position as possible (McEwen & Lloyd, 1990).

5. Provide the least amount of intervention needed to achieve the greatest level of function. It is important that the individual not be so rigidly supported in a seated position that he or she is unable to move. As the person's center of gravity changes with upper-body shifting (e.g., leaning forward, reaching, leaning back), his or her feet and arms must be free to move and compensate. In addition, most people both enjoy and need to assume a variety of positions throughout the day.

6. Provide support for resting. It is important to ensure that persons who become fatigued while using their AAC technology can rest with appropriate physical support. For

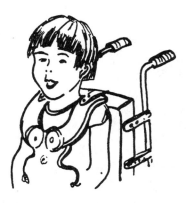

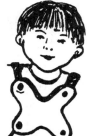

a

b

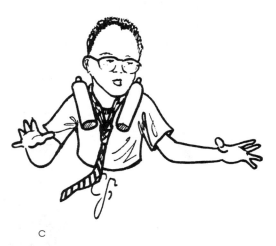

c

Figure 7.4.   Devices used for trunk and shoulder stability. a) Butterfly harness; b) Danmar harness; c) shoulder retractors. (From Goossens', C., & Crain, S. [1992]. *Utilizing switch interfaces with children who are severely physically challenged* [p. 32]. Austin, TX: PRO-ED; copyright © Carol Goossens'.)

example, individuals with weakness due to a degenerative disease such as amyotrophic lateral sclerosis need to be able to rest when they are not actively using their AAC technology (see Chapter 15).

Several general procedures are usually involved in the assessment of positioning and seating that is related to AAC use (Cook & Hussey, 2002; McEwen & Lloyd, 1990; Radell, 1997). First, the AAC team should observe the individual in his or her wheelchair or while he or she is seated in a standard chair. If the person's hips have slid down in the chair, the team should lift the individual so that his or her pelvis is centered on the back edge of the seat or on a custom insert. The person's feet and arms should be supported as needed for proper alignment and movement. If the person is likely to use an AAC device frequently in other positions, the team should observe the individual in these other situations as well. Second, if the person cannot assume or maintain a proper seated position independently, the AAC team should provide assistance in this regard while allowing as much participation by the individual as possible. The assessor(s) should provide firm support to

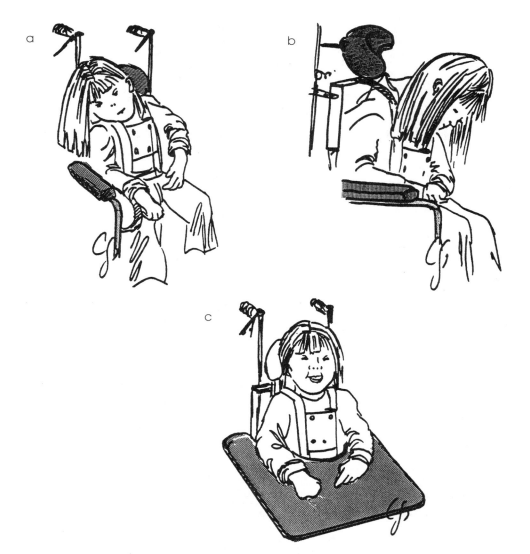

Figure 7.5.   a, b) Without a lap tray, the head and arms are unstable; c) the lap tray provides trunk, shoulder, neck, and head stability. (From Goossens', C., & Crain, S. [1992]. *Utilizing switch interfaces with children who are severely physically challenged* [p. 36]. Austin, TX: PRO-ED; copyright © Carol Goossens'.)

allow the person to achieve a stable and well-aligned position on his or her chair, beginning with his or her pelvis, which provides the base of support and, therefore, must be stable. Next, the AAC team should position the individual's lower extremities, followed by his or her trunk, upper extremities, head, and neck. In effect, the support provided by the hands of the team members simulates the type of support that might be sought through the use of assistive equipment. Third, the team should help the person under observation move out of the chair (if possible) so that team members can take note of the seat, back angles, and any adaptations already in place (e.g., a contoured seat back). Fourth, the team should assess the individual while he or she is out of the chair, looking for any deformities, pressure sores, contractures (i.e., shortening of certain muscle groups), and other physical problems.

Table 7.2.   Elements of an optimal seated position

Ideally, the **pelvis, hips, and thighs** should be positioned so that
- The sitting bones (i.e., ischial tuberosities) bear equal weight
- The pelvis is tilted slightly forward or in a neutral position
- The pelvis is centered in the back edge of seat
- The pelvis is not rotated forward on one side
- The hips are flexed to 90°
- The pelvis is secured to the chair with a belt at a 45° angle across the hips (not across the abdomen)
- The thighs are equal in length
- The thighs are slightly abducted (apart)

Ideally, the **trunk** should be positioned so that it is
- Symmetrical, not curved to the side
- Curved slightly at the low back
- Upright or leaning forward slightly

Ideally, the **shoulders, arms, and hands** should be positioned so that
- The shoulders are in a relaxed, neutral position (not hunched up or hanging low)
- The upper arms are flexed slightly forward
- The elbows are flexed in mid-range (about 90°)
- The forearms rest on a tray for support, if necessary to maintain alignment
- The forearms are neutral or rotated downward slightly
- The wrists are neutral or slightly extended
- The hands are relaxed, with fingers and thumbs opened

Ideally, the **legs, feet, and ankles** should be positioned so that
- The knees are flexed to 90°
- The feet are aligned directly below or posterior to the knees
- The ankles are flexed to 90°
- The feet are supported on a footrest
- The heels and balls of the feet bear weight
- The feet and toes face forward
- The feet can be moved backward behind the knees when the upper body moves forward (i.e., no straps or other restrictive devices unless needed)

Ideally, the **head and neck** should be positioned so that
- They are oriented toward the mid-line of the body
- The chin is slightly tucked (i.e., the back of the neck is elongated)

From York, J., & Weimann, G. (1991). Accommodating severe physical disabilities. In J. Reichle, J. York, & J. Sigafoos (Eds.), *Implementing augmentative and alternative communication: Strategies for learners with severe disabilities* (p. 247). Baltimore: Paul H. Brookes Publishing Co; reprinted by permission.

Once the AAC team has completed its observations, temporary changes can be implemented to improve the individual's positioning. Table 7.2 summarizes the elements of an optimal seated position, although not all of these elements may be attainable for every individual. After the team has properly positioned the person's pelvis, hips, and thighs and secured them to create a stable base, his or her trunk, upper extremities, lower extremities, head, and neck can also be supported. Rolled towels, foam inserts, heavy cardboard supports, temporary splints, Velcro straps, blocks, and other nonpermanent materials can serve as "mock-ups" for any supports that will eventually need to be custom made. The goal at this stage is simply to optimize positioning so that assessment of the motor skills necessary for AAC use can proceed. Over time, a variety of permanent supports may be needed to ensure that the individual has the efficiency and accuracy of movement needed for communication in a seated position. These permanent supports may be relatively simple in nature, such as floor sitters or seating orthoses that support chil-

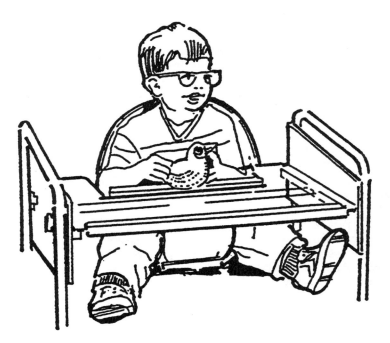

Figure 7.6. Floor sitter. (Source: Sunny Hill Health Centre for Children, Ministry of Health, and Ministry Responsible for Seniors. [1992]. *A conceptual model of practice for school system therapists* [p. 56]. Vancouver, British Columbia, Canada: Author.)

dren while they are seated on the floor, in the bathtub, or on other horizontal surfaces (see Figure 7.6). The supports can also be quite sophisticated, including those used to stabilize and align the pelvis, trunk, hips, thighs, legs, shoulders, and/or head. Figures 7.7–7.9 depict some of the most common permanent components used to support seating.

Assess Motor Capabilities

As was the case with assessment of seating and positioning, the involvement of physical and/or occupational therapists in the assessment of motor access is critical for individuals with severe motor impairments. There are two related motor assessment concerns: identifying a motor technique that the individual can use during the assessment process and identifying a technique that the individual can use for alternative access in the long term. (At this point, readers might wish to review the alternative access options presented in Chapter 4.) These two concerns might result in the selection of the same motor technique for both the assessment and for long-term access, or the team might choose two techniques that are quite different, depending on the individual who relies on AAC. Regardless, it is important to remember that the goal of an AAC motor assessment is to discover motor capabilities, not to describe motor problems.

Identification of Motor Skills for Assessment

The AAC assessment process requires identification of a number of cognitive, symbolic, language, literacy, and other skills related to communication. Therefore, whoever is involved in the assessment must ensure that the individual has a reliable and reasonably ef-

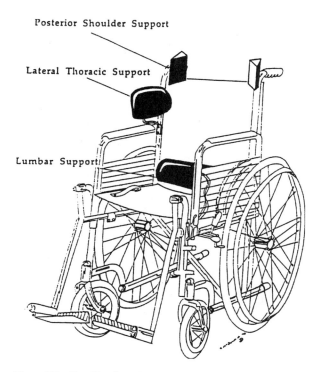

Posterior Shoulder Support

Lateral Thoracic Support

Lumbar Support

Figure 7.7. Shoulder, thoracic, and lumbar supports. (From Medhat, M.A., & Hobson, D. [1992]. *Standardization of terminology and descriptive methods for specialized seating: A reference manual* [p. 26]. Washington, DC: RESNA Press; reprinted by permission.)

ficient way to answer questions and provide other information during the assessment itself. The means of communication will need to be a direct selection technique because scanning appears to add cognitive difficulty to tasks (Mizuko, Reichle, Ratcliff, & Esser, 1994; Ratcliff, 1994; Szeto, Allen, & Littrell, 1993). In addition, Glennen (1997) noted that, when the team uses scanning for initial assessment, it is difficult to determine the source of errors—the individual may not understand how scanning works, may not be able to access the switch in time to select a desired response, may have forgotten the question while waiting for the scanning cursor to move to a desired response, or simply may not know the answer to the question! For these reasons, choosing one of the direct selection options is important, at least during assessment.

Temporary assessment of a direct selection technique can be quite straightforward and usually begins with assessment of the person's ability to answer yes/no questions because such a format can be used for adaptations most easily. It is important to ask questions that are developmentally appropriate, such as asking a child "Is your name Santa Claus?" or "Is this a car?" (while holding up a car or another item), asking an adult "Did you get here today in an airplane?" and so forth. Many individuals will be able to respond to such questions quite accurately with vocalizations; eye blinks; facial expressions; head shakes, turns, or nods; and other gestures. If the team plans to use a yes/no format during the remainder of the assessment, it is critical that the individual's responses be highly accurate and unambiguous. If the person's responses are vague, the team usually proceeds to examine finger/hand use as a second option. To do this, the assessor may place a vari-

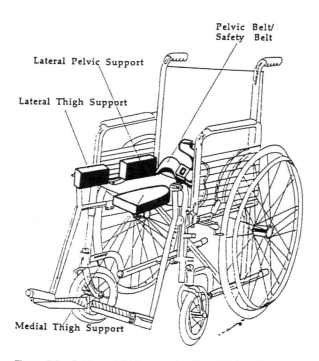

Pelvic Belt/
Safety Belt

Lateral Pelvic Support

Lateral Thigh Support

Medial Thigh Support

Figure 7.8. Pelvic and thigh supports. (From Medhat, M.A., & Hobson, D. [1992]. *Standardization of terminology and descriptive methods for specialized seating: A reference manual* [p. 26]. Washington, DC: RESNA Press; reprinted by permission.)

ety of food items, toys, or other motivating items on a table or lap tray. He or she can then encourage or ask the person under observation to reach for, pick up, or point to the objects while the assessor notes accuracy, range, and movement patterns (e.g., ability to cross the midline of the body). If the individual's hand and arm use are limited, the assessor can hold up items in front of the person at various distances and locations in the visual field in order to assess his or her eye gaze in a similar manner. Finally, if absolutely necessary, the team can provide the individual with a headstick or headlight pointer; however, this is usually the least desirable option because it requires the person to have some training and practice in order to use the headstick or pointer with sufficient accuracy.

It is important to allow adequate time for response during a preliminary direct selection assessment because individuals who do not regularly use these techniques may require considerable processing time before they can execute the necessary motor actions. For example, one woman we know had been deemed "unassessable" by two consecutive AAC teams because she could not demonstrate a reliable motor behavior during the initial screening. In reality, she could point to pictures and objects with her hand quite accurately—as long as assessors were willing to wait for up to 2 minutes so that she could slowly drag her hand across the lap tray to select an answer! Although this method was too slow to be useful as a permanent access technique, it was used successfully during assessment to identify this woman's language, symbol, and literacy skills, which were considerable.

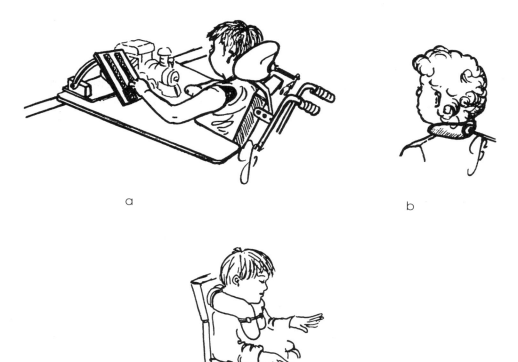

a

b

c

Figure 7.9. Head and neck supports. a) Curved headrest; b) neck ring; c) Hensinger head collar. (From Goossens', C., & Crain, S. [1992]. *Utilizing switch interfaces with children who are severely physically challenged* [p. 34]. Austin, TX: PRO-ED; copyright © Carol Goossens'.)

Identification of Long-Term Motor Skills

Once the team has identified a temporary response technique, the assessment may proceed to determining the best long-term technique. As we have seen, there are two approaches to indicating items in the selection display: direct selection and scanning. Because, in general, direct selection techniques can be more efficient for individuals with sufficient motor control and are generally preferred to scanning selection techniques, motor assessment usually focuses first on direct selection (Dowden & Cook, 2002). If direct selection techniques prove to be inaccurate, very slow, or fatiguing for the individual being assessed, the team will then initiate a scanning assessment. Of course, there are exceptions to this rule: consider, for example, a person who can communicate using direct selection in the morning but needs to change to scanning in the afternoon or evening as fatigue sets in. Or, consider an individual who can use a direct selection technique when she is properly positioned in a wheelchair, but must control her communication system or computer through scanning when seated in other types of chairs, when lying in bed, or when participating in personal care activities. In such cases, assessment will need to examine both direct selection and scanning abilities. Fortunately, because more and more AAC devices are manufactured with both scanning and direct selection options, individuals can incorporate both selection techniques into their systems as needed, while using the same or similar symbol representation, message formulation, and output strategies for both selection techniques.

Direct Selection   An assessment of direct selection capabilities generally occurs in the following stages: 1) assessment of hand and arm control, 2) assessment of head and orofacial control, and 3) assessment of foot and leg control. The individual's upper limbs are assessed first because the hand potentially provides the most discrete control and has the greatest social acceptance as an alternative access site (Dowden & Cook, 2002). Second, head, neck, and orofacial movements (e.g., eye pointing, head pointing) may be used. Third, the team usually assesses the individual's foot and leg control last because few people with physical impairments have the fine motor control of their lower extremities needed for direct selection techniques.

The form in Figure 7.10 has been developed to collect and summarize the information from a direct selection survey. Some of the techniques that teams may use to gather this information are summarized in the sections that follow. Additional forms for direct selection assessment can also be found in Cook and Hussey (2002).

Observation and Interview   A team usually begins an assessment of direct selection capabilities by observing the individual for a time to determine the types of movements he or she makes during communication or other routine activities. Interviews with the individual, family members, caregivers, and others also provide information about current movement patterns and activities. For example, some individuals may already point with their hands or their eyes to indicate items of choice. Such information is useful in guiding the assessment.

Assess Range and Accuracy of Movement   Next, the assessment generally involves testing the individual's range and accuracy of movements without using adaptations. The AAC team usually assesses hand (e.g., finger pointing) or headstick control by using a horizontal grid surface, while eye pointing or headlight pointing is assessed using a vertical grid surface (see Figure 7.11). Of course, the individual must understand the task requirements in order for the results to be valid; therefore, the team should try to minimize the cognitive, linguistic, and technical aspects of the assessment so that motor control can be isolated and studied. For this reason, the team usually does not use AAC symbols or ask people to formulate messages during the initial screening process. Rather, team members begin by placing various types of targets on the display surface and indicating that the individual is to touch, look at, or shine the light on each target. For adults with acquired conditions, individual numbers or letters might be used to mark locations to which they are asked to point. Coins often make excellent targets for children, especially when they are told they can keep each coin that they touch with their hands or feet, "hit" with a headstick or light pointer, or look at using eye gaze. We have found that even children with severe cognitive impairments often understand this task almost immediately. Alternatively, the team can use small edible items, toys, or other motivating items as targets. In some cases, individuals may be able to reach for items with their hands, but they lack the ability to point accurately and efficiently. If this is the case, the AAC assessors can provide a variety of manual supports or devices to facilitate pointing during assessment. These aids include, for example, temporary finger or wrist splints, hand-held

Movement pattern	Direct selection device	Adaptations used (e.g., splint, textured surface, keyguard)	Target (size, number, distance/ orientation to body)	Times hit/missed target	Negative impact (e.g., muscle tone, reflexes, postures, fatigue)	Comments
Right upper limb						
Left upper limb						
Head/neck	Headlight pointer					
Head/neck	Headstick/ mouthstick					
Eyes						
Other (e.g., lower limbs, sign of voice recognition)						

Augmentative and Alternative Communication: Supporting Children and Adults with Complex Communication Needs, Third Edition, by David R. Beukelman and Pat Mirenda. Copyright © 2005 Paul H. Brookes Publishing Co., Inc. All rights reserved.

Figure 7.10. Direct selection survey.

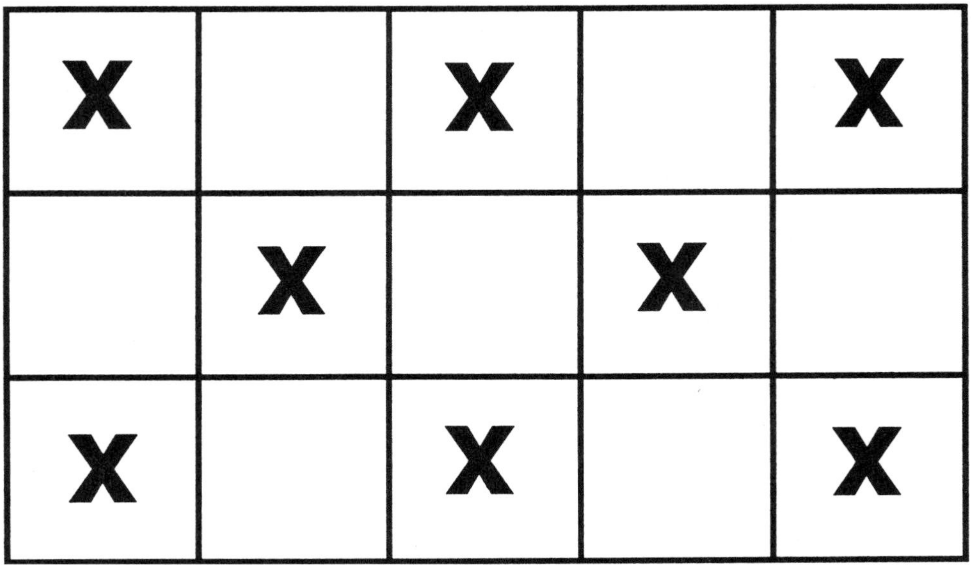

Figure 7.11. A targeting grid for motor assessment.

pointers (e.g., a pencil, a small flashlight), or mobile arm supports such as slings or hinged arm positioners.

The AAC team may need to enlarge targets to assess headlight (optical) pointing, at least initially, so that the individual experiences success. For adults who understand the task, colored circles of construction paper positioned on a large display surface, such as a light-colored wall, may be sufficient. For children, the assessment may include asking them to shine the headlight on large animal pictures or other motivating targets. Some children are also willing to try to play tag with the light pointer in an assessment. By "chasing" targets (the assessor's hand, toy animals, or large pictures) as they move slowly across a solid background, children may be able to demonstrate the range and accuracy of their head control. Many of these same techniques are useful for screening eye-pointing capabilities as well.

Optimizing Control   For motor techniques with which the individual was somewhat successful during screening, additional assessment can help to further define capabilities in areas such as 1) the degree of accuracy with which the person can use the technique to access targets of various sizes; 2) the maximum range and number of targets that he or she can access; and 3) the extent to which adaptations such as keyguards, various display surface angles, various textured surfaces (e.g., slick versus rough), head supports, and trunk supports can optimize his or her accuracy, efficiency, and range of motion. Because people with severe disabilities may have had little experience with the access options used in the assessment, the AAC team members should be quite conservative in their judgments about motor control. During an initial evaluation, an individual may demonstrate little of the ability that instruction and practice might produce. This is particularly true for techniques such as head pointing because few individuals are likely to have had any experience with this method of alternative access prior to an evaluation.

Therefore, the team should reassess options that appear even marginally viable—if possible, after the individual has practiced for a few weeks.

Assess Negative Impact   Throughout the motor control assessment, the AAC team should also focus on the overall impact each access technique has on the individual. For example, some direct selection control techniques can lead to unwanted consequences such as persistent abnormal reflexes, excessive muscle tone, abnormal postures, or excessive fatigue. In the assessment, the AAC team members must determine the extent to which they can minimize the negative impact of various alternative access options while preserving the potential benefits. Often, a compromise may be reached; however, the negative consequences associated with a particular alternative access option occasionally can be so detrimental that the team must abandon the option for the moment. Such techniques often can be considered later with additional instruction, practice, or adaptations.

Manual Signing   If manual signing is being considered for an individual, the AAC team may undertake assessment of the fine motor skills used for manual signs or formalized gestures, such as Amer-Ind. Dennis, Reichle, Williams, and Vogelsberg (1982) and Doherty (1985) reviewed a number of studies that examined the motoric dimensions that appear to be related to manual sign acquisition and retention; we have also reviewed these in Chapter 3. In addition, formal protocols for fine motor assessment related to the use of signs were developed by Dunn (1982) and described by Dennis et al. (1982).

Switch Assessment for Scanning   The AAC team will need to complete a switch assessment for scanning if an individual is unable to directly select items from a display. Switch assessment involves identification of body sites that the individual can use to activate one or more switches, as well as assessment of the individual's ability to use various scanning strategies and arrangements (see Chapter 4).

Screening for a switch activation site on the body is the first step of a scanning assessment. A note of caution: AAC teams have a tendency to utilize tasks that are too complex when identifying an individual's switch activation sites. The team should attempt to reduce the cognitive, visual, and communicative demands in a switch control assessment; for this reason, we rarely use AAC equipment to gather this information. We have found that asking an individual to activate a tape recorder and play music (or to turn on a battery-operated toy) is an effective way to provide a consequence during the scanning assessment. To perform the assessment, we attach a switch to the remote-control port of a tape recorder and insert an audiocassette tape appropriate for the age and interests of the person being assessed. A team can then try different switches as it assesses various motor control sites, such as fingers, hands, head, and feet.

Generally, we use a criterion-based assessment approach to identify a switch activation site. To this end, we begin a switch assessment with the most socially appropriate body site for switch control: the hands. If hand or finger control of a switch sufficiently allows accurate, efficient, and nonfatiguing alternative access, we do not continue the assessment with other body parts. If hand control seems insufficient, we usually assess the head next, followed by the feet, legs, and knees.

Components of Switch Control   There are essentially six components of switch control. To operate an electronic scanner, the individual must first be able to wait for the right moment in order to avoid inadvertently activating the switch. Some individuals have difficulty waiting because of cognitive or motor control problems. The second step in controlling a switch is activation, or closing the switch. During assessment, the team should determine whether the individual can activate a variety of switches, note the approximate length of time it takes for each activation to occur, and observe the efficiency with which the person completes the activation movements. The third step in controlling a switch is to hold it in an activated position for the required time. Some individuals who are able to activate the switch accurately and promptly are not able to hold or maintain switch closure. The fourth step in switch control is the ability to release the switch accurately and efficiently, a step that may be problematic for some people. Finally, the fifth and sixth steps involve the individual waiting and then reactivating the switch at the appropriate times.

The team can assess each of these components by using the tape recorder or toy strategy described previously. Members may ask the individual to turn the tape recorder on and off according to directions designed to assess each component, such as "Wait, don't play it yet," "Okay, play it now," "Stop," and "Play it again." The AAC team may need to observe individuals who are unable to follow verbal directions because of cognitive or other limitations while the individuals use switches to control appliances in natural environments. Regardless of the environment, this assessment should give the team an overall indication of the individual's ability to activate switches at various motor control sites. We provide a form to record the results of this assessment in Figure 7.12. Again, we remind readers that, although many body parts are listed on this form, it is often unnecessary to evaluate all of them.

Detailed instructions for switch assessment and mounting, as well as techniques for teaching scanning skills to young children, can be found in Goossens' and Crain (1992).

Cursor Control Techniques and Switch Control Capabilities   The choice of cursor control technique for scanning (e.g., automatic, directed, step scanning) is influenced by an individual's motor control capabilities. This match between techniques and capabilities is illustrated in Tables 7.3 and 7.4. The types of scanning are found across the top of Table 7.3, and the six components of switch control described previously are listed along the left side. The table includes the motor component skill-accuracy requirements for each type of scanning. Therefore, in the case of automatic scanning, in which the cursor moves automatically across the selection set and the person being assessed is required to stop it at a desired item, there is a high skill-accuracy requirement for the individual to wait until the cursor is in the correct location. There is also a high skill-accuracy requirement for the individual to activate the switch to stop the cursor. Because the item is selected at the moment of switch activation, it does not matter how long the person holds the switch closed, and the accuracy requirements for holding are low. The release phase also has a low skill-accuracy requirement because nothing is required during this phase of automatic scanning. Finally, the person requires high skill-accuracy for waiting and re-

Voluntary motor control (single switch)

	Is able to wait		Is able to activate		Is able to hold		Is able to release		Is able to wait		Is able to reactivate		Accuracy*
	Yes	No	Yes	No	Yes	No	Yes	No	Yes	No	Yes	No	
Fingers on left hand													
Fingers on right hand													
Left hand (palm? back?)													
Right hand (palm? back?)													
Left shoulder													
Right shoulder													
Head rotation (R? L?)													
Head flexion													
Head–side flexion (R? L?)													
Head extension													
Vertical eye motions													
Horizontal eye motions													
Tongue or chin													
Left outer leg/knee													
Right outer leg/knee													
Left Inner leg/knee													
Right inner leg/knee													
Left foot (up? down?)													
Right foot (up? down?)													

*Accuracy = rate of overall accuracy on a 0–4 scale in which 0 = never and 4 = always.

Augmentative and Alternative Communication: Supporting Children and Adults with Complex Communication Needs, Third Edition, by David R. Beukelman and Pat Mirenda. Copyright © 2005 Paul H. Brookes Publishing Co., Inc. All rights reserved.

Figure 7.12. Assessment of motor (switch) control for scanning.

Table 7.3. Skill accuracy requirements of cursor control techniques for scanning

Motor component	Cursor control technique		
	Automatic scanning	Directed scanning	Step scanning
Wait	High	Medium	Low
Activate	High	Low	Medium
Hold	Low	High	Low
Release	Low	High	Low
Wait	High	Medium	Medium
Reactivate	High	Medium	Medium
Fatigue value	Low	Medium	High

activating the switch. Automatic scanning relies on timing rather than on repeated movements or endurance, so it produces a low level of fatigue.

In directed scanning, the cursor moves to the desired item only when the switch is activated, and the individual must release the switch to make a selection. A review of Table 7.3 for this type of scanning indicates that waiting prior to activation has a medium skill-accuracy requirement. Although waiting does not affect accurate item selection directly, inadvertent activation at this point will initiate cursor movement before the individual is ready to begin. Switch activation has a low skill-accuracy requirement in directed scanning because activation does not involve precise timing. Holding in directed scanning has a high skill-accuracy requirement because the individual must hold the switch closed until the cursor is positioned at the desired item; therefore, a person's inability to adequately hold the switch closed will result in a selection error. During directed scanning the individual makes a selection in the switch release phase, requiring high skill-accuracy, whereas waiting and reactivation have medium skill-accuracy requirements. The fatigue value in directed scanning is medium because the individual must have some motor endurance to hold the switch closed for a period of time.

In step scanning, the cursor moves one step with each activation of the switch. Therefore, the individual's ability to wait has a low skill-accuracy requirement because it is not involved in item selection. Switch activation has a medium skill requirement because, although the activation does not have to be rapid, accurate, or well timed, it may be quite fatiguing. Holding in step scanning requires only low skill-accuracy because the cursor moves one step with each activation and therefore holding is not part of the selection process. For the same reason, releasing is also a low skill-accuracy requirement. Wait-

Table 7.4. Clinical illustrations of ease of motor control and capabilities for scanning

Motor component	Ease of motor control		
	Francesca (athetosis)	Isaac (spasticity)	Jin (weakness)
Wait	Difficult	Medium	Easy
Activate	Difficult	Medium	Medium
Hold	Medium	Easy	Difficult
Release	Easy	Difficult	Easy
Wait	Difficult	Medium	Easy
Reactivate	Difficult	Medium	Medium
Fatigue value	Medium	Medium	Difficult

ing and reactivation require medium motor control abilities because inadvertent switch activation at these phases will result in erroneous selections. Fatigue is high in step scanning because of the multiple, repeated switch activations.

The preceding discussion is based on clinical experience, not research—in fact, we are unaware of any research that exists to support this model. Nonetheless, professionals with whom we have worked tell us that generally applying these guidelines helps them achieve effective matching between an individual's motor control capabilities and a cursor control pattern for scanning. We illustrate clinical applications of these guidelines in the following sections by discussing three people who rely on scanning for alternative access.

Clinical Illustration: Francesca (Athetosis)

The results of a switch assessment for Francesca, a child with athetoid cerebral palsy, are illustrated in Table 7.4, in which we describe the ease or difficulty with which Francesca was able to accomplish the various components of switch activation. As is the case for many individuals with athetosis, accurate waiting was difficult for her. Because of involuntary motor movements ("overflow") associated with her athetosis, Francesca inadvertently activated the switch during the waiting phase. Similarly, accurate and efficient switch activation was also difficult because Francesca's overflow movements are accentuated in times of stress or anticipation. Therefore, she was unable to activate the switch quickly on command. We see that the holding phase was of medium ease for Francesca because she was able to maintain contact with the switch once she managed to activate it. In contrast to the difficulties associated with switch activation, the release phase was easy for this child, for she was able to release the switch efficiently and accurately. Finally, Francesca found that waiting and reactivation were again difficult because of her extraneous motor movements.

A comparison of Francesca's switch control profile with the requirements of cursor control in Table 7.3 suggests that directed scanning might be an alternative access mode for her. Directed scanning has high skill-accuracy requirements for holding and releasing, which match her capabilities. Conversely, automatic scanning has high skill requirements for waiting and activating, the two phases of switch activation that Francesca found most difficult. Step scanning would probably exacerbate her involuntary motor movements because it requires the greatest amount of actual motor activity and is quite fatiguing.

Clinical Illustration: Isaac (Spasticity)

Isaac is a young man with severe spasticity resulting from a traumatic brain injury; as in the case of Francesca, we provide a summary of his switch activation profile in Table 7.4. The assessment showed that Isaac had medium ease with waiting and switch activation, and that his activations were rather deliberate and slow. He found it easy to hold the switch closed briefly but difficult to release it in a timely and accurate manner. Release was difficult for Isaac because the spasticity prevented him from relaxing his contact with the switch when he wanted. He experienced medium ease with waiting and reactivation.

A review of the requirements of cursor control patterns suggests that Isaac's difficulty with switch release will probably make it difficult for him to use directed scanning successfully. Instead, automatic scanning might be a more appropriate choice for him because it has high waiting and activation requirements, activities that Isaac found moderately easy. Automatic scanning also has low skill requirements for switch releasing, the phase with which this young man has the most difficulty.

Clinical Illustration: Jin (Weakness)

Jin, a woman with ALS that causes severe weakness throughout her body, could operate a very sensitive switch affixed just above her eyebrow by raising her forehead slightly. Jin found waiting quite easy and was able to activate the switch with moderate ease when asked. She experienced difficulty holding the switch closed because of her weakness, but she could easily release it. She then had no difficulty waiting and could reactivate the switch with medium ease. As can be seen by consulting Table 7.3, the optimal cursor control pattern for Jin appeared to be automatic scanning because this option requires the greatest amount of waiting and causes the least fatigue, a major concern for someone like Jin who has little motor stamina.

We remind the reader that the clinical interpretations made in these case studies are illustrations only. In no sense do we mean to suggest that all individuals who experience athetosis, spasticity, or weakness will have switch activation profiles similar to those in this section. We simply present these examples to illustrate the process of matching an individual's capabilities with the motor control requirements for scanning. Readers should also note that the goal of the type of motor assessment described here is to screen an individual's motor capabilities so that intervention can begin. In addition to this initial process, the AAC team should continually assess an individual's motor control after an intervention is in place in order to further refine the alternative access technique and ensure that the person's performance becomes increasingly more accurate and efficient and less fatiguing.

Assess Cognitive/Linguistic Capabilities

In the Participation Model, assessment of an individual's current communication skills occurs at an earlier phase of assessment (see Chapter 6). At this point in the assessment process, we can use additional assessments to gather relevant information about specific cognitive, language, and related skills.

Cognitive/Communication Assessment

The purpose of cognitive/communication assessment in AAC is to determine how the individual understands the world and how the AAC team can best facilitate communication within this understanding. Rowland and Schweigert (2003) suggested six aspects of cognitive/communication development that are highly relevant to AAC: awareness, communicative intent, world knowledge, memory, symbolic representation, and metacognition. In addition, Wilkinson and Jagaroo (2004) suggested that a variety of visual perceptual skills are important to consider when making decisions about AAC devices or techniques.

Awareness involves a number of increasingly sophisticated understandings: 1) that "I" am separate and different from my surroundings; 2) that specific behaviors I perform (e.g., kicking, smiling at a familiar face) have specific consequences (e.g., a mobile moves, a person smiles and vocalizes back to me); and 3) that other people have thoughts, desires, and perceptions that may differ from mine (i.e., theory of mind). *Communicative intent*, an extension of social contingency awareness, involves behavior that is "purposefully directed toward another person with intended meaning . . . [and that] requires dual orientation—orientation to both the communication partner and the topic or referent" (Rowland & Schweigert, 2003, p. 251). Of course, communicative intentionality does not simply "happen" overnight—rather, it develops as caregivers respond positively to preintentional behaviors that become increasingly purposeful over time as a result. *World knowledge* includes general experience in the world that results in 1) expectations about how both people and inanimate objects should work, and (even more important) 2) the motivation to repeat pleasant experiences and avoid unpleasant ones. Motivation may be compromised in individuals who have repeatedly experienced failure in their attempts to communicate using conventional but nonsymbolic modes; this has been referred to as "learned helplessness" (Seligman, 1975). *Memory* involves a complex set of skills that are needed for all learning and that have profound implications for a person's ability to attend to, categorize, retrieve, select, and sequence messages that are represented through both unaided and aided symbols or codes (Light & Lindsay, 1991; Mirenda, 2003b; Oxley & Norris, 2000). Memory is also an important factor to consider when making decisions about many electronic communication devices, especially those that utilize dynamic displays or auditory scanning (Kovach & Kenyon, 2003). *Symbolic representation* involves an understanding of the relationship between symbols (e.g., manual signs, photographs, line drawings) and their referents. As noted in Chapter 3, a number of studies have demonstrated that the meanings of symbols that more closely resemble their referents are easier to learn and to deduce. *Metacognitive skills* allow people to consider their own cognitive experiences with regard to language use and learning (metalinguistics), memory strategies (metamemory), and self-regulation (executive functions). These more advanced cognitive skills are especially important for individuals who use electronic scanning as a selection technique (Light & Lindsay, 1991) and/or who use either low or high technology AAC devices with large vocabulary capacities organized in levels or categories (Oxley & Norris, 2000). Finally, *visual perceptual skills* related to an individual's ability to scan a grid, discriminate among symbols of various sizes and orientations, and perceive colors may also be important factors to consider in selecting an optimum AAC technique or mode (Wilkinson & Jagaroo, 2004).

Unfortunately, as of 2005 no empirically validated assessment tools were available to assess an individual's capabilities across all seven of these areas. However, some instruments are available to assess at least basic cognitive/communication skills such as contingency awareness, communicative intentionality, symbolic representation, and/or basic concepts related to world knowledge, using either observational, interview, or direct assessment methods. Table 7.5 presents a brief summary of some instruments that might be useful in this regard, including both those designed for general assessment and those specifically designed for individuals who use AAC.

Although several of these instruments may be useful for assessing individuals who are primarily nonsymbolic communicators, it is important to note that adaptations may be needed to accommodate motor or sensory impairments. For example, Iacono, Carter,

Table 7.5. Selected instruments for assessment of basic cognitive/communication skills related to AAC use

Instrument	Designed for AAC?	Skills assessed	Type(s) of assessment	Appropriate for . . .	Source
Augmentative Communication in the Medical Setting (Yorkston, 1992)	Yes	Comprehension, expression, cognition, motor/perceptual skills, partner needs, and others	Direct assessment, interviews, observations	Adults with locked-in syndrome, acquired brain injury, severe aphasia, and intensive care unit needs	PRO-ED, Inc.
Bracken Basic Concept Scale–Revised (Bracken, 1998)	No	Basic concepts and receptive language skills	Direct assessment with verbal directions and responses via pointing	Individuals ages 2 yr 6 mo through 7 yr who are unable to speak, read, or write English	Harcourt Assessment
Communication and Symbolic Behavior Scales (CSBS™; Wetherby & Prizant, 1993)	No	Communicative functions, gestural, vocal, and verbal communicative means; reciprocity, social-affective signaling, symbolic behavior	Caregiver questionnaire, interactive behavior sample with parent present	Individuals with developmental ages between 6 and 72 months, if cognitive delays are present	Paul H. Brookes Publishing Co.
Communication and Symbolic Behavior Scales Developmental Profile (CSBS DP™; Wetherby & Prizant, 2002)	No	Emotion and eye gaze, communication, gestures, sounds, words, understanding, and object use	Screening checklist, caregiver questionnaire, interactive behavior sample with parent present	Individuals with developmental ages between 6 and 72 months, if cognitive delays are present	Paul H. Brookes Publishing Co.
Communication Matrix (Rowland, 1996, 2004)	Yes	Symbolic abilities related to four functional categories of communication	Can be completed through observations, interviews, or direct elicitation	Individuals who are functioning at the earliest stages of communication	Design to Learn, Inc.
School Inventory of Problem-Solving Skills (SIPSS) and Home Inventory of Problem-Solving Skills (HIPSS) (Rowland & Schweigert, 2002)	Yes	Basic skills with objects (e.g., using simple actions, transferring), ability to gain access to objects (e.g., object permanence, tool use), and ability to use objects (e.g., functional use, matching)	Rating scale for each skill: mastered, mastered with limitations, emerging, not present	Nonverbal children with multiple disabilities (e.g., severe mental retardation or sensory impairments, including deaf-blindness)	Design to Learn, Inc.
Stages (Pugliese, 2001)	No	Cause and effect; receptive language; basic concepts; reading and math readiness; academic, money, and time skills; and written expression	Direct, computer-based assessment using software and printed materials	School-age individuals with cognitive and language delays	Assistive Technology, Inc.
Tangible Symbol Systems, Levels of Representation Pre-Test (Rowland & Schweigert, 1996)	Yes	Symbolic representation	Direct assessment using object–symbol matching tasks	Nonverbal individuals who do not already communicate clearly using AAC	Design to Learn, Inc.
The Triple C (Checklist of Communication Competencies) (Bloomberg & West, 1999)	Yes	Reflexivity and reactivity, contingency awareness, object use, imitation, object permanence, cause and effect, communicative intentionality, symbolic representation	Observational checklist and accompanying videotape	Adolescents or adults with severe or multiple disabilities	Scope Communication Resource Centre

188

and Hook (1998) modified the "communicative temptations" from the Communication and Symbolic Behavior Scales (Wetherby & Prizant, 1993) for individuals with cerebral palsy by providing repeated activity exposures to allow time for orientation and by adding a microswitch to facilitate self-activation of a toy or music activity. Snell (2002) made additional suggestions in this regard, and she also emphasized that formal measures are not appropriate for many nonsymbolic communicators because of the idiosyncratic form of their communication. As an alternative, she described the use of a process for dynamic assessment that is designed to accommodate individual needs in terms of tasks, materials, procedures, and assessors. Although dynamic assessments usually require more time than static (i.e., formal) assessments, they also provide much richer information about an individual's communication skills, the contexts and interaction methods that are most likely to facilitate his or her communication, and the types and amount of intervention that will be needed.

A parent-friendly version of the Communication Matrix (Rowland, 1996, 2004) is now available in two formats: printed and on-line! The free, on-line version enables parents to provide information about their child's skills and then—with the click of an on-screen button!—print out a profile of the results as well as a specific list of their child's communication behaviors and levels of communicative intent. The on-line version is available at http://www.communicationmatrix.org.

In addition, there are often situations—aside from those where the goal is to achieve a good match between an individual and an AAC technique—in which formal assessment of an individual's cognitive abilities may be necessary or useful. For example, we are frequently asked to suggest instruments that can be used in educational settings for cognitive assessment related to individual education planning, especially for individuals with severe and/or multiple disabilities. In the past few years, several reasonably reliable and valid standardized tests of cognitive ability have been used with children, adolescents, or adults who are unable to speak, as presented in Table 7.6. Many of these tests require no motor responses other than pointing. Alternatively, they can be adapted by, for example, cutting up test pages with pictures into separate items that can then be arranged on an eye-gaze display or individualized array for pointing; limiting the number of choices from which the individual is asked to choose; enlarging test stimuli (i.e., pictures) for individuals with visual impairments; and using a "yes/no" or multiple choice format instead of asking open-ended questions (Glennen, 1997). For example, if the original test question is "How are an orange and an apple the same?," the assessor might ask the question and then present a series of yes/no options in random order: "Are they both red?" "Are they both round?" "Are they both fruit?" "Are they both toys?" and so forth. Although such adaptations technically invalidate many cognitive assessments so that the scores obtained cannot be reported as "official" IQ scores, the modifications may have practical value in that they do allow the team to assess the cognitive skills that are measured by the test items.

Table 7.6. Selected instruments for nonverbal assessment of cognitive abilities

Instrument	Skills assessed	Direction and response modes	Appropriate for . . .	Source
Cognitive Abilities Test™, Form 6 (CogAT; Lohman & Hagen, 2001)	Verbal, quantitative, and nonverbal reasoning	Directions given verbally; responses via point to pictures	Individuals age 5–18 who are unable to speak, read, or write English	Riverside Publishing
Comprehensive Test of Nonverbal Intelligence (CTONI; Hammill, Pearson, & Wiederholt, 1996)	Nonverbal reasoning abilities	Directions given via gestures; responses via point or point/mouse click (Windows version)	Individuals ages 6–90 who are unable to speak, read, write, and/or understand English	AGS Publishing
Leiter International Performance Scale–Revised (Roid & Miller, 1997)	Visualization and reasoning (intellectual ability), attention, and memory	Directions given via pointing, gesture, and pantomime; responses via point, card match, or manipulatives	Individuals ages 2–20 who are unable to speak, read, write, and/or understand English	Stoelting Co.
Naglieri Nonverbal Ability Test–Individual (Naglieri, 2002)	Nonverbal reasoning and general problem-solving ability	Directions given via gestures; responses via point	Individuals ages 5–17 who are unable to speak, read, write, and/or understand English	Harcourt Assessment (Canada)
Pictorial Test of Intelligence–Second Edition (French, 2001)	General cognitive ability	Directions given verbally; responses via point	Individuals ages 3–8 who are unable to speak	PRO-ED, Inc.
Stoelting Brief Nonverbal Intelligence Test (Roid & Miller, 1999)	Nonverbal cognitive ability	Directions given in pantomime; responses via point or card match	Individuals ages 6–20 who are unable to speak, read, write, and/or understand English	Stoelting Co.
Test of Nonverbal Intelligence–Third Edition (TONI-3) (Brown, Sherbenou, & Johnsen, 1997)	Nonverbal intelligence, aptitude, abstract reasoning, and problem solving	Directions given in pantomime; responses via point, nod, or symbolic gesture	Individuals ages 6–90 who are unable to speak, read, write, and/or understand English	AGS Publishing
Universal Nonverbal Intelligence Test (UNIT) (Bracken & McCallum, 1998)	Memory, problem-solving, symbolic reasoning, nonsymbolic reasoning, overall intellectual ability	Directions given in pantomime and gestures; responses via point, paper and pencil tasks, manipulatives	Individuals ages 5–17 who are unable to speak, read, write, and/or understand English	Riverside Publishing

190

A new *Guide to Child Nonverbal IQ Measures* (DeThorne & Schaefer, 2004) provides a very useful summary of the psychometric properties (e.g., reliability, validity) of the most commonly used tests of this type in North America. It also contains descriptive tables summarizing the motor requirements and subtests contained in each test.

The fact is that the cognitive requirements of most AAC options have been described only minimally in the clinical and research literature, even though it is quite obvious that the operation of AAC techniques requires various types and degrees of cognitive abilities, ranging from basic to very sophisticated. Thus, in most cases, the AAC team must analyze the cognitive requirements of a particular approach, estimate the extent to which each individual will be able to meet these requirements, and then conduct intervention trials with one or more AAC techniques or devices to determine the optimal match. It is important to realize that thousands of successful AAC interventions have been instituted without formal documentation of cognitive abilities.

The Functional Assessment of Communication Skills for Adults (ASHA FACS; Ferketic, Fratalli, Holland, Thompson, & Wohl, 2004) is a reliable, valid, and sensitive measure that can be used with adults with aphasia resulting from either right or left hemisphere stroke and adults with cognitive communication disorders resulting from traumatic brain injury, dementia, or other acquired/progressive neurological disorders. It consists of 43 items and assesses functional communication in four areas: social communication; communication of basic needs; reading, writing, and number concepts; and daily planning. It is available from the American Speech-Language-Hearing Association.

Symbol Assessment

Symbols or codes represent a majority of the messages included in AAC systems. People who are unable to read or write may use one or more of the symbol options described in Chapter 3. It is not uncommon to see people who use AAC successfully employ a variety of symbol types. Thus, the goal of symbol assessment is not to identify a single symbol set to represent all messages. Instead, the goal of assessment is to select the types of symbols that will meet the individual's current communication needs and match his or her current abilities, as well as to identify symbol options that might be used in the future.

Assessment of an individual's ability to use symbols usually involves several steps. Before starting, the team members responsible for the symbol assessment should identify 10 or so functional items with which the individual is familiar, basing their selections on the recommendations of the individual's family members, teachers, or frequent communication partners (see Figure 7.13). These functional items might include a cup, brush, washcloth, spoon, and so forth. Next, the assessment team members should reach a consensus about the individual's familiarity with the selected items because one of the most com-

Format used: Direct request ("Show me what you do with this") _____   Caregiver interview _____

Assessor demonstration of correct usage _____

Instructions used _____

Response accepted as correct _____

List objects used	Confirmation of item knowledge by informant?

Indicate whether trial is correct or incorrect in appropriate column and describe responses

Trial no.	Object	Function correct? (describe)	Function incorrect? (describe)
1			
2			
3			
4			
5			
6			
7			
8			
9			
10			
11			
12			

Augmentative and Alternative Communication: Supporting Children and Adults with Complex Communication Needs, Third Edition, by David R. Beukelman and Pat Mirenda. Copyright © 2005 Paul H. Brookes Publishing Co., Inc. All rights reserved.

Figure 7.13.   Functional object use assessment.

mon errors is to attempt a symbol assessment using items that the individual does not understand or know. When the team reaches consensus on an item, it can indicate this in the appropriate column of Figure 7.13. Then, from a variety of sources, the team should compile symbols that represent the selected items. These symbols might include both color and black-and-white photographs, miniature objects, various types of line-drawing symbols (see Chapter 3), and written words. Figures 7.13–7.15, 7.18, and 7.19 contain spaces for recording the items and symbols selected for assessment.

Functional Use Format   At the most basic level of symbol use is the ability to understand the functional use of objects (Glennen, 1997). An AAC team can assess a child's level of functional understanding in a play context by giving him or her the items selected for the assessment and observing whether the child uses them functionally (e.g., trying to drink when presented with a cup). With older individuals, the team can make direct requests related to the uses of functional objects, such as "Show me what you do with this." Often, interviewing family members, teachers, or others reveals useful information in this regard—for example, a child's mother might report that he gets excited whenever she gets out his "going to the park" jacket, indicating that he recognizes its function. Finally, individuals with severe motor impairments that prevent them from manipulating objects can be assessed for functional understanding of object use if the assessor is willing to act as a "demonstrator." In this case, the demonstrator mimes both correct and incorrect uses of each object and observes the individual's reactions. For example, the assessor might brush her hair with a spoon or put a cup on her head as a hat, and then wait for the person under observation to give gestural or other indications that the demonstrated action is "wrong." The individual's responses should be quite different from those elicited by a "correct" mime (e.g., eating from a spoon, drinking from a cup). Success in one or more of these formats would suggest that the person recognizes that the test objects have specific uses. Figure 7.13 provides a format for assessing functional object use.

Receptive Labeling and Yes/No Formats   Observing an individual's receptive labeling ability is often the next step in symbol assessment because this is the most straightforward way to establish whether an individual can recognize a symbol as representing its referent. The person conducting the assessment presents the individual with two or more items or symbols of a particular type and asks him or her to "Give me/show me/point to the (label for one of the items)." Of course, obtaining the requested motor response depends on the person's motor abilities. Alternatively, the assessor can use a yes/no format, in which he or she holds up one item or symbol at a time and asks, "Is this a _____?" The assessor should arrange the trials so that yes/no questions are presented randomly for all target items. This testing format is only appropriate if the individual understands the concept of yes/no and has a clear and accurate way of answering yes/no questions. The team can assess several types of symbols, one type at a time, using any of these formats. The assessor records on a form (see Figure 7.14) whether the individual can identify target items from the various symbol sets.

Alternative Visual-Matching Format   In some cases, AAC team members cannot use the receptive labeling or yes/no formats because the person undergoing the symbol assessment does not understand either the task expectations or the verbal labels presented. However, there is evidence that a visual-matching format produces results similar

Format used: Receptive labeling _____   Yes/no _____

Number of items in array_____

Instructions used _____

Response accepted as correct _____

List items used   Confirmation of item knowledge by team?

_____

_____

_____

_____

_____

_____

_____

_____

_____

_____

Indicate whether trial is correct (+) or incorrect (−) in appropriate column

Trial no.	Target item	Real objects	Color photographs	Line drawings	Other (specify)
1					
2					
3					
4					
5					
6					
7					
8					
9					
10					
11					
12					

Augmentative and Alternative Communication: Supporting Children and Adults with Complex Communication Needs, Third Edition, by David R. Beukelman and Pat Mirenda. Copyright © 2005 Paul H. Brookes Publishing Co., Inc. All rights reserved.

Figure 7.14.   Symbol assessment: Receptive labeling and yes/no formats.

Format used: Standard matching _____   Sorting ____

Number of items in array _____

Instructions used _____

Response accepted as correct _____

List items used   Confirmation of item knowledge by team?

_____

_____

_____

_____

_____

_____

_____

_____

_____

_____

_____

Indicate whether trial is correct (+) or incorrect (−) in appropriate column

Trial no.	Target item	Real objects	Color photographs	Line drawings	Other (specify)
1					
2					
3					
4					
5					
6					
7					
8					
9					
10					
11					
12					

Augmentative and Alternative Communication: Supporting Children and Adults with Complex Communication Needs, Third Edition, by David R. Beukelman and Pat Mirenda. Copyright © 2005 Paul H. Brookes Publishing Co., Inc. All rights reserved.

Figure 7.15.   Symbol assessment: Visual-matching format.

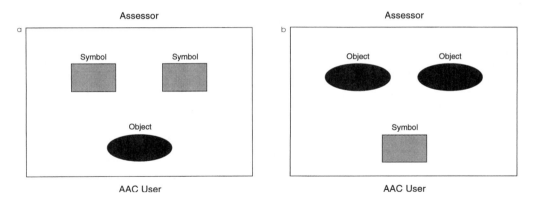

Figure 7.16.   a) Single-object-to-multiple-symbol matching format; b) single-symbol-to-multiple-object matching format.

to those elicited from the receptive labeling format, when used with 2- and 3-year-olds without disabilities and individuals of similar developmental ages with severe cognitive disabilities (Franklin, Mirenda, & Phillips, 1994). Thus, a visual-matching format similar to the one provided in Figure 7.15 may serve as a useful alternative to the receptive labeling option. In a standard matching assessment, the team provides the individual with a single object and places two or more symbols, one of which matches the object, on the table (see Figure 7.16a). The assessor then asks the individual to match the object to the corresponding symbol, using eye gaze, pointing, or another direct selection option. Alternatively, the team may give a single symbol to the individual, who then attempts to match the symbol to the correct object in an array (see Figure 7.16b). A study examining alternative symbol assessment strategies found these formats to be equivalent in difficulty (Franklin et al., 1994). The AAC team can also adjust the configuration, spacing, and number of items in the array in order to meet the needs of specific individuals. The goal is to make systematic adjustments that facilitate the acquisition of accurate and useful information about the person's ability to associate objects with their referents on the basis of perceptual characteristics.

Several cautions are in order with regard to the matching format. First, it is not essential for an individual to be able to match objects and symbols in order to learn to use symbols successfully (Romski & Sevcik, 1996). If a person *can* do this, he or she understands (at least at a visual level) the relationship between symbols and their referents; but if an individual lacks this understanding, it does not mean that he or she cannot learn to use symbols. Second, the matching assessment is not a standardized testing protocol; rather, it is a flexible format that the team can alter to suit the individual's abilities and interests. For example, many people with limited cognitive abilities may need to be taught to match items and symbols before actual assessment. The team can usually accomplish this instruction in a short time using a "teach–test" approach and discrete trial teaching (Lovaas, 2003). During the "teach" phase, team members can introduce and gradually fade out physical or other prompts in order to teach the person to match identical real objects. Once he or she can do this independently and accurately, the team can present various object–symbol matching tasks, as described previously (see Mirenda & Locke, 1989, for a more complete description of this approach).

Pulling It All Together   By this point in the symbol assessment, two things should be clear: 1) whether the individual understands the functional use of selected, familiar objects and 2) whether the person can either recognize the verbal labels for a variety of symbols or match them to their referents. If one or both of the latter skills is not evident, this may indicate that, at this particular time, the person will be best served by several "beginning communicator" strategies designed to build communicative skills while teaching symbol–referent associations. These strategies include schedule systems and "talking switch" techniques, as described in Chapter 11. The individual's ability to perform the assessment tasks successfully can be used to predict the type(s) of symbols with which he or she is most likely to be successful, at least initially. The initial symbol set(s) selected should enable accurate, efficient, and nonfatiguing communication with minimal instruction required. Over time, the individual can learn and use more sophisticated types of symbols, if needed. Symbol sets such as manual signs, Blissymbols, and others that require extensive learning and practice may be excellent choices for the future but may not be appropriate for initial use.

Because real communication rarely involves either receptive language labeling or symbol matching, we have found it useful to extend the assessment beyond these basic tasks to determine whether an individual can use symbols in a more communicative manner. The AAC team should include this portion of the assessment process regardless of whether the individual is successful during the initial symbol tasks because some individuals may find it easier to demonstrate symbolic understanding during natural interactions. Blockberger (1995) noted that typically developing children can talk for up to a year before they are able to use pictures symbolically, around 24–30 months of age. She commented that

> It may not be realistic for us to assume that the child with severe speech impairment will be able to use graphic symbols symbolically and communicatively at the same developmental age that a typical child begins to speak. When children are able to point to graphic symbols on request but do not spontaneously use that symbol communicatively, [it may be because] the child [has not] grasped the symbol's referential function. (1995, p. 225)

AAC team members can use one or both of the following formats to assess a person's symbol use in context.

Question-and-Answer Format   Figure 7.17 contains a form with which a team can assess whether an individual can use symbols to answer verbal questions. As in the basic assessment, the assessor should first identify items or concepts that are known to the individual by interviewing familiar communication partners and listing items on the form. The assessor should select two or more symbols of a specific type—such as objects, photographs, or line drawings—and present them to the individual, asking a question that the individual can answer correctly by indicating one of the symbols. Receptive labeling questions such as "Can you show me the car?" or "Where is the picture of your dog?" *should not* be used in this situation. Instead, the assessor may ask simple knowledge-based questions such as "What did you eat for breakfast?" while presenting symbol choices such as the person's favorite breakfast food, a car, and a dog; or questions such as "Who likes to ride in the car?" with symbol options such as a boy and a horse.

Number of items in array _____

Instructions used _____

Context: Out of context _____   In context (specify) _____

Response accepted as correct _____

List items used   Confirmation of item knowledge by informant? _____

_____

_____

_____

_____

_____

_____

_____

_____

_____

_____

Indicate whether trial is correct (+) or incorrect (−) in appropriate column

Trial no.	Question asked	Real objects	Color photographs	Line drawings	Other (specify)
1					
2					
3					
4					
5					
6					
7					
8					
9					
10					
11					
12					

Augmentative and Alternative Communication: Supporting Children and Adults with Complex Communication Needs, Third Edition, by David R. Beukelman and Pat Mirenda. Copyright © 2005 Paul H. Brookes Publishing Co., Inc. All rights reserved.

Figure 7.17.   Symbol assessment: Question-and-answer format.

In order to successfully complete this task, the individual must understand the task expectations, the questions, and the symbol options presented, and he or she must be motivated and cooperative during the evaluation. If the individual performs poorly in the assessment, it is important for the team to try to determine which of these aspects of the question-and-answer task is responsible for the individual's difficulties. Alternative formats, such as question-and-answer assessments in natural contexts, may be useful to counteract some factors contributing to poor performance, especially with people who have severe cognitive impairments. For example, many individuals may be able to answer the "breakfast" question if they are seated in the kitchen where they usually eat rather than in a classroom where meals never take place. The form in Figure 7.17 allows the assessor to provide relevant information related to context.

Requesting Format   Individuals with severe communication and cognitive limitations may be able to match symbols to objects and even answer simple questions using symbols, yet they may still be unable to use symbols to make requests. In Figure 7.18, we provide a form to guide the team's assessment of symbol use in a requesting format. An AAC team usually conducts this assessment in an appropriate natural context, such as during snacktime, a play activity, the performance of some domestic task (e.g., washing the dishes), or in any other context that is of interest to the person being assessed. As before, the team lists and confirms items that the person knows and that are available in the context. Then, the assessors provide symbols representing two or more of the available options, trying one type of symbol at a time. The structure of the interaction provides opportunities for the person to request objects or actions by selecting one of the available symbols without the assessor instructing him or her to do so. Indirect cues such as "I don't know what you want. Can you help me out?" may be used to elicit requests. Direct instructions such as "Touch the picture to tell me what you want" should be avoided because the purpose of this assessment is to determine whether the individual can make spontaneous, unprompted requests.

Pulling It All Together   The question-and-answer and requesting formats provide basic information about how the person can communicate with symbols; they do not indicate which symbols he or she recognizes linguistically or perceptually. Individuals who can do only one or neither task will need instruction to be able to use, in functional contexts, the symbols that were identified during the basic assessment. The strategies described in Chapter 11 for teaching requesting, rejecting, and so forth may be useful in this regard. Individuals who are able to answer questions or make requests using symbols may have the skills needed for more advanced symbol use, as assessed through the next two formats.

Advanced Symbol Use   Individuals who are adept at single-symbol use in communicative contexts may be able to use symbols for words other than nouns and/or chain two or more symbols together to construct messages. The team can assess both of these abilities through the use of an activity display with symbols that represent various syntactic elements—nouns, verbs, adjectives, and so forth. For example, we often use dual Go Fish displays with symbols representing the various elements of this simple card game because it is appropriate for individuals across the age range (see Figure 7.19). While playing the game, the assessor produces multiple one- and two-symbol messages using his or her display, thus providing models for advanced symbol use (e.g., DO YOU HAVE + KING or

Number of items in array _____

Instructions used _____

Were options: Visible? _____   Out of sight? _____

Context: Out of context _____   In context (specify) _____

Response accepted as correct _____

List items used _____   Confirmation of item knowledge by informant?

_____

_____

_____

_____

_____

_____

_____

_____

_____

_____

Indicate whether trial is correct (+) or incorrect (−) in appropriate column

Trial no.	Items available	Real objects	Color photographs	Line drawings	Other (specify)
1					
2					
3					
4					
5					
6					
7					
8					
9					
10					
11					
12					

Augmentative and Alternative Communication: Supporting Children and Adults with Complex Communication Needs, Third Edition, by David R. Beukelman and Pat Mirenda. Copyright © 2005 Paul H. Brookes Publishing Co., Inc. All rights reserved.

Figure 7.18.   Symbol assessment: Requesting format.

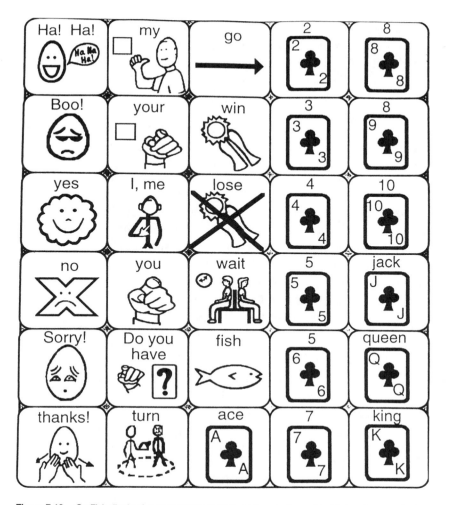

Figure 7.19. Go Fish display for assessment of advanced symbol use. (The Picture Communication Symbols © 1981–2004 by Mayer-Johnson LLC. All Rights Reserved Worldwide. Used with permission.)

MY + TURN). If the person being assessed learns how to use the display quite quickly, the assessor can then observe whether he or she uses any non-noun symbols or makes a sequence of two symbols when provided with opportunities to do so. For example, at appropriate times, the assessor can create opportunities for the individual to communicate two-symbol messages such as GO + FISH, YOU + LOSE, I + WIN, and so forth. The absence of one or both types of advanced symbol use suggests that the team should construct the initial system with single-symbol messages, keeping the goal of moving toward multiple-symbol messages. Of course, an individual with motor impairments that limit hand use will need to play the game with a partner who manages the cards, and he or she may need to use an eye-gaze display with the appropriate messages as well. Alternative activities, such as playing Space Invaders or another fun game with young children, can also be used during such assessments.

Symbol Categorization and Association Assessments   Some individuals might be able to use communication systems that depend on various symbol categorization strategies, or they might be candidates for iconic encoding. Teams can assess simple categorization skills with symbols of various items placed in two or more semantic categories, such as vehicles, foods, clothing, and animals. The individual is asked to sort the symbols into categories ("Put all of the animals in this box and all of the vehicles in that box") or is helped to do so using eye gazing ("Which box should I put this one in?"). Alternatively, a team can assess categorization abilities by asking the person to sort symbols for two very different activities, such as going to the beach and going to a birthday party ("Put the ones you'd use at the beach in this box and the ones you'd need at a birthday party in that box"). The results of this type of assessment can be useful to determine whether to incorporate categorization into AAC system design and in what manner to do so. For example, symbols in communication books or boards may be organized in semantic or activity category sections. Similarly, dynamic display devices require the ability to recognize and use categorization techniques. Individuals who cannot categorize will require additional instruction in this regard to use such AAC systems effectively.

The use of iconic encoding techniques such as Minspeak requires a related skill, that of association. Individuals need to be able to use various aspects of a symbol to "remind" them of associated concepts or words in a flexible manner. Several basic techniques for informal assessment of an individual's associative abilities with symbols have been developed for clinical use. Generally, the team provides an individual with a small set of colored symbols that he or she can already recognize by name (e.g., *sun, apple, car, clock*). The assessor then asks the person to use those symbols to answer questions requiring different types of associations. Assessment protocols designed by Elder, Goossens', and Bray (1989) and Glennen (1997) suggested that these questions should include associations such as the following:

- Object function (e.g., "What do you use to tell time?" CLOCK)

- Part/whole concepts (e.g., "Where is the wheel?" CAR)

- Similar item associations (e.g., "What goes together with rain?" SUN)

- Associations related to physical properties such as color, size, shape, texture or temperature, and substance (e.g., "Find something red" APPLE, "Find something hot" SUN, "Find something metal" CAR)

- Category associations (e.g., "What makes you think of food?" APPLE)

- Rhyming or "look-alike" associations (e.g., "What sounds like 'knock'?" CLOCK; "What looks like 'truck'?" CAR)

Assessors can ask individuals who make several types of associations correctly to select two- or three-symbol sequences to represent phrases such as "Let's walk the dog" (e.g., CAR + DOG) or "It's time to go eat" (CLOCK + CAR + APPLE). At issue is whether the person uses some kind of internal logic to select the sequences, not whether the assessor agrees with the selections made. Whether the individual uses internal logic will often be revealed by the team asking the person to recall the same sequences 10–15 minutes later— recall is more likely if the sequences were made logically than if they were selected arbitrarily. Thus, someone might choose the symbols APPLE + SUN for "What's for breakfast?" because he or she likes to eat fruit and drink orange juice—which is produced in sunny places—every morning—not a choice likely to be obvious to most assessors but one that may enhance recall for the person using the code! Success at one or more levels of an association assessment would suggest that an AAC strategy that incorporates iconic encoding might be appropriate for the individual.

Language Assessment

Language assessment should include an evaluation of the individual's single-word vocabulary capabilities as well as his or her use of common language structures (i.e., morphemes, syntax) (Roth & Cassatt-James, 1989). Basic strategies for assessment in these areas are discussed in the sections that follow.

Single-Word Vocabulary

Two types of language assessment typically are completed for AAC purposes. In the first assessment, the AAC team makes an attempt to measure vocabulary (i.e., single-word receptive language) comprehension in relation to the individual's overall level of functioning. Assessment instruments such as the Peabody Picture Vocabulary Test–Third Edition (PPVT-III; Dunn, Dunn, Williams, & Wang, 1997) may be used to assess nonrelational words, which researchers have defined as "words that have referents in the real world such as chair, dog, shirt, etc." (Roth & Cassatt-James, 1989, p. 169). Teams often prefer this test for AAC evaluations because they can modify it easily without sacrificing validity to meet the needs of individuals with motor limitations. Using a previous version of the PPVT (the Peabody Picture Vocabulary Test–Revised [PPVT-R]), Bristow and Fristoe (1987) compared scores that were obtained using the standard protocol with those obtained using six alternative response modes, including eye gaze, scanning, and headlight pointing. The results indicated that, with few exceptions, scores obtained under the modified conditions correlated highly with those obtained using standard test protocols. The MacArthur-Bates Communicative Development Inventory: Words and Sentences (Fenson et al., 1993), a parent report measure, can also be used to estimate single-word vocabulary comprehension (Romski & Sevcik, 1999).

In addition to assessing nonrelational words, it is important for the team to assess the individual's comprehension of action words; words for absent people or objects; and relational words (i.e., those that do not have real-world referents), such as *in* and *out* or *hot* and *cold* (Roth & Cassatt-James, 1989). The Bracken Basic Concept Scale–Revised (Bracken, 1998) is one instrument that assessors might use to assess this kind of comprehension. Romski and Sevcik (1999) also recommended the Clinical Assessment of Language Comprehension (Miller & Paul, 1995) and the Sequenced Inventory of Communication Development–Revised (Hedrick, Prather, & Tobin, 1984) as useful tools for assessing language comprehension. For individuals who are unable to complete formal tests, a team can often obtain an estimate of vocabulary comprehension by having family members, caregivers, and school personnel develop a diary of the words and concepts that the individual appears to understand.

Morphosyntactic and Grammatical Knowledge

In recent years, several AAC researchers have noted the importance of assessing morphosyntactic and grammatical knowledge of individuals who use AAC, since those who have not mastered skills in these areas are likely to have difficulty conveying ideas, fulfilling academic requirements, and securing or maintaining employment (Binger & Light, 2003; Blockberger & Johnston, 2003; Blockberger & Sutton, 2003). For people who can participate in formal testing, a number of standardized instruments that are based on simple multiple-choice or pointing formats and require no verbal output are available. These include selected subtests from one of the Clinical Evaluation of Language Fundamentals instruments (Semel, Wiig, & Secord, 2003; Wiig, Secord, & Semel, 1992), the Test for Auditory Comprehension of Language–Third Edition (Carrow-Woolfolk, 1999), the Test of Language Development (Hammill & Newcomer, 1996), and the Test for Reception of Grammar–Version 2 (Bishop, 2003). Although some adaptations may need to be made to accommodate the needs of specific individuals, such tests offer the advantage of empirical support related to reliability and validity.

In addition, a number of informal assessment techniques have been developed for language assessment of individuals who use AAC. For example, Blockberger and Johnston (2003) used three assessment tasks to examine children's acquisition of morphemes that included the past tense -ed (e.g., walk/walked), plural -s (e.g., boy/boys), and third person regular -s (e.g., I drink/he drinks). In a picture selection task, the child being assessed was presented with three similar pictures (e.g., pictures of 1) a baby with a dirty toy pig, 2) a baby with a dirty shirt, and 3) a dirty baby pig with a mother pig) and was asked to select the one that best matched a verbal utterance (e.g., *The baby's pig is dirty*). The task was adapted to a yes/no format for children who were unable to select a picture with a headlight pointer or their hands. In a structured writing task, the examiner read a short, illustrated story about a girl named Kate, her hats, and her teddy bears. The child was asked to print or type single words to "fill in the blanks" of the story. For example, one part of the story read as follows: "Yesterday Kate woke up. She ate breakfast. Then she pl_____ with her teddy bears."

In addition, several authors have used grammaticality judgment tasks for AAC assessment. In a study with adults who used AAC, Lund and Light (2003) verbally and visually presented correct and incorrect sentences and asked participants to indicate via a gesture whether or not each followed a specific grammatical rule (e.g., *Please give me the blue book* versus *Please give me the book blue* or *Please give me blue the book*). In a study with children who used AAC (Blockberger & Johnston, 2003), the child being assessed was introduced to a dog puppet that was described by the examiner as *just learning to talk*, and the child was asked to help the puppet practice saying some sentences. Two buckets were placed in front of the child, one containing dog biscuits and one containing rocks. The child was instructed to listen to a sentence that was "uttered" by the puppet and, if it was correct, to give the dog a biscuit; if the sentence was wrong, the dog was to be given a rock. For the third person regular -s, an example of a correct sentence was *Hockey players wear helmets* and an example of an incorrect sentence was *The cows eats the grass.* Children who were unable to pick up a biscuit or a rock used eye gaze or gestures to indicate which one the examiner should give to the puppet. A similar task was used by Redmond and Johnston (2001) with adolescents who used AAC, except that the dog puppet was replaced by two action figures—"moonguys"—and the participants were told that they were from outer space and were just learning to speak English, so they needed help to know when they talked "right" and "not so good."

Several more complex tasks have also been used to assess understanding and use of specific language forms in persons who use AAC. For example, Sutton and Gallagher (1995) used a task to assess understanding of past and future tense. One of two plastic figurines acted out a nonsense verb (e.g., *voll, meer, gling*) and the person being assessed was asked to point to or touch one of the figurines in response to the questions *Who (nonsense verb)ed?* and *Who will (nonsense verb)?* Sutton and her colleagues (Sutton, Gallagher, Morford, & Shahnaz, 2000; Sutton & Morford, 1998; Sutton et al., 2002) also used photographs of plastic figurines to assess both comprehension and production of relative clauses produced using graphic symbols, such as *the girl who pushes the clown wears a hat* versus *the girl pushes the clown who wears a hat.* The comprehension task requires the person being assessed to indicate a photograph corresponding to a graphic symbol utterance, whereas the production task requires the person to use graphic symbols to construct a sentence describing the photograph.

Finally, Sutton and Gallagher (1995) and Lund and Light (2003) both used language sampling in dyadic play or conversational contexts to examine the morphosyntactic abilities of individuals who use AAC systems to communicate. Others (e.g., Kelford Smith, Thurston, Light, Parnes, & O'Keefe, 1989) used written language samples toward the same end. Because both of these techniques require transcription and/or coding of utterances to be useful, they are more time-intensive than other tasks. However, they are also likely to yield richer and more broad-based information (Binger & Light, 2003; Sutton, Soto, & Blockberger, 2002). We refer readers to the March 1990 and September 1997 issues of the *Augmentative and Alternative Communication* journal for additional information about language assessment.

New technologies such as the Universal Language Activity Monitor (U-LAM; Hill & Romich, 2002; Romich et al., 2004), Performance Report Tool (PeRT; Hill, 2004), and Augmentative Communication Quantitative Analysis software (ACQUA; Lesher, Moulton, Rinkus, & Higginbotham, 2000) facilitate the collection and analysis of utterances that are produced using speech-generating devices (SGDs) and computers with serial ports. Such technologies can be useful for both initial and ongoing AAC assessment. The U-LAM and PeRT are available through the AAC Institute and ACQUA is available through the Rehabilitation Engineering Research Center on Communication Enhancement.

Pulling It All Together   Once again, it must be emphasized that the purpose of language assessment, both formal and informal, is not to assign a score or developmental age to the individual but rather to gather information that is needed for intervention planning. The goal is to develop a functional profile of the person's current language capabilities so that appropriate symbols, vocabulary items, and instructional procedures can be selected. There is no recipe for matching specific AAC strategies and techniques with the characteristics of the individual's language profile because this information must be considered in its totality along with information about the individual's motor, sensory, and other capabilities. For example, imagine a language profile for an individual with no motor or vision impairments indicating that she has a one-word vocabulary of 300 line-drawn symbols, produces no two- or three-word combinations, and initiates simple requests and answers questions with symbols. It is likely that the initial AAC intervention would involve either a low- or high-tech system with a large vocabulary capability that can be expanded easily and would include techniques aimed at encouraging multiword combinations and increasing communicative competence in conversational and other interactive contexts. Contrast this with the profile of an individual with severe motor and vision impairments who has a vocabulary of 10 manual signs, cannot make choices, and initiates no interactions. Clearly, the recommended intervention would be much different for the second individual than for the first one—not just because of differences in language ability but because of a combination of *many* factors. These two examples illustrate the importance of considering language assessment information as part of the "big picture" of all intervention information.

Assess Literacy Skills

Literacy encompasses a multitude of skills that, cumulatively, result in a person's ability to read, spell, and write (see Chapter 13). Literacy assessment is particularly important for people who use AAC, who may have received very irregular instruction in this area and may present with scattered profiles of ability as a result. The primary areas in which literacy assessment should be conducted are discussed in the sections that follow.

Print and Phoneme Recognition Assessment

Screening for recognition of letter names and sounds is useful as a beginning step in an overall literacy assessment. AAC teams can conduct such screening quite easily using simple letter boards, eye-gaze displays, or keyboards. Assessors can ask the individual to point to or look at specific letters by name ("Show me *A*, *S*, and *M*") and/or identify them by sound ("Show me the ones that sound like /ah/, /ssss/, and /mmm/"). Team members can ask individuals who can write to produce letters or their corresponding sounds by printing. It is important to note that some individuals who can read may be unable to recognize letters in either manner in isolation, so additional literacy assessment should proceed even in the absence of these basic skills.

Phonological Processing

Since the mid-1990s, an increasing number of AAC researchers have emphasized the importance of phonological processing skills, which are known to be critical for reading achievement in both persons without disabilities (Adams, 1990; Wagner & Torgeson, 1987) and those with severe speech and physical impairments (SSPI) (Dahlgren Sandberg, 2001; Dahlgren Sandberg & Hjelmquist, 1996a, 1996b; Foley & Pollatsek, 1999; Iacono & Cupples, 2004; Vandervelden & Siegel, 1999, 2001). Phonological processing is an umbrella term that encompasses two sets of abilities: 1) phonological awareness (PA), the ability to recognize and manipulate the phonemes (i.e., sounds) of spoken words; and 2) phonological recoding (PR), the ability to understand and make use of the relationships between phonemes and graphemes (i.e., printed sounds). Assessment of the latter often involves the use of nonword (i.e., pseudoword) tasks (Vandervelden & Siegel, 1999).

Most literacy researchers emphasize that assessment of both PA and PR skills should be part of any AAC assessment; the challenge is *how* to assess these in ways that are both accurate and useful in individuals who are unable to speak. A number of strategies may be employed in this regard. Iacono and Cupples (2004) reported the psychometric properties of a tool entitled the Assessment of Phonological Awareness and Reading (APAR) that was developed at Monash University (Australia) to assess phonological awareness and reading skills of adults with physical and/or intellectual disabilities who are unable to speak and/or write. The APAR includes both PA and PR tasks, as well as single-word vocabulary, sentence comprehension, and text listening comprehension tasks. Directions, stimulus cards, and scoring sheets for the APAR are available at no cost on-line, along with the Accessible Word Reading Intervention (AWRI) program that was designed to teach beginning reading skills (see Resource List for Web address). Additional formal measures of PA ability that can be used with individuals who are unable to speak are included in Table 7.7.

Foley and Pollatsek (1999) and Vandervelden and Siegel (1999) also utilized informal assessment batteries that were specifically designed to assess the PA and PR skills of children or adults with SSPI and thus require no verbal and minimal motor responding. Some of the tasks in these batteries that might be useful for clinical AAC assessments are summarized in Table 7.8. Blischak (1994) also summarized a number of PA tasks that have been used for research purposes, along with practical suggestions for how to adapt them for use with individuals with SSPI.

ABC-Link is an on-line, universally accessible alternative reading assessment battery for persons with severe speech and physical impairments that is under development through the Center for Literacy and Disability Studies at the University of North Carolina–Chapel Hill. It is complemented by ALL-Link, an integrated, Web-delivered set of reading and writing instructional materials at the beginning levels that will be available in both English and Spanish.

Word Recognition and Reading Comprehension Assessment

People who are even partially literate may be able to use their reading skills in AAC contexts. Assessment of reading skills for AAC usually involves checking both word recognition and reading comprehension, among other important skills. Subtests in several literacy assessment instruments that are commonly used in North America have been constructed to probe these skills and require only a yes/no response, simple pointing response, and/or can be easily adapted for use with alternative response modes. A selection of tests and subtests available in this area are summarized in Table 7.7.

It is often advisable to conduct an informal, interactive word recognition reading assessment as well, especially with individuals who demonstrate limited skills on standardized tests. For example, some people may recognize words visually either on flash cards or in natural contexts, perhaps because the words have been paired with symbols on their AAC displays. AAC teams can conduct informal assessments using words to which the individual has been exposed either formally or informally (e.g., *enter* or *exit, women* or *men,*

Table 7.7. Selected instruments for assessment of literacy skills that do not require verbal responding

Instrument	Skills assessed	Response Mode	Appropriate for . . .	Source
Gates-MacGinitie Reading Tests–Fourth Edition (MacGinitie, MacGinitie, Maria, & Dreyer, 2000)	Subtests for basic literacy concepts, phonological awareness, letter and letter–sound correspondences, initial/final consonants and consonant clusters, vowels, word decoding, reading comprehension, vocabulary	Pointing (multiple choice)	Kindergarten through adulthood; different tests available for different age ranges	Riverside Publishing
Group Reading Assessment and Diagnostic Evaluation (GRADE; Williams, 2001)	Subtests for phonological awareness; visual skills; concepts; early literacy skills; phoneme–grapheme understanding; word reading/meaning abilities; listening, sentence, and passage comprehension; vocabulary	Mark on paper; can be adapted easily to pointing for individual administration	Pre-K through adulthood, English and Spanish	AGS Publishing
Peabody Individual Achievement Test–Revised-Normative Update (Markwardt, 1998)	Subtests for recognition of printed letters, reading comprehension, correct spelling comprehension	Pointing (multiple choice)	Kindergarten through adulthood	AGS Publishing
Test of Phonological Awareness (Torgesen & Bryant, 1994)	Phonological awareness (initial and final sounds)	Pointing (multiple choice)	Kindergarten, grades 1–3 (ages 5–9 years)	PRO-ED, Inc.
Test of Reading Comprehension–Third Edition (Brown, Hammill, & Wiederholt, 1995)	Subtests for general vocabulary, syntactic similarities, paragraph comprehension, sentence sequencing, reading directions for school work	Marking or pointing (multiple choice)	Ages 7–17 years	PRO-ED, Inc.
Woodcock-Johnson III (Woodcock, McGrew, & Mather, 2001) (selected subtests)	Subtests for visual matching, reading fluency, listening comprehension, spelling, writing speed and ability	Pointing, yes/no; some subtests require writing	Preschool through adulthood	Riverside Publishing

Table 7.8. Examples of nonverbal tasks for assessment of basic reading/spelling, phonological recoding, and phonemic awareness skills in individuals with SSPI

Basic reading/spelling tasks	
Letter–sound recognition (VS)	Upper and lower case letters are presented, five at a time. The examiner sounds a letter (e.g., /oh/) and the person being assessed is asked to point to the corresponding sound.
Print-to-print matching (FP)	Pairs of printed word cards are presented. A yes/no response is required regarding whether the words are identical after the first letter. Half are positive examples (e.g., ball-call) and half are negative examples (e.g., moth-north).
Picture-to-print matching (VS)	Printed word cards are presented in sets of three (e.g., duck-soap-boot). A pointing response is required to identify the word that matches a picture shown by the examiner.
Speech-to-print matching (words) (VS)	Same as above, except the stimulus is a word said aloud by the examiner.
Speech-to-print matching (nonwords) (VS)	Printed nonword cards are presented in sets of three (e.g., fep-sut-pom). A pointing response is required to identify the word that matches the one said aloud by the examiner.
Word spelling (VS)	Examiner points to a body part or object and the person is asked to spell it, using an alphabet display.
Nonword spelling (VS)	Examiner dictates a nonword (e.g., dak, snom, skete) and the person is asked to spell it, using an alphabet display.
Phonological Recoding Tasks	
Rhyme judgment (VS)	Pairs of picture cards are presented. A yes/no response is required regarding whether the words in each pair rhyme. Half of the pairs rhyme (e.g., ghost-toast) and half do not (e.g., door-spoon).
Nonword rhyme judgment (VS)	A printed nonword card is presented (e.g., fum) along with a picture (e.g., black, drum). A yes/no response is required regarding whether the nonword and the name of the picture rhyme.
Alliteration (VS)	A printed nonword is presented (e.g., sut) along with a picture (e.g., heart, soap). A yes/no response is required regarding whether the nonword and the name of the picture start with the same sound.
Phonemic Awareness Tasks	
Consonant recognition (VS)	Example: The examiner says, "Listen for /s/. Does (/sock/-/boat/) have an /s/?" A yes/no response is required. Both initial and final (e.g., beet-bee) consonants are probed separately.
Complex consonant recognition (VS)	Same as above, except that some matches are initial and some are final consonants. The person is asked to indicate where the match occurs using a position grid requiring pointing.
Phoneme deletion (VS)	Example: The examiner says, "Listen! /hear/. Take away the /h/. What word is left?" Three pictures are presented (e.g., spoon, ear, car) and a pointing response is required. Both initial and final (e.g., beet-bee) consonants are probed separately.
Phoneme substitution (VS)	Example: The examiner says, "Listen! /ghost/. Change the /g/ to /t/ . What is the new word?" Three pictures are presented (e.g., turtle, toast, tire) and a pointing response is required. Both initial and final consonants and blends (e.g., skip-slip) are probed separately.

VS = Vandervelden & Siegel (1999)
FP = Foley & Pollatsek (1999)

stop, names of favorite foods or restaurants). Or, assessors may use multiple-choice questions of increasing difficulty to determine contextual reading abilities. For example, teams can construct sentences such as "I like to eat (pizza, chair, dog, shoe)," using information from family members or teachers. If the person succeeds at this level, assessors may gradually increase the similarity among options over subsequent trials, so that the answer sets for the above sentence might change to (doors, horses, donuts, arms [all plural]) and then to (come, cook, cane, cake [all with same initial letter]).

Spelling Assessment

Spelling abilities are also important targets during AAC assessment. Because various AAC techniques require different types of spelling skills, a nontraditional language or spelling evaluation may be necessary. Overall, three components of spelling ability should be assessed: spontaneous spelling; first-letter-of-word spelling; and, if necessary, recognition spelling.

Spontaneous Spelling   In spontaneous spelling, the individual is required to spell words letter by letter. Estimates of spontaneous spelling ability can be assessed either informally or by using the spelling subtests from measures such as the Wide Range Achievement Test (Wilkinson, 1993) or the Woodcock-Johnson III (Woodcock, McGrew, & Mather, 2001). Individuals who can spell, at least phonetically (e.g., *fon* for *phone*), can use these skills when operating dedicated or computer-based AAC devices that rely on orthography.

First-Letter-of-Word Spelling   Most word prediction techniques require first-letter-of-word spelling so that the individual can use word menus for each of the letters of the alphabet. Thus, it is important to evaluate the extent to which people can spontaneously indicate the first letters of words, even if their other spelling skills are minimal or nonexistent. This can be assessed by using the initial letter subtest from a measure such as the BRIGANCE® Comprehensive Inventory of Basic Skills–Revised (Brigance, 1999)[1] or the Gates-MacGinitie Reading Tests–Fourth Edition (MacGinitie, MacGinitie, Maria, & Dreyer, 2000). This skill is also quite easy to assess informally, using one of two procedures. The first (and more difficult) procedure involves showing the person pictures of common items and asking "What's the first letter of this word?" without saying the word out loud. The second procedure is to say the word while asking the question, such as "What's the first letter in *cat?*" In order to use first-letter-of-word spelling for AAC, individuals without speech need to be able to do the first of these tasks; however, it is also important to identify skills in the easier assessment task so they can be built on and expanded, if necessary.

Recognition Spelling   Many individuals who acquire literacy skills without appropriate writing systems may have learned to spell on a recognition basis—that is, they can recognize words that are spelled correctly but cannot spontaneously produce either those words or their first letters. They have, in effect, a "sight word vocabulary" in that they have memorized the configurations of certain words. Assessment of recognition spelling is only necessary if the individual can produce neither the first letters of words nor their correct spellings spontaneously. To assess recognition spelling, the individual is

---

[1]BRIGANCE is a registered trademark of Curriculum Associates, Inc.

asked to recognize either the correct or the incorrect word from a series of options. For example, assessors might present the words *esarar, eraser,* and *erisir* with a picture of an eraser, and the individual's task is to identify the word that is spelled correctly. A subtest from the Peabody Individual Achievement Test–Revised-Normative Update (Markwardt, 1998) also measures recognition spelling ability.

Pulling It All Together   AAC teams should incorporate any reading skills that are identified during assessment into the overall design of the AAC system at an appropriate level of difficulty. At the most basic level, printed words can be used as symbols instead of or in addition to pictorial symbols. Otherwise, displays using single-word options in a multiple-choice format can be provided, as reported for adults with aphasia in Chapter 16. In addition, reading assessment information can be used to design an appropriate literacy program of instruction. We discuss the importance of literacy instruction for individuals who rely on AAC in detail in Chapter 13.

It is not at all unusual for individuals who use AAC to have very uneven spelling and reading profiles; for example, individuals with fairly good reading skills are often unable to spell at the same level. Assessors should not overestimate the spelling skills of these individuals because the implications for each type of spelling skill with regard to AAC intervention differ considerably. For example, in order to learn Morse code, it appears that people need spontaneous spelling skills to at least the second-grade level (Marriner, Beukelman, Wilson, & Ross, 1989). Nevertheless, individuals who are not this proficient but who have first-letter-of-word spelling abilities and adequate reading abilities may be able to use a word prediction or word menu selection technique (e.g., Co:Writer or EZ Keys software). As with other types of assessments, it is important that the AAC team be aware of the available intervention options and the operational requirements to ensure a good client–system match.

Assess Sensory/Perceptual Skills

Because vision impairments accompany many of the developmental and acquired disabilities that are common in people who use AAC, an accurate vision assessment is quite important. Decisions about the type, size, placement, spacing, and colors of symbols will often be guided by the results of such an assessment. Assessment of hearing capabilities, although less critical, will also allow the AAC team to make decisions about output options (e.g., types of synthetic or digitized speech the person can hear) as well as options related to language input (e.g., whether to supplement speech with manual signs or symbols). Assessment in both of these areas is discussed in the sections that follow.

Vision Assessment

Vision is a three-stage system that involves *sight,* the reception of sensory stimulation through the eye; *transmission* of an image along the optic nerve; and *interpretation* of the image in the visual cortex of the brain. During interpretation, images are transformed into meaningful information. The interpretation of the image is a result of all that an individual brings to the task, including motivation, experience, and self-image, which are the tools of functional vision. How an individual actually uses and enhances his or her existing vision through various means is at least as important from a functional perspective as is the nature or severity of the visual impairment itself. This certainly applies to AAC system considerations; thus, it is important for intervention teams to consider the individual's impairment as well as perceptions of his or her visual abilities and disabilities.

Assessment of an individual's visual status involves evaluation of a number of components, including *visual acuity, visual field magnitude, oculomotor functioning, light and color sensitivity, visual stability*, and *functional visual competence*. Each element contributes to an individual's functional vision skills. Most of these components will require assessment by ophthalmologists, optometrists, or vision specialists either before or during the AAC evaluation process. Orel-Bixler (1999) provided an excellent summary of the strategies that comprise a clinical vision assessment for infants and very young children with multiple disabilities. These same procedures are also applicable to older individuals who are unable to understand complex language and/or respond to directions because of language and/or motor impairments.

Visual acuity, or clarity of vision, allows an individual to discriminate details. Visual acuity is expressed by notations that describe the size of a visual target and the distance at which the target is identified. Fractional notation is most commonly used, with the numerator indicating the testing distance and the denominator indicating the size of the test item that can be identified on an eye chart (see Figure 7.20). The designation for *normal vision* is 20/20 (Cline, Hofstetter, & Griffin, 1980). People with acuities of 20/70–20/200 are considered to be *partially sighted*, and those with less than 20/200 vision are labeled *legally blind*. When vision decreases to awareness of light only, visual level is referred to as *light perception*, and a person is considered to be *totally blind* in the absence of light perception.

Visual acuities should be measured close up and at a distance because visual performance may differ depending on the task, as well as on the person's overall abilities and the visual condition causing the impairment. Indirect tests, forced-choice preferential looking (FPL) procedures, and visual evoked potential tests can all be used to examine visual acuity in individuals who are unable to cooperate with standard "eye chart" exams (Orel-Bixler, 1999). Sobsey and Wolf-Schein (1996) described a simple FPL procedure that utilizes either two computer screens with the same illumination or one large split screen. Two images, one of which contains no pattern and the other of which is boldly striped, checkered, or has wavy lines, are displayed on the screen(s) over several trials in

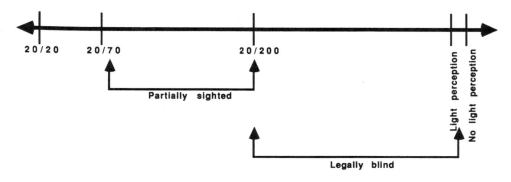

Figure 7.20.   Continuum depicting the range of visual impairments.

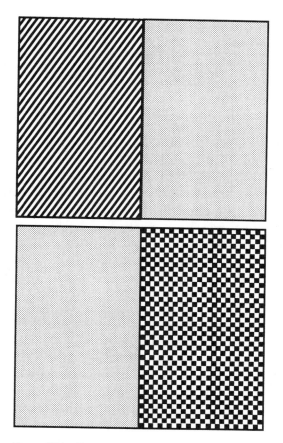

Figure 7.21. Examples of screens used for the forced-choice preferential looking (FPL) procedure for functional visual acuity.

alternating order (see Figure 7.21). Because most individuals will consistently look at the patterned screen, vision assessors can determine the person's ability to see at all. If the person orients toward the bold pattern, repeated pairings can then be presented with increasingly finer patterns until reaching the stage at which the person is unable to make a discrimination. Assessors can also vary the size of the squares systematically to approximate the size of potential communication symbols (e.g., $4'' \times 4''$, $2'' \times 2''$). In addition, the distance from the screen can be varied to determine the minimal and maximal distances within which the person demonstrates pattern preferences. Although the FPL procedure provides only an informal estimate of visual acuity, it can be useful in the absence of alternative tests.

AAC teams need information about visual acuity in order to decide whether to use aided symbols or unaided symbols (e.g., manual signs for someone with vision), and, if aided symbols are chosen, the type(s) of symbols to use, their size, their distance from the eyes of the person using AAC, and so forth. Even individuals who are considered legally blind often have some residual vision that they can use for communication. Utley (2002) described a number of simple procedures that can be used to assess distance and angle (e.g., horizontal, vertical) for optimal presentation of visual displays in AAC.

The *Technology Assessment Checklist for Students with Visual Impairments* and other forms for assessment related to assistive technology for individuals with visual impairments are available on-line through the Texas School for the Blind and Visually Impaired.

Visual field refers to the area in which objects are visible to the eye without a shift in gaze, normally extending in arcs of 150° horizontally and 120° vertically (Jose, 1983). The central visual field corresponds to the foveal and macular areas of the retina, which contain the cells most adapted to yield high visual acuity. Stimulation of these areas by visual impulses produces vision of the greatest clarity. Normal acuity decreases in proportion to the distance of the target from the fovea and macula. Thus, vision in the peripheral visual field is less clear than in the central visual field. The peripheral visual field detects movement and assists with vision in conditions of decreased illumination (Cline et al., 1980).

There are many impairments associated with the visual field, including 1) decreased vision in either the central or the peripheral field; 2) depressed visual sensitivity in specific areas; 3) blind spots (also referred to as opacities or scotomas) of varying shapes and sizes; 4) hemispheric losses; and 5) field losses that may occur subsequent to acquired brain injury, stroke, or other causes, in which entire segments of the visual field are missing. These losses can occur in one or both eyes. An individual with a *central visual field loss* has difficulty seeing a visual target presented at the midline of the body. This person must shift his or her focus off center to bring a target into view, generally by moving the head or eye horizontally or vertically. Individuals with *peripheral visual field losses* tend to experience difficulties when moving because they may be unable to detect movement or locate objects to their sides or beneath them. *Depressed sensitivity* results in areas of decreased acuity, which affect functional vision depending on the location of the affected areas and their shape and size (Harrington, 1976). Similarly, *blind spots* or *hemispheric losses* in the visual field can create a variety of problems that require adjustment of the point of visual fixation, head position, and the placement of materials. Such adjustments are often difficult to achieve for individuals with visual impairments who use AAC because they may experience additional physical impairments that interfere with their ability to move, maintain head control, or precisely direct their eye gaze. A qualified professional should make a careful assessment of visual field impairments in order to ensure proper placement and arrangement of communication symbols and devices for such individuals.

Oculomotor functioning refers to the operation of the eye muscles that enable the eyes to move together smoothly in all directions. These muscles allow the eyes to move into position and to place and maintain the image of an object on the optimal area of the retina. Oculomotor functioning includes movements that allow the eyes to establish and maintain visual fixation, locate and scan for objects, and follow moving objects. Problems with oculomotor functioning impair an individual's ability to direct precisely his or her gaze and may result in *double vision* or other problems. For example, a person with *strabismus* is unable to maintain the eyes in a position of binocular fixation because of weak eye muscles, and, thus, the eyes either converge (i.e., cross) or diverge. *Nystagmus*, another oculomotor disorder, is characterized by various involuntary movements of the eye and results in significantly reduced visual acuity. Individuals with this oculomotor disorder often attempt to compensate for it by repositioning their eyes, their head, and/or the materials they are examining. Thus, the detection of oculomotor disorders is of particular importance when an intervention team designs AAC systems for an individual with physical disabilities because the individual may lack the ability to freely adjust his or her body positions in order to compensate for the oculomotor disorder. Decisions regarding the positioning of an AAC device, the configuration of a symbol array, and the spacing of items on the display are all affected by the person's ocular motility and coordination. In addition, an individual with oculomotor problems may have great difficulty using scanning devices that require him or her to track moving lights on a display (see Utley, 2002, for additional information).

Light sensitivity must also be considered when evaluating an individual's visual status. Some disorders necessitate reduction or intensification of ambient light in order to achieve optimal visual functioning. For example, individuals with retinal problems may demonstrate abnormal sensitivity to light and require low light conditions for maximum performance. Individuals with conditions such as *degenerative myopia* (nearsightedness) require significantly increased levels of illumination in order to see. In addition to various disorders affecting light sensitivity, *glare* is a consideration for all but those individuals with the most severe visual impairments. Glare is the dazzling sensation that is caused by bright light or the reflection of bright light, and it produces discomfort and interferes with optimal vision (Cline et al., 1980). Glare is a concern for all individuals who communicate by using displays that are laminated or are otherwise covered by plastic because such coverings heighten the reflection of light off the surface of the page. In addition, glare may be a problem for people who use AAC devices with computer screen displays, especially those that are highly reflective. Attention to ambient light sources used for illumination, as well as to the positioning of displays with reflective surfaces, are important in order to minimize glare.

Color perception occurs when certain eye structures are stimulated by specific wavelengths of light and may be impaired in ways that affect accurate visual discrimination of contrast and detail. Generally, problems occur in the ability of the eyes to interpret particular (but not all) wavelength frequencies, so total color blindness is quite rare. People can learn to accommodate color vision problems, but the problems may be difficult to identify in very young children or in those who have difficulty labeling or matching. Nonetheless, AAC teams need to identify color impairments accurately to ensure that functional implications are minimized. For example, color codes using color wavelengths involved in an individual's particular impairment may serve only to reduce communication accuracy and increase frustration. Colors used on AAC displays for organizational or coding purposes must be discriminable and helpful to the person using the display and must be used in ways that enhance communication accuracy rather than detract from it (see Bailey & Downing, 1994).

Another visual component affecting AAC use is *visual stability*. Some individuals have eye conditions that are stable and relatively unchanging over time. Others have conditions that fluctuate, sometimes daily, depending on the individuals' physical status or on environmental factors. In addition, some conditions deteriorate over time, with variability in both the rate of deterioration and the final visual outcome. For example, individuals with *retinitis pigmentosa* (a progressive genetic visual impairment) experience a gradual reduction in the size of their visual field, along with night blindness, abnormal sensitivity to light, and color impairments. They may retain some vision throughout life, or they may eventually lose most or all vision. Because the condition is progressive and unpredictable and because it cannot be treated, these individuals must consider their current and potential visual status when making long-term decisions. Teams should consider AAC techniques for both current and future use even at the point of initial assessment.

In addition to the measures mentioned previously, either formal or informal functional vision assessment procedures may provide AAC team members with useful strategies for gathering information relevant to *functional visual competence*. This term refers to how an individual actually uses and enhances his or her existing vision through various means and is at least as important from a functional perspective as is the nature or severity of any visual impairments that may exist. For example, consider two individuals with the same eye condition that results in identical visual acuities of 20/200 (the limit for legal blindness). One person lives a typical life: She uses adaptations to perform certain tasks but continues to work, raise a family, and generally function independently in society. Her counterpart functions much less independently and is unable to perform basic tasks, including those necessary for employment. The major difference between these two individuals is in the functional use of the vision they have, not in their impairments. This variation in functional use of vision certainly affects AAC system considerations because it is important to consider not only the individual's impairments but also his or her perceptions and ability to compensate for them.

Topor (1999) offered a number of excellent suggestions for conducting functional vision assessments with infants and young children, including a list of important questions to ask family members. Another useful reference is a recent book on functional vision assessment by Lueck (2004), which contains numerous sample forms and practical assessment strategies that can be used with young children, school-age individuals, and adults, including those with multiple disabilities. Finally, the computerized EvaluWare assessment tool (Assistive Technology, Inc.) includes a number of tasks for examining functional "looking skills" that are directly relevant to AAC. On-screen tasks are provided to assess an individual's visual tracking skills as well as the optimal target, border, and text sizes; number of targets in an array; complexity of contextual screen displays; and foreground/background coloring. All of the tasks can be accessed using mouse, switch, keyboard, and motor techniques.

An excellent videotape called *Functional Vision: A Bridge to Learning and Living—Functional Vision Assessment* is available from the American Printing House (APH) for the Blind, Inc. The APH also publishes Braille versions of many popular tests that measure overall cognitive ability and academic achievement.

Pulling It All Together   Throughout this section, we suggest how information in each area might be useful in the overall design of an AAC system. In our experience, it is not at all uncommon for inadequate vision assessment or inadequate application of assessment information to cause individuals to abandon using their systems. Information about a person's visual *abilities* is far more important for AAC application than information about his or her visual *impairments.* Some of the most important questions to ask include the following: What *can* the person see accurately? How close to the person and how large do stimuli need to be? How far apart should they be arranged? Would colored or dark backgrounds help accommodate for problems of contrast? Are there blind spots or areas of reduced vision, and, if so, where in the visual field is vision most accurate? How should displays be positioned to allow maximal visual efficiency? If oculomotor problems are present, how are they best minimized or accommodated? Which colors can be seen? What lighting is required for optimal vision? If additional visual losses will occur over time, what is the time line and predicted progression? The answers to such questions are often implicit in formal vision assessments but may not be addressed explicitly by an examiner without prompting from other team members. It is up to the AAC team to ensure that information needed for system design is made explicit to the person conducting a vision assessment, and we have found that most vision specialists are able and willing to provide such information if it is requested.

Hearing Assessment

Assessment of hearing capabilities is important, especially if the selection set is displayed auditorily, as with auditory scanning. AAC teams usually select auditory display systems for people with severe visual impairments, and these systems require that the person using them be able to hear and understand the items in the selection set as they are announced. If interventionists consider auditory scanning via synthetic or digitized speech as an option, the hearing assessment should also serve to determine the individual's ability to comprehend the particular type of synthesized speech used in the system. In many electronic devices, feedback is also auditory and may be in the form of a beep to indicate that an item has been selected or a spoken echo produced via synthetic or digitized speech. Finally, many AAC devices utilize speech synthesis or digitization for output. Although such output is provided primarily for the benefit of the communication partner, not the person using the device, auditory comprehension of the output signal by the latter is generally desirable.

Assessment of hearing capabilities is usually straightforward and can be conducted by a qualified audiologist who does not necessarily have experience with AAC. If needed, evaluation of a person's ability to understand synthetic or digitized speech may be requested as an additional service. Of course, for some individuals, examiners may need to employ alternative response modes, a number of which were described by Abdala (1999) and by Sobsey and Wolf-Schein (1996). People with severe cognitive impairments may require considerable instruction prior to formal testing in order to establish a reliable operant response to sound. The empirically validated procedures developed by Goetz, Gee, and Sailor (1983) may be useful during such instruction. In addition, examiners may need to test individuals who cannot participate actively in audiological assessment using an auditory brain-stem response procedure (Abdala, 1999).

CONCLUSIONS

The goal of assessment is to gather a sufficient amount of information for the AAC team—the person who relies on AAC, family members, professionals, and other facilitators—to make intervention decisions that meet both the individual's current and future communication needs. Because of the many complex issues that must be considered in such assessments, there is a widespread tendency to overassess capabilities. Too much testing of an individual's motor, cognitive, linguistic, and sensory performance can actually interfere with AAC intervention because it takes so much time and places so many demands on the family and the person who will use AAC to communicate. In this chapter, we have provided a framework for completing assessments that are broad-based in scope but not necessarily exhaustive. Additional details regarding the assessment of people with acquired communication impairments appear in Chapters 15–19.

CHAPTER 8

Principles of Decision Making, Intervention, and Evaluation

Once the assessment process has been completed, the augmentative and alternative communication (AAC) team can finalize decisions about intervention and evaluate the outcomes. In Chapter 5, we discussed the importance of using a team approach to both AAC assessment and intervention planning, and in Chapters 6 and 7 we presented additional guidelines in this regard. During implementation, the person who relies on AAC, his or her family, and the interventionists involved must continue to work together to share information about preferences and strategies. In this chapter, we discuss a number of general principles that can be used during the intervention phase and thereafter. Chapters 9–19 contain specific intervention guidelines and techniques for people with various types of disabilities who rely on AAC.

OPPORTUNITY BARRIER INTERVENTIONS

The reason for assessing the nature of opportunity barriers in the first place is to facilitate appropriate interventions at this stage of the process. *Policy barriers* in the form of "official" written laws, standards, or regulations that govern the contexts in which people who use AAC find themselves will need to be resolved through advocacy efforts aimed at changing the restrictive legislation or regulations. For example, in the United States, the passage of the Assistive Technology Act of 1998 (PL 105-394) and the Americans with Disabilities Act (ADA) of 1990 (PL 101-336) resulted in the dissolution of many barriers that formerly made AAC services inaccessible to many people who needed them. Until 2001, the policy of Medicare (the U.S. federal health insurance program for people over age 65 and those with disabilities) was that AAC devices were "convenience items" and were not eligible for funding. After many months of work by a coalition of dedicated AAC professionals, this policy was changed in 2001, and speech-generating devices (SGDs) are now considered to be "durable medical equipment" and are funded by Medicare (see Blackstone, 2001, and the AAC-RERC Web site for more information). Remediation of policy barriers will almost always require the efforts of collaborative groups of parents and professionals working together to institute change.

Table 8.1. A communication bill of rights

All persons, regardless of the extent or severity of their disabilities, have a basic right to affect, through communication, the conditions of their own existence. Beyond this general right, a number of specific communication rights should be ensured in all daily interactions and interventions involving persons who have severe disabilities. These basic communication rights are as follows:

1. The right to request desired objects, actions, events, and persons, and to express personal preferences, or feelings.
2. The right to be offered choices and alternatives.
3. The right to reject or refuse undesired objects, events, or actions, including the right to decline or request all proffered choices.
4. The right to request, and be given, attention from and interaction with another person.
5. The right to request feedback or information about a state, an object, a person, or an event of interest.
6. The right to active treatment and intervention efforts to enable people with severe disabilities to communicate messages in whatever modes and as effectively and efficiently as their specific abilities allow.
7. The right to have communicative acts acknowledged and responded to, even when the intent of these acts cannot be fulfilled by the responder.
8. The right to have access at all times to any needed augmentative and alternative communication devices and other assistive devices, and to have those devices in good working order.
9. The right to environmental contexts, interactions, and opportunities that expect and encourage persons with disabilities to participate as full communicative partners with other people, including peers.
10. The right to be informed about people, things, and events in one's immediate environment.
11. The right to be communicated with in a manner that recognizes and acknowledges the inherent dignity of the person being addressed, including the right to be part of communication exchanges about individuals that are conducted in his or her presence.
12. The right to be communicated with in ways that are meaningful, understandable, and culturally and linguistically appropriate.

From the National Joint Committee for the Communication Needs of Persons with Severe Disabilities. (1992). Guidelines for meeting the communication needs of persons with severe disabilities. *Asha, 34*(Suppl. 7), 2–3; reprinted by permission.

Practice barriers refer to procedures or conventions that have become common in a family, school, or workplace but that contradict official policies that allow for service provision. Advocacy efforts are often needed to address practice barriers, but they should almost always be combined with educational and sensitization efforts as well. A good example of an intervention aimed at remediating practice barriers is the *Communication Supports Checklist for Programs Serving Individuals with Severe Disabilities*, which was developed by the National Joint Committee for the Communication Needs of Persons with Severe Disabilities to help AAC teams "develop a shared understanding and vision" for their programs (McCarthy et al., 1998, p. 7). The book contains a Communication Bill of Rights, originally published in *Asha*, which is presented in Table 8.1, as well as numerous self-assessment checklists that AAC teams can use to assess their current practices and plan related interventions, as needed. In general, practice barriers are easier to eliminate than policy barriers, especially if policies are already in place to support the need for change.

Since the summer of 1998, the Quality Indicators for Assistive Technology (QIAT) Consortium has focused its efforts on developing a set of descriptors that can serve as guidelines for assistive technology service delivery in schools (McCloskey & Zabala, 2003; Zabala et al., 2000). The most recent version of these descriptors (QIAT, 2003) can be downloaded from the QIAT Web site.

Knowledge barriers stem from a lack of information on the part of someone other than the person who uses AAC that results in limited opportunities for participation. Knowledge barriers can occur even when policies and practices in support of communication are in place. These barriers are best remediated through educational efforts such as in-service training, courses, workshops, directed readings, and so forth. Related to these are *skill barriers*, which occur when team members have difficulty with the actual implementation of an AAC technique or strategy despite even extensive knowledge. Educational efforts need to be directed toward additional practice, the provision of technical assistance, and other individualized and "hands-on" efforts. Skill barriers are what all of us have experienced after coming back from an exciting course or workshop only to realize that actually implementing all of the new information is a formidable task! Working with other colleagues who have more experience in the area or asking someone to brainstorm about strategies for translating theory into practice are two good examples of appropriate skill-building strategies.

Finally, some opportunity barriers are related to *attitudes* that restrict or prevent communication participation. Sometimes, the beliefs held by an individual are problematic; at other times, the culture of a service delivery agency or school system acts as a barrier. Often, attitude barriers persist even when policy and practice barriers do not. For example, we know of a group home run by a very progressive agency that had clear policies related to the importance of providing supports to enable the men who lived there to make choices and control their own lives as much as possible. In fact, in this group home, the general practice was in compliance with this policy; the men were encouraged to participate in designing meal menus, decorating their home, determining their own activity schedules, and so forth. However, one particular staff member's attitude presented an opportunity barrier in that he did not believe that the men should be "allowed to have" as much control and choice as they did. The result was that he limited their communication opportunities by failing to both provide them with choices and honor the choices they made. Clearly, this was not an issue for which advocacy efforts were appropriate. Instead, attitude barriers are best approached with such strategies as providing information about the issue of concern, arranging to have the person talk with or visit colleagues with more appropriate attitudes, providing time for open discussion of ideas about the issue, and modeling appropriate practices. In other words, it is easier to reduce attitude barriers with personalized educational efforts directed at change rather than with administrative or legislative solutions. In the preceding example, the "problem" staff member at the group home was provided with readings about choice and empowerment of people with disabilities, instruction related to how to facilitate choice making, and ample opportunities to discuss his feelings and concerns with other staff. Over time, his attitude barriers fell away as he was able to incorporate a new way of thinking into his existing repertoire.

PLAN AND IMPLEMENT
INTERVENTIONS FOR TODAY AND TOMORROW

Once a plan is in place to deal with the identified opportunity barriers over time, team members can compile and access assessment information and use it to make decisions about AAC interventions that best match the individual's profile of capabilities and constraints. Such decisions should be made using the principles of evidence-based practice (EBP), "the integration of best and current research evidence with clinical/educational expertise and relevant stakeholder perspectives to facilitate decisions for assessment and intervention that are deemed effective and efficient for a given stakeholder" (Schlosser & Raghavendra, 2003, p. 263). EBP does not mean that either clinical reasoning or the perspectives of persons who use AAC and their families are discounted when making decisions about optimal AAC techniques and strategies. It does mean that, in addition to these important components, a third component—current research evidence—is added to the mix. Thus, AAC teams who claim that they use EBP must be familiar with and consider the results of research when making clinical decisions.

Providers must not only do the right thing, they must do the right thing right. (Parnes, 1995)

Fortunately, one of the positive outcomes of the emphasis on EBP has been the generation of a number of integrative reviews of AAC research in recent years. In such reviews, authors examine existing research related to a specific type of intervention (e.g., communication aids with voice output), using either statistical (e.g., meta-analysis) or quantitative techniques. They also provide summary statements regarding (for example) the type(s) of individuals for whom the intervention has been shown to be effective, the benefits that have been shown to result from use of the technique, the optimal conditions for generating positive outcomes, and so forth. This information can be used fruitfully by AAC teams during intervention planning. For example, if research suggests that a specific technique is likely to be successful when implemented with some types of communicators but not others, the team can use this information to determine the likelihood of a positive outcome for the individual to whom they are providing support. Some examples of integrative reviews that have appeared in recent years are provided in Table 8.2.

Schlosser (2003b) noted the difference between efficacy and effectiveness, as follows: Efficacy pertains to the "probability of benefit [of an AAC intervention] to individuals in a defined population . . . under *ideal* conditions of use," while effectiveness pertains to the "probability of benefit [of an AAC intervention] . . . . under *average* conditions of use." (pp. 16–17)

The EBP process described by Schlosser and Raghavendra (2003) can be used to make decisions about the intervention components that are most likely to lead to positive outcomes for a given individual. The six steps or phases of this process are as follows: 1) ask a well-built question (e.g., Should we introduce aided or unaided symbols to teach requesting to this beginning communicator with autism? Should we use a computer-based

Table 8.2.   Integrative reviews of research evidence in AAC

Topic of review	Author(s)	Type of review
Functional communication training and/or visual schedule interventions for persons with developmental disabilities	Bopp, Brown, & Mirenda, 2004; Mirenda, 1997	Quantitative
Behavior chain interruption strategy	Carter & Grunsell, 2001	Quantitative
Graphic symbol techniques and/or manual signing for individuals with autism	Goldstein, 2002; Mirenda, 2001, 2003b	Quantitative
Efficacy of AAC interventions with persons with chronic severe aphasia	Koul & Corwin, 2003	Quantitative
Effects of AAC on natural speech development	Millar, Light, & Schlosser, 2002; Schlosser, 2003a	Meta-analysis
Presymbolic communication interventions	Olsson & Granlund, 2003	Quantitative
Effectiveness of aided and unaided AAC strategies for promoting generalization and maintenance	Schlosser & Lee (2000)	Meta-analysis
Selecting graphic symbols for requesting	Schlosser & Sigafoos, 2002	Quantitative
Use of speech-generating devices in AAC	Schlosser, Blischak, & Koul, 2003	Quantitative
AAC strategies for beginning communicators	Sigafoos, Drasgow, & Schlosser, 2003	Quantitative

system to support this man with severe global aphasia?); 2) select evidence sources (e.g., textbooks, research databases, and journals); 3) search the literature; 4) examine the evidence systematically; 5) apply the evidence to make decisions on behalf of the specific individual who requires AAC; and 6) evaluate the outcome of the decisions over time. As noted previously, integrative research reviews (see Table 8.2) can be very useful to AAC teams who have limited time or resources with regard to executing steps 2 and 3 of this process.

Numerous Web sites provide information about EBP in general or for specific fields of practice. Blackstone (2002) summarized many of the most relevant sites that pertain, at least in part, to AAC decision making.

In general, two sets of AAC-related decisions should be made from the outset: those aimed at "today" and those aimed at "tomorrow" (Beukelman, Yorkston, & Dowden, 1985). The relationship between decisions for today and decisions for tomorrow is depicted in Figure 8.1. The "today" decisions should meet the person's immediate communication needs and match the current capabilities and constraints identified during the assessment process. The "tomorrow" decisions are based on projections of future opportunities, needs, and constraints, as well as capabilities that result from instruction. Both decisions are critical to the long-term success of an intervention plan. Typically, communication interventions for persons who use AAC consist of three components: 1) interventions designed to increase natural abilities, 2) interventions that utilize environmental adaptations, and 3) interventions that incorporate AAC strategies and techniques.

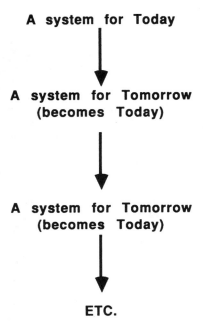

A system for Today

**A system for Tomorrow
(becomes Today)**

**A system for Tomorrow
(becomes Today)**

ETC.

Figure 8.1.   The longitudinal nature of AAC interventions.

Natural Ability Interventions

The first decision that the team must make often involves the relative emphasis to be placed on natural ability interventions and adaptive approaches. Of course, this consideration depends on the origin, stage, and course of an individual's communication disability. For example, an individual with end-stage amyotrophic lateral sclerosis (ALS) will not benefit from interventions designed to increase natural speech, whereas a preschool child with autism is likely to require extensive attention in this area.

A common issue for families of persons who use AAC is their concern that AAC interventions will inhibit the individual's natural ability development. For example, the family of a young adult with traumatic brain injury (TBI) whose limited speech cannot be understood by unfamiliar people may perceive a team's recommendation to provide an AAC system as an indicator that the team will no longer exert therapeutic efforts to improve the young adult's speech. Or, the family of a young child with severe cerebral palsy may perceive the recommendation of a single-switch scanning device with a head switch as an indication that the team will discontinue current therapeutic interventions to improve the child's upper-extremity motor function.

Clearly, the first step in resolving such concerns is to provide both reassurances and concrete evidence that natural ability interventions will not be discontinued. In reality, the evidence for one position and the accuracy of predictions concerning future improvements in natural abilities are often weak at best (see Schlosser, 2003b). Thus, compromise is a reasonable solution in most cases, considering a combination of both natural ability and augmented communication approaches. Often, we approach compromise with the analogy of an investment portfolio, in which negotiable percentages of professional time are allocated to (for example) natural speech and AAC investments, respectively. Thus, the team might decide to invest 50% of available intervention time in therapies to increase natural speech and motor skills and 50% of its time to AAC system development and use, or 10% to natural ability areas and 90% to the area of AAC, or whatever reasonable compromise can be reached by the team. When a compromise is reached, it is critical that the team follow through with the negotiated plan and meet regularly to share progress or lack thereof so that adjustments can be made in the "investment portfolio" accordingly. In Chapters 9–19, we discuss natural ability interventions in more detail as they pertain to specific disabilities across the lifespan.

Environmental Adaptation Interventions

The second intervention component in the access strand of the Participation Model (see Figure 6.1) involves resolving communication difficulties through environmental adaptations. These adaptations can be divided into two main categories: space/location adaptations and physical structure adaptations.

Space/location issues are specific to each intervention and should be solvable by the AAC team without major policy-level changes, assuming that consensus building has been effective, as discussed previously. Space adaptations may be necessary for removing physical barriers that interfere with use of an AAC system. For example, a woman with a brain-stem stroke who lives in a residential care home may be unable to bring her communication device into the cafeteria because the tables and chairs are too close together for the device to pass when mounted on her power wheelchair. Or, a college student with spinal cord injury may not be able to install his speech recognition computer system in his dormitory room because there is not enough space. In the first case, the necessary adaptations are simple: move the chairs and tables farther apart; in the second case, more complex space accommodations will be necessary.

Location adaptations are more related to the location of the person who uses AAC than to the equipment. For example, we know of a young girl with a low-tech AAC system who was seated in the back of the classroom, making it difficult for her to interact regularly with the teacher. This problem was resolved by moving her toward the front of the room.

Physical structure adaptations go beyond space and location adjustments and are necessary for accommodating the communication system or for facilitating its use. Obvious examples include adjusting tables or classroom desks to accommodate a student and his or her AAC system, adapting beds with adjustable swing arms in order to mount AAC systems for individuals who are partially bedridden, and widening doorways to allow passage of wheelchair-mounted equipment. Physical structure adaptations related to making public places accessible are required in the United States by the ADA.

AAC Interventions

The third intervention component in the access strand of the Participation Model (see Figure 6.1) involves the use of specific AAC strategies and techniques. In Chapters 9–19, we discuss this component in detail as it pertains to individuals with both developmental and acquired disabilities.

Interventions for Today

It is important to first consider the AAC technique(s) that meet the person's immediate needs within the available opportunities and are accurate, efficient, and nonfatiguing. An *accurate* system is one that the individual can use to produce intended messages with a minimal number of communication breakdowns and errors. An *efficient* system enables an individual to produce messages in an acceptable amount of time, without unduly extensive practice or training. A *nonfatiguing* system enables the person to communicate for as long as necessary without becoming excessively tired or experiencing significantly reduced accuracy or efficiency. An AAC system that is accurate, efficient, and nonfatiguing must match the person's *current* linguistic, cognitive, sensory, and motor abilities as closely as possible. It should also be selected in consideration of existing constraints and unresolved opportunity barriers. The "system for today" should require a minimum of training and practice in order for the individual to use it effectively to communicate messages about his or her most important and immediate needs. Of course, some initial instruction or training will need to occur in most situations, but both the length and complexity of training should be minimized.

> When we first got the [AAC device], Ana had very poor head control. Getting the light to hit the right squares became a daily battle. But she carried on with a determination I found extraordinary. She must have known that this device was eventually going to liberate her, at least from the confines of speechlessness. I have never been so proud of my daughter as I was during those times. (Cy Berlowitz, describing his daughter who has severe cerebral palsy, in Berlowitz, 1991, p. 16)

Interventions for Tomorrow

Decision making for tomorrow should be concurrent with decision making for today, under most circumstances. That is, as the AAC team institutes a communication system that matches the individual's *current* abilities and immediate needs, it should also develop plans for broadening the individual's skill base in preparation for a system for tomorrow. These plans might involve providing instruction to improve specific motor, symbol recognition, pragmatic, or literacy skills. They might involve remediating identified barriers that limit the quantity or quality of communication opportunities. For individuals with degenerative conditions such as ALS, Parkinson's disease, or Rett syndrome, plans need to anticipate the future loss of motor, communication, and other skills and prepare the person accordingly. Whatever the focus of planning for tomorrow, the goal should be to institute an intervention that will enable more of the person's communication needs to be met and/or to maintain or increase the accuracy, efficiency, and ease of use of the current system.

The system for tomorrow may be an expansion or extension of the system for today, or it may involve a different device or technique. For example, a component of the system for today for a young man with TBI early in recovery may be a series of eye-gaze communication boards with color photographs that represent the major choices available in his day. An expansion of this system for tomorrow might introduce printed words or Picture Communication Symbols (PCS) for the same messages by placing them next to the photographs and then fading the photos as he becomes able to accurately eye point to the new symbols. As another example, perhaps the photographic eye-gaze system for today was intended as a temporary measure to allow the motor therapists to develop the adaptations and skills needed for more effective hand and arm use. If this is the case, the eye-gaze system might be discontinued when motor control is sufficient and can be replaced with a lap-tray communication board containing the same printed words or photographs. In either case, once the system for tomorrow has been instituted, it becomes the new system for today, and planning can begin immediately for yet another tomorrow. Thus, a longitudinal AAC plan should always be two-pronged by including plans for both today and tomorrow—although the time between successive "tomorrows" is likely to lengthen as the AAC system comes closer and closer to meeting all of the person's communication needs.

In some cases, it might be fairly obvious what the system for today should be but not at all clear how to plan for tomorrow logically. This is often the case if the individual's motor impairments are very severe and not easily remediable. In such cases, it is often advisable to institute multiple and simultaneous training programs for tomorrow, each designed to improve the person's ability to control and use a different motor site. For example, consider a young man with severe athetoid cerebral palsy and good literacy skills. It was apparent from assessment that a simple orthographic eye-gaze system (Goossens' & Crain, 1987) combined with dependent auditory scanning (a 20-questions approach) was the best match for his current abilities. It was also apparent that in order for him to gain access to a more efficient and comprehensive system, he would need to achieve increased control of at least one motor movement sequence. It was not at all clear, however, which motor movement sequence could be taught best. Therefore, training programs designed to increase his ability to operate a single switch using his head, right hand, and left foot, respectively, were instituted at the same time. It became apparent that his head control was improving at the fastest rate, and after 6 months of work, he was able to use a head switch to control a single-switch scanner accurately, efficiently, and without undue fatigue. When the logical direction for tomorrow is not clear, such a multiple target approach is vastly preferable (and certainly less frustrating!) to one in which single training targets are tested in succession until the best one is selected.

PROVIDE INSTRUCTION TO PERSONS WHO RELY ON AAC AND THEIR FACILITATORS

Both persons who use AAC and their facilitators are likely to require at least minimal instruction in the use of the AAC system for today and more extensive instruction in skill-building for tomorrow. Instruction in AAC techniques has come a long way from the days when one or two professionals did the majority of such work in isolated therapy rooms (Musselwhite & St. Louis, 1988). It is now well established in the AAC literature that much, if not most, of the focus of intervention should take place in natural contexts such as classrooms, homes, community environments, and workplaces. Instructional plans that emphasize natural context interventions appear to result in better response generalization (to novel targets within the same response class) and better stimulus generalization (to novel people, environments, materials, and situations) than do instructional plans that emphasize isolated skill training (Reichle, York, & Sigafoos, 1991).

Facilitators (i.e., regular communication partners of people who use AAC) will also require various types of training, depending on the AAC system itself and the person who uses it. For example, facilitators may require training in partner-assisted scanning techniques or in how to interpret specific communicative gestures and vocalizations. Facilitators may also need to learn how to program and maintain electronic AAC devices, or how to set up a microswitch or head mouse for someone who uses these access techniques. In Parts II and II, we present facilitator training programs and strategies that can be used with individuals who rely on AAC because of specific conditions or disabilities.

Alliance '95 was the first AAC conference focused on efficacy research and outcome evaluation (Blackstone & Pressman, 1995). Panels of international experts on these topics were also convened at the 1997 convention of the American Speech-Language-Hearing Association and the 1998 conference of the International Society for Augmentative and Alternative Communication (Bedrosian, 1999). In 1999, a special issue of the *Augmentative and Alternative Communication* journal focused on efficacy research, followed four years later by a book on AAC efficacy and strategies for measuring it in meaningful ways. (Schlosser, 2003a)

MEASURE AND EVALUATE INTERVENTION OUTCOMES

Over the past decade, outcome evaluation has received increased attention in the AAC field. Schlosser (2003b) defined outcomes research in AAC as "the process of demonstrating, under average or less-than-average conditions, . . . the acquisition, maintenance, and generalization of behavior change (i.e., effectiveness) . . . " (p. 22). In the Participation Model (see Figure 6.1), we emphasize that outcomes evaluation should measure parameters that are important to both the person who uses AAC and to his or her family. Thus, we are less concerned about establishing precise, cause-and-effect relationships between specific intervention components and specific changes than about answering the more general questions, "Can the person participate successfully in specific activities and contexts that are common to his or her peers without disabilities?" and "Has the person's social network expanded in meaningful ways as a result of the AAC intervention?" (Blackstone & Hunt Berg, 2003a, 2003b; Calculator, 1999a; Schlosser, 2003c). Thus, an evaluation of intervention effectiveness in the Participation Model requires an examination of the person's ability to participate successfully in the specific activities and contexts that were identified as important during the initial needs assessment. If the desired level of participation is not achieved, the Participation Model requires reexamination and remediation of the opportunity and access factors that may be barriers (see Figure 6.1).

Several other approaches to outcome evaluation are also available and may be useful as an adjunct to the Participation Model process. These include specific measures of functional limitations as well as general measures of consumer/communication satisfaction and quality of life.

Functional Limitations

Functional limitations refer to "limitations in performance at the level of the whole . . . person" (Nagi, 1991, p. 322). Measurements of the impact of AAC interventions at this level seek to judge improvements in specific, functional skills. Culp referred to a number of "interaction parameters" (1987, p. 174) that might be measured in this regard, such as which modes of communication an individual uses and how many times a person who uses AAC initiates or responds to a partner's message, repairs communication breakdowns, makes choices, engages in social conversations, and so forth (Calculator, 1999a). Parameters such as these can be measured by frequency counts and traditional language sampling procedures. Automated systems such as the Language Activity Monitor (LAM) can also be used to record language samples for analysis from persons who use electronic AAC devices (see Romich et al., 2004). In the United States, the National Center for Treatment Effectiveness in Communication Disorders developed a series of Functional Communication Measures (FCMs) that are designed to be administered before and after intervention by speech-language pathologists. Goal Attainment Scaling (GAS) can also be used to measure an individual's progress toward specific, functional communication goals (see Calculator, 1991; Granlund & Blackstone, 1999; Schlosser, 2003d). Finally, a number of informal evaluation tools have also been developed to measure the impact of AAC interventions on a person's functional limitations (e.g., Culp, 1987, 1989; Culp & Carlisle, 1988; Romski and Sevcik, 1988a).

Consumer Satisfaction

Measuring consumer satisfaction with AAC services and interventions is regarded as a key means of obtaining outcome data (Cook & Hussey, 2002; Weiss-Lambrou, 2002). In this context, satisfaction refers to a person's opinion of the impact of a service, specific AAC technique, or overall AAC intervention. Perhaps the most widely used measure in this regard is the Quebec User Evaluation of Satisfaction with Assistive Technology (QUEST 2.0; Demers, Weiss-Lambrou, & Ska, 1996). QUEST 2.0 was the first standardized tool designed specifically for assistive technology services and consists of questions in 12 areas; it is intended for use by adults regardless of disability and can be either self-administered or completed with assistance (Weiss-Lambrou, 2002).

The QUEST has been field tested at research centers in Canada, the United States, and the Netherlands and has been translated into Danish, Dutch, Italian, Japanese, Norwegian, Swedish, and Portuguese. It assess satisfaction with factors such as simplicity of use, effectiveness, durability, repairs and servicing, and various aspects of service delivery. The QUEST 2.0 can be ordered through the Institute for Matching Person and Technology, Inc. Web site.

A related approach is the measurement of perceived "communication satisfaction" that results from an AAC intervention. This can be achieved by asking facilitators (e.g., parents and teachers) about how well the person who relies on AAC is able to communicate as a result of intervention (e.g., Bruno & Dribbon, 1998; Culp & Ladtkow, 1992). A preferable approach is to ask people who use AAC themselves to provide ratings of their own communication satisfaction either before and after intervention or over longer periods of time. For example, Slesaransky-Poe (1997) developed the Consumer Survey on Communicative Effectiveness, which asks people who use AAC to rate their level of satisfaction regarding communication, independence, productivity, and community inclusion. Hamm and Mirenda (2004) developed the Communication Survey, which examines both the degree of importance of and a person's satisfaction with various communication contexts, partners, and functions.

> Outcomes measurement should be consumer driven, flexible, and enduring. The result of AAC interventions should be an improved quality of life for people who use AAC. The results of outcomes measurement also should be used to improve cost-effectiveness and to improve the quality of equipment and services. (Consensus statement developed by participants in Alliance '95, an international conference on AAC outcome evaluation, in Blackstone & Pressman, 1995)

Quality of Life

Outcome evaluation related to quality of life (QOL) focuses on the impact of the AAC intervention on a person's ability to access and participate in preferred school, community, home, recreational, and vocational environments. The importance of outcome evaluation at this level has become increasingly recognized since the mid-1990s (Blackstone & Pressman, 1995; DeRuyter, 1995; Heaton, Beliveau, & Blois, 1995). QOL evaluations can be used to answer questions about whether an AAC intervention has resulted in (for example) increased self-determination, social inclusion, independence, participation in the community, gainful employment, academic achievement, and/or educational inclusion (Blackstone & Pressman, 1995).

Structured interviews can be used to elicit information related to QOL, as exemplified by the work of Cambridge and Forrester-Jones (2003) in the United Kingdom. Several formal QOL measures have also been used in the AAC field to measure this construct. For example, the Psychological Impact of Assistive Devices Scale (PIADS; Day & Jutai, 1996; Jutai & Day, 2002) and the Matching Person and Technology instruments (Galvin & Scherer, 1996) were both developed specifically to measure QOL as a result of assistive technology use. The ASHA Quality of Communication Life Scale (Paul et al., 2004) provides information about the psychosocial, vocational, and educational effects of communication impairment in adults. It can be used to assist with treatment planning, prioritization of goals, counseling, and documentation of outcomes. Hamm and Mirenda (2004) and Lund (2001) used the Quality of Life Profile: People with Physical and Sensory Disabilities instrument (QOLP-PD; Renwick, Rudman, Raphael, & Brown, 1998) to measure long-term outcomes for people who use AAC. The QOLP-PD asks individuals to rate the importance of various aspects of their lives as well as their degree of satisfaction with each. Scores on the QOLP-PD are reported on a 21-point scale ranging in value from +10 to −10, with lower scores indicating a less satisfying life for that individual. Schlosser (2003d) reviewed a number of additional QOL instruments as well that were developed for various groups of people with disabilities.

> The Quality of Life Profile: People with Physical and Sensory Disabilities (QOLP-PD) can be obtained from the Quality of Life Research Unit at the Canadian Center for Health Promotion. The Quality of Communication Life Scale is available from the American Speech-Language-Hearing Association.

FOLLOW-UP

According to the principle of interventions for today and tomorrow discussed previously, most AAC interventions never end! That is, once an individual has mastered a device or system for today, parallel training and practice can begin to prepare for one that is even more accurate, efficient, and nonfatiguing for tomorrow. Once these new skills are acquired, today becomes yesterday, tomorrow becomes today, and planning can begin for a new tomorrow!

If the person using AAC is a child, this cycle is likely to require repetition at each transition—from preschool to kindergarten, from elementary school to junior high, from junior high to senior high, and from senior high to either employment or post-secondary schooling. Adults with either congenital impairments (e.g., cerebral palsy) or acquired, nondegenerative impairments (e.g., stroke) are likely to need system alterations less frequently, unless their employment, residence, or family status changes markedly. Adults with degenerative illnesses (e.g., ALS, MS), however, may require frequent system changes as their abilities deteriorate and living situations change. Finally, most individuals who use AAC will require additional modifications to their systems as they approach retirement age, begin to shift priorities, and experience changes in ability that occur as a result of aging (see Light, 1988).

> Whose outcome is it anyway? Is it the outcome of the people that control the money, the persons who want the quickest intervention at the lowest price? Is it the outcome of the program administrator who is always looking to put up good numbers in order to make his program look effective? Or might it be the outcome of the potential user of AAC? Will he receive and be trained in an AAC system he can use effectively so he can go forth and do battle . . . ? Isn't this the outcome we all could be working towards? (Williams, 1995, p. 2)

AUGMENTATIVE & ALTERNATIVE COMMUNICATION INTERVENTIONS FOR INDIVIDUALS WITH DEVELOPMENTAL DISABILITIES

AAC Issues for People with Developmental Disabilities

This chapter provides a context for the information presented in Part II, which addresses the communication needs of individuals who are acquiring communication and language skills for the first time. These individuals have disabilities that were either present since birth or before the age of 22 and that affect one or more aspects of development (e.g., physical, sensory, cognitive). Augmentative and alternative communication (AAC) techniques are used quite routinely with people who experience such developmental disabilities, including cerebral palsy, intellectual disability (i.e., mental retardation), autism and the associated spectrum disorders, and developmental apraxia of speech. In this chapter, each of these conditions is defined and explained briefly in terms of its description, prevalence, and major characteristics. An overview of the AAC issues most pertinent to each impairment follows.

CEREBRAL PALSY

A healthy mind holds no boundaries or limitations. We, as non-speaking people, are likely to be more expressive or vocal than people who can speak. If we write out who we are as individuals and keep writing about our own identities, then others will see who we really are . . . . (Tony Diamanti, a man with cerebral palsy, in Diamanti, 2000, p. 98)

Definition, Prevalence, and Causes

The term *cerebral palsy* is typically used to refer to a developmental neuromotor condition that is the result of a nonprogressive abnormality of the developing brain (Hardy, 1983). It is estimated that the incidence of cerebral palsy is approximately 1 in 500 (Winter, Autry, Boyle, & Yeargin-Allsopp, 2002) and varies little across industrialized countries. It appears that the overall prevalence of cerebral palsy has not changed significantly since the mid-1990s, despite improved neonatal intensive care (Winter et al., 2002). Despite the multiplicity of problems associated with cerebral palsy, most children with this condition will live to adulthood. These individuals, however, do have a significantly lower life expectancy compared with the general population (Strauss & Shavelle, 1998).

There are a number of etiologies that result in early lesions or malformations of developing brain tissue. Until the 1980s it was thought that most cases of cerebral palsy were caused by a lack of oxygen to the brain during the birth process; however, it is now clear that this is rarely the case (Moster, Lie, Irgens, Bjerkedal, & Markestad, 2001). Data compiled by Pellegrino (2002) indicated that, among children born prematurely, the primary cause is damage to the white matter of the brain that occurs after birth as a result of cerebral hemorrhage or other problems (54%). In children born at term, brain malformations occurring during intrauterine development account for the majority of known causes (33%). In approximately 38% of people with cerebral palsy (whether they were born prematurely or at term), there is no identifiable cause.

The Augmentative Communication Online User's Group is an Internet discussion group open to all people who communicate through AAC. To subscribe, e-mail acolugrequest@vm.temple.edu.

Characteristics

Motor Skills

Individuals with cerebral palsy primarily experience difficulty with motor skills, which vary depending on the location of the brain lesion. The most common condition, spastic cerebral palsy, results in hypertonia (increased muscle tone). It may manifest as diplegia, in which the legs are affected more than the arms; hemiplegia, in which one side of the body is primarily affected; or quadriplegia, in which there is diffuse and severe damage affecting all four limbs as well as the trunk and oral-motor structures (Pellegrino, 2002). A second condition, dyskinetic cerebral palsy, is characterized by involuntary movements as well as changing patterns of muscle tone across the day (often, spasticity when awake and normal or even decreased tone when asleep). One subtype, dystonic cerebral palsy, involves rigid posturing of the neck and trunk; whereas another subtype, athetoid cerebral palsy, is marked by the presence of abrupt, involuntary movements of the extremities that result in difficulty regulating movement and maintaining posture. Finally, ataxic cerebral palsy, which can be associated with either increased or decreased muscle tone, causes problems with balance and positioning the trunk and limbs in space. Individuals with ataxia have a characteristic wide-based, unsteady gait when walking. In addition, some individuals have mixed cerebral palsy, which includes more than one type of motor pattern (e.g., spastic-athetoid cerebral palsy). Needless to say, the wide diversity of motor problems associated with cerebral palsy presents significant challenges to AAC teams serving this population.

Associated Conditions

A number of associated conditions are also common in people with cerebral palsy. Pellegrino (2002) stated that approximately one half to two thirds of all children with cerebral palsy also have some degree of mental retardation; individuals with hemiplegia and spastic diplegia are the least likely to be affected. In addition, it is not uncommon for individuals with cerebral palsy to have visual problems that may include eye muscle imbalances (e.g., strabismus), visual field cuts, visual-perceptual problems, and/or loss of visual acuity (especially farsightedness), any of which can significantly affect educational and communication programming. The incidence of hearing, speech, and language impairments has been estimated to occur in approximately 30% of individuals with cerebral palsy, and the underlying brain injury precipitates seizure activity in roughly 40%–50% of these individuals (Pellegrino, 2002).

Speech and Communication Skills

Problems with speech are also common sequelae to this neurological condition, with the incidence of dysarthria estimated to occur in a significant portion (estimates range from 31% to 88%) of all people with cerebral palsy (Yorkston, Beukelman, Strand, & Bell, 1999). The speech problems are associated with poor respiratory control as a result of muscular weakness and other factors, laryngeal and velopharyngeal dysfunction, and oral articulation difficulties that result from restricted movement in the oral-facial muscles. The incidence of dysarthria varies in relation to the type and degree of motor impairment. Other communication characteristics (e.g., overall language delay) may be associated with the problems of intellectual disability, hearing impairment, and learned helplessness that often co-occur with cerebral palsy.

> I do not like when people pity me. Like those ladies in the shops or people on the streets. They stare at me as if I were a weirdo. I really hate that look. I want people to accept me as I am. Sometimes, I just want to stick my tongue out at them. But I never do. I think to myself, it's not worth it. Often, I ask myself the question, why don't people want to understand me, isn't it so simple? (Magdalena Rackowska, a woman from Poland with cerebral palsy, in Rackowska, 2000, p. 88)

Unique AAC Issues

Team Approach to Intervention

Communication interventions with individuals who experience cerebral palsy require the expertise of a team of professionals from a number of disciplines, perhaps more so than with any other developmental disability. The wide variety of motor impairments in this population necessitates the involvement of professionals such as occupational and physical therapists, orthotics specialists, and rehabilitation engineers in the assessment process for determining the appropriate communication system for each individual. Professionals should be familiar with positioning and seating adaptations that must be developed on an individual basis in order to ensure optimum stability and the movement efficiency necessary to access a communication system. The team should also be familiar with the wide range of communication options available as well as with the special considerations necessary to achieve the optimal client–system match. The importance of such individualization was emphasized in a U.S. study by Lafontaine and DeRuyter (1987), in which they reported that, across 64 individuals with cerebral palsy who were assessed and fitted with AAC devices, a total of 17 different types of communication devices were prescribed. These included several different types of nonelectronic devices such as picture or word boards and 13 different types of electronic devices. Although 47% of the individuals in Lafontaine and DeRuyter's study were able to access their devices through the use of a finger, the remainder used a number of alternative access techniques, including optical indicators, chin pointers, joysticks, and a variety of switches for scanning. Similarly diverse patterns of AAC system use have been reported in other developed countries such as Scotland (Murphy, Marková, Moodie, Scott, & Boa, 1995), Australia (Balandin & Morgan, 2001), and Israel (Hetzroni, 2002). In developing countries such as South Africa (Alant, 1999), this diversity may not be seen because the types of available AAC systems are more restricted.

In addition, visual acuity and visual-perceptual problems will affect decisions regarding the size and figure–ground contrast of the symbol system chosen for communication, and comprehensive assessment by a pediatric ophthalmologist or another team member trained to assess these issues is often required (DeCoste, 1997a). Perceptual impairments (e.g., hearing loss) can impede the process of learning to read or spell in those individuals who have this capability, requiring input from professionals such as speech-language pathologists or educators who specialize in remediation of these problems. Finally, but certainly of no less importance, the input of speech-language pathologists and both general and special educators will be necessary during the assessment process to train those who rely on AAC and their facilitators and to manage the intervention process.

> For an AAC user, the development of one's voice poses [a] . . . . challenge because AAC devices can be limiting. A symbol or word might not appear on a board. A voice synthesizer might not have the right intonation. All of this can limit or change what is trying to be said . . . . Because I rely on AAC, it has taken me many years to learn how to communicate effectively. I now use a combination of "agencies," including speech, written words, telecommunications, a word board, and a voice output device. All of these devices allow my "voice" to be heard. (Nola Millin, a young woman with cerebral palsy, in Millin, 1995, p. 3)

Balanced Approach to Intervention

Beukelman (1987) emphasized the need for a "balanced approach" to communication programming for people with severe expressive communication disorders. In the case of people with cerebral palsy, emphasis on AAC needs to be balanced with motor development training, speech therapy, and academic instruction, as necessary. For example, some individuals will require extensive motor training in order to use adaptive access techniques such as headlight pointing or scanning. However, in the search for a technique that an individual can use immediately, a frequent mistake is to abandon such motorically demanding options. The result is that long-term efficiency is often sacrificed for short-term gains. Instead, a longitudinal program designed to meet the person's immediate communication needs with a number of readily accessible approaches, which also "invests in the future" through a systematic motor or speech therapy program to train more complex skills, may be more fruitful and, ultimately, more balanced (see Treviranus & Roberts, 2003, for additional discussion of this issue).

This principle also applies to the selection of multimodal communication systems for individuals with cerebral palsy. A number of augmentative techniques may be used in different contexts and with different people to communicate a variety of messages (see Light, Collier, & Parnes, 1985a, 1985b, 1985c). In addition, although speech, gestures, and facial expressions may be severely affected as a result of motor impairment, this does not mean that people with cerebral palsy should be discouraged from using these natural modes for communication (Hustad & Shapley, 2003). Rather, a balanced approach calls for efforts to encourage and support the use of such multimodal systems, including training of both individuals and their communication partners concerning the most effective techniques to use in various situations. For example, the individual may be able to communicate with family members very effectively using natural modes, whereas he or she may need to rely on AAC techniques with unfamiliar partners (Blackstone & Hunt Berg, 2003a, 2003b).

> The silence of communication is never golden. We all need to communicate and connect with each other—not just in one way, but in as many ways as possible. It is a basic human need, a basic human right. And much more than this, it is a basic human power. (Bob Williams, an augmented communicator, in Williams, 2000, p. 248)

INTELLECTUAL DISABILITY

People who are labeled as having intellectual disabilities have only been recognized as appropriate candidates for AAC interventions since the mid-1980s. Indeed, many school districts, adult services agencies, and residential facilities still inappropriately maintain "candidacy" criteria to ascertain whether such individuals are likely to qualify for AAC services (National Joint Committee for the Communication Needs of Persons with Severe Disabilities, 2003a, 2003b). Nonetheless, since the mid-1980s, important positive changes have occurred in societal and professional attitudes toward these individuals. People with intellectual disabilities increasingly are being provided with the opportunities and technology needed to assist them to communicate in inclusive, dynamic environments.

Definition and Causes

According to the most recent definition by the American Association on Mental Retardation (AAMR), intellectual disability (also known as mental retardation) is characterized by

> Significant limitations both in intellectual functioning and in adaptive behavior as expressed in conceptual, social, and practical adaptive skills. This disability originates before age 18. (Luckasson et al., 2002, p. 5)

The AAMR definition deemphasizes ability-level (or IQ-based) classifications (mild, moderate, severe, profound) in favor of a focus on the level(s) of support a person needs (Luckasson et al., 2002). Thus, an individual with intellectual disability may be described as requiring intermittent, limited, extensive, or pervasive supports in one or more areas. This new descriptive system acknowledges that appropriate supports can have a significant impact on the ability of individuals with intellectual disability to live, work, recreate, and learn successfully in community environments typical of their same-age peers.

Most intellectual disability requiring intermittent supports (formerly referred to as "mild" intellectual disability) is associated with lower socioeconomic status and inadequate environmental stimulation, including prenatal exposure to drugs and/or alcohol, infection or asphyxia soon after birth, and minor chromosomal and congenital anomalies (Batshaw & Shapiro, 2002). A large number of conditions related to intellectual disability requiring more extensive supports (i.e., moderate to profound intellectual disabilities) are the result of either chromosomal or genetic disorders (43%). Down syndrome, fragile X syndrome, and fetal alcohol syndrome together account for almost one third of all intellectual disability whose cause is known (Batshaw & Shapiro, 2002), although literally hundreds of other conditions and syndromes are also associated with this diagnosis. As is the case with cerebral palsy, intellectual disability can co-occur with hearing, vision, motor, seizure, and communication disorders.

> What is retardation? It's hard to say. I guess it's having problems thinking. Some people think that you can tell if a person is retarded by looking at them. If you think that way you don't give people the benefit of the doubt. You judge a person by how they look or how they talk or what the tests show, but you can never really tell what is inside the person. (A man labeled as having mental retardation, in Bogdan & Taylor, 1994, pp. 90–91)

Prevalence

According to the World Health Organization (2001), the prevalence of intellectual disability is believed to be between 1% and 3% worldwide, with higher rates in developing countries because of the higher incidence of injuries and anoxia around birth, and early childhood brain infections. A common worldwide cause is endemic iodine deficiency, which constitutes the world's greatest single cause of preventable brain damage and intellectual disability (Delange, 2000). In the United States, the prevalence of intellectual disability in the noninstitutionalized population is estimated to be approximately 1% or 7.8 per 1,000 (Lee et al., 2001); this figure also applies to the school-age population (U.S. Department of Education, 2000).

A demographic study conducted in the state of Washington indicated that people with intellectual disability comprise the largest percentage of the school-age population of individuals who are unable to speak (Matas, Mathy-Laikko, Beukelman, & Legresley, 1985). This study estimated that 4%–12% of school-age children with intellectual disability requiring intermittent to limited support and 92%–100% of children with intellectual disability requiring extensive to pervasive support could potentially use AAC. It is becoming increasingly accepted that AAC teams can and should deliver communication services of some type to these individuals regardless of the degree of impairment (National Joint Committee for the Communication Needs of Persons with Severe Disabilities, 2003a, 2003b).

Unique AAC Issues

Opportunity Factors

When designing communication interventions for people with intellectual disability, it is vital to address their lack of naturally occurring communication opportunities. Such opportunities can exist only when responsive communication partners interact in inclusive home, school, and community environments (Mirenda, 1993). Unfortunately, many people with intellectual disability continue to live, work, and recreate in segregated environments where the only people available to them as communication partners are other individuals with communication impairments or paid staff members. In addition, the notion persists in many places that AAC instruction with this population should be conducted in highly structured settings until some arbitrary criterion is reached; only then is the individual exposed to natural situations in which communication skills are actually required. Unfortunately, given the generalization difficulties common in people with intellectual disability, this approach is usually futile. In an extensive discussion of this issue, Calculator and Bedrosian noted that "there is little justification for conducting communication intervention as an isolated activity because communication is neither any more nor less than a tool that facilitates individuals' abilities to function in the various activities of daily living" (1988, p. 104). The presence of integrated, natural communication opportunities will directly affect the vocabulary selected as well as the instructional techniques used and must be considered an integral part of any AAC intervention.

Do not try to control me. I have a right to my power as a person. What you call non-compliance or manipulation may actually be the only way I can exert some control over my life . . . (Kunc & Van der Klift, 1995)

Problem Behavior

Most people with intellectual disability do not engage in socially inappropriate behaviors. Behavior problems, however, do occur in these individuals more often than in people without disabilities (Batshaw & Shapiro, 2002), for reasons that should be quite obvi- ous—a lack of preferred and functional places to go, people to be with, things to do, and ways to communicate. For decades, the primary strategies that have been used to "man- age" the behavior of people with intellectual disabilities include incarceration (i.e., insti- tutionalization), medication, and the use of aversive (i.e., punitive) behavior modification techniques. Since the mid-1980s, the emphasis has shifted to the use of proactive, eco- logical strategies to prevent behavior problems, as well as numerous strategies for teach- ing functional communication skills as alternatives for problem behavior (Carr et al., 1994; Durand, 1990; Reichle & Wacker, 1993; Sigafoos, Arthur, & O'Reilly, 2003; Wacker, Berg, & Harding, 2002). This shift has great relevance to AAC because many individuals with intellectual disabilities do not use speech as their primary mode of communication. It is critically important that AAC facilitators working with individuals who engage in problem behavior familiarize themselves with the literature on communication ap- proaches for behavior support so that they can act as both facilitators and advocates in this regard (see Bopp, Brown, & Mirenda, 2004, and Mirenda, 1997, for reviews).

The journal *Down Syndrome Research and Practice* and the newsletter *Disability Solutions* are both excellent sources of information about AAC interventions for people with Down syndrome. Best of all, both of these resources are available on-line! For example, Foreman and Crews (1998) reported the results of a study in which aided and unaided AAC techniques were used with young children with Down syndrome; Mirenda (1999) and Reed (1998) provided suggestions for AAC use at home and in school; and Gee (1999) discussed language and communi- cation interventions for children with both Down syndrome and autism spectrum disorders.

Different Strokes for Different Folks

As noted previously, the term "intellectual disability" is really an "umbrella" term that encompasses a large range of syndromes and conditions that result in, among other things, cognitive impairment. Individuals with some of the conditions that fall under this umbrella (e.g., Down syndrome and congenital deafblindness) commonly experience sig- nificant problems with communication in addition to cognitive impairments, whereas in- dividuals with other conditions (e.g., Williams syndrome and Prader-Willi syndrome) do not (Dykens, Hodapp, & Finucane, 2000). Furthermore, even those individuals who do have difficulty with communication are not necessarily alike with regard to the nature of their impairments. For example, individuals with Down syndrome usually develop ade- quate speech for functional communication (Dykens et al., 2000), but those with Angel- man syndrome often do not (Jolleff & Ryan, 1993).

Given this diversity, the nature of remedial interventions directed at both natural speech development and AAC will vary considerably among persons with intellectual disabilities, depending on the specific disability involved. Thus, AAC team members should be alert to the importance of understanding the language, communication, and social-relational characteristics; learning strengths; and overall developmental patterns that are typical for individuals with specific intellectual disabilities, so that intervention can be staged and implemented with these characteristics in mind. It is also important to remember that many individuals with developmental disabilities may have multiple diagnoses (e.g., Down syndrome and autism; see Rasmussen, Börjesson, Wentz, & Gillberg, 2001), which can further complicate both their developmental profiles and the nature of their intervention needs. On the other hand, it is also important to remember that most AAC strategies and techniques can be applied to individuals across the range of specific syndromes and conditions; we will discuss these generic approaches in Chapters 10–14.

I think in pictures. Words are like a second to me. I translate spoken and written words into full-color movies, complete with sound, which run like a VCR tape in my head. When somebody speaks to me, his words are instantly translated into pictures. (Temple Grandin, a professor with autism, in Grandin, 1995, p. 19)

AUTISM AND PERVASIVE DEVELOPMENTAL DISORDERS

Definition, Prevalence, and Causes

It is increasingly accepted that autism and a number of related pervasive developmental disorders (PDDs) occur as a spectrum of impairments (Wing, 1996). On the one end of the spectrum are individuals with autism who also have intellectual disabilities requiring extensive to pervasive support. On the other end are socially eccentric or "odd" individuals who may get married, hold down jobs, and are never diagnosed as having a disability. For example, individuals with Asperger syndrome (high-functioning autism) may have no cognitive or language impairments but exhibit a number of unusual social and behavioral characteristics. Between the extremes are individuals with autism without intellectual disability; PDD not otherwise specified; or one of the other, less common disorders under the PDD "umbrella" (e.g., Rett syndrome).

All of the diagnostic systems commonly used to describe autism agree that there are three main diagnostic features: 1) impairments in social interaction; 2) impairments in communication; and 3) restricted, repetitive, and stereotypical patterns of behaviors, interests, and activities (American Psychiatric Association, 1994; World Health Organization, 1992). Although the cause of autism is not known, a large body of research is available to demonstrate that it is not caused by family, emotional, or environmental factors (Wing, 1996). Considerable research is currently focused on identifying a number of genetic and neurological factors that may cause the syndrome. The prevalence of all PDDs is estimated to be between 1 in 150 (Chakrabarti & Fombonne, 2001) and 1 in 500 (Fombonne, 1999). It is well established that focused educational and related interventions from an early age can make a real difference with regard to outcome (National Research Council, 2001).

For additional information about current North American research on the causes of autism and other PDDs, visit the Web sites of the National Alliance of Autism Research (NAAR), the Autism Spectrum Disorders–Canadian American Research Consortium (ASD-CARC), the Studies to Advance Autism Research and Treatment (STAART) network, and Cure Autism Now (CAN).

Characteristics

Cognitive Impairments

Recent research offers conflicting information about the co-occurrence of intellectual disabilities and autism. Fombonne (1999), in a review of past epidemiological studies, found that approximately 75% of people with autism also have intellectual disabilities. However, the results of a recent study from the United Kingdom suggest that only about 25% of people with autism have co-occurring intellectual disabilities (Chakrabarti & Fombonne, 2001). This suggests that the relationship between these two impairments is not as straightforward as previously thought (Bölte & Poutska, 2002), possibly due to changes in how autism is manifested in general, the positive impact of early intervention, or a combination of the two.

As she grew, the problem of her speech took precedence over all the others. It was through speech that she must join the human race. (Clara Claiborne Park, referring to her daughter with autism, in Park, 1982, p. 198)

Social/Communication Impairments

Because autism is, by definition, primarily a social/communicative impairment, a comprehensive description of the communication characteristics is beyond the scope of this book (see Wetherby & Prizant, 2000, for more complete descriptions and intervention implications). Nevertheless, individuals with autism experience a wide range of complex issues related to both the means and the forms of language and communication. In the absence of appropriate early intervention, approximately 50% of people with autism never develop sufficient speech as a means for communication (National Research Council, 2001). There is some evidence that some individuals with autism have increased difficulty producing the oral-motor movements necessary for speech, which may account, at least in part, for their lack of speech development (Adams, 1998). If speech and language do develop, certain abnormalities are common, including echolalia, repetitiveness, literalness of meaning, monotonous intonation, and idiosyncratic use of words or phrases.

Most striking in individuals with autism are a number of verbal and nonverbal impairments of social interaction. Researchers have documented several core symptoms that, if noted before 12 months of age, are usually good predictors for a later diagnosis of autism. These include failure to look at other people (i.e., decreased eye contact), failure to orient to name, reduced reciprocal social smiling, atypical sensory behavior, difficulty initiating visual tracking and disengaging visual attention, difficulty with imitation, and a general lack of social interest (Osterling, Dawson, & Munson, 2002; Roberts & Brian, 2004). Impairments in nonverbal communication, including an inability to "read" the facial expressions or take the perspective of others, are also central features of the syndrome (Frith, 2003).

Language Impairment

People with autism often have language impairments as well, and substantial delays in receptive language ability are not uncommon. These problems may be masked, however, by unusual skills in other areas that make it seem that people with autism understand everything that is said to them. Indeed, many people with autism have visual-spatial and visual-memory skills that far surpass their apparent abilities in the language area, which may account for reports of unusual reading and spelling abilities (hyperlexia) (Tirosh & Canby, 1993). In fact, it appears that at least some individuals with autism may have relatively intact language systems despite appearances to the contrary, as evidenced by reports of some who have progressed from typing with assistance to typing independently through use of facilitated communication (Biklen, 1993; see Chapter 11). Other individuals with autism may use such visuospatial splinter skills to compensate for a lack of linguistic understanding by memorizing routines and attending to the subtle situational cues that accompany spoken language (Mirenda & Erickson, 2000).

> As a child, the "people world" was often too stimulating to my senses. Ordinary days with a change in schedule or unexpected events threw me into a frenzy, but Thanksgiving or Christmas was even worse. At those times our home bulged with relatives. The clamor of many voices, the different smells—perfume, cigars, damp wool caps or gloves—people moving around at different speeds, going in different directions, the constant noise and confusion, the constant touching, were overwhelming . . . . This is not unusual for autistic children because they are over-responsive to some stimuli and under-sensitive to other stimuli . . . . [They] have to make a choice of either self-stimulating like spinning, mutilating themselves, or escape into their inner world to screen out outside stimuli. Otherwise, they become overwhelmed with many simultaneous stimuli and react with temper tantrums, screaming, or other unacceptable behavior. (Temple Grandin describing her experience as a child with autism, in Grandin & Scariano, 1986, pp. 24–25)

Processing Impairments

Underlying the speech/language/communication impairments of autism are a number of developmental and cognitive processing issues that directly affect social and communication interventions. For example, researchers in the United Kingdom have provided evidence that people with autism lack a "theory of mind"—the ability to attribute independent mental states to oneself and others, in order to explain behavior. This could account for the inability of even the most capable individuals with Asperger's syndrome to take the perspective of others into account in social situations. In addition, Prizant (1983) described people with autism as "gestalt processors," referring to their tendency to process the gestalt, or "whole," of a situation or utterance rather than its component parts; this could account for much of the echolalic language frequently observed in these individuals, at least during the early stages of language development. Overall, it is clear that autism spectrum disorders are extremely complex and varied both within and across individuals and present numerous challenges with regard to both speech-based and AAC interventions.

Unique AAC Issues

Early Intervention

There are several elements that research has shown to be critical in intervention programs for individuals with autism. The most important of these are

1. Start early

2. Start early

3. Start early

4. Start early

5. Start early!!

In their comprehensive report issued in 2001, the National Research Council's Committee on Educational Interventions for Children with Autism strongly recommended that entry into intervention programs should begin as soon as a diagnosis is seriously considered (not necessarily confirmed). As noted previously, such a "presumptive" diagnosis is now possible in children as young as 6–12 months of age. The Committee also concurred that "active engagement in intensive instructional programming" (p. 219) should be provided to children at least up to age 8 years for a minimum of 25 hours per week on a year-round basis and should consist of "repeated, planned teaching opportunities" (p. 219) conducted in both one-to-one and very small group sessions. They also recommended that emphasis be placed on the use of evidence-based instructional techniques in six main areas: 1) functional, spontaneous communication using verbal and/or AAC modalities; 2) developmentally appropriate social skills with parents and peers; 3) play skills with peers; 4) various goals for cognitive development, with emphasis on generalization; 5) positive behavior supports for problem behaviors; and 6) functional academic skills, as appropriate.

The Committee acknowledged that a wide range of instructional approaches may be used to accomplish these goals, including discrete trial teaching (Smith, 2001), incidental teaching (McGee, Morrier, & Daly, 1999), and other structured teaching approaches based on applied behavior analysis (e.g., Leaf & McEachin, 1999; Sundberg & Partington, 1998); the Developmental, Individual-Difference, Relationship-Based (DIR) model (Greenspan & Weider, 1999); the SCERTS™ Model (Social Communication, Emotional Regulation, and Transactional Support; Prizant, Wetherby, Rubin, & Laurent, 2003; Prizant, Wetherby, Rubin, Laurent & Rydell, 2005a, 2005b), and many others. Although they did *not* recommend a specific curriculum or approach, they stressed the importance of goal-directed, evidence-based, individualized programs that meet the needs of both children with autism and their families. It is beyond the scope of this chapter to either summarize or critique the various autism intervention approaches; however, we emphasize that families are continuously faced with the task of deciding what to do for their child with autism and how best to do it. Some of the decisions that may drastically affect the extent to which AAC techniques of various types will be accepted and used by the family (e.g., in a "verbal behavior" approach, manual signing may be accepted but graphic symbols may not be; see Mirenda, 2003b, and Sundberg, 1993). Thus, AAC interventionists may need to work with other professionals whose views are quite divergent from (and perhaps even incompatible with) their own; this may require considerable skill at negotiation and collaboration.

> How peaceful it is to withdraw from the complicated world of human relationships! I do however enjoy the presence of a friend and feel so content in the company of one who is willing to take me as I am. My friends have been willing to see me this way and I am so grateful to have been given the opportunities to discover life in the real world. (A man with autism, in Lawson, 1998, p. 100)

Communication in a Social and Developmental Context

Because autism profoundly affects the very nature of communication as a social mediator, it is critically important that interventions emphasize the pragmatic aspects of communication rather than merely aspects related to form (Duchan, 1987). To quote Rees, "morphology plus syntax plus semantics does not equal communication" (1982, p. 310) for most individuals with autism. Especially for beginning communicators with autism, the development of spontaneous communication as a dynamic, interpersonal process is critical. Related to this is the need to teach the individual to use communication skills in the context of naturally occurring routines related to functional activities in daily life.

It is also important that interventions start at the individual's level of social/communicative/cognitive development and build skills in a natural developmental progression. A number of researchers have demonstrated that the developmental profiles of children with autism, unlike those typically found in children with mental retardation, are characterized by an uneven distribution of skills; this is often referred to as "developmental discontinuity" (Fay & Schuler, 1980). On a sensorimotor assessment battery, for example, children with autism tend to perform markedly better in the areas of object permanence and tool use (causality) than in areas requiring interpersonal interaction, such as gestural or vocal imitation, use of adult-as-agent (means–ends), symbolic understanding, or language comprehension (Curcio, 1978; Wetherby & Prutting, 1984). This information has direct implications for AAC interventions, as it is important to gear such interventions to the child's social and linguistic abilities rather than object abilities. For example, it is not unusual to see manual sign language or other formalized communication systems (e.g., pictorial systems) recommended for children with autism who do not speak. This presumes that the problem is simply lack of an output mode and that communicative intent or language is intact. In fact, many such children have neither the language nor the social base on which communication must be built, even though they demonstrate substantial abilities in nonlanguage areas such as fine and gross motor skills or areas that involve object manipulation (e.g., puzzle assembly). Formal language or communication approaches with children who show evidence of significant developmental discontinuity should be preceded by interventions designed to build imitation, joint attention, and natural gestural communication skills. Premature initiation of formal language-based AAC (or speech) approaches will often result in nonfunctional, stereotypical behavior, with resulting frustration on the part of both the child and his or her facilitators.

Through the AAC-RERC, Howard Shane and his colleagues at Children's Hospital Boston are exploring the use of "intelligent agents" (IAs)—computer characters designed to model for or direct those interacting with computer software—with individuals with autism. In 2002, he and a colleague reported that six boys with autism attended to a task and followed simple directions significantly better when directed by an IA than a live human (Douglas & Shane, 2002). In the future, IAs may be used to teach communication and other skills to people with autism.

Speech Output

Historically, the use of speech output technologies (i.e., "talking" computers and SGDs) with individuals with autism spectrum disorders has been a subject of some debate, for a variety of reasons (see Mirenda, 2001, 2003b, and Schlosser & Blischak, 2001). However, in recent years, a number of studies have demonstrated that these technologies can be used effectively with individuals with autism to teach literacy skills (Heimann, Nelson, Tjus, & Gillberg, 1995; Schlosser, Blischak, Belfiore, Bartley, & Barnett, 1998; Tjus, Heimann, & Nelson, 1998); communication skills for requesting access to preferred objects or activities (Brady, 2000; Durand, 1999; Dyches, 1998; Schepis, Reid, Behrmann, & Sutton, 1998; Sigafoos, Didden, & O'Reilly, 2003; Sigafoos & Drasgow, 2001), and communication skills for responding to questions and social commenting (Schepis et al., 1998). Speech output technologies have also been shown to have positive effects with regard to object labeling skills (Brady, 2000); reduced frequencies of problem behavior (Durand, 1999); and (perhaps most important), natural speech production (Hetzroni & Tannous, 2004; Parsons & LaSorte, 1993; Sigafoos, Didden, et al., 2003). Girls with Rett syndrome, one of the less common of the autism spectrum disorders, have been shown to benefit from speech-output technology as well, with regard to skills such as labeling and commenting during storybook reading (Koppenhaver, Erickson, Harris, et al., 2001; Koppenhaver, Erickson, & Skotko, 2001; Skotko, Koppenhaver, & Erickson, 2004); symbol-to-word matching (Hetzroni, Rubin, & Konkol, 2002); and requesting access to preferred objects or activities (Van Acker & Grant, 1995). Finally, there is some evidence from case studies and retrospective reports that SGD use can have a generally positive effect on the day-to-day communication abilities of individuals with autism (Bornman & Alant, 1999; Light, Roberts, Dimarco, & Greiner, 1998; Mirenda, Wilk, & Carson, 2000).

Cumulatively, this growing research base is encouraging and should alleviate previous concerns about the appropriateness of speech-output technology with this population (see Schlosser, 2003c, for additional information about research on the use of SGDs in general).

DEVELOPMENTAL APRAXIA OF SPEECH

Description and Characteristics

The term *developmental apraxia of speech* (DAS; also known as childhood apraxia of speech, childhood verbal apraxia, and childhood dyspraxia, among other terms) has been used since the 1970s to refer to children with articulation errors who also have difficulty with volitional or imitative production of speech sounds and sequences (Bernthal & Bankson, 1988). Aram and Nation (1982) listed a number of behavioral symptoms commonly attributed to children with DAS. These include a difference between voluntary and involuntary use of speech articulators, difficulty in selection and sequencing of phonological articulatory movements, slow improvement with traditional articulation treatment, fine and gross motor incoordination and nonfocal neurological findings, and frequent oral apraxia. Some researchers view DAS as "just another motor problem" (Robin, 1992, p. 19; see also Guyette & Diedrich, 1981, and Nijland, Maassen, & van der Meilen, 2003) that requires treatment focused on teaching the child to use the articulators consistently and accurately. Others suggest that DAS is an impairment of immature lexical stress (Shriberg, Aram, & Kwiatowski, 1997a, 1997b, 1997c) or emphasize a range of motor, phonological, and/or linguistic symptoms, suggesting that a "multifocal" intervention be directed at several aspects (e.g., Aram & Nation, 1982; Velleman & Strand, 1994).

To further complicate matters, DAS is often associated with other impairments, including intellectual disability and neuromuscular disorders (Hall, Jordan, & Robin, 1992). Individuals with DAS often have deficits in both receptive and expressive language even when speech improves as a result of either maturation or treatment (Lewis, Freebairn, Hansen, Iyengar, & Taylor, 2004). In addition, the difficulties with motor planning during volitional nonspeech activities may account for the disorders found in many of these children in areas such as reading, spelling, and writing (Aram & Nation, 1982; Lewis et al., 2004). Shriberg (1994) estimated the incidence of speech delay plus DAS as 1–2 cases per 1,000, with 80%–90% of these being males. They often come from families with a history of speech and/or language problems (Lewis et al., 2004). Because the speech of children with severe DAS may not be intelligible enough to meet their daily communication needs at home or in school, they may be candidates for communication augmentation.

A series of brief "Letters to Parents" of children with DAS was published in the April 2000 issue of *Language, Speech, and Hearing Services in Schools*. In plain language, the letters explain the speech characteristics, nature, and causes of DAS, as well as associated problems and treatment approaches (Hall, 2001a, 2001b, 2001c, 2001d).

Unique AAC Issues

AAC as a Secondary Strategy

The goal of AAC is to support the child's attempts to communicate successfully, until such time as (hopefully) speech is adequate to meet ongoing communication needs. One of the major concerns voiced by parents and others is whether the provision of AAC techniques to individuals with DAS will inhibit their speech production. A number of case studies have offered evidence that should alleviate this concern (Bornman, Alant, & Meiring, 2001; Culp, 1989; Cumley, 1997; Cumley & Swanson, 1999). While speech may not improve as a result of AAC use (Bornman et al., 2001), it does not appear to decrease to a significant degree and may improve over time. For example, Cumley (1997) reported the results of an activity-based AAC intervention directed at young children with DAS during play activities with an adult. He analyzed the level and type of comprehensible communicative behaviors across different modalities, among other variables. He found that the children who used their AAC displays most frequently were those who had the most severe speech disorders, relative to the entire group. The availability of the AAC displays did not inhibit speech production but replaced the children's use of gestures with a more symbolic form of communication, thus raising their likelihood of being more comprehensible. When AAC displays were provided to the children with "less severe DAS," they continued to use either spoken words and/or gestures as their primary modes of communication and used the AAC displays only as secondary strategies.

Of course, it goes without saying that intensive work to improve natural speech production should be part of every intervention for children with DAS. As Blackstone noted, "Every intelligible word/phrase is worth it" (1989c, p. 4). Speech therapy is often focused on teaching children with DAS to put sounds together into fluent, smooth utterances and remediating the incorrect prosodic elements of speech (see Huntley Bahr, Velleman, & Ziegler, 1999). Several natural speech treatment approaches for DAS incorporate AAC techniques such as gestures in conjunction with speech. These include movement techniques such as arm swinging (Yoss & Darley, 1974) and conventional gestures (Klick, 1985). Klick (1994) described the successful use of what she termed an *adapted cuing technique*, in which manual cues that reflect the shape of the oral cavity, the articulatory placement and movement pattern, and the manner in which a sound is produced are presented with the speech sounds. Similarly, a touch cue method (Bashir, Grahamjones, & Bostwick, 1984) and the Prompts for Restructuring Oral Muscular Phonetic Targets (PROMPT©) system (Hayden & Square, 1994) incorporate systematic manual-tactile cues to the face concurrent with speech to elicit specific sounds in therapy sessions.

Additional information about speech interventions for DAS is available through Apraxia-Kids and PROMPT© Institute Web sites. Information about DAS and Down syndrome is available in the December 2002 issue of *Disability Solutions* (Kumin, 2002).

Manual signing has also been used to promote speech development. For example, the efficacy of "melodic intonation therapy" was reported for two children with DAS (Helfrich-Miller, 1994). This multiphasic technique involves the use of manual signs (in this case, Signed English) with intoned phonemic sequences, and the technique was reported to result in a gradual decrease in articulation and sequencing errors over the course of training. Similarly positive results were reported as a result of "signed target phoneme" therapy, in which fingerspelled letters from American Sign Language are paired with difficult sounds during therapy (Shelton & Garves, 1985).

Multimodal Communication

As noted previously, children whose speech is largely unintelligible may benefit, at least in a practical sense, from an intervention package that includes AAC techniques. Children with DAS may show evidence of significant language delays that can be traced (at least hypothetically) to their inability to "practice" language in their early years (Stromswold, 1994). Delayed language development is a high price to pay while either waiting for speech to develop naturally or devoting 99% of the available therapy time to speech intervention. Rather, it is critically important to provide children with DAS with one or more appropriate AAC modalities from an early age so that they have ample opportunities to use and "play" with language. For example, Cumley and Swanson (1997) provided a case study example of a preschool child with DAS whose mean length of utterance increased from 2.6 words per utterance without AAC to 4.6 words per utterance with AAC supports. These included a speech-generating device (SGD) with Picture Communication Symbols on activity displays.

From the outset, multimodal AAC systems for individuals with DAS are likely to include at least gestures and visuospatial (i.e., pictorial) symbols in addition to manual signs, if these are appropriate. Children whose fine motor abilities are not compromised (i.e., children without accompanying limb apraxia) may benefit from a total communication approach (speech plus manual signs) or one that incorporates the use of highly iconic gestures, such as Amer-Ind (Crary, 1987). Motivation for communicating may also be increased through the use of pictures or other symbols that are visual and concrete in nature (Haynes, 1985).

Nonelectronic communication/conversation books, miniboards, wallets, and other formats are often useful as well (Blackstone, 1989c; Bornman et al., 2001). The advantage of these techniques, particularly if they incorporate line drawings or orthographic symbol output, is that they are often more intelligible to unfamiliar communication partners than are manual signs. The main disadvantages are the vocabulary and portability constraints that they can impose on the person communicating through AAC. Kravitz and Littman (1990) emphasized the importance of providing an adequate number of vocabulary items, noting that for many DAS individuals with whom they have worked, communication books are often nonfunctional unless they have 400–500 items. In terms of motor ability, individuals with DAS can almost always manage multiple overlays and pages, so extensive vocabulary displays can be carried, worn, or strategically placed in the environment.

Careful, flexible combinations of aided and unaided approaches can be effective in enhancing the advantages and minimizing the disadvantages of each approach. For example, Blockberger and Kamp (1990) reported the use of multimodal systems consisting of natural speech, gestures, manual signs, and SGDs with school-age children with DAS. The children and their families generally preferred to use unaided approaches and only resorted to aided techniques when communication breakdowns occurred. Kravitz and Littman (1990) provided another example in their discussion of an adult with DAS, among other impairments. This woman used sign language to exchange basic information rapidly, whereas she used her communication book primarily to achieve social closeness and to engage in more elaborate conversational interactions. She also used a simple SGD in specific situations such as introducing herself to new people, asking for assistance at the bank, or ordering at fast-food restaurants.

It is important to remember to plan ahead to make aided AAC techniques portable and easy to manage because most individuals with DAS are ambulatory. One child with DAS who was provided with a multimodal system consisting of natural speech, gestures, manual signs, and a communication book relied primarily on the first three of these techniques, largely because of the lack of portability of her communication book (Culp, 1989). Some alternative techniques that may help to circumvent the lack of portability include communication miniboards mounted on walls, mealtime place mats, car dashboards, refrigerators, bathtub tiles—in short, mounted in any and all of the places the child may go, so that opportunities and vocabulary for communication are abundantly available (Blackstone, 1989c). SGDs can be transported using shoulder straps, carrying cases, or briefcases.

I wanted to let everyone know how wonderful Kennedy is doing. A few weeks ago, she had said a few two-word phrases, but then I never heard them again. This past Tuesday she started talking in two-word phrases (*want, more,* and *got,* combined with every single word she has). We have no more single words now. She is now talking in all two-word phrases! She still struggles a little and the apraxia is obvious, but she does NOT need a visual or auditory cue to produce the phrases . . . . I cannot stress enough how important it is to be doing the right type of therapy with an apraxic child. We had almost no progress for a year with language stimulation therapy. Now, with visual, tactile, and auditory cues and lots of repetition, we are on our way to sentences! We are so very proud of her! (Traci, Kennedy's mother, in the *Apraxia-Kids Monthly* newsletter, January 2003, p. 7)

Social Competence

Once a multimodal AAC system has been provided, most individuals with DAS will require specific instruction to develop specific skills related to social competence, in order to use the system efficiently and effectively (see Iacono, 2003; Light, 1989b; and Light, Arnold, & Clark, 2003). Three sets of skills are especially important for conversational interactions: strategies for topic setting, strategies for clarification and repair, and strategies for decision making about when to use which communication modality.

Strategies for topic setting are usually related to the use of natural speech, which is almost always the child's mode of choice even when intelligibility is poor. The difficulty is that when the child attempts to introduce a new topic of conversation with one or more poorly articulated words, the communication partner is required to guess what the word is from a virtual universe of possibilities. If the child can narrow the range of possibilities by referring to a topic card, conversation book, or other option (see Chapter 11), his or her communication partner may find it easier to guess the spoken words that are difficult to understand.

Clarification and repair strategies include repetition, rephrasing, adding or changing communication modes, using a cuing display (e.g., first sounds, rhyming words), gesturing, using body language/pantomime, and pointing to environmental cues (Blackstone, 1989c). Instructions for communication partners concerning useful ways to resolve breakdowns are often necessary and beneficial as well (e.g., "Try asking me the question another way"). Finally, the child may need to learn a decision-making strategy regarding when to use manual signs, a communication book, or an electronic aid. For example, Reichle and Ward (1985) taught an adolescent to point to the orthographic message "Do you use sign language?" when asked a question by an unfamiliar person and then to use either manual signs or his SGD, depending on the partner's response.

I just wanted to let everyone know that my son Samuel, 10 years old, just gave his first ever oral report in school. It was on the planet Mercury, and he had a wonderful model and used cards for guidance, but didn't read word-for-word off the cards. I wish I had been there! I can tell he was very proud of himself and was waiting for people to come by at the planet fair and ask him questions. The school principal spent some time giving him attention, too. By contrast, last year in third grade his oral biography project was taped sentence-by-sentence at home, and then he played the tape to the class, and gave the oral report just to the speech therapist. What a difference in a year! He has grown and matured so very far. Now, as long as he speaks loudly enough, he is clear enough to be understood almost all the time. With more time and confidence, I now feel that he may not automatically present as someone with a speech disorder the rest of his life. (Trina, Samuel's mother, in the *Apraxia-Kids Monthly* newsletter, March 2004, p. 5)

Parent Support

As noted previously, parents (and some clinicians) are often reluctant to augment verbal communication "too soon," for fear that speech will fail to progress if other communication modes are available. Furthermore, parents may assume that a decision to augment communication is tantamount to "giving up on speech" or may be unable to understand why AAC interventions are recommended for an otherwise healthy, intact child. Sensitive but systematic parent counseling is often necessary to adequately discuss these issues and to assure family members that the intention is to augment communication in the truest sense of the word rather than to replace speech. It may be useful to have parents visit classrooms where other children are using AAC systems so that they can see for themselves how various components can be integrated into efforts to enhance natural speech. In addition, parents and other primary communication partners will usually require input related to strategies that facilitate communication interactions once the decision to augment speech has been made. Such efforts may require considerable time and energy on the part of the clinician and should be geared to increasing the parents' understanding of the nature of communication and the importance of supporting the child's efforts in this regard. Blackstone (1989c) provided additional suggestions about parent support strategies.

Closely related to the issue of parent counseling is that of when intervention should begin. If the family or clinician views the decision to augment communication for a child with DAS as a last resort, there will almost always be great reluctance to initiate such an intervention with very young, preschool-age children (see Cress & Marvin, 2003). Unfortunately, the child may enter kindergarten or first grade unequipped to deal with the extensive written and spoken communication demands of an academic setting. For example, because many of these children also exhibit fine motor planning problems that affect handwriting abilities, they may be at risk for problems with learning to read and spell because these areas appear to be closely intertwined (Gloeckler & Simpson, 1988). Obviously, if the child with DAS is mildly affected, augmentative writing or verbal expression techniques may not be necessary. However, AAC teams should consider providing children who have more severe conditions with augmentation in these areas even prior to entering school, to ensure that their verbal and fine motor planning problems do not stand in the way of academic proficiency.

CHAPTER 10

AAC STRATEGIES FOR BEGINNING COMMUNICATORS

Opportunity and Nonsymbolic Interventions

In this chapter and in Chapter 11, we use the term *beginning communicators* to refer to individuals *across the age range* who have one or more of the following characteristics:

- They rely primarily on nonsymbolic modes of communication such as gestures, vocalizations, eye gaze, and body language. Use of these modalities may be either intentional or unintentional.

- They are learning to use aided or unaided symbols to represent basic messages for communicative functions such as requesting, rejecting, sharing information, and engaging in conversations.

- They use nonelectronic communication displays or simple technologies (e.g., switches and electronic devices with limited message capabilities) for participation and communication.

Beginning communicators may be young children with various types of disabilities whose communication is developing in accordance with their chronological ages. They may be children, adolescents, or adults with one or more developmental disabilities such as cerebral palsy, autism, dual sensory impairments, intellectual disabilities, or developmental apraxia of speech. They may be individuals who are in the early stages of recovery following acquired brain injury or some other neurological trauma. Regardless of their ages or the etiologies of their communication impairments, they require support to learn that, through communication, they can have a positive impact on their environments and the people around them. In this chapter, we discuss interventions for beginning communicators that are related to opportunity barriers and nonsymbolic communication; in Chapter 11, we discuss strategies for symbolic communication.

Many terms have been used in the child language literature to refer to what we term "nonsymbolic communication." These include partner-perceived communication (Wilcox, Bacon, & Shannon, 1995), non- or prelinguistic communication (Wetherby, Warren, & Reichle, 1998), perlocutionary communication (Bates, 1979), and early AAC behaviors (Siegel & Cress, 2002). What these terms have in common is that they refer to both intentional and unintentional signals, and to both conventional and unconventional behaviors, that do not involve the use of symbolic modes of communication such as pictures, manual signs, or printed words.

Relationship Between Communication and Problem Behavior

It is not unusual for individuals who are beginning communicators to engage in non-symbolic behaviors that create unique challenges for those with whom they live, learn, play, and/or work. These might include problem behaviors such as tantrums, hitting, screaming, pushing, various forms of self-injurious behavior, and many others. Numerous authors have suggested that most problem behavior can be interpreted as communicative in nature and treated as such (Carr et al., 1994; Donnellan, Mirenda, Mesaros, & Fassbender, 1984; Durand, 1990; Reichle & Wacker, 1993). Throughout this chapter, communication interventions related to individuals who exhibit problem behavior are discussed in the context of other communication interventions.

Three important principles are common to both nonsymbolic and symbolic communication interventions for problem behavior. First is the *principle of functional equivalence:* Often, the most appropriate intervention involves teaching the individual an alternative behavior that serves the same function as the problem behavior. This means that interventionists must undertake a comprehensive, functional behavior assessment to identify the current function(s) of the behavior(s) of concern, so that they can design and teach appropriate alternatives (see Carr et al., 1994; Durand, 1990; and O'Neill et al., 1997, for examples of functional assessment procedures). For example, if the function of the behavior is to get attention, the new behavior must result in attention; or if the current behavior allows the individual to avoid nonpreferred events, the new behavior must also allow the individual to accomplish this.

A number of Internet resources on functional behavior assessment are available through the Center for Effective Collaboration and Practice, the Elearning Design Lab, and the Rehabilitation Research and Training Center on Positive Behavior Support.

The second principle, called the *principle of efficiency and response effectiveness*, states that people communicate in the most efficient and effective manner available to them at any given point in time. This means that the alternative behavior must be at least as easy for the individual to produce as is the problem behavior and must also be as effective in obtaining the desired outcome. If the new behavior is more difficult or less effective, the old behavior will persist. Finally, the third principle is the *principle of goodness-of-fit*, which says that sometimes the most appropriate response to problem behavior is to create a better "fit" between the person and his/her environment. This usually requires altering relevant aspects of the environment, based on the results of the functional assessment described previously. A recent published example of this principle involved a man named Christos, who was labeled as having autism, seizure disorders, and rapid-cycling bipolar mood disorder, in addition to complex communication needs (Magito-McLaughlin, Mullen-James, Anderson-Ryan, & Carr, 2002). He engaged in frequent, highly disruptive problem behaviors including self-injury, aggression toward others, property destruction, and running away. A functional behavior assessment revealed that virtually all of Christos's behaviors were aimed at enabling him to escape or avoid nonpreferred environmental or social events (e.g., crowding; overheating; large, male staff; lack of access to community activities). When Christos's environment was altered to achieve a better "fit" with his needs and preferences, the rate and intensity of his problem behaviors decreased dramatically. Some of the interventions used in this regard included moving him to his own apartment with support, hiring Greek-speaking staff who shared his interests, teaching him self-control and communication skills, providing him with a visual schedule so he could predict upcoming events, and getting him more involved in preferred activities with his family and community.

Unfortunately, many people with severe disabilities—like Christos—live in isolated, noninteractive environments; engage primarily in boring, nonpreferred tasks; and are forced to adhere to rigidly structured schedules over which they have no control or choice on a daily basis (see Brown, 1991). As Carr, Robinson, and Palumbo (1990) noted in their eloquent discussion of this issue, the appropriate response in such situations is to focus on changing the environment or the sequence of events, not the person. As we learn more and more about the relationship between behavior and communication, it becomes increasingly important to remember that it is critical to provide opportunities for communication and control in the context of meaningful, interactive activities and environments.

The Participation Model and a Tri-Focus Framework for Intervention

Siegel and her colleagues have described a *Tri-Focus Framework* of interactive influences that affect interactions involving individuals who communicate nonsymbolically (Siegel & Bashinski, 1997; Siegel & Cress, 2002; Siegel & Wetherby, 2000). This framework as it relates to intervention is represented in Figure 10.1, and consists of environmental, partner, and learner components. Within the Participation Model, these correspond to communication opportunities (environmental contexts), facilitator skills (partners), and AAC interventions for supporting and building intentional, nonsymbolic communication (learners).

Both the communication opportunity component of the Participation Model (see Figure 6.1) and the environment component of the Tri-Focus Framework (see Figure 10.1) refer to the contexts in which communication occurs. Within the Participation Model, AAC planning and implementation require assessment of the individual's participation and communication needs in natural contexts such as community, home, and school environments. As we discussed in Chapter 6, the Participation Model requires that

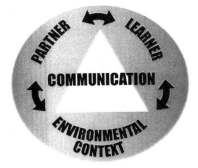

Figure 10.1. Tri-Focus Framework of interactive influences that affect interactions involving individuals who communicate non-symbolically. (Copyright © 2001 Ellin B. Siegel, used with permission.)

the participation patterns of typically developing peers in relevant environments first be assessed for comparison. The participation patterns of the target individual are then assessed in the same contexts and compared with those of the peer. Finally, interventions are designed to increase the participation levels of the target individual to match peer levels more closely. For infants and toddlers, this requires analyzing the interaction patterns of peers in home and community settings. When dealing with preschoolers and school-age children, teams also need to conduct this kind of examination in the classroom. When dealing with adults who are beginning communicators, teams should perform participation analyses in home, community, and work environments. In the sections that follow, we provide specific strategies for minimizing or eliminating opportunity barriers that were identified during assessment; and, in the spirit of Siegel's Tri-Focus Framework, the optimal environmental arrangements to support beginning communicators across the age range.

> I am eternally grateful that M could get [his speech-generating device, SGD] one year before entering grade one, although I wish it was one year earlier. I would like to recommend that children start with the [SGD] from at least the age of three years. The earlier they experience themselves speakers, the better . . . .
> (M's mother, in Bornman, Alant, & Meiring, 2001, p. 631)

YOUNG CHILDREN

Early Intervention Philosophy

A number of principles guide augmentative and alternative communication (AAC) interventions for young children. First, AAC teams should be aware that norm-referenced assessment tools cannot accurately and meaningfully measure the abilities of children with complex sensory, motor, and speech problems. Thus, it is important not to put undue credence in the results of such assessments, especially if observation provides information and impressions that are contradictory to the test results. Second, it is critical to build on young children's strengths rather than focus on their impairments. Finally, AAC interventions with young children should operate under the assumption that *all* children have the potential to make significant skill gains.

In addition to following these basic principles, AAC teams should conduct communication interventions with the view that long-term outcome predictions are almost always inappropriate when addressing the needs of young children. Thus, without exception, strategies for supporting the development of natural speech should *always* be included in communication interventions for this age group. Similarly, teams should include strategies for supporting the development of literacy skills (e.g., reading, writing) in all intervention plans, even for children who may seem unlikely to acquire such skills. In addition, AAC professionals should base their intervention strategies on the assumption that general kindergarten placement is the goal for *all* young children, although some may need supports in order to participate optimally in this setting. This aggressive approach can result only in positive outcomes for the child and will guard against the all-too-frequent later realization that a child with many skill deficits might have been able to develop a number of skills if he or she had received communication opportunities in the early years. Interventions designed to increase communication opportunities as well as those designed to teach specific communication and social interaction skills are usually necessary for positive outcomes.

Early Intervention Services

During the first few years of a child's life, his or her primary caregivers usually deliver early intervention services in the home. Family members generally learn to provide appropriate inputs and supports, including those related to communication, from teachers and therapists who visit the home regularly. Starting at approximately 3 years of age, the child usually attends a preschool program for at least part of the day, where he or she receives direct services from professional staff. The type of preschool program may vary greatly; for example, it may accommodate only children with disabilities or may serve primarily typically developing children.

> For young children with disabilities, "peer-related social competence is clearly aligned with issues of personal independence and . . . . personal choice. The ability to achieve successfully and appropriately interpersonal goals involving one's peers is empowering in perhaps the most meaningful sense of the term." (Guralnick, 2001, p. 496)

There is no doubt that preschool environments that include at least some typically developing children are vastly preferable to segregated classrooms for social interaction and communication (Romski, Sevcik, & Forrest, 2001). In this chapter and subsequent chapters, we assume that some amount of regular, systematic integration with peers without disabilities exists in the preschool setting, and, if it does not, this should be recognized as an opportunity barrier and targeted for remediation. We also use the generic term *children* to refer to the people targeted for early intervention, although this may include infants, toddlers, and preschoolers, depending on the intervention discussed.

Communication Opportunities

Table 10.1 displays an example of a participation analysis and intervention plan for a preschool-age child's daytime activities. In this example, the AAC team identified discrepancies between the participation patterns and teachers' expectations of the target student and other children. The team then designed assistive device and environmental adaptations to reduce discrepancies at certain times in the child's day, such as during music and pretend-play time. The team identified the need for both adaptations and instructional modifications (e.g., adapting toys with Velcro) during a range of activities. In all cases, the basic principle of the Participation Model is reflected: The first step to increasing communication is to increase meaningful participation in natural contexts.

Table 10.1.   Sample participation analysis and intervention plan for a preschool-age child

Activity	How do peers participate? (What is expected?)	How does child participate?	Intervention plan
Music (group)	Choose songs, sing repetitive parts of songs, put record on player, do hand or body movements to songs	Does not choose or sing, does not put on record, does hand and body movements with aide's assistance, mostly sits and watches/listens	Provide taped songs that child can turn on with a switch to sing along, provide picture symbols representing songs so she can choose, continue to imitate hand/body movements with aide
Snacktime (group)	Wash hands with help, sit down, ask for snack item, ask for drink, ask for help as needed, eat/drink appropriately, take dirty plate/cup to sink and rinse, wash hands/face with help	Washes hands and sits with help; does not ask for snack, drink, or help; needs help to eat and drink; does not take or rinse plate/cup at sink; hands and face washed by aide	Provide real object choices of two snacks and drink options; look for eye gaze or reach to indicate choice; talk to physical therapist about facilitating standing at sink so she can participate in cleanup routine
Pretend-play time (solo or small group)	Doll play in kitchen or grooming area, block and car play, dress up play: children expected to play appropriately with peers while teacher encourages verbal language according to IEP goals	Tues. & Thurs.: sits in wheelchair and watches peers play in an area; Mon., Wed., & Fri.: practices switch use with battery-operated toys (solo)	Encourage peers to use her lap tray as a play surface, adapt toys with Velcro so she can pick up with adapted Velcro glove, use Fisher-Price stove and sink on lap tray instead of large play kitchen furniture, adapt battery-operated blender and mixer for switch activation, use activity frame to display small items within reach

Some of the basic strategies for accomplishing this in preschool settings are summarized in the sections that follow.

Creating Predictable Routines at Home and in the Preschool Classroom

Daily living routines can provide many opportunities for communication, if caregivers help structure them with this purpose in mind. In most homes and classrooms, routines such as dressing, bathing, eating, and changing the child's position occur at regular times and intervals throughout the day. If this is not the case, these routines should be regularized as much as possible so that the child can begin to anticipate their occurrence. In addition, caregivers should perform routines in roughly the same sequence each time so that the child can begin to anticipate what happens next. Whenever possible, caregivers should allow sufficient time to carry out the routine so that contextual communication instruction can occur concurrently with the activity. Specific strategies for using regular, predictable routines to teach communication skills (e.g., using scripted routines) are discussed later in this chapter.

Adaptive Play

Because the primary "business" of young children is play, their primary communicative opportunities occur in play contexts. By increasing participation in play activities, we automatically increase the quality and quantity of communication opportunities (Brodin, 1991). Play is an intrinsic activity that is "done for its own sake, rather than as a means to achieving any specific end . . . . [It is also] spontaneous and voluntary, undertaken by choice rather than by compulsion . . . . Play includes an element of enjoyment, something that is done for fun" (Musselwhite, 1986, pp. 3–4). Unfortunately, when play skills are taught in classrooms, these characterizations of play are often ignored—and play becomes, quite literally, the child's "work." This is not to imply that educators cannot use play as a vehicle to promote the development of gross motor, fine motor, social, cognitive, self-help, and (of course) communication skills. In fact, whenever possible, it is desirable to "telescope" goals and activities by working on one primary and one or more secondary goals simultaneously in a play context. For example, a "dress the doll" activity might provide a context within which a child can practice fine motor skills related to dressing, as well as social and communication skills with peers. What is critical is that the activity remain *playful* and not become one in which toys are used as vehicles for work. This requires careful selection of play materials and the ways they are used.

In order for play activities to foster the development of communication skills, parents and educators must select toys and play materials with interaction goals in mind. For example, some types of toys (e.g., blocks, balls, toy vehicles, puppets) have been found to be more facilitative of peer interactions than others that are primarily used in solitary play (e.g., books, paper and crayons, play dough, puzzles) (Beckman & Kohl, 1984). Other important considerations in selecting a toy include safety, durability, motivational value for children with various types of disabilities, attractiveness, and reactivity (Musselwhite, 1986). Reactivity refers to the extent to which the toy "does something" (e.g., produces sound, sustains movement, creates a visual display). Research has demonstrated that young children with severe disabilities engage in longer periods of manipulative play with reactive toys than with nonreactive toys (Bambara, Spiegel-McGill, Shores, & Fox, 1984). Finally, parents and teachers should select toys for realistic and imaginative play so that children have opportunities to engage in both concrete and pretend (i.e., symbolic) play.

Another way to increase the probability that children will play with toys is to make them easy to hold, carry, and manipulate. This is particularly important for children with motor impairments because the quality of early communication and the motor ability to manipulate objects appear to be related (Granlund & Olsson, 1987). Numerous play adaptations can be made at home or at school, including activity frames, adjustable easels, learning boxes, play boxes, and other means of stabilizing and presenting manipulable toys so that they are accessible to children with limited hand and arm control. Toys can also be attached to lap trays with Velcro or elastic cords so they are within reach. Books can be adapted with small foam or carpet tape squares pasted on the corners to separate pages for easier turning (these are often called "page fluffers"). Small magnets or squares of Velcro can be attached to toys so that the child can then pick them up with a headstick or mitten affixed with the same material. Toys with movable parts (e.g., levers, knobs) can be adapted with plastic or Velcro extenders for children with sensory or motor impairments. Figure 10.2 illustrates some of the many possible toy adaptations.

The World Wide Web features a number of excellent on-line resources focused on adapting toys and increasing meaningful communication participation in pre-school settings for young children with disabilities. Some of these include Creative Communicating, AAC Intervention, Let's Play!, Do2Learn, and Simplified Technology.

If a child with motor impairments has access to battery-operated toys and appliances (e.g., blenders, slide projectors), these also will require adaptation so that he or she can operate them successfully. Parents and school staff can either purchase the switches through commercial distributors or manufacturers or construct them inexpensively at home or at school using readily available components (e.g., see http://www.lburkhart.com/handouts.htm). Playing with battery-operated toys should serve as the means to an end (i.e., participation), not as an end in itself. All too often, children with motor or other impairments can be found sitting in the corner of a classroom with a paraprofessional, playing with a battery-operated toy and a microswitch while the other preschoolers are having fun playing house, garage, or dress-up! Unfortunately, this poor practice is often compounded when teachers provide a child with only one or two battery-operated toys for switch activation, apparently under the assumption that a monkey (or a bear, or a dog) hitting a drum (or crashing a pair of cymbals, or riding a car) is so fascinating that it will sustain the child's attention for an extended period of time, day after day! None of these practices reflect an understanding of the principles of child development in general, the Participation Model, or the appropriate use of microswitch technology, and they are almost certain to result in the widespread lament, "We spent all that money to buy a switch

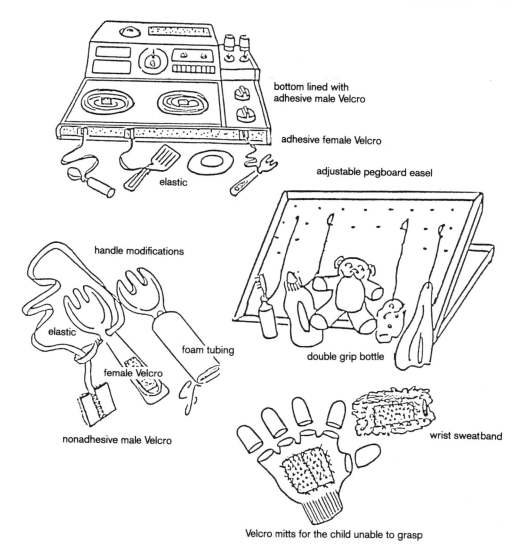

bottom lined with
adhesive male Velcro

adhesive female Velcro

adjustable pegboard easel

elastic

handle modifications

elastic

female Velcro

foam tubing

double grip bottle

nonadhesive male Velcro

wrist sweatband

Velcro mitts for the child unable to grasp

Figure 10.2.   Examples of toy play adaptations that can be made at home or at school. (From Goossens', C. [1989]. Aided communication intervention before assessment: A case study of a child with cerebral palsy. *Augmentative and Alternative Communication, 5,* 17; reprinted by permission of Taylor & Francis Ltd, http://www.tandf.co.uk/journals.)

and a toy and the child is bored with it after 2 minutes!" Table 10.2 summarizes some suggestions for using microswitches to enhance participation in home and preschool activities for children.

Communication opportunities can also arise or be created in the context of music, movement, puppetry, acting, and other fine arts activities for young children. Like other play activities, these may require adaptations in order to be accessible to children with disabilities. For example, many songs can be adapted so they are easily represented through manual signs or pictorial symbols and incorporated throughout the preschool day. Music-movement activities (e.g., fingerplay songs such as "Where Is Thumbkin?") and gross

Table 10.2. Suggestions for using microswitch technology to enhance participation of preschoolers

Environment	Activity	Participation via microswitch technology
School	Transition from one activity to another	Child activates switch attached to a cassette tape recorder with a recorded tape of the teacher singing the cleanup song or saying, "Time to get ready for x," or whatever the verbal transition routine usually is.
	Snacktime	Child uses a switch to operate a toy car or truck that "delivers" the snack of the day to each of his or her friends at the table.
	Free playtime	Child uses a switch to operate simple computer game with a peer (e.g., Interaction Games, Don Johnston, Inc.). Child controls a battery-operated toy in play interaction with a peer.
Home/school	Playtime	Child in a crib accidentally activates a switch placed near a mobile body part to turn on a toy that provides stimulating and enjoyable feedback (e.g., a light display, a music tape, a mobile).
	Music time	Child activates a switch to turn on a sing-along tape or a prerecorded tape of a same-gender child singing his or her part in a song.
	Pretend-play time	Child uses a switch to activate a battery-operated car, truck, robot, toy blender, or toy mixer, depending on the theme of the pretend play.
	Art time	Child uses switch to operate a broken record player (no arm or needle) with paper affixed to the turntable and a blob of paint placed on the paper to make a swirly design pattern. Child provides power for electric scissors used by a peer or adult to cut paper.
	Storytime	Child uses a switch to operate a recorded tape of an adult reading the "story of the day," as he or she looks at the book to read along.
	Cooking	Child operates a blender with a switch to make a milkshake, uses a mixer to make cake batter, or uses a food processor to make salad.

motor games (e.g., Red Light, Green Light) are also excellent vehicles for teaching basic cognitive/communication skills such as following directions, imitation, sequencing, and concept development. However, many standard movement activities and songs require one or more of the following modifications to be used for communication purposes: 1) simplifying target movements so that the child can participate meaningfully (this is also a good place to incorporate movement goals identified by motor therapists); 2) slowing the speed of the song/activity; 3) making directions shorter, simpler, and more repetitive; 4) simplifying the vocabulary; 5) pairing words with manual signs; 6) accompanying movements with sounds or words to encourage speech; and 7) including visual aids or concrete materials for children who do not yet engage in pretend play (Musselwhite, 1985). Arts activities such as acting (Stuart, 1988) and puppetry (Musselwhite, 1985) can also serve to create communication opportunities. For example, the teacher can attach a puppet to the child's foot or wrist rather than to his or her hand, or the child's wheelchair can be decorated so that it can be used as a prop or stage in a play or puppet show.

Sherazad is a 4-year-old Indo-Canadian girl who lives with her mother, father, and brother. She is ventilator-dependent as a result of a high spinal cord injury from a fall when she was 2 years old. She cannot speak and depends on others for all of her personal care needs. She is learning to use a sip-and-puff switch in the context of daily activities at home and in her preschool. For example, with her switch she can turn the lights on and off in the classroom; turn music on and off during music time; help to make blender drinks daily during snacktime; and play adapted versions of Candy Land, Chutes and Ladders, and other children's games using a battery-operated "spinner" attached to her switch. Paper templates with colored or numbered sections are fitted under the spinner dial. When she sips on her switch, the spinner spins around and when she puffs, it stops. Her game partner then moves her token to the color or the number of spaces selected (Canfield & Locke, 1997). She can also play computer games with her friends; operate a battery-operated toy mixer, blender, and microwave during "house play" time; tell the teacher to turn the pages of a book during storytime by activating a small communication device with a single recorded message; and operate electric scissors and a hot glue gun to make art projects with a helper during art time. Once Sherazad enters kindergarten, she will use the switch to type letters and words with an AAC device at the same time that her classmates learn to write letters with pencil and paper.

SCHOOL-AGE INDIVIDUALS

Where do typically developing children and adolescents find communication opportunities, meet communication partners, and learn to communicate in a variety of ways? As most parents know, these opportunities all occur primarily at school, when children interact with classmates and other peers. However, a number of studies have shown that communication opportunities for beginning communicators may be severely limited even in schools, especially when students with significant disabilities are placed in self-contained classrooms with similar students (e.g., Rowland, 1996; Sigafoos, Roberts, Kerr, Couzens, & Baglioni, 1994). Since the mid-1980s, the school reform movement in North America and elsewhere has emphasized the importance of including students with disabilities in general education classrooms along with their typically developing peers. Research indicates that inclusive education with appropriate supports greatly increases the likelihood that students with disabilities will have numerous, daily opportunities for natural communication with a variety of partners (Hunt, Alwell, Farron-Davis, & Goetz, 1996; Katz & Mirenda, 2002).

Of course, there is no guarantee that just because students are enrolled in general education classrooms, they will be included in the educational and social milieu of the school in ways that promote communication. Sigafoos (1999) noted several factors that may limit communication opportunities, including: 1) potential communication partners may fail to recognize or make use of naturally occurring events related to communication; 2) partners may preempt communication by anticipating students' wants and needs; and 3) students with disabilities may have limited repertoires of communicative behaviors, making it less likely that others will offer them opportunities to communicate (Sigafoos, Roberts, et al., 1994). As a result of these factors, it may be necessary to engineer school environments and support teachers and paraprofessionals to create explicit opportunities for communication. Some simple strategies that can be used in this regard include withholding an item needed to complete or engage in an activity, so that the student has an opportunity to request it; interrupting an ongoing activity to create an opportunity for requesting or protesting (e.g., "Get out of my way"); providing a wrong or incomplete item in response to a request (e.g., providing part of a toy, so the child has to ask for the rest); and delaying assistance, to create the need to ask for help (Sigafoos, 1999; Sigafoos & Mirenda, 2002; Sigafoos, O'Reilly, Drasgow, & Reichle, 2002). If such strategies are used, it is important that they be incorporated as unobtrusively as possible in general education activities and contexts.

It is also important to acknowledge that inclusive education presents considerable challenges to those who provide classroom support, in that students in general education classrooms usually have a broader range of communication needs than do students in segregated situations. In general education classrooms, students need to be able to ask and answer questions on a number of topics, give reports, participate in instructional groups, and participate in a wide variety of social exchanges (Kent-Walsh & Light, 2003; Nelson, 1992). In social environments, students encounter communication opportunities that go beyond simple requesting, rejecting, and identifying wants and needs as they interact with classmates and friends. For example, if an adolescent is sitting in the cafeteria with his high school friends and one of them is helping him eat lunch, he probably does not have to communicate many wants and needs messages because his needs are already being met. Instead, he may be asked by his friends to share information about what he did last weekend or about a musical group or athletic team that he and his facilitator found on the Internet; or he might be expected to contribute to the conversation by sharing the latest teenage joke. In order for students to be fully included in social as well as educational activities, it is critically important that they have strategies for communication in areas such as information sharing, social closeness, and social etiquette (Light, 1988).

Across North America, a number of models for inclusion have been developed to assist administrators (Villa & Thousand, 2000), educators (Downing, 2002; Jorgensen, 1998), and AAC teams (Giangreco, 1996b, 2000; Rainforth & York-Barr, 1997) to accomplish these goals. The following sections summarize the primary approaches to inclusion that are especially relevant for students who communicate through AAC.

MAPs, Circles of Friends, and PATH

MAPs (Making Action Plans), Circles of Friends, and PATH (Planning Alternative Tomorrows with Hope) (Falvey, Forest, Pearpoint, & Rosenberg, 1994) are three related models that have been used primarily to facilitate the inclusion of school-age individuals with disabilities into general classroom settings, although they certainly can be used to create inclusive neighborhoods, workplaces, and other settings as well. When applied to school inclusion, these dynamic processes involve family members, school principals, both general and special education teachers, paraprofessionals, support personnel, and general class peers. The processes involve strategies for building school communities in which an individual with disabilities can be supported and develop friendships (Pearpoint, Forest, & O'Brien, 1996; Vandercook, York, & Forest, 1989). MAPs is a "collaborative planning process for action that brings together the key factors in a child's life" (Pearpoint et al., 1996, p. 68). These people can use MAPs to carefully consider a student's strengths, lifestyle, and dreams and develop a concrete plan of action for helping the student reach his or her dreams. Interventionists often use the Circles of Friends process in conjunction with MAPs to support the development of friendships among classmates and peers. Finally, PATH is an in-depth, eight-step process for helping people assist a student by solving complex individual, family, or system problems through focused planning (Pearpoint, O'Brien, & Forest, 2001). These three approaches have been used widely in many countries around the world to facilitate social inclusion in general education classrooms and in the community for children and adults.

Social Networks

A recent addition to the list of inclusion support tools is the "Social Networks" approach (Blackstone & Hunt Berg, 2003a, 2003b) that was designed specifically for use with students who use AAC. The approach is based on the Circles of Friends model (Falvey et al., 1994) and is aimed at helping educational teams to collect and interpret information that is relevant to planning AAC interventions in inclusive settings. A central element of the model involves identifying communication partners across five "circles" that constitute the social network of the person using AAC: 1) life partners (e.g., family members); 2) good friends (i.e., people with whom the person enjoys spending time and has a close relationship); 3) neighbors and acquaintances (e.g., classmates, co-workers); 4) people who are paid to interact with the individual using AAC (e.g., teachers, classrooms assistants); and 5) unfamiliar partners with whom the individual interacts occasionally (e.g., shopkeepers, community helpers). This tool provides a comprehensive approach for both recognizing areas of strength and identifying areas that require skill development across the five "circles."

COACH and VISTA

COACH (Choosing Outcomes and Accommodations for Children, Second Edition; Giangreco, Cloninger, & Iverson, 1998) and VISTA (Vermont Interdependent Services Team Approach; Giangreco, 1996b) are two related approaches for developing individual education plans (IEPs) and assisting educational teams to develop collaborations for implementing IEPs in inclusive classrooms. COACH is a process in which family members and others are interviewed by a member of the educational team to identify a long-term vision for the student as well as annual educational goals. Interventionists then identify members of the educational team who will implement the plan, and program content is defined in a format that facilitates implementation in general classrooms and other settings. VISTA picks up where COACH leaves off and provides alternative ways for the student's educational support team to integrate related services (e.g., speech-language pathology, occupational and/or physical therapy) in general education classrooms. Research on COACH indicates that it is highly rated by parents, teachers, and educational "experts" along a number of dimensions, when it is used as intended. In particular, use of COACH appears to facilitate the provision of natural supports by peers (see Giangreco, 1996a, for a summary of COACH research). A number of studies examining VISTA provide support for its usefulness in assisting educational teams to work together collaboratively, increase parent and general education teacher involvement, and avoid service gaps and overlaps, among other outcomes (Giangreco, 2000). When used together, these tools can be very useful in assisting professionals in creating meaningful communication opportunities for students who use AAC in general education classrooms.

> If she needs something, if she needs help opening the paint, she'll tap one of the other kids and hand them the jar like, "You know, I can't get this cover off." And they have gotten so they've been as excited as I have. "Hey, Holly wants me to open it! Holly asked me to do it! She's communicating!" (A mother whose daughter was supported in an general education classroom using COACH, in Giangreco, 1996a, p. 252)

ADULTS

Since the mid-1970s, a number of authors have argued that adults who are beginning communicators, like other citizens, should be fully included in the community and should participate in the same types of vocational, recreational and leisure, and other activities as typical adults (Meyer, Peck, & Brown, 1991). In order to accomplish this, these adults must have access to a community-referenced support model, within which they can learn the skills needed to participate in activities that are age appropriate, functional (i.e., directly useful in their daily activities), taught in the actual community or vocational environments where they are needed, and taught with reference to the cues and corrections that are naturally available (Falvey, 1986; Ford & Mirenda, 1984). Such activities may occur in home, recreational and leisure, community, vocational, or school environments.

Adoption of a community-referenced approach to instruction has a direct, positive impact on the quantity and quality of the participation and communication opportunities that are available to adults who communicate through AAC. Because of increased involvement in the community, an individual may, for example, need to order food in a restaurant, cheer for the local basketball team, ask for help at the library, or chat with co-workers at break time—the list of natural opportunities for things to say and people to say them to becomes endless! Careful analysis of the settings in which the individual participates helps to identify the opportunities available for communication and to ensure that necessary adaptive and AAC techniques are included in an intervention.

The "ecological inventory" process has been used successfully for this purpose for many years, and Reichle, York, and Sigafoos (1991) described it as it applies to communication interventions. In brief, the ecological inventory process is similar to the first few steps in the Participation Model and involves the following:

- Observe a peer without disabilities engage in the activity of interest

- Write a step-by-step list of the skills required

- Assess the target individual against the skill inventory to identify discrepancies

- Design communication supports and instructional programs to teach needed skills

Figure 10.3 provides excerpts from an ecological inventory completed for an adult in a community environment, along with suggested participation and communication adaptations in discrepancy areas. AAC teams can apply this basic format to activities at home, in the workplace, or in the community. If the individual is not supported to participate in functional, age-appropriate activities in a wide variety of settings, this restriction clearly should be considered an opportunity barrier and targeted for remediation.

InterAACtion Strategies for Intentional and Unintentional Communicators (Bloomberg, West, Johnson, & Caithness, 2001) is a videotape aimed at facilitators who support adults with developmental or multiple disabilities who use AAC techniques. It is available through the Scope Communication Resource Centre in Australia.

Communication Partners

Who is there to talk to? For most adults with significant disabilities, the answer is family members; adults who are paid to be communication partners; and, perhaps, other people with disabilities. These are all perfectly *acceptable* communication partners—but they should not be the *only* communication partners. Imagine what it would be like, day after day, to communicate only with your parents, teachers, and other people who have at least as much difficulty as you do in getting messages across!

The PATH and Social Networks models that were described previously can be used very effectively with adults who use AAC to identify opportunity barriers and develop plans to address them systematically. One additional model, Person-Centered Planning (O'Brien & Lyle O'Brien, 2002), is described in the next section.

In the next decade, with advancements in knowledge and availability of AAC technology, a generation of children who successfully communicate using AAC will grow into adults with developmental disabilities . . . There will be an obligation from AAC professionals and program administrators to [ensure] that the communication gains made in childhood transfer into successful integration of AAC into the adult community. (Delsandro, 1997, p. 672)

Person-Centered Planning

The person-centered planning process emphasizes assisting supporters to "focus on opportunities for people with severe disabilities to develop personal relationships, have positive roles in community life, increase their control of their own lives, and develop the skills and abilities to achieve these goals" (Mount & Zwernik, 1988, p. 1). It can be used to facilitate community integration of individuals of all ages, but it has been particularly successful in assisting adults with disabilities to make successful transitions from institutional to community settings and from segregated community settings to more integrated ones.

Environment: Prendle's Drug Store
Target Individual: Sarah, age 20
Activity: Purchasing personal care items
Set-up: In the store with a friend who also needs to do some shopping, friend is wheeling Sarah in wheelchair

Skill (as performed by a peer without a disability)	Participation (person with a disability)			Possible participation or communication adaptations
1. Enter store.	−			Pause before entering, wait for signal indicating anticipation/acceptance.
2. Greet salesperson at jewelry counter, if present.	+ (vocalized)			In addition, consider single message loop tape with greeting that can be activated with microswitch by left hand.

	Items to Purchase			
	1	**2**	**3**	
Repeat for each item:				
3a. Walk/wheel along front of store, looking down each aisle until desired aisle is identified.	−	−	−	Encourage Sarah to look down aisle, pause and look for accept signal, proceed down aisle after signal.
3b. Walk/wheel down aisle.	−	−	−	Friend can wheel her slowly down aisle.
3c. Locate correct section.	−	−	−	As she wheels past the sections, look for an accept signal and stop.
3d. Examine options.	P	P	P	Friend can hold up two options at a time to make this easier.
3e. Choose desired item.	P	P	P	Look for eye gaze or arm movement toward one of the two options presented. If none, try another two options.
3f. Converse with friend as desired/needed.	P	−	P	Consider a multiple message loop tape with topic-setter statements that can be activated with microswitch by left hand: "Have you seen any good movies lately?"
3g. Check to see if next item is in the aisle. If yes, go to step 3a. If no, go to step 2.	−	−	−	Friend can push her down aisle again slowly, looking for signal to stop.

4. Locate checkout stand.	−			Wheel to front of store and pause within view of stand, pause and wait for a signal to proceed.
5. Greet cashier.	P (smiled slightly)			Consider single message loop tape as in Step 2.

Figure 10.3. Excerpts from an ecological inventory with suggestions for participation and communication adaptations. (Key: + = performed independently by target individual; − = not attempted by target individual; *P* = attempted.)

Skill (as performed by a peer without a disability)	Participation (person with a disability)	Possible participation or communication adaptations
6. Put items on counter.	–	Friend can do this.
7. Get out money.	–	Friend can do this.
8. Give cashier money when requested to do so.	–	Place a Velcro strap around her left hand and tuck bills under it. Have her extend her left hand toward the cashier, who can then remove the money.
9. Receive change.	–	Friend can do this.
10. Put change away.	–	Friend can do this.
11. Take bag with purchases.	–	Take bag from counter and hold in front of Sarah, and pause. Look for an accept signal and place bag on lap.
12. Exit store.	–	Pause before door, look for an accept signal, and leave store.

Person-centered planning is as much a process for organizational change as for individual planning, and consists of several basic steps. First, a "vision plan" is developed from a group interview of the "focus person" and all of the people involved in his or her life ("supporters") to gather information about past events, relationships, places, preferences, choices, ideas about the future, obstacles, and opportunities. The goal of this first step is to develop a collective vision of the future that emphasizes the person's capacities and gifts, rather than his or her impairments and problems (O'Brien & Pearpoint, n.d.). Next, the group develops both short- and long-term goals based on the vision plan. Finally, supporters make commitments of various types and levels to help the individual carry out the plan over time. Additional activities may include interactive problem solving; strategic redesign of the support system or agency to facilitate the vision plan; and other activities that facilitate harmony among the person's vision, the community opportunities available, and the system resources.

A variety of written materials and training videotapes on Circles of Friends, MAPs, PATH, and person-centered planning are available from the Marsha Forest Centre/Inclusion Press in Toronto, Ontario, Canada.

THE BOTTOM LINE

Over and over again, friends, parents, professionals, and community members have documented the incredible impact of inclusive communication opportunities—or lack thereof—on the communication abilities of people who are beginning communicators. There is simply no doubt about it: The availability of genuine and motivating communication opportunities in inclusive settings is *at least* as important to the success of a communication intervention as the availability of an appropriate access system. This is perhaps more true for people who are just learning the basics of communication than for anyone else because these individuals are among those with the fewest personal resources and the most need for assistance from others. If the communication partners of these individuals do not include a substantial number of people who are not paid to interact with them, who are not likely to leave for a new job next year, and who do not believe that their primary task is to make the individual more like everyone else, the communication interventions are almost certainly going to have a limited impact!

Once the AAC team has created communication opportunities and contexts and has identified communication partners, it can begin to plan a multimodal and multi-element approach for building communication skills. For many beginning communicators, initial interventions may be aimed at strengthening their repertoires of nonsymbolic communication behaviors.

Support Helps Others Use Technology (SHOUT) is a nonprofit society in the United States that was organized primarily to help adults who use AAC to overcome barriers related to employment. SHOUT sponsors the annual Pittsburgh Employment Conference for Augmented Communicators. In Canada, Speaking Differently is a society aimed at improving the quality of life of people who use AAC, and Speak Up is an organization devoted to giving people with complex communication needs the information, education, and means to communicate about healthy sexuality and sexual abuse. The Web sites for all three organizations are listed in the Resource section of this book.

SENSITIZING AND TRAINING FACILITATORS TO STRENGTHEN NONSYMBOLIC COMMUNICATION

The second and third components of the Tri-Focus Framework (see Figure 10.1) refer to providing supports to communication partners so that they, in turn, can better facilitate and support the nonsymbolic communication of people with complex communication needs. As mentioned in Chapter 2, we use the term *facilitator* rather than partner to refer to an individual who assumes or is assigned responsibility for supporting a person's communicative attempts.

Several studies have highlighted the importance of teaching facilitators to identify and respond to emerging communication signals of beginning communicators. For example, Houghton, Bronicki, and Guess (1987) observed 37 students with severe multiple disabilities across 12 classrooms. They coded the frequency of student initiations related to expression of preferences, as well as facilitator responses to these initiations. The results indicated that body movements and facial expressions were the most frequently observed communicative behaviors produced by the students. The students initiated such behaviors approximately once per minute in both structured and unstructured situations, but facilitators responded to these communications only 7%–15% of the time! Unfortunately, the authors of subsequent studies involving preschoolers with dual sensory impairments (Rowland, 1990) and students with severe, multiple disabilities in self-contained classrooms (Sigafoos, Roberts, et al., 1994) reported similarly dismal data. In general, these studies suggest that, in many cases, 1) facilitators may be largely unaware of or insensitive to individuals' attempts to communicate and/or 2) the constraints imposed by various contextual demands may preclude the level of facilitator attentiveness that is desirable. Regardless, the critical need for sensitization training in this area is obvious.

Another issue of concern is that facilitators who support beginning communicators may neglect to establish a strong communicative foundation before instituting AAC interventions to teach the use of symbols. When this occurs, initial interventions usually involve introducing a formal symbolic communication system that uses manual signing or pictures, even though the individual may not understand many of the basic elements of communication such as turn taking, joint attending, and the role of other people as communication partners. In typical development, early forms of communication such as gestures and vocalizations are gradually augmented by new forms and eventually result in an integrated multimodal system, which includes speech (Capone & McGregor, 2004). With a developmental model as the basis, facilitators should promote the use of natural gestures and vocalizations in a variety of natural contexts with individuals of any age who show little evidence of intentional communication. The goal of such nonsymbolic communication interventions is to build a strong foundation for the development of speech and/or symbolic AAC techniques.

Professionals at The Hanen Centre in Toronto, Ontario, have developed a number of parent/facilitator training programs with the goal of supporting communication, beginning with the earliest stages of development. For example, *More than Words* (Sussman, 1999) was designed for facilitators of children with autism spectrum disorders and *Allow Me* (Ruiter, 2000) was designed for staff and others who support adults with developmental disabilities. Information and additional resources (e.g., videotapes) are available through The Hanen Centre Web site.

Distinguishing and Responding to Intentional and Nonintentional Signals for Communication

Individuals who communicate primarily through gestures and vocalizations initially do so when the need arises, rather than in response to queries or directives from their communication partners. Initially, an individual's spontaneous signaling behavior is not intended to be communicative but simply occurs at random. When facilitators consistently interpret and respond to such behaviors as if they were intentional, the individual gradually learns to initiate them intentionally. Interpretation and responsiveness continue to be important facilitator techniques to expand communication repertoires, even after individuals begin to attach meaning to their gestures and vocalizations.

Unfortunately, although most adults are attuned to conventional gestures and vocalizations of typical children and adults, they often either ignore or misinterpret many of the more idiosyncratic behaviors exhibited by children and especially adults with disabilities (Rowland, 1990). In particular, facilitators may find it difficult to distinguish intentional from unintentional behaviors (Carter & Iacono, 2002; Iacono, Carter, & Hook, 1998), since these distinctions are often quite subtle. However, these distinctions are important so that facilitators can respond differentially to intentional rather than unintentional behaviors in order to strengthen the former, a process often referred to as *shaping*. Siegel and Cress (2002) and Carter and Iacono (2002) summarized some of the indicators of intentionality that have been noted by a number of investigators; these are displayed in Table 10.3.

> Parents rely heavily on their own intuition and ability to interpret their child . . . . [This] involves a great degree of guesswork . . . . Parents are often regarded with suspicion about the validity of their interpretations. They often hear from other people that they over-interpret the child and that their comprehension is only an expression of wishful thinking . . . . Parents have a unique competence in knowing their children and understanding their children's communication. (Brodin, 1991, p. 237)

Three of the essential building blocks of communication are spontaneous signals for getting attention, accepting, and rejecting. Even individuals who have a limited repertoire of gestural or vocal behaviors can usually be taught to communicate using signals for these purposes. Attention-getting signals are those the individual uses primarily to initiate social interactions with others, such as laughing, crying, or making eye contact. Questions such as "How does Liz let you know that she wants you to pay attention to her?" or "What does Maurice do to let you know he wants you to talk to him?" will often elicit

Table 10.3. Indicators of intentional communicative behaviors

1. Is there alternating gaze between an object (i.e., goal) and a facilitator?
2. Is there body orientation to indicate that the signal is being directed toward a facilitator?
3. When a signal is produced, is there a pause before it is repeated that might indicate the communicator is awaiting a response from a facilitator?
4. When a signal is produced and the facilitator responds, does the signal terminate?
5. When a signal is produced and the facilitator responds, does the communicator show either satisfaction or dissatisfaction with the response?
6. When a signal is produced and the facilitator fails to respond, does the communicator persist by repeating or changing the signal?
7. Is the signal ritualized (i.e., the same every time) or does it have a conventional form (e.g., pointing, shaking head)?

Sources: Siegel and Cress, 2002, and Carter and Iacono, 2002.

examples of behaviors that serve this function. Acceptance signals are those used to communicate that whatever is currently happening is tolerable, okay, or enjoyable. Familiar communication partners are usually able to describe these behaviors if asked questions such as "How do you know when Joey likes something?" or "How do you know when Quinta is happy?" Rejection signals are used to communicate that the individual finds his or her current status unacceptable, not enjoyable, or intolerable for some reason. Partners will often describe these behaviors when asked questions such as "How do you know when Leon doesn't like something?" or "How do you know when Shawna is unhappy or in pain?" Note that the ability to signal "acceptance" and "rejection" is not the same as the ability to respond to yes or no questions—the latter involves a much more sophisticated set of skills. Accept and reject signals may be overt and obvious, such as smiling, laughing, frowning, or crying, or may be very subtle, such as averted eye gaze, increased body tension, increased rate of respiration, or sudden passivity.

Most individuals are able to signal acceptance and rejection in some way, although this may be quite idiosyncratic. If clear, intentional, and socially appropriate attention-seeking, acceptance, and rejection signals are not part of an individual's communication repertoire, initial interventions should include strategies for developing these behaviors.

There's more to life than cookies. (Light, Parsons, & Drager, 2002, p. 187)

Attention-Seeking Signals for Social Interaction

Without a repertoire of behaviors for social interaction, beginning communicators may have limited opportunities to establish relationships, enjoy the company of other people, and provide others with ways of getting to know them as individuals with unique personalities and preferences. Light et al. (2002) noted that this requires parents and other caregivers to learn a number of related skills, including how to structure activities and contexts to promote social interaction; recognize and interpret the (often subtle) initiation, turn taking, and interaction behaviors of presymbolic communicators; and interact with them in mutually enjoyable, age-appropriate ways.

It is particularly important that facilitators be attuned to attention-seeking behaviors initiated by the individual. Initially, facilitators should respond to *any* intentional behaviors that are socially and culturally acceptable and appear to function to get attention, so that the person can repeatedly experience the communicative results of his or her efforts (Smebye, 1990). For example, a facilitator might respond to a behavior such as pounding on a lap tray or vocalizing loudly as an indicator of a desire for attention (Baumgart, Johnson, & Helmsteter, 1990). After a repertoire of acceptable attention-seeking behaviors has been established and is used intentionally, facilitators can then begin to limit their responses to the most desirable and frequent behaviors only.

Simple technology can serve to enhance the salience of attention-getting behaviors, especially for individuals whose behaviors are quite subtle and easily missed. For example, one study investigated the use of switch-activated attention-getting devices such as call buzzers and a single-message tape recording that said *Come here please* (Gee, Graham, Goetz, Oshima, & Yoshioka, 1991). The study used an "interrupted behavior chain" intervention to teach use of the devices to three children with significant intellectual, sensory, physical, and medical disabilities who were extremely limited in their ability to participate in daily school routines (a more extensive discussion of this teaching technique appears in Chapter 11). Teachers identified three or four routines that could be interrupted to provide opportunities during the school day for the students to use their attention-getting devices. For example, one such opportunity occurred during a transfer activity when a student, Erik, was told it was time to get out of his wheelchair, had his straps loosened and tray removed, but was not then moved. Erik's teacher waited for him to initiate a gestural or vocal behavior to call attention (e.g., extending his arms, making agitated noises, whimpering) and then prompted him to activate a switch mounted in an appropriate location and connected to one of the attention-getting devices described previously. When the device was activated after teacher prompting, the routine continued as planned (i.e., Erik was moved from the wheelchair). Over time, instructional prompts for switch activation were gradually faded using a time-delay procedure (see discussion in Chapter 11). All three students learned to activate their attention-getting switches independently across several such routines within a maximum of 63 instructional opportunities. This study demonstrated clearly that well-planned instruction using appropriate contexts and technology can result in the acquisition of at least simple communicative behaviors even by individuals with very severe disabilities.

Relationship to Problem Behavior   Unfortunately, attention-getting signals for many individuals take the form of socially unacceptable (i.e., problem) behaviors, such as screaming, grabbing, hitting, throwing tantrums, performing self-injurious behaviors, and others. Since the 1980s, a technique known as functional communication training (FCT) has been used widely in response to such behaviors. FCT involves a set of procedures designed to reduce problem behaviors by teaching functionally equivalent communication skills. FCT requires a thorough functional behavior assessment to identify the function (i.e., message) of the behavior of concern, as well as systematic instruction to teach new communicative behaviors. Mirenda (1997) and Bopp, Brown, and Mirenda (2004) reported that a large number of FCT interventions involving people who use AAC to communicate have focused on teaching alternative attention-getting behaviors. This has been accomplished by teaching use of nonsymbolic communicative behaviors such as a hand/arm tap/wave (Kennedy, Meyer, Knowles, & Shukla, 2000; Lalli, Browder, Mace, & Brown, 1993; Sigafoos & Meikle, 1996), activating a microswitch with the taped message PLEASE COME HERE (Northup et al., 1994; Peck et al., 1996), and activating an electronic communication device with messages such as I WANT TO BE WITH THE GROUP (Durand, 1993) or WOULD YOU HELP ME WITH THIS? (Durand, 1999). The AAC techniques and the specific messages that were taught varied, to match the context of the problem behaviors. Systematic teaching strategies such as prompting and fading were used to teach the new attention-getting behaviors in natural contexts, and brief attention was provided in all cases as a response. Bopp et al. (2004) provided a useful description of the key steps required to plan and implement FCT/AAC interventions for individuals with developmental disabilities.

First Things First: Early Communication for the Pre-Symbolic Child with Severe Disabilities (Rowland & Schweigert, 2004) is a manual designed for parents and professionals. It includes strategies for assessment as well as for teaching basic communication messages such as asking for more, gaining attention, and making choices. It is available from Design to Learn.

Accept/Reject Signals

The basic principles of contingent interpretation and responsiveness are also the cornerstones for building communicative signals that serve the functions of acceptance or rejection (Sigafoos & Mirenda, 2002; Sigafoos et al., 2002). Often, these signals are quite subtle; for example, an individual might not display behavior changes when he or she is content but might whimper slightly when distressed or uncomfortable. In other cases, a person might exhibit more overt indicators such as limb movements, smiling, or crying. Initially, it is necessary for facilitators to respond to and comply with any communicative behaviors that can be socially and culturally tolerated, in order to strengthen the behaviors over time and teach the power of communication. Occasionally, facilitators express concern about the implications of this strategy, worrying that people will become "spoiled" if they always "give them what they want." This need not be a concern if facilitators are attuned to the amount and level of responsiveness the individual needs so that they can decide when to begin to respond intermittently to these signals and/or shape them into less subtle forms.

Relationship to Challenging Behavior   Some individuals utilize unconventional gestural behaviors to signal acceptance or rejection, or to engage in social interactions with others. For example, both self-stimulatory behaviors (e.g., spinning objects, rocking back and forth) and aggressive behaviors (e.g., tantrums, self-injurious behaviors) can be interpreted as rejection messages that serve an escape function (Durand & Carr, 1987, 1991; Kennedy et al., 2000). Other individuals may flap their hands, squeal repetitively, or become aggressive when they are happy or excited, which are two clear occasions for sending acceptance messages. Individuals may also initiate and maintain social interactions with a variety of socially inappropriate behaviors.

As is the case with inappropriate forms of attention getting, FCT can be used to teach alternatives to inappropriate acceptance, rejection, and social interaction signals. For example, Monica used to bang loudly on her wheelchair lap tray when she did not want to eat the food her mother offered to her. Her mother began to watch to see whether Monica produced more subtle rejection cues before she started banging. She noticed that occasionally Monica would purse her lips and turn her head away first, so Monica's mother started to respond to this behavior whenever it occurred by removing the rejected food. At the same time, when Monica banged on the lap tray, her mother would prompt her to turn her head instead. Over a 2-month period, Monica's lip pursing behavior increased and she stopped banging on the tray almost completely because she now had another way to tell her mother "No, thanks!"

When it is time to go out to recess, the paraprofessionals in Mrs. Hennessey's grade 3 classroom make sure everyone is dressed properly in coats, gloves, and hats. Sarah, one paraprofessional, directs Ken (a student with trisomy 13) toward the coat rack. She holds his hand and they swing their arms back and forth slightly as they walk. While smiling at Ken, Sarah's voice is warm as she says to him, "It's almost time for recess now, what do you need to do?" Ken returns the smile and looks delighted as he reaches for his coat. He obviously enjoys the attention Sarah pays him and uses his nonsymbolic behaviors (e.g., reaching, smiling) to communicate with her. (Siegel-Causey & Guess, 1989, p. 28)

Parent/Facilitator Training Programs

A number of instructional programs are available to teach parents and other facilitators who support beginning communicators across the age range to use the social-pragmatic-developmental principles reviewed in the previous sections. In general, these programs share a number of intervention techniques that can be summarized as follows (Siegel & Cress, 2002):

- *Optimize the person's behavior state (i.e., degree of alertness and responsiveness):* Provide adapted seating and other supports to decrease the energy expenditure needed to stay upright and stable; provide interesting, novel, accessible materials and activities (see Ault, Guy, Guess, Bashinski, & Roberts, 1995, for more information on behavior state).

- *Be person-oriented:* Respond to the person's focus of attention, follow the person's lead, match the person's style and abilities, organize the environment to promote communication, and maintain face-to-face interaction with a positive affect.

- *Recognize and interpret early communicative behaviors:* Apply clear criteria for intentionality (see Table 10.3) and respond in a manner consistent with the interpreted intent (both acceptance *and* rejection!)

- *Promote interaction:* Create predictable routines for interaction, take one turn at a time, wait with anticipation, and signal for turns.

- *Model language:* Comment on the ongoing activity; use contingent labeling; use repetition and short, simple utterances; and expand or extend the person's turn.

Examples of social-pragmatic-developmental communication training programs for parents and facilitators who support individuals with autism and other special needs include the Communicating Partners model (MacDonald, 2004), and the SCERTS™ Model (Social Communication, Emotional Regulation, and Transactional Support; Prizant, Wetherby, Rubin, & Laurent, 2003; Prizant, Wetherby, Rubin, Laurent, & Rydell, 2005a, 2005b).

Another approach for facilitator training is based on the work of Dr. Jan Van Dijk (1966) and his colleagues at the Institute for the Deaf in Sint Michielsgestel, the Netherlands.

Van Dijk and his colleagues first described this approach for enhancing the social and communicative abilities of young children with deafblindness. The van Dijk technique and its adaptations are based on the principle that "learning through doing" enables people to acquire concepts, form social relationships, and influence the environment as communicators. Thus, these approaches emphasize movement as a way for the individual to be actively involved in the ongoing activities of daily life.

It is perhaps not surprising that movement-based techniques were first developed for use with individuals who can neither see nor hear and for whom movement in its many forms, such as touch, motion, or object manipulation, represents the most viable way of learning about the environment. This approach has been successfully adapted and used since the 1960s with individuals with intellectual disabilities requiring extensive to pervasive support, multiple disabilities, autism, and other disabilities in addition to sensory impairments (e.g., Rowland & Schweigert, 1989, 1990; Siegel-Causey & Guess, 1989; Sternberg, 1982; Stillman & Battle, 1984; Writer, 1987). The approach provides strategies organized around six levels: nurturance, resonance, coactive movement, nonrepresentational reference, deferred imitation, and natural gestures.

Catherine Nelson and Jan van Dijk (2001) have collaborated to produce an interactive CD-ROM entitled *Child-Guided Strategies for Assessing Children Who Are Deafblind or Have Multiple Disabilities*. It features more than 40 video clips to demonstrate strategies for determining how best to teach communication and other skills to children who require pervasive supports. Using an interactive question-and-answer format, the viewer can view assessments and then design an individualized education program for two children. It is available in the United States and Canada through the National Information Clearinghouse on Children Who Are Deaf-Blind and in Europe from AapNootMuis.

Scripted Routines

One strategy taught in many facilitator training programs is the use of scripted routines that provide structured opportunities for beginning communicators to practice using attention-getting, acceptance, and rejection signals in the context of naturally occurring activities (e.g., Keen, Sigafoos, & Woodyatt, 2001; Siegel & Wetherby, 2000). Table 10.4 displays part of a scripted routine created for Adam, a young man with dual sensory impairments (i.e., deafblindness) and severe physical disabilities, to use while preparing for swimming. As can be seen from this example, scripted routines usually consist of five elements, depending on the type of routine and the person's disability. These five elements—touch cue, verbal cue, pause, verbal feedback, and action—are described with reference to Table 10.4.

1. Touch cue: Touch cues are information provided in addition to spoken words and should be provided before each step in the routine. The touch cue for a step should be the same each time, and all facilitators should use the same cues. Touch cues are critical for individuals with one or more sensory impairments (e.g., vision, hearing, or both) and

Table 10.4. Example of a scripted routine

Touch cue (how you give nonverbal information)	Verbal cue (what you say)	Pause (wait for at least 10 sec., and look for a response)	Verbal feedback (what you say while performing the action)	Action (what you do after the person accepts or the second pause is over)
1. Rub seat belt under Adam's elbow. Release buckle so that a sound is made.	"Time to get ready for a swim."	Pause, observe	"Okay, I hear you *making a noise*; let's put on your swimsuit."	Continue to Step 2.
2. Rub the waist band of swimsuit against his wrist.	"It's time to put on your swimsuit."	Pause, observe	"Oh, *you moved your foot*; okay, let's get undressed."	Continue to Step 3.
3. Unzip coat/sweater.	"It's time to take off your coat/sweater."	Pause, observe	"I *see you moved your arm*; here, I'll help you take off your coat."	Continue to Step 4.
4. Rub Adam's back.	"Let's lean forward now."	Pause, observe	"I *hear you make a noise*; good, you can lean forward now."	Lean him forward.
5. Tug coat collar behind Adam's head and rub your hand on the back of his head.	"Going to pull this over your head now, Adam."	Pause, observe	"You *moved your head*, so I'll help you take off the sweater."	Pull up back of coat all the way and over Adam's head.
6. Pat his first arm where the sleeve ends.	"Time to take off your sleeve."	Pause, observe	"I see you *trying to move your hand*; I'll help you get your hand out."	Remove hand from sleeve.
7. Pat his second arm where the sleeve ends.	"Let's take off the other sleeve now."	Pause, observe	"Good for you, you're *trying to get the other hand out.* Let's take it out."	Remove hand from sleeve.
8. Tap his first shoe, hard.	"Time to take off your shoes."	Pause, observe	"I *hear you making a noise* to tell me to take off your shoe."	Untie shoe, and remove.
9. Tap second shoe, hard.	"Time to take off your other shoe."	Pause, observe	"You *moved this foot*; I guess you want the other shoe off."	Untie shoe, and remove.

280

are often useful with other individuals as well. For example, in Step 2 of Table 10.4, the touch cue associated with putting on Adam's swimsuit is the suit brushing against his wrist.

2. Verbal cue: The verbal cue is a general description of what the facilitator should say while providing the touch cue. For example, while rubbing Adam's swimsuit against his wrist before putting it on, the facilitator might say, "It's time to put on your swimsuit" (Step 2, Table 10.4). Facilitators should not be rigid about the precise structure of verbal cues and should provide necessary information as naturally as possible. Facilitators should always use verbal cues, even with individuals who have hearing impairments, because most of these individuals have at least some residual hearing.

3. Pause: After each touch cue and verbal cue pair, the facilitator should pause for 10–30 seconds and observe the person for a response. A response means any motor movement or vocalization that appears to be deliberate or can be interpreted as deliberate. If the person responds with a signal that can be interpreted as an acceptance signal after the pause, the facilitator should continue the routine. If the individual gives a rejection signal, the facilitator may stop the routine briefly and then try again, explore an alternative way of proceeding, or terminate the routine altogether. If neither type of signal is produced, the facilitator should repeat the paired touch and verbal cues and wait 10–30 seconds again for a signal. If the individual still gives no signal, the facilitator should continue the routine. The length of the pause depends largely on the individual's level of responsiveness and the extent of motor involvement. Individuals with severe disabilities require much longer pauses in order to have time to formulate and produce signals.

4. Verbal feedback: After the individual's acceptance signal, verbal feedback in the form of a comment about what the person did and what action the facilitator will do in response should be provided in conjunction with the appropriate action. For example, after pausing (Step 2, Table 10.4), Adam's facilitator might say, "Oh, you moved your foot; okay, I'll unzip your coat first" or "I see you moved your arm; here, I'll help you take your coat off."

5. Action: For each step in the scripted routine, the facilitator performs an action at the same time as the verbal feedback. An action is the actual step in the routine that is identified through a task analysis. The facilitator may have to assist individuals who are unable to perform the action independently. The facilitator should adjust the amount of assistance provided to the individual's needs. It is important to remember that the point of a scripted routine is *not* to teach the person to perform the action; rather, it is to facilitate the development of communicative signaling within the context of a familiar activity.

To teach scripted routines for play to young children, facilitators can utilize a simplified format similar to the one used for the dressing/undressing routine, but without the touch and verbal cues. For example, the facilitator can create an interactive routine for singing "Row, Row, Row Your Boat" by sitting on the floor facing the child while holding his or her hands. As the facilitator sings the song, he or she rocks to and fro in a boat-like motion with the child. Once the routine has been established and the child is seen to enjoy it, the facilitator pauses after every 1–2 lines in the song and watches for any indication that the child wants to continue the game. The facilitator can apply this basic format—action, pause, action—to other interactive games and songs as well. Individuals older than

Table 10.5.   Examples of scripted routine segments for older individuals

Touch cue (how you give nonverbal information)	Verbal cue (what you say)	Pause (wait for at least 10 sec., and look for a response)	Action (what you do after the person accepts)
Swimming			
1. Move an inner tube up and down when the person is safely seated in it.	"Get ready to float. 1, 2, 3. . . . "	Pause, observe	Verbally acknowledge, and push the inner tube gently across to a partner, 2–3 feet. Repeat.
2. Float the person in a life jacket under the spray fountain in the middle of the pool. Let the water spray on his or her body.	"Getting wet, going under the water. . . . "	Pause, observe	Verbally acknowledge, and keep the person in the spray for 2–3 minutes. Repeat.
Video or pinball game			
1. Place hand on video joystick or pinball lever.	"Okay, it's time to fire/shoot. Here we go."	Pause, observe	Verbally acknowledge, and use hand-on-hand assistance to fire/shoot. Repeat.
Going to a school dance			
1. Wheel the person onto the dance floor and spin around once or twice.	"What great music for dancing!! Let's go for it!"	Pause, observe	Verbally acknowledge, and dance around with chair for 2–3 minutes. Repeat.
2. Go to the refreshment table and get some punch. Brush the cup along the person's lower lip.	"Here's some punch. I bet you're thirsty from all that dancing."	Pause, observe	Verbally acknowledge, and give a sip of punch. Repeat.
Relay race			
1. As each team member runs and the line moves forward, the person's team partner shakes the wheelchair slightly before moving up in line.	"Okay, here we go, we need to move closer to the front to take our turn."	Pause, observe	Verbally acknowledge, and move the chair forward. Repeat.
2. Before taking a turn in the race, place the baton in the person's hands.	"Ready, on your mark, get set. . . . "	Pause, observe	Push wheelchair, and run as required, then go to the back of the line when finished.

5 years of age can engage in scripted routines in the context of age-appropriate social/recreational activities such as swimming, playing video or pinball games, going to school dances, participating in relay races, and so forth. Table 10.5 illustrates some adaptations that can be made to these activities for scripted routines.

Over a 6-month period, Adam gradually began to participate in the dressing and undressing routine for swimming by moving his left arm or leg or by vocalizing during the pauses in the routine. At first, these movements occurred infrequently, but they gradually became more common as his support staff responded to them. Additional scripted routines were introduced during meal-times, position changes, and bath time in the evening. Now, 12 years later, Adam has changed from a 27-year-old man who spent 99% of his day either sleeping or passively allowing people to care for him to a 39-year-old man who spends most of his day actively involved in home and community activities. He operates a large switch positioned by his head to activate an attention-getting buzzer and uses over 50 tangible symbols to make choices and express his preferences. His communication skills continue to develop as his social network expands and as he is increasingly included in his community.

It is important to note that communication interventions need to "match" the characteristics of both beginning communicators themselves and their facilitators. For example, one variation of scripted routine instruction, Prelinguistic Milieu Teaching (PMT; Yoder & Warren, 1998), has been found to be more effective for teaching nonsymbolic accept/request behaviors to toddlers *without* Down syndrome than to those *with* this disorder (Yoder & Warren, 2002), although the reasons for this remain unclear. Young children who produce many vocalizations that contain at least one vowel and one consonant (e.g., *ba, da*) and who often use nonsymbolic behaviors such as pointing to "comment" to their facilitators also appear to benefit from PMT instruction (Yoder & Warren, 1999, 2002). Finally, it appears that PMT produces better outcomes in toddlers whose mothers are better educated and more responsive to their children's communication acts prior to intervention (Yoder & Warren, 1998, 2001). On the other hand, responsiveness parent education via the Hanen curriculum (Pepper & Weitzman, 2004) appears to be more effective with toddlers whose mothers are less educated and less responsive (Yoder & Warren, 2001, 2002). From this, it seems clear that the type of parent/facilitator training should be selected carefully, based on both communicator and facilitator characteristics.

Scripted routines have also been referred to as joint action routines (McLean, McLean, Brady, & Etter, 1991; Snyder-McLean, Solomonson, McLean, & Sack, 1984), Prelinguistic Milieu Teaching (Yoder & Warren, 1998, 2001, 2002), and planned dialogues (Siegel & Wetherby, 2000; Siegel-Causey & Guess, 1989). Additional examples for creating scripts and adapting activities for communication can be found in these publications.

Gesture Dictionaries

By the time facilitators have instituted interventions successfully to teach signals for attention, acceptance, and rejection, the individual has probably developed a fairly large repertoire of vocalizations and gestures for communication. Many of these signals may be idiosyncratic, so that only a few familiar facilitators (e.g., parents, support workers) are able to understand and respond to them consistently, whereas people less familiar with the person may have difficulty understanding and interpreting the messages. This may result in unnecessary, problematic communication breakdowns. For example, a child's babysitter may not know that the child's way of asking someone to change the channel on the television is to walk over to the television and bang on it repeatedly with moderate force. If the sitter tries to dissuade the child from engaging in this seemingly destructive act, the child's efforts may intensify until both individuals are frustrated and dissatisfied!

The gesture dictionary has also been called a "communication diary" (Bloomberg, 1996), "communication dictionary" (Siegel & Wetherby, 2000), and "communication signal inventory" (Siegel & Cress, 2002). All of these consist of three components: what the person does (communicative behavior), what it means (function or message), and how facilitators should react (consequence).

Such communication breakdowns may be avoided by using a "gesture dictionary," in which descriptions of the person's gestures, along with their meanings and suggestions for appropriate responses, are compiled. The dictionary may take the form of a wall poster in the classroom or home or may be an alphabetized notebook with cross-referenced en-

Table 10.6.   Example of a gesture dictionary

What Shawn does	What it means	What you should do
Manual sign for *T* to chin	Wants to go to the bathroom	Give him permission, and help him to door.
"Sshh" sound	"Yes"	Respond according to situation.
Shakes head back and forth	"No"	Respond according to situation.
Reaches out his hand to other person	"I want to shake your hand." [Greeting]	Shake his hand.
Clapping other's hand when offered	"I'm feeling sociable/ affectionate."	Respond according to situation.
Puts both arms around his stomach	Wants a hug	Encourage him to shake your hand by prompting, or give him a hug, if appropriate.
Hands crossed at chest and tapping both shoulders		
Pulls your hand to bring you close to him		
Tapping his opposite shoulder with one hand		
Hand flat across mouth	Wants food	If mealtime or near mealtime, help him to table or ask him to wait a few minutes.
Hand sideways to mouth	Wants a drink	If between meals, provide small amount of milk or bland food (ulcer).
Hand to mouth with grinding teeth	"I'm *really* hungry!"	
Jumping up and down	In a good mood	Respond in kind.
	Needs to go to the bathroom	Give permission, and take to the door.

tries. For example, in the previous situation, the babysitter might look in the child's gesture dictionary under *B* for banging or *T* for television. Under either (or both), he or she might find a description of the banging behavior, its meaning, and how to respond (e.g., "Banging means he wants you to change the channel on the television. Get him to try to say 'Help me,' and then change the channel for him"). Table 10.6 displays a portion of a gesture dictionary created for Shawn, an adolescent with visual and cognitive impairments. The gesture dictionary can also be used for individuals well beyond preschool age. In fact, this technique has been used effectively as a method of orienting new staff to the communication patterns of residents with severe disabilities in group homes and other adult residential environments that have a high staff turnover.

Augmentative Communication Empowerment Supports (ACES) is a year-long support and training program established in 1988 at Temple University in Philadelphia. The purpose of ACES is to increase the communication effectiveness of adults with complex communication needs. ACES participants learn how to become effective communicators by learning how to use voice output communication systems. The participants also learn about resources available to assist them in developing a vision and plan for their future. For information about ACES, contact the Institute on Disabilities at Temple University.

CHAPTER 11

AAC Strategies
for Beginning Communicators

Symbolic Approaches

In Chapter 10, we introduced strategies for establishing communication opportunities and encouraging the development of nonsymbolic communication. The strategies in that chapter are meant to include beginning communicators in communicative interactions and build a foundation for symbolic communication. In this chapter, we describe some of the most common techniques for teaching functional communication skills using symbols and a range of instructional approaches that have been reported in the augmentative and alternative communication (AAC) literature.

INTRODUCING SYMBOLIC COMMUNICATION: VISUAL SCHEDULES AND "TALKING SWITCH" TECHNIQUES

A number of strategies for communication participation are particularly applicable to individuals who have developed the basic skills of attention getting, accepting, and rejecting and are being introduced to symbolic communication. It is important to expand the repertoires of these individuals to include basic skills such as following a symbol schedule and engaging in simple social routines. We summarize briefly a few of the most prevalent or innovative introductory symbol techniques.

Visual Schedules

A visual schedule (also known as a calendar system, schedule system, or activity schedule) represents each activity in the person's day with symbols and may serve several purposes: 1) to introduce the individual to the concept of symbolization, which is the idea that one thing can stand for another; 2) to provide an overview of the sequence of activities across a day; 3) to provide specific information about what will happen next in the day; 4) to ease transitions from one activity to the next; and 5) to serve as one component of a behavioral support plan for individuals who have a high need for predictability (Flannery &

Horner, 1994). The visual schedule strategy originally came from the work of Stillman and Battle (1984) and other practitioners supporting individuals with deafblindness. It has also been used with people who have visual, developmental/cognitive, or multiple disabilities (see Bopp, Brown, & Mirenda, 2004; Hodgdon, 1996; McClannahan & Krantz, 1999; Mesibov, Browder, & Kirkland, 2002; Rowland & Schweigert, 1989, 1990, 1996; Vicker, 1996). Schedule systems can be effective in home, school, and community settings for beginning communicators across the range of age and ability (see Bopp et al., 2004). Table 11.1 outlines how to create and use a basic visual schedule.

Visual schedules can incorporate real objects or tangible symbols as well as photographs or line-drawing symbols in age-appropriate daily appointment books, wall displays, or other formats (see Glennen & DeCoste, 1997; Hodgdon, 1996; McClannahan & Krantz, 1999, for examples). Schedules can also be created to take advantage of com-

---

Table 11.1.   Creating and using a visual schedule

Organizing the visual schedule

The *first step* in putting together a schedule system is to identify the individual's daily schedule across relevant home, school, and community environments. This schedule should include all of the activities he or she does every day or during a relevant portion of the day. Make a list of the activities in order as they occur.

Second, symbols that can be used to represent each of these activities should be identified. For most beginning communicators, these symbols will probably be real object or partial object symbols, although they may be photographs, line drawings, or any other type of symbol the individual can recognize. Once you have identified the appropriate types of symbols, you should gather symbols representing each of the activities in the schedule. For example, if you use real objects, a brush might represent morning grooming activities, a milk container might represent eating breakfast, and socks might represent getting dressed. Collect the symbols in one place (such as a cardboard box) so that they are readily available. The same objects should represent the activities every time.

Third, a container for the schedule system should be constructed. You can place real objects in a series of shallow containers arranged in a left-to-right order. These can be a series of empty shoe boxes or cardboard magazine holders taped together, a series of transparent plastic bags hung on cup hooks, or maybe just a long cardboard box with cardboard dividers taped into it at intervals. If you chose photographs or other graphic symbols, you can place them in the slots of a slide projector page, on the pages of a photo album, or in some other portable carrier. Figure 11.1 depicts a schedule box system with real objects laid out in order to represent eight activities in one day.

Fourth, you should devise a system for identifying finished activities. If you use real objects, this system can be a "discard box" into which the individual can deposit each object after finishing the activity. If you selected photographs or other graphic symbols, the individual can simply turn them over at the end of each activity.

Using the visual schedule

Before each activity, you should prompt the individual to go to the schedule box or to open the schedule book. The symbol for the first activity should be selected or identified. If real objects are used, the object should be taken to the related activity and used during the activity. For example, the symbol for breakfast (a milk container) might have been selected because the first thing that happens at BREAKFAST is that someone pours the milk. Perhaps the individual could be assigned this task as his or her way of participating in breakfast preparation. This will help him or her make the connection between the symbol and the activity.

When the activity is completed, the person should discard the symbol in the manner determined. The discarded symbols should be readily accessible to the individual at all times. He or she thus has the option of going to the box and taking out a symbol of an activity that has been completed if he or she wants to do that activity again. If this ever happens, facilitators should make *every attempt* to respond to the request—let the individual do the activity the symbol represents, if at all possible!

Positive signs that might indicate that the person is making the connection between a symbol and the activity it represents include 1) taking a symbol and then wheeling or walking to the room or area where the activity typically occurs (e.g., to the bathroom for grooming, to the table for eating) and 2) smiling or laughing when the individual picks up a symbol for something he or she likes to do.

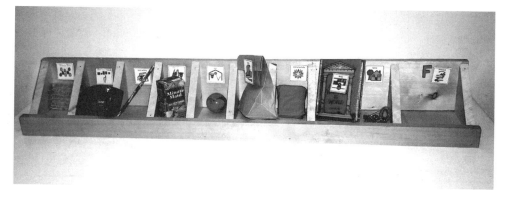

Figure 11.1. Object schedule used at home and in the community by a preschooler.

puter technologies such as Microsoft Powerpoint and various software programs for digital videotape editing (Rehfeldt, Kinney, Root, & Stromer, 2004). Instruction in the use of a visual schedule is generally conducted in loosely structured naturalistic formats, with a hierarchy of prompts that are gradually faded. Figure 11.1 provides an example of a schedule used at home and in the community by a preschooler who has Down syndrome and Figure 11.2 provides an example of one used by an adolescent with autism.

A CD and book entitled *Schedule It! Sequence It!* (Baker & Chaparro, 2003) are available from Mayer-Johnson Inc. The CD is intended to be used with Mayer-Johnson's Boardmaker software and contains pre-made (but changeable) visual schedules for a wide range of domestic, community, and recreation-leisure activities represented with Picture Communication Symbols. The book and the CD both include templates for making various types of schedules, and the book includes step-by-step directions in this regard.

"Talking Switch" Techniques

Burkhart (1993) referred to a number of "talking switch" devices with which facilitators can introduce symbolic communication and provide limited context communication using voice output. One such device is the BIGmack (or its companion, the LITTLEmack), a small, battery-powered communication aid that can be programmed with a single, short message. The BIGmack has a built-in microswitch that, when activated, plays a recorded message. A more cumbersome alternative involves multiple, single-message cassette tapes and a tape recorder operated with a microswitch (Fried-Oken, Howard, & Prillwitz, 1988). In either case, the facilitator can record human voice messages, music, or other sounds (e.g., a dog barking), and the person using the device can play the recording with a simple switch activation. Ideally, the person who records the message should be the same age and gender as the persons who relies on AAC technology. Activation may be direct (i.e., the individual with sufficient fine motor skills activates the BIGmack or turns on the tape recorder) or remote. In the latter case, some type of switch (e.g., one

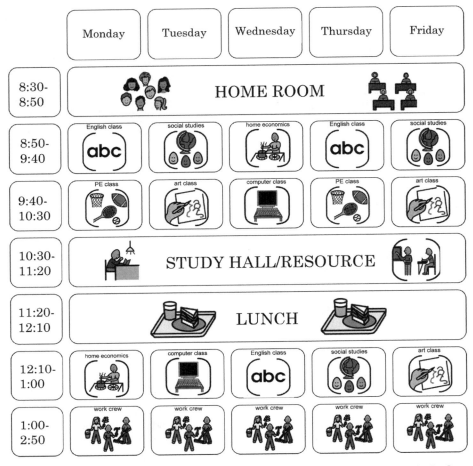

Figure 11.2.   Visual schedule for school used by an adolescent with autism. (The Picture Communication Symbols © 1981–2004 by Mayer-Johnson LLC. All Rights Reserved Worldwide. Used with permission.)

that is operated by the head) is connected to the device in some way (e.g., through a latch timer or other adapter). Such simple voice-output techniques might be particularly appropriate for beginning communicators who use wheelchairs and who are learning to employ microswitches to participate in communication (see Rowland & Schweigert, 1991). Because devices like the BIGmack are lightweight and transported easily (a carrying strap for the BIGmack is available from the manufacturer), they can also be used by ambulatory individuals in a variety of settings.

The most obvious context for using a single-message talking switch technique is one in which the individual can participate in a preferred activity. In this case, a single symbol representing the message should be fastened to the switch prior to use. The type of symbol (e.g., real object, tangible symbol) can vary, depending on the needs and abilities of the individual (see Chapter 7 for assessment information). For example, a talking switch technique might be used in a preschool or elementary school classroom

- During opening "circle time" (e.g., the child activates a message to sing his or her part in the greeting song)

- At transition times (e.g., the child activates a recording of someone singing the cleanup song or of a voice saying "Time to clean up!")

- Whenever a request for continuation or turn taking is appropriate (e.g., the child plays a recording that says "More, please" or "My turn")

- Any time the schedule dictates that a specific activity take place (e.g., in the morning the child plays a recording that says "Take my coat off, please")

- During any activity that requires a leader to announce movements to be performed by the other children (e.g., while singing "The Hokey Pokey"; while saying, "Simon says clap your hands")

- Any time an interjection during an activity is appropriate (e.g., "Wowee!" "Cool!")

Older individuals who use AAC can employ talking switch techniques for similar purposes in age-appropriate contexts during activities such as the following:

- Participating in specific events that require contextual messages (e.g., singing "For He's a Jolly Good Fellow" to a co-worker, singing "Happy Birthday" at a party)

- Cheering (or booing) a favorite sports team on television or in person

- Conversing on the telephone by activating a single message—a nice way for beginning communicators to keep in touch with friends and relatives

- Greeting (e.g., "Hi, how are you today?") or saying farewell (e.g., "Good-bye," "Good to see you," "Let's get together soon")

- Making single requests in predictable situations (e.g., "I'd like a cheeseburger and small fries, please")

- Initiating conversations or introducing topics (e.g., "So, how was your weekend?")

- Making introductions (e.g., "Hi, my name is George; what's yours?")

In some cases, beginning communicators might be able to understand all of the words in such messages, although in other cases, they may participate beyond their level of receptive language understanding. For example, Jeremiah is a young man with multiple disabilities who communicates primarily with facial expressions and body language. When he uses his talking switch to say the blessing before dinner with his family, he does not understand all of the words, nor does he recognize the *pray* symbol on his switch. However, Jeremiah smiles broadly when it is time for him to hit his switch and lead this ritual and appears to enjoy participating in it. As he leads his family in the blessing, he also learns about basic concepts such as cause and effect (hit the switch and your whole family talks!) and using symbols to participate in a meaningful communication context.

A slightly more advanced type of talking switch device is capable of multiple recorded messages in a fixed sequence. For example, the Step-by-Step Communicator can be used to record any number of series of sequential messages up to 75 seconds in total. The messages are then played one-at-a-time by simply hitting the switch. This type of simple device might enable a person to (for example)

- Tell his or her half of a knock-knock joke, waiting in between each switch hit for the partner to take a turn

- Recite a series of scripted lines in a class play

- Dictate the words in a spelling test to the rest of the class, one at a time

- Engage in simple, predictable conversations that involve turn taking, and

- Participate in singing a predictable song with repeated lines (e.g., Old Macdonald had a horse . . . a pig . . . . a cow . . .)

Like single message talking switches, such multiple message devices are only as limited as the opportunities provided to the person communicating with them and the imagination of his or her facilitators!

Many types of talking switches (with both single and multiple message capacity) are available from AbleNet, Inc.; Adaptivation, Inc.; and Enabling Devices.

INTRODUCTION TO CHOICE MAKING AND REQUESTING

Do you remember our discussion about teaching people to accept and reject in Chapter 10? The development of nonsymbolic behaviors to signal acceptance and rejection shows an implicit awareness of *preference*. Preference is evident when an individual indicates acceptance and rejection after he or she is offered options *one at a time*. For example, when Maxwell's dad tries to help him put on his red shirt, he squirms around and begins to whine. When his dad gets the message and offers his Vancouver Canucks shirt instead, Max smiles and cooperates with dressing.

In the above example, Maxwell showed that he preferred the Canucks shirt and could communicate his preference with gestures. The development of preferences and a way to communicate them through nonsymbolic means is a necessary first step to choice making. People who don't have preferences find it difficult to make choices—think of the last time you went shopping and couldn't find anything you really liked! You might have bought something anyway, but it was more difficult to make the choice because nothing really caught your eye! The same thing applies to people who are learning to make choices, at least in the beginning of instruction—if they don't have preferences, they will find it hard to make choices. In particular, this applies to older individuals who have spent years in institutional settings in which they were provided with few opportunities to express their preferences or make choices. As these individuals begin to move into communities, they may need to be exposed to many, many new activities, environments, foods, drinks, and people before they begin to develop preferences and communicate them through "accept" and "reject" behaviors. (See Chapter 10 for a discussion of opportunity strategies related to this concern.) Once they have developed such preferences, they can learn to make choices among them or requests for them.

A Continuum of Choice Making and Requesting

You may be wondering how choice making and requesting are related. *Choice making* occurs when an individual selects a preferred item or activity from *two or more options*, either independently or when someone else offers them. Thus, choice making is not always self-initiated and does not always occur in the context of a communicative interaction. For example, when Estrella goes to the store to buy new shoes, she may use one of several strategies to make her choice:

- She may wait until the clerk approaches her to offer help and then tell the clerk what type of shoe she has in mind. She might then wait until the clerk shows her some options ("Which of these do you like?"), try them on, and make her selection from the offered options (an elicited choice);

- She may look around the store, try on a few pairs of shoes, and then decide to purchase one pair instead of another without consulting anyone (a self-initiated, independent choice).

In both of these scenarios, Estrella made a choice by the time she left the store with her new shoes. She *never*, however, made a request, since one of the two essential components of a request interaction did not occur. The first of these is that another person must be inclined to provide mediation or assistance if asked to do so; in Estella's case, the shoe store clerk potentially fulfilled this role. The second component is that the individual who attempts to gain access to a specific activity or item (e.g., new shoes) must be *unable to do so without the assistance or mediation of another person* (Sigafoos & Mirenda, 2002). Because it was possible for Estrella to purchase new shoes without asking for help or advice from the clerk, this component was not fulfilled. *Requesting* always involves a communication interaction between two people, while choice making does not.

Both choice making and requesting behaviors can be conceptualized as occurring on a continuum defined by 1) the amount of partner support that is needed and 2) the memory requirements that are involved in the task (Sigafoos & Mirenda, 2002). Table 11.2 summarizes one version of this continuum, which arranges formats for choice making and requesting from those that are easier to those that are more difficult in terms of the demands placed on beginning communicators. Although there is no direct empirical evidence in support of the continuum outlined in Table 11.2, there is considerable research that supports the logic underlying it. For example, both elicited (i.e., "offered") choices and elicited requests, which do not require initiation on the part of beginning communicators, appear first on the continuum on the basis of research that suggests that learning to initiate communication is quite difficult for many beginning communicators (Carter, Hotchkis, & Cassar, 1996; Halle, 1987). The remaining three formats are arranged according to the extent to which the available options require independent performance and place demands on short-term memory (Light & Lindsay, 1991) since it appears that the more profound the intellectual disability, the more limited the short-term memory capacity (e.g., Evans & Bilsky, 1979; Siegel & Linder, 1984). Hence, requests that simply require an individual to choose an item from an array (e.g., make an "offered" choice or an independent choice from an array, Table 11.2) can be thought of as having lower memory requirements than those that require the individual to retrieve a symbol from memory (e.g., a request initiated by the individual using AAC with no array, Table 11.2). The point of the continuum is to emphasize that an individual's ability to make one type of request in a specific context does not guarantee his or her ability to make a different type of request in a different context. Hence, exemplary strategies for teaching requesting must consider a number of important variables, depending on the type of request and context. These will be reviewed in detail in a later section.

Table 11.2. Continuum of formats for requesting

Type of choice/request	Partner support	Array	Example	Initiation/knowledge demands
Elicited (offered) choice	Partner initiates (What do you want?) and offers two or more explicit choice options	Array of two or more explicit options	Alfred's teacher offers him a red crayon and a blue crayon and asks, "Which one do you want?"	No demands for either initiation or independent knowledge of available options
Elicited request	Partner initiates (What do you want?) and person using AAC makes request	No explicit array available	Fred's classmate asks him what he wants to do at recess; Fred makes the manual sign for swing	No demands for initiation; demands independent knowledge of available options
User-initiated request, offered choice	Person using AAC initiates generic request (want) and partner offers two or more explicit choice options	Array of two or more explicit options	Jordan approaches his mother with a want symbol; she offers him a cracker and an apple and asks, "Which one do you want?"	Demands initiation, but access to array is supported and requires no memory of available options
User-initiated request, independent choice from array	Person using AAC initiates and makes choice without partner support	Array of two or more explicit options	Alisha scans a catalog, selects the blouse she wants to order, and points it out to her roommate	Demands initiation and ability to independently access information about available options from array
User-initiated request, no array	Person using AAC initiates and makes request without partner support	No explicit array available	Jared approaches a clerk and points to his help symbol to ask for assistance getting a desired item from a high shelf	Demands initiation and memory of available options

Source: Sigafoos and Mirenda, 2003.

TEACHING ELICITED CHOICE MAKING

As noted previously, both elicited choices and elicited requests are initiated *by a facilitator* rather than by the person using AAC. The following three examples involving Alison, a teenager with autism, and her facilitator Maura illustrate the difference between an elicited choice, an elicited request, and a self-initiated request:

Maura: Alison, where shall we go first today—to the store (holds up a wallet) or to the library (holds up a book)?

Alison: [takes the book] *(elicited choice)*

Maura: Okay, library first, then store. Let's go!

Maura: Alison, where shall we go first today?

Alison: [gets her library book and brings it to Maura] *(elicited request)*

Maura: Okay, library first, then store. Let's go!

Maura: Alison, it's time to go out now. Remember to bring your wallet!

Alison: [gets her library book and brings it to Maura] *(self-initiated request)*

Maura: Oh, you want to go to the library first. Okay, we can do that, and then we'll go to the store.

From these examples, it should be clear that, because they do not involve initiation by the person using AAC, the skills needed to make elicited choices and requests can be easier to teach (and to learn!) than those for self-initiated requests. In this section, we will examine some of the major issues involved in teaching elicited choice making.

Choice-Making Opportunities

People who are learning to make elicited choices need frequent, meaningful opportunities to control their environments in this way. Thus, the AAC team's first step in teaching choice making is to identify when, where, and by whom choices can be offered to an individual throughout the day. Some occasions for choice making are obvious: deciding which food to eat or drink, which music to listen to, which television shows to watch, and which clothes to wear. Other instances may be less obvious, such as choosing whom to sit next to (or avoid!) during an activity, how to complete an activity, and the order in which to complete a multicomponent task (e.g., a personal care routine in the morning). Still other choice-making opportunities depend on the extent to which the individual is included in school and community life. These instances include, for example, choices about what brand of beer to order in the pub, which team to cheer for, which store to shop in, whom to call on the telephone, or whom to invite to a slumber party. Without exception, the number of choices available in the course of a day directly reflects the quality and quantity of integrated opportunities in an individual's life. Sigafoos and his colleagues, who successfully developed strategies to increase choice-making opportunities in both classroom and group home settings, demonstrated this in a series of Australian studies (Sigafoos, Kerr, Roberts, & Couzens, 1994; Sigafoos, Roberts, Couzens, & Kerr, 1993; Sigafoos, Roberts, Kerr, Couzens, & Baglioni, 1994). Thus, facilitators should focus initial choice-making interventions toward expanding opportunities rather than toward new and more sophisticated ways to teach the person who relies on AAC the essential skills involved.

Age Appropriateness

Options available in choice-making instruction for beginning communicators should be appropriate for people of the same age who do not have disabilities. With sufficient exposure and encouragement from friends and others, most adolescents and adults with disabilities will acquire sensitivity to age-appropriate cultural norms. Unfortunately, many of these individuals may have had limited exposure to age-appropriate experiences, and when presented with such unfamiliar options, they may express no interest or may continue to choose options that are age inappropriate. This presents communication facilitators with a dilemma: Do we offer *age-inappropriate* options when teaching choice making because these are more motivating for the individual, or do we offer only *age-appropriate* options, although the person shows little interest in them?

The principle of *today and tomorrow* discussed in Chapter 8 offers a solution to this dilemma. According to this principle, decisions for today should meet immediate communication needs and match current capabilities and constraints identified during assessment. Decisions for tomorrow should be based on projections of future opportunities, needs, constraints, and capabilities as a result of instruction. In terms of the choice-making dilemma, the principle of today and tomorrow suggests that for today, choice-making options presented should be those that are valued by the individual, regardless of their age appropriateness. Nevertheless, the principle also *demands* that the facilitator take concurrent steps to expose the individual to a variety of age-appropriate options so that the facilitator can incorporate them into the individual's choice-making repertoire for tomorrow. Although the "today decision" may be necessary to provide motivation, it is certainly not an acceptable long-term solution.

An international team of researchers is investigating the use of microswitches for choice making by individuals with complex multiple disabilities requiring pervasive supports. For example, in one study, an adolescent who had never before participated in choice making learned to choose first between food and drink options and then between two specific foods or drinks, using a series of microswitches (Singh et al., 2003). In two more recent studies, nonsymbolic communicators with significant disabilities learned to associate spoken words with specific microswitches to activate preferred leisure media (e.g., music, tape recorded stories) (Lancioni, Singh, O'Reilly, & Oliva, 2003a; Lancioni, Singh, O'Reilly, Oliva, Dardanelli, & Pirani, 2003). Summaries of this important and innovative work are available in Lancioni, Singh, O'Reilly, and Oliva (2003b) and Lancioni, O'Reilly, and Basili (2001).

Choice-Making Arrays

In addition to arranging for multiple choice-making opportunities throughout the day, the facilitator must select the types of choices that will be available and how many to offer at one time. Usually, initial choice arrays often utilize two options, progressing gradually to three, four, and so forth, as the individual learns to visually scan and select from more options. Large choice arrays for individuals with physical impairments may require aids such as an eye-gaze board, scanning device, or other system for displaying the options so that they are motorically accessible.

With regard to the nature of the choices available, the facilitator has several options: He or she 1) may select two preferred options (Rowland & Schweigert, 2000a), 2) may opt for one preferred and one nonpreferred option (DePaepe, Reichle, & O'Neill, 1993; Frost & Bondy, 2002), or 3) may use one preferred option and a "nothing" or "distractor" option for teaching initial choice making (Reichle, York, & Sigafoos, 1991; Rowland & Schweigert, 2000b). (Note that a fourth option promoted by some in the past, which involves using one preferred and one disliked or aversive item, does not appear in our list of acceptable strategies.) No empirical data are available to guide decisions in this area, and reasonable arguments can be made in support of each option (Sigafoos & Mirenda, 2002). Our preference, particularly when teaching individuals to choose between two real items, is to start out with two preferred options (i.e., items known to be acceptable to the individual) because this is the most natural choice format (Rowland & Schweigert, 2000a). If there are indications that the person is having difficulty making choices—for example, if he or she frequently chooses an option and then rejects it, or if he or she always chooses the item on one side of the array—one of the other array formats might help to clarify the task. Other strategies to consider for individuals who seem to find initial choice making difficult include spacing options closer together or farther apart, aligning them vertically rather than horizontally, and holding them out of reach from individuals who are impulsive (Mirenda, 1985).

Choice-Making Items or Symbols

During choice-making interventions for individuals who are just learning the concept of "choice," facilitators should initially employ real, meaningful items (e.g., drinks, foods, toys) rather than symbols of those items. For example, a facilitator might offer a girl or woman who is learning to make choices both a toothbrush and a washcloth and ask, "What should we do first?" during a personal care routine. The facilitator could then help her to use whichever object she chooses. There is no correct or incorrect answer during such early choice-making interactions because the person is learning that "what you point to/reach for/look at, you get." Even this basic concept may be quite novel for many individuals, especially those who have lived in segregated or institutional settings, because they have not been provided with opportunities to make choices in the past. Facilitators may need to offer such individuals simple, motivating choices many times each day before they begin to understand what choice making is all about.

People who can make choices using real items can begin to learn the use of symbols for elicited choice making. As with all AAC interventions, those that pertain to choice making should incorporate symbols with which the individual is likely to have the most success. This may require the facilitator to provide real object symbols (e.g., an empty cola can to represent *soda* or *pop*) or tangible symbols for people with vision impairments.

Or, the facilitator may furnish more abstract aided symbols such as color photographs, line drawings, or written words, depending on the person's symbol abilities. Individuals who use manual signs as their primary symbol system may find it easier to learn about initial choice making with aided symbols because they can offer and manipulate these symbols more easily. Some evidence also indicates that augmented choice making—that is, choice making using aided symbols—can result in greater accuracy for individuals who can speak but have difficulty with behavioral regulation (Vaughn & Horner, 1995; Wood, Lasker, Siegel-Causey, Beukelman, & Ball, 1998). (See Chapter 7 for a discussion of symbol assessment strategies related to this issue.) When in doubt, it is probably better for facilitators to err on the side of caution by selecting a more concrete rather than a more abstract type of symbol during the introductory stages of teaching symbol use for choice making.

Darcy is a 23-year-old with cerebral palsy who lived in a hospital setting where she attended school for 15 years. She now lives in a group home with four other women. When she moved into the community, she had no formal communication system at all, although she could communicate her preferences quite well through facial expressions, vocalizations, and body language. Darcy's family wanted her to be able to make choices and communicate her wants and needs more spontaneously and with greater clarity. To accomplish this, Darcy's support staff first made decisions about her daily schedule and provided her with real objects in a visual schedule system to represent each of the activities in her day. Through repeated exposure and practice over a 6-month period, she learned to recognize the objects as representing specific activities. Then her support staff offered Darcy choices among activities using the object symbols and constructed her daily schedule based on those choices. Once she made a choice between two object symbols, they showed a large Picture Communication Symbol (PCS) corresponding to her choice as feedback. They did this to expose Darcy to the PCS symbol for tomorrow. She learned to make elicited choices with objects within about 3 months and also began to recognize PCS symbols. Over the next 3 months, her support staff faded out the object symbols, and Darcy began making elicited choices using only PCS symbols, which facilitators offer to her in pairs in appropriate contexts.

Instructional Techniques

AAC specialists have a variety of opinions about how to best teach choice making, once symbols are introduced. One of the most common approaches employs a "comprehension check" procedure such as that described by Rowland and Schweigert (2000b). First, the facilitator offers the person a choice of one preferred and one nonpreferred item (e.g., a puzzle and a sock) and asks, "What do you want?" After the person chooses one of the items (in this case, the puzzle), the facilitator offers two symbols, one of which corresponds to the item selected (i.e., a picture of the puzzle) and one of which does not (i.e., a picture of a sock). A "correct" response occurs if the person selects the symbol that represents the chosen item (i.e., the puzzle), whereas an "incorrect" response occurs if the person selects the opposite symbol (i.e., the sock). Alternatively, facilitators may implement the reverse version of this procedure in which the person first selects a symbol representing a desired item, and the facilitator then provides him or her with a corresponding and a distractor item. Again, a "correct" response occurs if the person selects the item represented by the selected symbol. Regardless of which option is used, the person should always receive the chosen item following a successful comprehension check. Unsuccessful comprehension checks can be followed by a second trial in which the facilitator provides an appropriate type of prompt to elicit a correct response (e.g., Kozleski, 1991b) or uses an error correction procedure of some type (e.g., Sigafoos & Couzens, 1995).

Another approach to teaching choice making employs prompts such as verbal cues, gestures, modeling, and/or physical assistance within an errorless learning paradigm to teach the person to select the symbol for a preferred item from an array of two; the item is then provided. The size of the array is then increased gradually over time. In errorless learning, facilitators provide a prompt *before* the individual has a chance to make a "mistake," and then fade the prompt as quickly as possible (e.g., Locke & Mirenda, 1988; Sigafoos, Couzens, Roberts, Phillips, & Goodison, 1996). This approach is similar to that used during the initial stages of instruction in the Picture Exchange Communication System (Frost & Bondy, 2002), which will be discussed in a later section of this chapter.

As of 2005, there were no empirically validated guidelines regarding the selection of one instructional approach over another, either in general or for individuals who rely on AAC. Thus, facilitators can only employ whichever approach seems to "best fit" the person involved and switch to another approach if this is not fruitful within a reasonable amount of time. Regardless of the instructional technique selected to teach elicited choices, it will always be critical for the facilitator to provide natural consequences following a selection.

Natural Consequences

As stated previously, beginning communicators need to experience natural consequences in order to learn, even if this means that sometimes they do not get what they want because they were not paying sufficient attention or failed to weigh the options adequately. A common mistake that facilitators make is to offer the individual two options and then to provide corrective input if the individual selects the option that the facilitator presumes or knows to be less preferred. The following scene in a kitchen illustrates this mistake:

Tom: Do you want milk [shows empty milk carton] or juice [shows juice container]?

Nan: [looks at and points to milk]

Tom: [suspects that Nan doesn't really want milk]: Do you want *milk*?

Nan: [looks at and points to juice]

Tom: Yes, okay, you want the juice.

Providing corrective feedback in this way almost certainly ensures that problems will occur later in instruction. Nan will learn that it is not necessary to pay attention or think about her response because Tom will always "make it better" in the end. Instead, it would be preferable for Tom to let the natural consequence of a bad choice occur and then offer an opportunity for Nan to try again, as illustrated in the following scene in a fast-food restaurant. In this example, Nan has just chosen to eat a portion of her hamburger, but Tom suspects that she really wants a french fry:

Tom: [gives Nan the hamburger that she selected]

Nan: [pushes the hamburger away and begins to whine, cry, and scream]

Tom: Oh, you don't want hamburger now? Okay, we'll try again in a minute. [removes the hamburger, pauses at least 30–60 seconds, and presents a new opportunity to choose between the hamburger and french fries]

Facilitators commonly make another feedback error when they check an individual's response for correctness by providing a second or even a third opportunity to make the same choice. The following scene in a video arcade illustrates this kind of mistake:

Mark: Do you want to play Mario [points] or Donkey Kong [points]?

Zack: [gestures toward Mario]

Mark: Okay, let's try it again. Do you want to play Donkey Kong [points] or Mario [points]?

Zack: [assumes he must have misunderstood the first time and gestures toward Donkey Kong]

Mark: You need to start paying attention. Do you want to play Mario [points] or Donkey Kong [points]?

Zack: [does not respond because there seems to be no way to win this game!]

The "massed trial" approach to choice making shown in this example is inappropriate and almost certainly will confuse the individual because the consequence of the choice is unclear. Instead, a natural consequence should follow *each* choice-making opportunity so that the individual can gradually learn the effects of his or her actions.

Alternative Access

Individuals with severe motor impairments may have difficulty making choices or engaging in other basic communicative interactions because they are unable to point to, reach for, or otherwise indicate a choice. Of course, many of these individuals can use eye gazing as a motor access technique, and AAC teams can adapt any of the aforementioned techniques for teaching elicited choice making in this response modality. In addition, many dedicated communication devices allow multiple-switch input and can be used to make elicited choices. If this option is appropriate, facilitators should label each switch with an appropriate object, tactile, or pictorial symbol representing the associated choice. For example, a support worker offers Sophie a choice of two activities after dinner: listening to taped music or making popcorn for a movie later on that night. Head switches with symbols for each activity are attached to Sophie's communication device. After showing her what each switch activates, her support worker in the group home asks, "Which one do you want to do?" Sophie uses her head to activate the popcorn popper switch and make her choice, and later experiences the consequences as the popcorn begins to shoot out of the popper chute.

Communication devices such as the Supertalker and iTalk2 (AbleNet, Inc.), VoicePal (Adaptivation, Inc.), Cheap Talk 4 Inline with Jacks and Cheap Talk 4 Square with Jacks (Enabling Devices), and ChatBox Deluxe (Saltillo Corp.) can be used by persons with significant motor impairments for choice making via external switches.

It should be clear from this lengthy discussion that teaching elicited choice making to beginning communicators involves careful planning and decision making. Since the ability to make elicited choices lays the foundation for the ability to make both elicited and self-initiated requests, it is important to take the time to teach this skill systematically. Once the skills for elicited choice making are in place, instruction for requesting can commence.

TEACHING BASIC REQUESTING

Requesting is clearly one of the most basic and essential communication skills, and facilitators need a systematic approach of some sort to teach this skill in many cases. The sections that follow summarize some of the most common techniques that facilitators have used to teach either elicited or self-initiated requesting. Facilitators may use some methods such as the Picture Exchange Communication System (PECS) (Bondy & Frost, 2001; Frost & Bondy, 2002) and the generalized requesting approach (Reichle et al., 1991) to teach specific forms of requesting, whereas others may be used to teach more than one form.

Relationship to Problem Behavior

The ability to make self-initiated requests is a behavior skill as well as a communication skill. It is not uncommon for beginning communicators to use socially unacceptable behaviors to initiate requests for desired items or activities (Durand, 1990). Mirenda (1997) and Bopp et al. (2004) found that one third to one half of published interventions in which AAC techniques were used to treat problem behavior were related to inappropriate requesting behaviors. Interventionists taught participants in these interventions to make generic (e.g., *want, more, please*) and/or specific requests for desired items or activities using gestures (Wacker et al., 1990), manual signs (e.g., Day, Horner, & O'Neill, 1994; Drasgow, Halle, & Ostrosky, 1998; Kennedy, Meyer, Knowles, & Shulka, 2000), tangible symbols (e.g., Durand & Kishi, 1987; Gerra, Dorfman, Plaue, Schlackman, & Workman, 1995), photographs or pictographic symbols (e.g., Frea, Arnold, & Vittemberga, 2001; Lalli, Browder, Mace, & Brown, 1993; Peck Peterson, Derby, Harding, Weddle, & Barretto, 2002), a speech-generating device (SGD) (Durand, 1993), and/or a microswitch and taped message (Steege et al., 1990; Wacker et al., 1990). Clearly, learning some form of self-initiated requesting was important to these beginning communicators.

Teaching Generalized and Explicit Requesting and Use of an Attention-Getting Signal

In this section and those that follow, we discuss a number of the most commonly used procedures that can be used to teach requesting behavior. It is important to remember that the issues related to opportunity, age-appropriateness, type of symbol, and other factors discussed in the section on choice making are equally relevant here. Readers may want to review those sections of this chapter before proceeding to read about specific instructional techniques.

One of the most well-researched instructional approaches involves teaching both generalized and explicit requesting within natural contexts using a behavioral framework (Reichle et al., 1991; Sigafoos & Reichle, 1992). Generalized requesting is accomplished when the individual uses a single, uniform symbol (e.g., WANT or PLEASE) to initiate requesting and then makes elicited choices among two or more options that involve real items (e.g., two or more toys, two or more drinks). Use of a generalized request symbol requires no symbol discrimination skills because only one symbol is used.

In order to make *self-initiated* generalized requests, the individual must first be able to gain the attention of his or her communication partner. Thus, facilitators should always teach attention getting as part of the generalized requesting routine. Keogh and Reichle (1985) noted that learners initially may use the attention-getting signal frequently until the novelty has worn off. They emphasized the importance of the facilitator's response to these initiations, even if the individual does complete the request sequence. Table 11.3 summarizes the instructional steps for teaching generalized requesting and the use of an attention-getting signal. This approach has been demonstrated to be effective with many individuals with developmental disabilities, including those with whom AAC interventions are often unsuccessful (e.g., Rett syndrome; Sigafoos, Laurie, & Pennell, 1995, 1996).

Naturalistic Teaching Interventions

Naturalistic teaching interventions, also known as milieu teaching (Kaiser, Yoder, & Keetz, 1992) and incidental teaching procedures (Sigafoos & Mirenda, 2002), consist of a set of strategies for teaching functional language skills in the context of everyday activities and routines. All naturalistic teaching strategies have several elements in common. First, a facilitator arranges the environment to create communication opportunities that will be motivating to the person learning to make requests. Second, the facilitator initially provides support in the form of verbal, gestural, modeling, or physical prompts to assist the person learning to make requests to do so effectively. Third, requests are always followed by consequences (i.e., responses) that are functionally related rather than artificial in nature (Goodman & Remington, 1993). Table 11.4 summarizes seven naturalistic procedures that have been used successfully to teach the use of both aided and unaided AAC symbols for requesting.

Table 11.3.   Teaching generalized requesting and use of an attention-getting signal

Teaching self-selection

1. *Provide* an assortment of potentially reinforcing items (e.g., toys, food, drinks) on a cafeteria tray.
2. *Hold tray* within the target individual's reach for 10–20 seconds, and encourage him or her to select an object.
3. *Accept* the individual's reach or point as an indicator.
4. When an item has been selected, *remove* the tray, *provide* the item, and *record* the selected item as data.
5. If no response occurs within 10–20 seconds, remove the tray, wait, and try again.
6. Repeat Steps 1–6 until Step 4 occurs three times in a row.
7. Repeat over 3–4 days to determine what the individual's preferences are and how long each practice session should last.

Teaching use of a generic want symbol with arranged cues

1. *Place* a *want* symbol (e.g., a Picture Communication Symbol for *want*) on a large cardboard in front of the individual within reach.
2. *Offer* the cafeteria tray with various items on it and ask, "What do you want?"
3. When the individual attempts to reach for a desired item:
    a. *Note* the item for which he or she was reaching.
    b. *Slide* the tray well out of reach.
    c. Physically (not verbally) *prompt* the individual to touch the *want* symbol.
4. After the *want* symbol has been touched, *provide* the desired item.
5. Over subsequent trials, gradually *fade* the physical prompt until the individual is consistently and independently touching the *want* symbol in response to "What do you want?"
6. Practice Steps 1–5 in a variety of natural contexts with a variety of items (e.g., at breakfast with food items, at the library with books, during a grooming session with self-care items). *Do not* practice in one context only, or the individual will fail to learn that *want* can be used anytime, anyplace.

Teaching use of an attention-getting signal to initiate requests

1. Be sure the *want* symbol is readily available to the individual.
2. Identify a manual or aided attention-getting signal that will be taught. Some possibilities include tapping a listener's arm or shoulder (manual), raising a hand until attended to (manual), ringing a bell (aided), and activating a call buzzer (aided).
3. If an aided call signal is selected, be sure it is accessible to the individual.
4. Use a physical prompt to teach the individual to use the signal to get a partner's attention.
5. When the partner's attention has been gained, the partner approaches the individual and repeats Steps 2–6 of "Teaching use of a generic *want* symbol."
6. Be sure to fade the prompt used to teach the attention-getting signal.
7. Make the attention-getting signal available to the individual during as much of the day as possible to encourage spontaneous requests.

Sources: Keogh and Reichle, 1985; Reichle et al., 1991.

It is important to note that effective requesting involves much more than simply responding to directives such as "Tell me what you want" or questions such as "What do you want?" For example, some individuals may not automatically recognize when they can access desired items or activities by themselves and when they need to make requests in order to do so. This has been referred to as "conditional requesting" and can be taught systematically (see Reichle & Johnston, 1999; Sigafoos, 1998; and Sigafoos & Mirenda, 2002). In addition, some individuals may be unable to make requests spontaneously (i.e., in the absence of verbal questions or directives to do so) without specific instruction (Halle, 1987). For example, Carter (2003a, 2003b) observed 23 beginning communicators who attended self-contained classrooms for students with severe and multiple disabilities, and found that more than two thirds (67.9%) of the students' communicative interactions were requests. However, he also found that more than half (57.9%) of students' communicative acts were preceded by a teacher question, directive, or physical/gestural

Table 11.4.   Naturalistic instructional strategies to teach requesting

Strategy	Description
Expectant time delay	Preferred items or activities are present but access is delayed until a request occurs. For example, a person's grocery bag is placed in sight on the table but access to it is delayed for 10–60 seconds, to create an opportunity for the individual to ask for it (Halle, Baer, & Spradlin, 1981; Kozleski, 1991a)
Missing/out of reach item	An item needed for a preferred activity is missing. For example, during dinner preparation, salad ingredients are laid out but no bowl is provided or the bowl is kept out of reach on a shelf, thereby creating a need to ask for it (Cipani, 1988)
Incomplete presentation	An initial request is followed by incomplete presentation of the requested item. For example, after requesting toast with jam, an adult is provided with bread but no jam or butter, and needs to request these separately (Duker, Kraaykamp, & Visser, 1994)
Interrupted behavior chain	An ongoing activity is interrupted to create a need for requesting. For example, as an adult is proceeding through a cafeteria line, she must ask the attendant for certain items before proceeding to the next station (Carter & Grunsell, 2001; Goetz, Gee, & Sailor, 1983)
Verbal prompt-free strategy	A symbol representing a preferred item is placed in proximity to the person, but no verbal cues (e.g., "What do you want?") are used to refer to it. If the person touches the symbol, either intentionally or unintentionally, the item is provided (Mirenda & Dattilo,1987; Mirenda & Santogrossi, 1985)
Delayed assistance	Required assistance is delayed until a request occurs. For example, if the person needs help to open a jar, the facilitator refrains from providing it until the person asks for help (Reichle, Anderson, & Schermer, 1986).
Wrong-item format	The individual is provided with a wrong item following a request. For example, after asking for a cup of tea, and adult is provided with a cup of coffee instead, creating the need to use a repair strategy to clarify the original request (Sigafoos & Roberts-Pennell, 1999)

Source: Sigafoos and Mirenda, 2002.

prompt. Thus, the rate of spontaneous communication was quite low, suggesting the need for naturalistic strategies that are designed to minimize the use of prompts, such as time delay, the verbal prompt-free strategy, and behavior chain interruption (see Table 11.3). PECS also uses instructional techniques that encourage communicative spontaneity from the outset.

Picture Exchange Communication System (PECS)

PECS is another behavioral approach that facilitators may employ to teach self-initiated requesting with aided symbols. The method teaches requesting as the very first skill in the person's communicative repertoire, without requiring the individual to have skills such as eye contact, imitation, facial orientation, match-to-sample, or labeling as prerequisites (Frost & Bondy, 2002). In PECS, learners are taught to exchange symbols for desired items rather than point to them on a communication display; the communication partner then provides the requested item or activity. PECS instructional techniques are similar to (and partially derived from) both the verbal prompt-free (Locke & Mirenda, 1988; Mirenda & Datillo, 1987; Mirenda & Santogrossi, 1985; Mirenda & Schuler, 1988) and the expectant delay strategies (Kozleski, 1991a).

Instruction in PECS begins after an assessment of potential reinforcers for the person learning to communicate. In the first phase of PECS, the person learns to pick up a single symbol (e.g., photograph, line drawing) and hand it to a facilitator, who gives the person the associated item (e.g., food, drink, toy). At first, an assistant to the facilitator provides physical and gestural prompts but *no* verbal prompts (e.g., "What do you want?" "Give me the picture") to enable the learner to initiate this exchange. Over time, the assistant gradually fades the prompts until the exchange is made unassisted. In phase 2, the assistant gradually moves away so that the person learns to find the picture and take it to the facilitator to exchange it for the desired item independently. In phase 3, the number of symbols available is increased and procedures for teaching symbol discrimination are implemented using one of the comprehension check procedures described previously. Once the individual has mastered basic requesting, the facilitator may extend the program in phases 4–6 to build sentence structures (e.g., teaching the person to chain an I WANT symbol and a specific referent symbol), teach the person to answer yes/no questions in a request context, and label items (e.g., "What is this?") (see Frost & Bondy, 2002, for additional information).

Bondy and Frost (1998) reported on the use of PECS with 66 preschool-age children with autism. Of those children who used PECS for more than 1 year, 39 developed independent speech (59%), 20 others used speech plus PECS (30%), and the remaining 7 used only PECS (11%). Of the children who used PECS for less than 1 year, 2 acquired independent speech and 5 developed some functional speech; the remaining 12 used PECS as their sole communication modality. Bondy and Frost (1994) noted that speech tended to develop once the children were able to use 30–100 symbols to communicate.

In addition to these anecdotal reports, several empirical studies have also demonstrated the positive impact of PECS. For example, Charlop-Christy, Carpenter, Le, LeBlanc, and Kellet (2002) documented a clear increase in both spontaneous and imitative speech production in three young children with autism who learned to use PECS. All three children had some imitative abilities prior to PECS instruction, but none was able to produce speech without prompting. Similarly, Schwartz, Garfinkle, and Bauer (1998) reported that 6 of 11 children with autism (55%) developed independent speech following 12 months of PECS use. Interestingly, the children's pre-intervention communication abilities in this study did not appear to be related to whether they developed speech. In a study that involved a 6-year-old girl with autism, researchers also documented significant increases in the frequency of both spontaneous speech and symbol use following PECS training, although the range of spoken vocabulary (i.e., the number of different words) did not increase (Kravits, Kamps, Kemmerer, & Potucek, 2002). Finally, PECS instruction had a positive effect on both appropriate requesting behavior and elimination of severe aggressive behavior in a preschooler with autism (Frea et al., 2001).

General Case Instruction

Facilitators have relied on general case instruction since the early 1980s to teach functional living skills to people with severe disabilities (Horner, McDonnell, & Bellamy, 1986). However, only since the early 1990s have facilitators applied the method to teach communication skills such as requesting (e.g., Chadsey-Rusch, Drasgow, Reinoehl, Halle, & Collet-Klingenberg, 1993; Chadsey-Rusch & Halle, 1992; Halle & Drasgow, 1995; Reichle & Johnston, 1999). General case instruction involves analyzing the relevant stimulus and response classes associated with particular tasks or situations and teaching individuals both when to respond and when *not* to respond under a variety of conditions

(Chadsey-Rusch et al., 1993). General case instruction can be used in conjunction with any of the instructional techniques discussed previously for teaching requesting.

As an example of general case instruction, consider Cay, a young woman with cerebral palsy who uses a wheelchair for mobility and has great difficulty with fine motor skills. In order to teach Cay to request assistance by pointing to a generic HELP, PLEASE symbol on her lap tray, her facilitator first identified a number of diverse situations across relevant environments in which she would be likely to require assistance (i.e., positive exemplars). Such situations included, among others, a food preparation activity during which Cay would need assistance to open tightly closed containers; a shopping outing when she would encounter doors that she could not open herself; and a dressing activity in which she would require someone to fasten buttons and snaps on her clothes. Cay's facilitator also identified specific situations in which Cay would *not* require assistance (i.e., negative exemplars); some of these included opening loosely closed containers during food preparation, entering stores with electronic doors that opened automatically, and putting on clothes with Velcro fasteners. Next, her facilitator conducted a task analysis to identify the steps involved in the task of asking for help (e.g., recognizing the need for help, gaining a listener's attention, asking for help, and saying thank you) as well as some of the task variations that Cay might encounter at each step. For example, "recognizing the need for help" would require Cay to recognize various types of containers, doors, and clothing items for which she both *would* and *would not* require assistance.

Once Cay's facilitator completed these preparatory steps, instruction was conducted across a number of additional facilitators in order to enhance generalization. Her facilitators all provided verbal and modeling prompts that they faded quickly to teach Cay to use her HELP, PLEASE symbol in the situations that were identified as positive exemplars and to refrain from doing so when she encountered negative exemplars. Both positive and negative exemplars were intermixed from the outset of instruction. Once Cay acquired the basic skill of asking for help in the contexts identified as positive exemplars, her facilitators arranged opportunities for her to practice her new skill across the day in novel settings and situations. Although the general case technique requires more time and instructional effort than teaching in only one or two restricted contexts, research suggests that it is also more likely to result in spontaneous use and generalization of newly acquired communication skills (see DePaepe, Reichle, & O'Neill, 1993, for additional examples of the use of this approach).

Aldo is 17 years old and attends a local high school. Two years ago, his educational team met to brainstorm about how to encourage Aldo to make decisions for himself because it seemed like he always waited to be told what, when, with whom, and how to do things. He could choose between two objects or color photographs when they were offered to him, but he never initiated decisions on his own. The team decided to first teach Aldo to make requests from more than two options. They constructed five choice displays for Aldo, each with five photographs representing preferred foods, drinks, school activities, friends, and recreation activities. They identified contexts during the day when they could ask him to use the displays, and they began to ask questions such as "What do you want?" to elicit requests in those contexts. They also implemented the interrupted behavior chain strategy to teach him to make spontaneous requests in natural contexts such as going through the cafeteria line, checking out books from the library, and getting equipment in gym class. Aldo gradually learned to use the displays to make choices when people asked him to do so and when opportunities occurred within structured activity chains. Later, the facilitators provided Aldo with the displays in natural contexts but refrained from asking him what he wanted. Instead, they used a time-delay procedure to encourage him to initiate requests. At first, Aldo made slow progress, but once he caught on that he could ask for things by himself, he began to use the displays spontaneously in numerous contexts. During the next school year, facilitators expanded his choice displays in type, quantity, and size. Aldo now makes both elicited and spontaneous requests using PCS symbols representing more than 150 options.

TEACHING BASIC REJECTING

Communicative rejecting is defined as "the use of behavior that works through the mediation of a listener and enables the person to escape from or avoid objects, activities, or social interactions" (Sigafoos, Drasgow, Reichle, O'Reilly, & Tait, 2004, p. 33). Communicative rejecting functions as an escape (i.e., leave taking) response when it is used to terminate an ongoing event. For example, Olivia screams when the evening news comes on the television and she wants her mother to change the channel. Communicative rejecting functions as an avoidance (i.e., refusal) response when it allows an individual to evade an event that has not yet occurred. For example, when told that it is time to go to school, Yasmeen sits down on the floor in her living room and refuses to get up. As can be seen in both of these examples, rejecting behavior—like requesting behavior—is often expressed through problem behavior.

Relationship to Problem Behavior

Many individuals are highly motivated to escape or avoid undesired items or activities and often use problem behaviors such as aggression, tantrums, and self-injury to do so. Mirenda (1997) and Bopp et al. (2004) found that between one third to one half of studies in which communicative alternatives to problem behavior were taught involved the escape function. Interventions that have incorporated numerous AAC techniques to teach communicative rejecting, including gestures (Lalli, Casey, & Kates, 1995), a tangible symbol for "break" (Bird, Dores, Moniz, & Robinson, 1989), manual signs (e.g., Drasgow, Halle, Ostroksy, & Harbers, 1996; Kennedy et al., 2000; Peck et al., 1996), picture symbols (Wacker et al., 2002), a card with the word *break* or *done* printed on it (e.g., Brown et al., 2000; Peck et al., 1996; Peck Peterson et al., 2002), a microswitch with a taped message such as "STOP!" (Hanley, Iwata, & Thompson, 2001; Steege et al., 1990), and an SGD (Durand, 1993, 1999). There is no doubt that functional communication training to teach communicative rejecting is critically important in almost all situations when problem behavior is used for the purpose of escape, avoidance, or both.

Teaching Generalized and Explicit Rejecting

Communicative rejecting can be taught in both generic and specific forms using AAC techniques. The generic form involves teaching the individual to indicate "no" by gesturing, producing a manual sign, pointing to or giving a picture symbol, activating an SGD, or using other modalities. The advantage of teaching a generalized rejecting behavior is that it can be used in a variety of situations to indicate both escape (i.e., "I don't want to do this anymore") and avoidance ("I don't want to do this at all!"). The disadvantage is that it might not be easy to interpret exactly what the person is trying to reject or why (Sigafoos, O'Reilly, Drasgow, & Reichle, 2002). For example, Trina and her classmates are following an obstacle course during physical education class in the school gymnasium. When Trina signs NO while navigating the course, her teacher does not know whether Trina wants to 1) take a short break from the *current* obstacle (escape), 2) refrain from engaging in an *upcoming* obstacle (avoid), 3) leave the gymnasium altogether for the rest of the class (escape), or 4) escape or avoid in some other way. On the positive side, Trina's signing NO is vastly preferable to her previous rejecting behaviors, which involved loud screaming and having a tantrum.

There are five main steps involved in teaching generalized rejecting (Sigafoos et al., 2002). First, an appropriate AAC modality is selected to suit the beginning communicator who is involved in the intervention. Second, nonpreferred items or activities are identified across a wide range of routines and contexts. As with requesting, a general case approach may be used here which also requires identification of situations in which rejecting will *not* be required. Third, the need for rejecting is created in each of the identified positive exemplar situations by, for example, providing a nonpreferred item or activity (Duker & Jutten, 1997; Reichle, Rogers, & Barrett, 1984), or providing a wrong item (e.g., Sigafoos & Roberts-Pennell, 1999; Yamamoto & Mochizuki, 1988). If general case instruction is used, negative exemplars also can be interspersed. Fourth, prompts are provided to enable the person to make the desired rejecting response, and the prompts are faded gradually over time. Finally, the fifth step is to remove the nonpreferred item or activity following the appropriate rejecting behavior. Initially, this should occur immediately, every time the new rejecting behavior is produced. Furthermore, once an individual learns a rejecting behavior, it is important for facilitators to honor it even in situations that may not be clear cut, such as when the individual rejects a preferred item because he or she does not wish to have *more* (e.g., rejecting a third cup of coffee although the first two were accepted) (Sigafoos et al., 2002, 2004).

Once the new rejecting behavior is well-established, systematic modifications and extensions can be made as needed. For example, increasingly longer delays (e.g., "Jeff, do just one more problem and then you can take a break" or "Two more peas and you're done!") can be inserted between the communicative rejecting behavior and removal of the nonpreferred item or activity (Hanley et al., 2001; Lalli et al., 1995). Similarly, instruction for teaching appropriate rejecting may need to be combined with instruction in other communicative domains, especially when escape or avoidance of specific activities are not in the person's long-term best interests (Sigafoos et al., 2002). For example, even when an individual uses an appropriate communicative form (e.g., a picture symbol) to refuse to take a needed medication or to refuse to go to school, it may be impossible for facilitators to comply. In such cases, use of a visual schedule to ensure predictability, clarify the non-negotiability of specific activities, and remind the person about upcoming preferred activities may be helpful. For example, Mirenda (2003c) described the successful use of a visual schedule with Alec, a 17-year-old with autism, in which symbols representing required, non-negotiable activities (e.g., taking his medication, attending a scheduled class at school) were marked with a large red dot in the upper left corner to signify "no choice," while symbols representing activities over which Alec had some control were marked with a green dot. Finally, the same basic procedures used to teach generalized rejecting can be used to teach the person to chain two responses together for explicit rejecting (e.g., in Trina's case, NO + CLIMB or NO + GYM).

TEACHING "YES" AND "NO"

It should be obvious from the preceding discussions that teaching individuals to respond to yes/no questions—which some authors have referred to as "teaching conditional use of requesting and rejecting" (Sigafoos et al., 2004, p. 35)—is yet another skill set that may be relevant for some beginning communicators. It is important to note that 1) this seemingly simple task is actually quite complex and 2) very few studies have been done to examine the best ways of teaching yes/no skills to individuals who communicate through AAC.

Regarding the issue of complexity, consider the following yes/no questions:

- Do you want to go to the park? (yes/no requesting/rejecting)

- Do you like to go to the park? (yes/no communication of preference)

- Is this the park? (yes/no labeling)

- Have you ever been to the park? (yes/no information sharing)

It should be evident from these examples that the apparently simple act of "teaching yes/ no" actually involves teaching an individual how to use both of these words to respond to a *wide range* of linguistically diverse questions. Sometimes, the result is that the person will receive a preferred item or will engage in a preferred activity—but this is not usually the case! In fact, there is no reason to anticipate that individuals who learn to use yes/no appropriately for requesting or rejecting will automatically generalize this usage to answer other types of questions (Sigafoos et al., 2004).

In addition, yes/no instruction has received very little research attention, especially with beginning communicators who use AAC. In the few studies that do exist, yes/no was taught in response to highly preferred and highly nonpreferred items or activities only but not to less discriminable stimuli. Furthermore, yes/no was not always taught explicitly. For example, Reichle et al. (1984) taught an adolescent who required extensive supports to respond to two questions: 1) "What do you want?" plus presentation of a tray of preferred items and 2) "Want one?" plus presentation of a tray of nonpreferred items. The adolescent was taught to produce a manual sign for WANT in response to the first question and a manual sign for NO in response to the second. Although she learned to differentially respond to the two questions accurately, this is not the same as learning to sign YES or NO in response to a single, generic question (e.g., "Do you want this?"), as is typically the case.

More recently, Duker and Jutten (1997) taught three men who required pervasive supports to first use a gesture for either *yes* or *no* in response to highly preferred or nonpreferred items, using prompting, fading, and reinforcement (i.e., either providing or removing the item, depending on the first word taught). They then taught a gesture for the opposite word in the same manner, intermixing preferred or nonpreferred items while providing prompts and appropriate reinforcement for each trial. Although the three men all learned to use yes/no to answer requesting/rejecting questions, accurate responding did not generalize to a novel environment without additional instruction in the new environment. As these two studies indicate, there is a real need for focused research examining exemplary practices for teaching both yes/no for requesting/rejecting and yes/no for other question forms to beginning communicators who use AAC.

Having the power to speak one's heart and mind changes the disability equation dramatically. In fact, it is the only thing I know that can take a sledgehammer to the age-old walls of myths and stereotypes and begin to shatter the silence that looms so large in many people's lives. (Bob Williams, a disability advocate and author who uses AAC, in Williams, 2000, p. 249)

TEACHING CONVERSATION SKILLS TO ENHANCE COMMUNICATIVE COMPETENCE

In 1989, Light proposed a definition of communicative competence for people who use AAC. She argued that the development of communicative competence is a complex process that relies on knowledge, judgment, and skills in four domains: operational, linguistic, social, and strategic (Light, 1989b). Operationally, individuals who use AAC must learn to apply the necessary motor (Treviranus & Roberts, 2003), cognitive (Rowland & Schweigert, 2003), and visual/auditory skills (Kovach & Kenyon, 2003) needed for operation of their AAC systems, whether the systems are manual sign-based, low tech, or electronic. Linguistically, persons who use AAC need to learn the linguistic code(s) of their AAC systems (e.g., Blissymbols, manual signs) as well as the semantic, morphosyntactic, pragmatic, and other skills required by the language(s) spoken in their homes and social communities (Blockberger & Sutton, 2003; Mineo Mollica, 2003; Romski & Sevcik, 2003; Smith & Grove, 2003). Social competence skills include those related to discourse strategies such as initiating, maintaining, repairing, and terminating conversations as well as those needed for choice making, requesting, and rejecting (Brady & Halle, 2002; Iacono, 2003; Light, Parsons, & Drager, 2002; Sigafoos & Mirenda, 2002; Sigafoos et al., 2002). Social domain skills also include those that relate to interpersonal dynamics, such as knowing how to put partners at ease, actively participate in conversations, and so forth (Light, Arnold, & Clark, 2003). Finally, strategic skills are those that allow people who use AAC to "make the best of what they do know and can do" (Light, 1996, p. 9; see also Mirenda & Bopp, 2003). There is no doubt that Light's description of these four domains and their importance for persons who communicate with AAC led the field in a new direction that resulted, 14 years later, in an edited book entitled *Communicative Competence for Individuals Who Use AAC: From Research to Practice* (Light, Beukelman, & Reichle, 2003). In this book, AAC researchers and clinicians from around the world described the four components of communicative competence in detail, along with implications for practice.

All of the skills required for communicative competence, and almost all of the research that has examined these skills, are directly applicable to conversational interactions between individuals who use AAC and their communicative partners. At a minimum, conversational interactions require an individual who communicates through AAC to be able to 1) initiate a topic; 2) maintain the topic by asking questions, answering questions, acknowledging others' contributions, and commenting; 3) repair communication breakdowns when they occur; and 4) terminate the conversation appropriately. In the following sections, we review common instructional techniques and clinical strategies for facilitating operational, linguistic, social, and/or strategic competence with regard to these basic conversation skills.

No longer can we select communicative target behaviors for both the AAC user and partner from a magician's hat without considering the effects of these behaviors on perceptions of the AAC user's communicative competence. (Bedrosian, Hoag, Calculator, & Molineux, 1992)

Instructional Techniques

Four empirically supported instructional techniques for teaching conversation skills are described in this section. They include the adapted Strategic Instruction Model (A-SIM), structured practice, conversational coaching, and graduated prompting.

Adapted Strategic Instruction Model (A-SIM)

A considerable body of research has demonstrated the effectiveness of instructional strategies developed in conjunction with the Strategic Instruction Model (SIM) for teaching a wide range of skills to students with learning disabilities (Deshler & Schumaker, 1988). Light and Binger (1998) adapted SIM instruction to teach a variety of conversation skills to individuals who communicate through AAC. The adapted SIM procedures consist of the following steps:

1. Define the specific goal (i.e., target skill) to be taught to the person using AAC.

2. Explain the skill to the person and why it is important.

3. Demonstrate how to use the skill or have the person observe someone else applying the skill while saying "think-aloud" statements that explain when to use the skill.

4. Ask the person or significant others (as appropriate) to think of a situation in which he or she might use the skill.

5. Set up situations for the person using AAC to learn the skill, either during natural interactions or during a combination of role playing and actual interactions. Use several different settings, partners, and sets of materials during instruction. Start instruction in situations that are less demanding and, as the individual develops competencies, introduce more demanding situations.

6. Provide guided practice for the person to use the target skill in naturally occurring situations or role playing. Always give the person an opportunity to use the skill spontaneously, and prompt only as required using a least-to-most cuing hierarchy (natural cue, expectant pause, general point and pause, and model). Provide feedback on both appropriate use of the skill and problem areas after each instructional session.

7. Evaluate progress regularly to measure the effects of instruction. Practice until the individual uses the skill spontaneously in 80% of opportunities during instructional sessions on at least two consecutive occasions.

8. Conduct probes in novel settings with novel partners to evaluate the generalized effects of instruction; offer "booster sessions" of role playing and practice, as needed, to facilitate generalization.

Light and her colleagues have used this approach to teach a variety of conversational initiation, maintenance, repair, and termination skills that we will describe later in this chapter.

Structured Practice

Experimenters have also used a structured practice approach to teach the linguistic and social aspects of conversation either sequentially (Dattilo & Camarata, 1991) or simultaneously (Spiegel, Benjamin, & Spiegel, 1993). In the Dattilo and Camarata (1991) study, experimenters first taught a number of Minspeak icon sequences to two adults with cerebral palsy (a linguistic competence skill). They then provided the adults with a variety of leisure materials and encouraged them to use their AAC systems to ask for or talk about the materials (social competence skills). In the Spiegel et al. (1993) study, experimenters offered two types of concurrent instruction to an adult with cerebral palsy: instruction related to production of icon sequences and instruction related to conversational role playing. During the practice sessions, a facilitator provided narrative cues to set the stage for the participant's selection of pre-programmed sentences. In both studies, the facilitator provided expectant pauses and minimal verbal prompts to facilitate initiation and commenting on the conversational topics. All three individuals showed marked improvement of their conversational skills and evidence of generalization to nontraining settings within four to six practice sessions. The results suggest that, for some individuals, the acquisition of basic conversational skills may require structured practice opportunities in natural contexts.

Conversational Coaching

Hunt, Alwell, and Goetz (1988, 1990, 1991a, 1991b) and Storey and Provost (1996) introduced another strategy that holds real promise for teaching individuals to use AAC displays in conversational interactions. This strategy requires a facilitator to provide unobtrusive conversational coaching to the person using AAC and to communication partners (e.g., friends, parents, co-workers) during instructional sessions. The facilitator provides gestural, physical, indirect verbal, and direct verbal prompts to teach the basic conversational skills of turn taking, commenting, question asking and answering, and using "fillers" (e.g., head nods, smiles, vocalizations indicating interest) and fades these cues gradually. First, the person using AAC is prompted to initiate the conversation by pointing to a picture, remnant, or other topic-setter on a communication display, to either ask a question or make a comment. The partner then responds to the question or comment, makes additional comments about the topic, and ends his or her turn by asking a question about something else represented on the display. The facilitator then prompts the person using AAC to answer the question, comment as desired, and ask another question. A loose form of this cycle (depicted in Figure 11.3) is repeated until the conversation reaches its natural end point. Several studies regarding this strategy have indicated that many individuals with developmental disabilities who use AAC can learn to initiate and maintain augmented conversations independently after several weeks of instruction (Hunt, Alwell, & Goetz, 1988, 1991a, 1991b; Storey & Provost, 1996).

Facilitators can implement a similar coaching strategy to introduce conversation displays during play interactions between young beginning communicators and their peers (Rao, 1994). First, using the communication display while speaking during activities, the facilitator acts as an active communicator, play partner, and model for the beginning communicator and at least one peer without a disability. The facilitator encourages peers without disabilities to use the display and also assumes the role of translator for nonsymbolic communicative behaviors, as needed (e.g., "Look, Grace pointed to the picture of

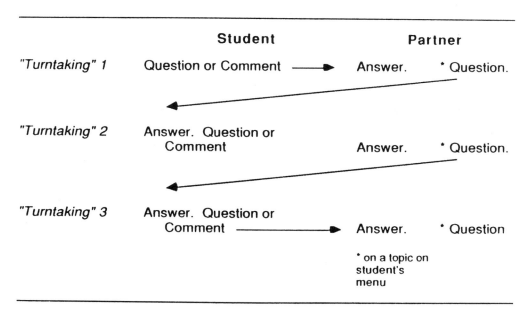

Figure 11.3. Basic conversational strategy. (From Hunt, P., Alwell, M., & Goetz, L. [1991]. Interacting with peers through conversation turn taking with a communication book adaptation. *Augmentative and Alternative Communication, 7,* 120; reprinted by permission of Taylor & Francis Ltd, http://www.tandf.co.uk/journals.)

the horse. She's telling us that she wants to talk about horses"). Gradually, the facilitator transfers the role of translator to the peers, while continuing to prompt and model as needed (e.g., "Grace is showing us the picture for *hot*. What do you think she's telling us?"). The facilitator's goal is to fade out of the interaction altogether (or at least fade out but remain within earshot), as the peers become capable of both understanding the messages of and interacting with the beginning communicator.

Graduated Prompting

Graduated prompting is an instructional technique in which a facilitator provides increasingly directive cues to elicit a desired communicative response. All three of the instructional techniques described previously involve different graduated prompting strategies. Step 6 in the A-SIM approach employs graduated prompts consisting of a natural cue, expectant pause, general point and pause, and model. The structured practice approach employs only an expectant pause and verbal prompt; while conversational coaching employs gestural, physical, indirect verbal, and direct verbal cues. Another commonly used graduated prompting hierarchy in AAC conversation research consists of a verbal model (e.g., "After you answer me, I want *you* to ask *me* something. Like this: 'News. You?' Go ahead, you do it"); a verbal model plus a model using an SGD or a communicative gesture; and a verbal model, an SGD/gesture model, and physical assistance (i.e., hand-over-hand prompting) to produce the desired behavior (O'Keefe & Dattilo, 1992). Regardless, the idea here is to predetermine the order of the prompts that will be provided in a least-to-most-intrusive hierarchy and then to fade them as quickly as possible.

Conversation Skills

One or more of the aforementioned instructional techniques (or variations thereof) can be used to teach a variety of skills needed for conversational interactions. In the sections that follow, we describe the use of an introduction strategy, initiation and topic-setter strategies, partner-focused questions, nonobligatory turns and comments, regulatory phrases, conversational repairs, and termination strategies for conversational interactions.

Introduction Strategy

Most of us introduce ourselves briefly when we meet someone new. Similarly, individuals who communicate through AAC need to both have a way to introduce themselves and the skills required to do so. For someone who uses AAC, an introductory message usually requires three components: 1) basic information about who the person is, 2) information about the person's means of communication, and 3) information about what the partner can do to facilitate the interaction. Light and Binger (1998) provided an example of an introduction strategy produced by Maureen, a 44-year-old woman with cerebral palsy, using an SGD:

> HI. MY NAME IS MAUREEN KRAMER. I UNDERSTAND WHAT IS SAID TO ME. I USE THIS COMPUTER TO COMMUNICATE; I JUST TYPE IN MY MESSAGE AND THE COMPUTER SPEAKS IT OUT. YOU CAN READ THE SCREEN IF YOU DO NOT UNDERSTAND. PLEASE WAIT PATIENTLY WHILE I AM TYPING ON THE COMPUTER. WHEN I SEND YOU A MESSAGE, TRY TO GUESS WHAT I AM COMMUNICATING. CHECK WITH ME TO SEE IF YOU ARE CORRECT. I NOD MY HEAD TO SAY "YES" AND SHAKE MY HEAD TO SAY "NO." IF YOU DO NOT UNDERSTAND, PLEASE LET ME KNOW. THANKS! (Light & Binger, 1998, p. 104)

Light, Binger, Dilg, and Livelsberger (1996) reported that use of an introduction strategy positively influenced perceptions of communicative competence, as rated by 30 adults and 30 adolescents without prior AAC experience and by 30 AAC professionals. In a related study, experimenters successfully used A-SIM instruction to teach the use of introductory strategies to five individuals who communicated through AAC (ages 12–44 years) with cerebral palsy, autism, acquired brain injury (ABI), or developmental delays (Light & Binger, 1998). The participants in this study communicated via a variety of AAC techniques including eye gazing, gestures, some speech, and various SGDs.

Bedrosian, Hoag, and McCoy (2003) found that sales clerks rated individuals who sought specific information using SGDs as more communicatively competent when their messages were entirely rather than partially relevant to the topic at hand, even when the entirely relevant messages required more time to deliver. In this case, relevance appeared to be more important than rate of communication. However, Todman & Rzepecka (2003) found that, in "getting-to-know-you" social conversations, individuals who used their SGDs at a faster speed (i.e., with less pause time between utterances) were judged to be more competent than those who communicated more slowly. This suggests that the importance of rate and relevance differs depending on the communicative context.

Initiation and Topic-Setting Strategies

Initiation and topic-setting strategies allow beginning communicators to start and establish topics of conversation using various types of basic symbols. We discuss six initiation and topic-setting approaches: visual supports, collections, topic-setting or remnant books, topic-setting cards, joke cards, and conversation displays.

Visual Supports   Simple visual supports for various types can be used to help children in particular initiate interactions with peers. For example, two 10–12-year-old boys with cerebral palsy and severe intellectual disabilities were provided with communication "badges" that they used to initiate play activities (Jolly, Test, & Spooner, 1993). During free-play time at school, four badges that featured photographs of preferred activities were attached to the boys' lap trays with Velcro. They were taught to pull off a badge and hand it to a peer who did not have a disability in order to initiate play activities. Similarly, three preschoolers with autism and their peers were each given a colored PCS symbol representing the message CAN I PLAY?, which was glued to a large key-shaped form and laminated (Johnston, Nelson, Evans, & Palazolo, 2003). The symbol could be worn as a necklace or attached to each child's belt loop or pocket. Through structured teaching, the children with autism learned to show the symbol to their peers to gain entry to play groups, and they also showed evidence of reduced off-task behavior. Simple visual supports such as badges and initiation cards have the advantage of being both effective and easy to teach (Johnston et al., 2003).

Collections   Many individuals of all ages enjoy collecting various objects. Even preschoolers may begin to accumulate collections of items such as Pokemon cards, bracelets, toy cars, squirt guns, or stuffed animals. Older individuals may collect stamps, hockey cards, political buttons, or baseball caps—the possibilities are endless! If facilitators systematically encourage them and display them appropriately, such collections can be used to stimulate interactions between individuals who communicate through AAC and their peers across the ability range. For example, a teenager could wear a different message button from her collection to school every day or a teacher could display a child's toy robot collection on a bulletin board at school. Facilitators could remind both adults and children to comment on the newest addition to the collection and could encourage the child's peers to look at the collection items and talk with the child about them. Items in some collections may also be shared as play or personal materials (e.g., toy cars, jewelry).

Remnant Books   A book or album made up of "remnants" or scraps saved from activities provides a way for individuals who are just beginning to use symbols and have limited verbal skills to tell people about past events, such as those that occurred during the school day or over the weekend. The remnant book allows the individual to answer questions such as "What did you do at school/work/home today?" or "What did you do over the weekend?" and to settle on a topic of conversation about an interesting past event. Determining the topic of conversation may be a particularly useful skill for individuals who can talk somewhat but who have poor articulation, such as those with developmental apraxia of speech (Cumley & Swanson, 1999). Once such an individual has narrowed down the topic of conversation by referring to a remnant in the book, his or her communication partner may find it easier to guess the parts of the individual's speech that are difficult to understand. Table 11.5 displays a strategy sheet that facilitators can use at home or school to establish a remnant book.

Work by Marvin and Privratsky (1999) compared the effects of child-focused materials (e.g., stickers, art products, mementos) and parent-focused materials (e.g., newsletters, journals, teacher memos) on conversations between young children without disabilities and their parents immediately after leaving preschool settings. The results indicated that the preschoolers initiated considerably more conversations and talked about more school-related events when they brought child-focused materials home. This suggests that remnant books might similarly facilitate such interactions, because the types of materials that facilitators and people who use AAC place in them are usually person focused.

Musselwhite (1990) included suggestions for teaching the use of remnant books, including a sequenced partner training approach, which consists of three steps. She suggested that after the individual and the facilitator select a remnant and place it in the book, they rehearse using the remnant to introduce a topic through role playing or through puppets (with young children). Next, a third person begins interacting with the individual, and the facilitator coaches the individual to use the remnant with the third person. Finally, the third person is asked to facilitate an interaction with another person. Musselwhite also suggested that the facilitator provide written cues with the remnants to assist literate communication partners to engage in turn-taking conversations with the individual using a remnant book. For example, a cue card might read "Ask me what I did this weekend," "Ask me who I went with," or "Ask me what funny thing happened there."

Topic-Setter Cards   Topic-setter cards are simple drawings or symbols on self-adhesive notes or index cards that present topics of interest (Musselwhite & St. Louis, 1988). Topic-setter cards may be used in conjunction with collections, remnant books, or

Table 11.5.   Starting and using a remnant book

Putting things in the book

1. When you go somewhere in the community with the individual, *save a remnant* of the place you went. *Remnant* is a fancy word for something that the person used or encountered during the activity. The remnant should be something that is meaningful *to the individual* and that he or she will be able to associate with the place from which it came. Let the person help to select the remnant, if possible.

Examples

- If you go to a movie, you might save a ticket stub, or the popcorn container, or the candy box—whichever one the individual prefers and finds most meaningful.
- If you go out to eat, you might save a napkin, or the hamburger wrapper, or the styrofoam chicken box, or the empty paper cup from pop—whichever one the individual prefers and finds most meaningful.
- If you do something interesting or special at home, save a remnant of that as well—such as birthday parties, watching a video, having a friend come for tea.

2. Help the individual to put the remnant in his or her communication book on the page marked with the correct day of the week (Monday, Tuesday, and so forth). You may have to flatten the remnant to put it on the page under a plastic page cover. It will be bulky, but there's not much to do about that.

General strategies for using the book

Don't

- Ask the person "accuracy questions" with the book—"Show me where you went first on Monday," "Show me what you did next," and so forth—in which there is a "right" and "wrong" answer. This is not much fun for the individual and will make him or her hate the book very quickly!

Do

- Make interactions fun and casual.
- Use the book when the person indicates that he or she is interested.
- Encourage the person to try to say the words for the place or activity the remnant represents.
- Make the book readily available at all times so that the individual can initiate interactions by simply opening the book and pointing to one or more remnants. When he or she does this, have a conversation about the place or activity the remnant represents.
- Ask the person what happened today/last night/over the weekend, and encourage him or her to get out the book. Talk about the places and activities the remnants represent (e.g., "Oh, I see you went to the basketball game. Did you have a good time?").
- Get out the book and go through it with the person to talk about what he or she has been up to lately—sort of like reading a story together, but it's a personal story that's being read!

---

other techniques. For example, a card fastened to a wheelchair lap tray might display a symbol of a television along with a written message that faces the communication partner (i.e., upside down to the persons relying on AAC) stating, "My favorite television show is *The Simpsons.* Do you have a favorite show? Do you like *Will and Grace?*" A facilitator can also place the cards in a communication book or program an electronic device to speak the message (Musselwhite, 1990). The person relying on AAC simply points to the card in order to initiate the interaction.

Joke Cards   Individuals who have a sense of humor may enjoy initiating interactions with joke cards. We like to use 5″ × 7″ file cards with a riddle on one side and the answer on the other. For example, one side might have a picture or symbol of a chicken with the caption, *Why did the chicken cross the road?* and the directions on the bottom *Please turn over for answer.* The other side would bear a picture of a chicken across the road and the punch line, *To get to the other side.* The facilitator can teach the person to approach an appropriate partner and hand him or her the card, riddle-side up (color coding the correct side might be helpful). Some individuals may use joke cards without really understanding the language of the joke themselves—but who understands the chicken joke anyway?! The person is learning how to initiate an interaction and (most important) how to make a friend laugh and share a positive exchange—both valuable communication skills for beginning communicators.

Facilitators can make a slightly more advanced form of the joke card by using either low tech or electronic "knock, knock" jokes. The format of this joke (with which most people in North America are familiar) lends itself readily to simple conversational turn taking. In the low-tech version, a series of pictures representing the parts of the joke facilitate the telling of the joke. For example, Tomas first touches a picture of someone knocking on a door accompanied by a written label such as WANNA HEAR A COOL JOKE? KNOCK, KNOCK . . . . After his partner Rajinder responds "Who's there?" Tomas touches the next picture (e.g., a picture of plates and bowls labeled DISHES). Rajinder responds "Dishes who?" and Tomas touches the final picture, which is a photo of himself with the caption DISHES ME, WHO IS YOU? and everyone groans together! As noted previously in the section entitled "Talking Switch Techniques," simple communication devices such as the Step-by-Step Communicator (AbleNet, Inc.) or the Chipper (Adaptivation, Inc.) can also be used to tell knock-knock jokes and riddles.

Symbol dictionaries consist of pages of symbols accompanied by written words or short phrases. They can be used in several ways to support communication. For example, Haley, a girl with autism who was also profoundly deaf, had invented many manual signs over the years; unfortunately, most of them were not readily understood by her facilitators, resulting in frequent (and frustrating!) communication breakdowns. Haley was provided with a dictionary of PCSs representing foods, activities, places, animals, people, colors, emotions, and action words. Whenever she used an invented sign, she was directed toward the dictionary and asked to *find it in the book.* She quickly learned to flip through the pages, locate a symbol that at least approximated the word she wanted to communicate, and point to it. Her facilitator then provided her with the real manual sign for the word (Mirenda, MacGregor, & Kelly-Keough, 2002). In another application, three young, deaf adults with intellectual disabilities requiring intermittent support learned to use symbol dictionaries to communicate with co-workers. They were taught to locate the symbols for needed words or phases in their books, copy the associated words, tear the printed message out of a notepad, and hand it to another person. All three individuals preferred this system over a traditional symbol-based communication display (Cohen, Allgood, Heller, & Castelle, 2001).

Conversation Displays   If we want individuals to initiate conversations with their AAC systems, the systems must be constructed and designed with this goal in mind. Toward this end, conversation displays (e.g., books, boards, wallets, electronic overlays) should contain messages related to favorite people, pets, places, activities, and other items important in the person's life. Past and upcoming events should also be represented. For example, one individual we know had a plastic bag containing grass clippings in his communication book, so that he could tell his friends that he learned to mow the lawn over the weekend. Hunt, Alwell, and Goetz (1990) described a teenager who had a few pieces of dry cat food taped in her communication book to help her initiate conversations about taking care of her cat at home. The point is to provide those who use AAC, through a combination of media, with symbols and messages that promote topics of conversation that are interesting and motivating both to them *and to their communication partners.* Facilitators should change and expand these regularly so that communication displays reflect current events in the person's life. Of course, the format and the content of the displays should also reflect age-appropriate interests. Polite though they may be, the co-workers of an adult with a developmental disability are not going to be interested for very long in photos of dolls or in cut-out pictures from the movies *Bambi* and *Snow White!*

Dual Communication Boards   Another technique for conversational initiation and interaction involves the use of dual communication boards (e.g., Heller, Allgood, Ware, Arnold, & Castelle, 1996; Heller, Ware, Allgood, & Castelle, 1994). The individual using AAC and his or her conversational partner receive identical boards with symbols on them that both persons can understand and use appropriately. A facilitator then uses graduated prompting and conversational coaching to teach the person using AAC to initiate, take turns, ask and answer questions, and so forth. The dual display format has been shown to decrease communication breakdowns by promoting natural turn taking and allowing both partners to interact at natural distances. Some evidence also suggests that communication partners who are not familiar with AAC prefer dual displays to the more typical single-display format (Heller et al., 1994). AAC teams have implemented this technique successfully with individuals who have severe to profound hearing loss and reduced vision in community-based vocational sites.

The Yooralla Society of Victoria, Australia, developed an excellent videotape entitled *prAACtically speaking*. The tape, designed for staff who support adults with developmental disabilities in community settings, features gesture dictionaries, conversation books, visual schedule systems, and community request cards, as well as basic techniques for interaction. An information booklet accompanies the video, which is available from the Scope Communication Resource Centre.

Partner-Focused Questions

Partner-focused questions consist of questions about the conversational partner and his or her experiences. They might include, for example, questions such as "How was your weekend?" "What do you think?" "What's up?" "How about you?" and so forth. Light, Corbett, Gullapalli, and Lepowski (1995) reported that use of partner-focused questions was positively related to perceptions of communicative competence in observers both with and without prior AAC experience. In a related study, Light, Binger, Agate, and Ramsay (1999) used A-SIM instruction to teach the generalized use of partner-focused questions to six individuals who used AAC and ranged in age from 10 to 44 years. The study included individuals with cerebral palsy, intellectual disability, or ABI who used various combinations of eye gazing, speech, gestures, a communication board with line drawings, and SGDs.

Another form of a partner-focused question is the response-recode (R-R) strategy (Farrier, Yorkston, Marriner, & Beukelman, 1985). When an interactant responds to a question and then asks a related question in return (e.g., "My favorite coffee drink is cappuccino; what's yours?"), he or she has used the R-R form. O'Keefe and Dattilo (1992) taught the R-R strategy to three adults with developmental disabilities who used AAC techniques in conversations about preferred leisure activities. Two participants used communication boards and one used an SGD; in addition, all three used gestures, facial expressions, and a few spoken words. During instruction, a facilitator initiated a topic by asking a question and then provided the participant with graduated prompts to elicit the R-R form. All three individuals learned to produce generalized R-R forms that were maintained over time. Family members and caregivers reported lasting changes in the participants' conversational repertoires and agreed that the R-R skill was "fundamental to true conversational involvement" (O'Keefe & Dattilo, p. 231).

Bedrosian, Hoag, and their colleagues examined the impact of aided message length (i.e., one word vs. two to four words) on perceptions of the communicative competence of persons who used AAC. In two studies, message length did not affect the perceptions of either adults who were unfamiliar with AAC or of adults with cerebral palsy (Bedrosian et al., 1992; Bedrosian, Hoag, Johnson, & Calculator, 1998). However, in two other studies, individuals who used longer messages were perceived by unfamiliar adults to be more competent than those who used one-word messages (Hoag & Bedrosian, 1992; Hoag, Bedrosian, Johnson, & Molineux, 1994).

Nonobligatory Turns and Comments

Nonobligatory turns follow a partner's comment or statement (but not a question) and include interjections such as "Cool," "No way," and "Awesome!" as well as more substantive comments on the conversational topic. Light, Binger, Bailey, and Millar (1997) found nonobligatory turn taking to be related to positive perceptions of communicative competence and taught this skill to six individuals (4–21 years of age) with developmental delays, intellectual disabilities, cerebral palsy, or autism. The participants' communication systems consisted of speech, gestures, communication boards with line drawings and/or printed words, manual signs, and assorted SGDs. Following instruction using the A-SIM technique described previously, five of the six individuals were able to take nonobligatory turns in conversations with new people in new settings.

In a related study, Buzolich, King, and Baroody (1991) reported the successful use of graduated prompting plus time delay to teach conversational commenting to three students who used SGDs. The comments consisted of phrases such as "This is fun," "Sounds good," "Yuck!" and "I didn't like it." Experimenters provided instruction in the context of a regular communication group that occurred daily in the students' classroom. All three students learned to produce the comments appropriately using a range of SGDs, and two students generalized this ability to novel contexts.

> Partner reauditorization occurs when a speaking partner repeats and expands an aided message without rising intonation. For example, an individual using AAC in a conversation with her friend says "TV." Reauditorization occurs when her partner then says, "Oh, you were watching TV last night, were you?" Four studies have provided evidence that reauditorization does *not* affect perceptions of the communicative competence of persons using AAC, either positively or negatively (Bedrosian et al., 1992; Bedrosian et al., 1998; Hoag & Bedrosian, 1992; Hoag et al., 1994).

Regulatory Phrases

Regulatory phrases allow individuals who communicate using AAC to manage and control aspects of interactions that are related to the operation of their AAC systems. Such phrases might provide directions to the communication partner with regard to positioning (e.g., CAN YOU COME OVER HERE WHERE I CAN SEE YOU?), effective use of the AAC system (e.g., SAY EACH LETTER AS I POINT TO IT), obtaining and securing conversational turns (e.g., I HAVE SOMETHING TO SAY), and signaling the need to repair a communication breakdown (e.g., WAIT, LET ME SAY IT DIFFERENTLY). Buzolich and Lunger (1995) provided a case study in which a clinician taught Vivian, an adolescent who used AAC, to interact with classmates without disabilities by using a variety of regulatory phrases preprogrammed into her SGD. Instruction was provided through both role playing and conversational coaching with peers. Although Vivian did not use more regulatory phrases during postintervention probes, she did initiate more topics, repair more conversational breakdowns, and use a wider variety of conversational strategies after instruction.

> Grammatically complete messages include all of the content words as well as the functional words required by the grammar of the language (e.g., "The boy and his dog went to the lake"). They differ from telegraphic messages, which contain the content words but not the functors (e.g., "Boy dog go lake"). Light, Beer, et al. (1995) found that the use of grammatically complete messages was *not* consistently related to positive perceptions of communicative competence. They suggested that the grammatically complete message strategy interacts with the communication rate such that the positive impact of the former might be "counterbalanced" by the added time required to produce the messages.

Conversational Repairs

Conversational repair strategies are sometimes needed to resolve communication breakdowns that occur during interactions. Such breakdowns may occur during conversations with beginning communicators who use AAC because of difficulties related to message intelligibility or comprehensibility, conversational timing, partner unfamiliarity with AAC, and numerous other factors (Brady & Halle, 2002). The need for a repair strategy by a person using AAC may be signaled when the communicative partner requests clarification (e.g., "What?" "Pardon me?"), responds to a communicative attempt inappropriately (e.g., by changing the topic or providing erroneous information), or fails to respond to a communicative attempt at all (Bedrosian et al., 2003; Brady & Halle, 2002).

Halle, Brady, and Drasgow (2004) described two basic types of repair strategies, repetitions and modifications; the latter type can be further subdivided into additions, reductions, and substitutions. Repetition (i.e., saying, signing, or pointing to the same message again) may be the least effective strategy, especially when the source of the breakdown is poor intelligibility. Additions involve adding a new element to the original message (e.g., signing JUICE again + pointing to a glass) while reductions involve deleting an element (e.g., pointing emphatically to a single symbol for HELP rather than to the symbols I + WANT + HELP). Substitutions involve using a completely different message form than in the original utterance (e.g., activating LEAVE ME ALONE on an SGD rather than the more polite CAN I HAVE SOME TIME TO MYSELF?).

Halle et al. (2004) emphasized that beginning communicators often use problem behavior to repair communication breakdowns. For example, consider an interaction between Mrs. Sherman, a teacher, and Henry, a student who uses vocalizations, gestures, body language, and pictures to communicate. Mrs. Sherman is sitting at her desk in the morning, talking to Jelissa, one of Henry's classmates, when Henry enters the room:

Henry: [stands by Mrs. Sherman's desk and hums quietly)

Mrs. S: [fails to notice Henry and continues talking to Jelissa]

Henry: [taps his hand softly on the side of the desk]

Mrs. S: [fails to notice Henry and continues talking to Jelissa]

Henry: [grabs a handful of Mrs. Sherman's hair and pulls]

Mrs. S: Henry, NO!!!! That hurts! You must not pull my hair! You need to go to the principal's office so he can call your mother and tell her what you did!

Of course, readers have the advantage of having "insider information" about the subtle communicative messages underlying Henry's humming and tapping behaviors that was not available either to Mrs. Sherman or to Henry. It seems clear to us that Henry's humming was an attempt to initiate a "Good morning!" conversation with Mrs. Sherman, and that the tapping was a repair strategy that he used when she ignored his humming. However, Mrs. Sherman would surely be surprised with this analysis, since both behaviors were so subtle that she failed to recognize them at all. She only "heard" Henry when he finally resorted to the more blatant (but less socially acceptable) behavior of hair pulling which, unfortunately, did not have a positive communicative outcome. This is a typical example of a situation in which instruction in the use of one or more appropriate repair strategies is urgently needed. Fortunately, Henry received such instruction using graduated prompting to teach him to tap Mrs. Sherman gently on the shoulder if she failed to notice his humming. This served two purposes: it resolved the hair pulling problem and it resulted in Henry learning a generic substitution strategy for failed communicative initiations.

Unfortunately, aside from common sense and a few case studies such as Henry's (see Brady & Halle, 2002, and Halle et al., 2004), little research is available to provide guidance about how to teach repair strategies to beginning communicators who use AAC. However, Halle et al. (2004) offered a number of suggestions that are based on research outcomes related to functional communication training in general, including:

1. Identify current and future situations in which use of a repair strategy might be relevant because of communication breakdowns.

2. Select two or more forms to teach as repairs. These authors suggested that teaching *at least* two forms is important so that (as was the case with Henry) if the first is unsuccessful, the person has an alternative. All of the repair strategies taught should be both socially appropriate and sufficiently transparent to communicative partners to communicate the intended message.

3. Teach the repair strategies using graduated prompting procedures in naturally occurring routines and contexts. As much as possible, ignore problem behaviors that occur in response to communication breakdowns.

4. Encourage communication partners to respond to appropriate repairs as soon as they occur with the behavior indicated by the repair.

5. Monitor use of the new repair strategies and teach additional ones as needed.

A conversional "floorholder" (e.g., PLEASE GIVE ME A MINUTE TO COMPOSE A MESSAGE) can be thought of as an anticipatory repair strategy that is used by a person who communicates through AAC to signal that a message is forthcoming but will take some time to compose. Bedrosian et al. (2003) found that the use of floorholders positively affected sales clerks' perceptions of the communicative competence of persons who communicated slowly using an SGD.

FACILITATED COMMUNICATION

Sharisa Kochmeister is a person with autism who at one time had a measured IQ score somewhere between 10 and 15 (Biklen, 1996; Kliewer & Biklen, 1996). She does not speak. When she first began using facilitated communication (FC) several years ago to type on a keyboard, she required an FC facilitator to hold her hand or arm as she hunted for letters on a keyboard. No one thought she could read, write, or spell. She can now type independently (i.e., with no physical support) on a computer or typewriter. Sharisa addressed the 1994 conference of The Association for Persons with Severe Handicaps by typing, with a facilitator sitting nearby for emotional support. When asked what has made the biggest difference in her life now that she can type independently, Sharisa responded, OTHER PEOPLE KNOWING I'M SMART AND SELF-CONTROL AND ESTEEM (Kliewer & Biklen, 1996).

Sharisa joins a small group of people around the world who began communicating through FC and are now able to type either independently or with minimal, hand-on-shoulder support. There can be no doubt that, for them, FC "worked," in that it opened the door to communication for the first time. In addition, hundreds (or even thousands) of individuals use FC with physical support. To many observers, it does not seem clear whether these individuals are authoring their own messages. Thus, FC has become controversial and hotly contested as a valid and reliable technique (e.g., Calculator, 1999b; Duchan, 1999; Green & Shane, 1994). We include FC here because of Sharisa Kochmeister (1997), Lucy Blackman (1999), Jamie Burke (Broderick & Kasa-Hendrickson, 2001), Sue Rubin (1998), and others who now communicate fluently and independently, thanks to FC. For them, the controversy has ended.

> Before I began to type, I did not think . . . . What was amazing was that no one had taught me how to read or spell, but I was able to do both . . . . I believe I picked up this information from the environment and stored it away. It was only after I started typing that the information was accessible. (Sue Rubin, a former facilitated communicator who now types independently, 1998, p. 5)

What Is Facilitated Communication?

Crossley (1988, 1990, 1991) first used FC in 1977 with Anne McDonald, a young woman with cerebral palsy, who was diagnosed as having profound disabilities and was institutionalized in Australia. The story of Anne's progress with FC and her eventual release from the institution was described in detail in *Annie's Coming Out*, which she and Crossley wrote (Crossley & McDonald, 1984). Crossley used the approach subsequently with individuals at the Dignity, Education, and Language (DEAL) Communication Center in Melbourne, Australia, many of whom were diagnosed as having autism. The approach was introduced to a North American audience with the publication of a paper by Douglas Biklen, a professor of special education at Syracuse University, who spent several months in Australia observing Crossley's work and interacting with 27 facilitated communicators who had autism (Biklen, 1990). Biklen and his colleagues have implemented the approach in his community with children and adults with autism and have reported impressive results (Biklen, 1993; Biklen & Cardinal, 1997).

> MY LIGHTWRITER IS A WONDERFUL TOOL TO HELP MY BRAIN FIGURE OUT THE CONNECTION BETWEEN WORDS SOUNDING AND MEANING . . . IT'S SEEING AND HEARING TOGETHER. (Jamie Burke, a young man who developed functional speech after using FC for 8 years, in Broderick & Kasa-Hendrickson, 2001)

FC assumes communicative competence rather than impairment. FC facilitators are encouraged to expect that their communication partners with autism will produce meaningful, even complex, communicative messages with the proper supports. The technique involves the use of a keyboard communication device of some type (e.g., an alphabet display, a small portable typewriter). The FC facilitator physically supports the individual's forearm, wrist, and, if necessary, index finger. The individual is introduced to the keyboard device gradually and is initially physically prompted to touch the correct letter keys in response to simple questions (e.g., "Where is the letter *m?*" "Show me which letter 'dog' starts with"). The FC facilitator provides errorless teaching, including positive verbal feedback for correct responses, so that the person experiences successful interactions. Gradually, the FC facilitator asks the individual to type more complex responses, such as his or her name, simple questions, or fill-in-the-blank statements. Eventually, the individual is encouraged to initiate typing communicative messages and to carry on conversations with facilitation. Gradually, prompts and other supports are faded, although the FC facilitator may provide physical arm, wrist, and hand support as long as the individual indicates a need for it.

What Is the Controversy?

The central controversy has to do with the issue of authorship: Who is typing the messages, the individual relying on FC or the facilitator? Multiple experimental studies have been unable to confirm authorship by the person using FC when experimenters controlled facilitator knowledge (e.g., when the person using FC and facilitator were shown different pictures and the person using FC was asked to type what he or she saw). In addition, multiple studies provide unequivocal documentation of instances in which facilitators have controlled the communicative content of messages, presumably without intending to do so. Some experimental studies, however, have provided preliminary evidence of communicative competence by persons using FC, although the degree of experimental control across these studies has varied widely (e.g., Cardinal, Hanson, & Wakeham, 1996; Sheehan & Matuozzi, 1996; Weiss, Wagner, & Bauman, 1996). In response to the predominant evidence against the validity of FC, numerous professional organizations in the United States have issued position statements urging members of their professions to consider FC an experimental intervention at best.

I spent in excess of 11 years (ages 1 to 13+) with no way to communicate because I was and still am, almost completely non-verbal . . . . Although I readily understand spoken and written language . . . I couldn't speak, or use sign language effectively . . . . People fully believed I was "hopelessly retarded" since I couldn't express myself or respond well. When I started to type, I needed my hand held and index finger supported. Over time, I moved to wrist support, elbow support, a hand on my shoulder, and just having someone's hand "shadowing" mine. All these kinds of "facilitation" made it easier to overcome my inertia; but they also caused people to question whether it was my hand or that of my "facilitator" actually typing. I finally became an independent typist because of those doubts that became the ultimate motivator . . . (Sharisa Kochmeister, 1997, p. 10)

Where Does This Leave Us?

Overall, the "FC debate" leaves FC proponents in North America more cautious than they were after Biklen's 1990 article yet still determined to fight for the right of people with communication impairments to try FC and to continue to use it if their communication with the technique is validated. FC critics have been largely silent since the mid-1990s, perhaps because the preponderance of evidence appears to support their position that FC is not a valid technique. Indeed, the use of FC in North America appears to have decreased markedly since the mid-1990s, and the intense media attention it once warranted has also faded.

Where all of this leaves people who use AAC is the more critical issue. Clearly, some individuals eventually become independent typists through FC and find it to be a useful technique. Others develop speech concurrent with FC and are able to use one or both modalities for communication (Broderick & Kasa-Hendrickson, 2001). However, we do not believe that FC works for everyone. We believe that FC facilitators must obtain informed consent from the individual and his or her family, which includes making them aware of all of the potential problems associated with FC and the lack of empirical support available (see State of New Hampshire, Dept. of Health and Human Services, 1999; http://soeweb.syr.edu/thefci/8–3new.htm). We believe that FC facilitators and AAC experts who promote FC should obtain signed release forms from the individual and his or her legal representatives before instituting the intervention. FC facilitators must receive appropriate training about all aspects of the technique, including validation techniques and the importance of using them. FC facilitators must also address seating, positioning, and other support issues (e.g., assuming competence, providing emotional support, exerting backward resistance to the hand or arm during typing) on an ongoing basis, in order to give the technique a fair test. Critical decisions about legal, financial, and health matters, as well as those pertaining to residential, vocational, and educational placements, should not be made on the basis of FC messages unless multiple sources of evidence confirm that the individual constructed the messages without influence. Finally, interventionists should conduct regular, systematic attempts to verify messages produced through FC, starting from the beginning of intervention (see Shevin & Schubert, 2000).

Ethical guidelines and training standards for the use of FC have been developed by the Facilitated Communication Institute (see http://soeweb.syr.edu/thefci/8–4toc.htm); and by the Communication Aid Users Society of Australia (see http://soeweb.syr.edu/thefci/9–1cau.htm).

Autism is a World is a documentary about Sue Rubin, a young woman with autism who types independently on a keyboard. Sue began to communicate using FC. The documentary was nominated for a 2005 Academy Award.

CHAPTER 12

Language Learning and Development

Dig in, get the support of both the school and the social services agencies, get the devices funded, and [then] make us work our little tails off until we master enough language to become competent communicators. (Advice to AAC interventionists from Gus Estrella, a man who relies on AAC, in Estrella, 2000)

In this quote, Gus Estrella reminds us that successful use of AAC requires more than symbol displays, selection techniques, and voice output. These are some of the tools of AAC, to be sure—but they are not at the heart of the matter, any more than a basketball is at the heart of what Michael Jordan needs to be a star NBA player! Once AAC tools are in place, a person's ability to use language interactively is critically important for communicative competence. In this chapter, we summarize what we know about language development and people who rely on AAC.

LANGUAGE DEVELOPMENT IN PERSONS WHO RELY ON AAC

Language is what allows us to talk, read, write, understand what others say, and learn about the world. When we have language, we can combine symbols in unique ways and describe our perceptions, thoughts, and experiences using spoken or written phrases and sentences. Regardless of the cultural, cognitive, social, and other factors that influence language development, all languages are composed of five domains: pragmatics, phonology, semantics, morphology, and syntax. Summaries of current knowledge about the capabilities of people who use AAC in each of these domains are provided in the sections that follow.

Pragmatics

Pragmatics refers to the communicative functions of language and the rules for using language contextually for social purposes such as conversation (Iacono, 2003). Communicative functions include, for example, the ability to request, comment, repair/clarify, reject/ protest, and solicit information by asking questions. Numerous studies from around the world have indicated that the range and general patterns of communicative functions produced by individuals who use AAC tend to be restricted to responses and requests, regardless of the observational context (e.g., Basil, 1992; Carter, 2003a, 2003b; Iacono, 2003; Light, Collier, & Parnes, 1985b; Sutton, 1999; Udwin & Yule, 1991; von Tetzchner & Martinsen, 1992).

Pragmatics also has to do with knowledge of the rules of language use in a social context. For example, one of the pragmatic rules for conversations in North American culture is that when two strangers greet each other (a communicative function), they do not typically kiss or hug. It is not unusual to find reports suggesting that people who communicate through AAC have impaired pragmatic skills, especially in conversational interactions, which researchers have studied the most. Research suggests that, during interactions with speaking partners, people who use AAC tend to occupy a respondent role; they seldom initiate conversations, respond primarily when obliged to do so, and produce utterances that are only as long as they need to be to get a message across (Calculator & Dollaghan, 1982; Collins, 1996; Light, Collier, & Parnes, 1985b; von Tetzchner & Martinsen, 1996). Naturally speaking partners, on the other hand, tend to control conversational topics, ask many questions (especially those requiring yes/no and single word responses), and spend a significant amount of time repairing and/or averting breakdowns during conversations with people who use AAC (Basil, 1992; Iacono, 2003; Light et al., 1985b). However, Müller & Soto (2002) found that when two people who use AAC interacted with *one another*, their conversations were much more "equal" than when they interacted with natural speakers. Thus, it appears that the phenomenon of conversational asymmetry is a function of an imbalance in conversational "power" rather than of pragmatic deficits per se in people who use AAC.

By now, my speech is virtually gone, except for the occasional short phrase. I am heavily reliant on my [speech-generating device, SGD]. In social situations, the computer functions very well. . . .In restaurants, I've learned to modulate the volume to a point where the voice is audible but unobtrusive to others, although I've grown accustomed to inquisitive looks . . . I use [my SGD] on the telephone and, when I need to discuss or authorize work in process, it's a simple matter to disconnect the cords . . . and carry the computer around with me. . . .I am confident that with planning, forethought, and assistance . . . my . . . journey. . . .will never be a silent one. (Michael Olshan, a man with amyotrophic lateral sclerosis, in Olshan, 2000, p. 5)

Phonology

Phonology refers to the rules of the sounds of language. A person with phonological awareness can "manipulate the sounds of spoken language with or without alphabet knowledge" (Blischak, 1994, p. 246). So, for example, such a person could hear the difference between /pa/ and either /po/ or /ba/. Phonological awareness for individuals with little or no speech relates primarily to learning to read, spell, and write. Although much is known about the development of phonological awareness in speaking children (e.g., Bishop, Rankin, & Mirenda, 1994; Blischak, 1994), researchers have conducted relatively few studies in this area for individuals with severe speech impairments. These studies, which have primarily focused on children and youth with severe speech and physical impairments (SSPI; e.g., cerebral palsy), involve the administration of a variety of phonological awareness and phoneme discrimination tasks that do not require speech. Uniformly, the results indicate that although at least some individuals with SSPI are able to analyze and manipulate phonologic information successfully, they score well below control participants on research tasks, regardless of whether other language problems are present (Bishop, Byers Brown, & Robson, 1990; Bishop & Robson, 1989a, 1989b; Dahlgren Sandberg, 2001; Dahlgren Sandberg & Hjelmquist, 1996b, 1997; Foley & Pollatsek, 1999; Vandervelden & Siegel, 1999, 2001). In addition, the same positive relationship between phonological awareness and reading that has been found for individuals without disability appears to exist for those with SSPI (Iacono & Cupples, 2004). This suggests strongly that many individuals who are candidates for AAC are at risk for delays in the area of phonology and hence reading acquisition, at least in the absence of intervention.

Semantics

Semantics refers to understanding words and how they relate to one another. For example, a school-age child with intact semantic knowledge would know that the words *pin*, *pan*, and *pen* each refer to a different object and could discriminate among them. In Chapter 2, we discussed semantic development in terms of "messaging" or vocabulary development for persons who rely on AAC. A substantial body of research suggests that children who use AAC often experience delays in this area because

- They may be talked to less than children who do not have disabilities, for a variety of reasons (Blockberger & Sutton, 2003). The landmark work of Hart and Risley (1995, 1999) clearly indicates that young, typical children who are talked to more by adults, especially in the context of mutual or parallel activities that are social/playful rather than goal-directed, develop larger vocabularies.

- There is an asymmetry between language input and output such that children "receive" and process words in one modality (i.e., speech) but communicate through another (e.g., manual signs or graphic symbols; Oxley & von Tetzchner, 1999; Smith & Grove, 1999, 2003)

- They cannot select their own lexicon (i.e., the corpus of words from which a word can be chosen) for their AAC displays but must depend instead on adults to do so for them. Hence, a child's external lexicon (i.e., the words on his or her communication display) may not reflect his or her internal lexicon (i.e., the words in his or her head; Blockberger & Sutton, 2003; Nelson, 1992; Smith & Grove, 1999, 2003; Sutton, 1999).

- As they select words from their communication displays, they do not receive symbol feedback from their partners, particularly if they overextend words. For example, if a child uses the symbol COW to refer to a dog, she might be told the correct word verbally ("No, that's not a cow, that's a dog") but she is unlikely to be shown the correct symbol on her communication display, even if it is there (Smith & Grove, 2003; von Tetzchner & Martinsen, 1992).

• There may be less "convergence" between semantic and conceptual organization in some graphic symbol sets and systems (Blissymbolics) than others (e.g., Picture Communication Symbols; Schlosser, 1999a, 1999b).

Of course, one of the assumptions underlying these concerns is that children who use AAC learn new words through processes that are quite similar to those used by children without disabilities. If this is the case, the challenge for AAC teams in building semantic knowledge is primarily one of providing individuals with sufficient access to new vocabulary via some type of symbol system and then providing ongoing input to build semantic knowledge through the use of that system. However, this is true only if those who use AAC are able to "fast map"—that is, learn new words with minimal exposure (Carey & Bartlett, 1978). Dollaghan (1987) demonstrated that most children without disabilities as young as 12–15 months of age are able to learn new words after as little as one exposure. Most children with Down syndrome who can speak are also able to do this at a level commensurate with age-matched and language-matched children (Chapman, Kay-Raining Bird, & Schwartz, 1990). This accounts partially for the rapid growth in vocabulary size of young children; by one estimate, they learn an average of nine new words each day and know at least 14,000 words by the time they are 6 years old (Carey, 1978)! Clearly, the ability to fast map would greatly enhance the semantic learning process of children who use AAC as well.

Fast mapping is one behavioral demonstration of the *novel name–nameless category principle* (N3C) that guides children's learning of words. The N3C principle states that "when a child hears a novel word in the presence of an unknown object, he or she will immediately map the novel name onto the novel entity" (Romski, Sevcik, Robinson, Mervis, & Bertrand, 1995, p. 391). Interested readers can refer to Crais (1992) for a comprehensive discussion of N3C as it relates to fast mapping.

Can children who use AAC fast map? If so, how can AAC teams best facilitate this process? A study by Romski, Sevcik, and their colleagues (Romski et al., 1995) provides some information in this regard. The study involved 12 youths with little or no functional speech and intellectual disabilities requiring limited to extensive support. Each participant received four exposure trials in one sitting to each of four novel objects labeled with both nonsense words and abstract symbols (i.e., lexigrams) on an SGD. After four exposures, researchers tested the participants' ability to both comprehend and produce the lexigrams immediately as well as 1 day and 15 days later. Seven of the participants fast mapped the symbol meanings and retained their comprehension of some of the words for up to 15 days. Furthermore, they generalized their knowledge from comprehension to production. Four of the five participants who did not fast map had historical symbol achievement patterns characterized by slower symbol acquisition and less generalization than those who did fast map. Thus, it appears in this case that at least some individuals who use AAC are able to fast map, despite moderate to severe cognitive impairments.

Morphology

The rules for building and changing words are referred to as morphology. For example, knowing that *pin* refers to one object and *pins* refers to more than one object or that *walk* describes a current action whereas *walked* describes a past action indicates an individual's morphological awareness. Most studies have demonstrated that individuals who use AAC experience marked difficulties with grammatical morphology (e.g., Berninger & Gans, 1986; Kelford Smith, Thurston, Light, Parnes, & O'Keefe, 1989; Sutton & Gallagher, 1993). A 2003 study by Blockberger and Johnston is particularly illustrative in this regard. They assessed mastery of three grammatical morphemes (possessive -*'s*, third person singular -*s*, and past tense -*ed*) in children who used AAC (5–17 years of age) and in children who were typically developing. The children were matched by Peabody Picture Vocabulary Test–Revised (Dunn & Dunn, 1981) scores and had comparable chronological ages. They found that participants without disabilities of all ages scored significantly higher on three tasks that probed acquisition of morphological understanding and use: a comprehension task involving picture selection, a grammaticality judgment task, and a structured written word (fill-in-the-blank) task. Sutton and Gallagher (1993) found similar results with regard to the past tense -*ed*.

It is not clear why people who use AAC regularly experience problems with morphology, but at least five explanations are possible:

- The symbols needed to indicate (for example) plural, possessive, or past tense are not available on most communication displays, so children do not have experience with using them (Blockberger & Johnston, 2003).

- Individuals who communicate through AAC choose efficiency over accuracy as a strategy for enhancing the speed of communication (Blockberger & Sutton, 2003; Light, 1989a; Mirenda & Bopp, 2003).

- Individuals who use AAC are not taught the morphological rules that apply to various situations (Blockberger & Johnston, 2003; Sutton & Gallagher, 1993).

- The AAC modality itself influences output and precludes the need for conventional English morphemes (Smith, 1996; Smith & Grove, 1999, 2003). Smith (1996) provided an example by referring to the Picture Communication Symbol (PCS) symbol for SIT, which is a line drawing of a person sitting on a chair. When asked to symbolize the sentence "The girl is sitting on the chair," one of Smith's research participants simply pointed to the symbol for sit, rather than combining the PCS symbols GIRL, SIT, ON, and CHAIR. In fact, this participant was correct—the form of the PCS symbol for SIT itself precludes the need for constructing the utterance word-by-word! It is likely that similar occurrences contribute to other difficulties with grammatical morphology, but research to examine this issue is in its infancy.

An American movie titled *Field of Dreams* was about a man building a baseball field in his cornfield. A voice told him, "If you build it, they will come." The same voice is speaking for people using augmentative and alternative communication. It says, "If you build language, effective and independent communication will come." (Van Tatenhove, 1996)

Syntax

Syntax refers to the rules for putting words into sentences; for example, if a person understands English syntax, then he or she would know that "I like this cake" is preferable to "Like I this cake," even though listeners might comprehend both. We actually know quite a bit about the syntactic difficulties of individuals who communicate with graphic symbols. Blockberger and Sutton (2003) summarized the most commonly reported expressive syntactic characteristics identified in the literature:

- A predominance of one- or two-word messages, both in spontaneous and elicited conditions (e.g., Nakamura, Newell, Alm, & Waller, 1998; Soto, 1999; Sutton & Morford, 1998; Udwin & Yule, 1990)

- A prevalence of simple clauses (e.g., "I like cake"), with limited use of complex structures such as questions, commands, negatives, and auxiliary verbs (Soto & Toro-Zambrana, 1995; van Balkom & Welle Donker-Gimbrère, 1996)

- Use of constituent orders that differ from the individual's spoken language background, regardless of the AAC modality used. For example, individuals using AAC whose native language is English have been noted to produce subject-object-verb orders (e.g., GIRL + HOUSE + GO), verb-subject-object orders (GO + GIRL + HOUSE), or even object-verb-subject order (HOUSE + GO + GIRL; e.g., Sutton, Gallagher, Morford, & Shahnaz, 2000; Smith & Grove, 1999, 2003). Even individuals with more advanced language skills often have difficulty with word orders in compound sentences (e.g., GIRL BLUE BOX HELP BOY IN SHOPPING CAR for *The girl helps the boy putting the blue box in the shopping cart*; Smith & Grove, 2003)

- Omission of words that appear frequently in the individual's language, such as verbs and articles, even when these are available on the communication display (Soto & Toro-Zambrana, 1995; van Balkom & Welle Donker-Gimbrère, 1996)

- Extensive use of multimodal combinations (e.g., gesture + symbol, vocalization + symbol), word overextensions (e.g., *dog* instead of *cow*), and other metalinguistic strategies that compensate for a lack of needed symbols (Light et al., 1985c; Mirenda & Bopp, 2003; Sutton, Soto, & Blockberger, 2002)

Why do these unusual syntactic patterns occur in the messages of people who use AAC? Three primary explanations have been put forward over the years. The first and earliest explanation, the deficit hypothesis, suggested that most individuals who use AAC systems have underlying language deficits, a notion that has since been disabused (see Kraat, 1985, for the most notable review of evidence against this assumption). The second, the compensation hypothesis, suggests that atypical "graphic symbol utterance structures reflect compensatory strategies used to circumvent the cognitive, physical, and linguistic constraints involved in aided communication" (Sutton et al., 2002, p. 195). Thus, the message BOY WILL PUSH TO STORE GIRL might be produced to mean *The boy will push the girl to the store* (van Balkom & Welle Donker-Gimbrère, 1996, p. 165) by someone who does not have the word *the* on her communication display. The third, the modality-specific hypothesis suggests that unusual graphic symbol utterance structures reflect the asymmetry between what individuals who use AAC hear (i.e., spoken language) and how they communicate, and are a function of the differences between the two (Sutton et al., 2002; Smith & Grove, 2003). For example, AAC messages are often co-constructed by a communicator and his or her facilitator, while spoken messages are not. Thus, the PCS message ME SISTER BOY FISH MOVIE FUNNY might be produced to mean "My sister and I went to see the movie *Finding Nemo* [a movie about a boy fish who gets lost] and we thought it was funny" even by someone who has intact language ability, with the expectation that the communication partner will either know the required background information or ask clarifying questions to assist with co-construction (Sutton et al., 2002). It is probable that both the compensatory and modality-specific hypotheses contribute to the differences seen in the language patterns of persons who use AAC, but more research is needed to develop a comprehensive theoretical model of language development that can be tested systematically.

Summary

In summary, we can make several statements about language learning and development in individuals who communicate through AAC. First, many of these individuals show evidence of both receptive and expressive language impairments. However, it is important to note that many individuals who have never been able to use natural speech have written and spoken eloquently about their experiences and their lives using AAC—clearly, they mastered the intricacies of language and are now able to pass their knowledge on to others. For example, people from around the world who use AAC shared their poems, stories, and narratives in a book entitled *Beneath the Surface* (Williams & Krezman, 2000). Second, and perhaps most important, the language difficulties experienced by many individuals who use AAC are undoubtedly influenced by the fact that their language-learning experiences are so very different from those of individuals who can speak. As Nelson so eloquently noted,

> How can [we] assess what words and structures a young child knows if the only words and structures available [to] the child . . . have been provided by someone else? How can [we] know whether a preliterate child might actually have a variety of words in mind to express a concept or communicate a feeling, but cannot because the words are inaccessible for expression? . . . How can [we] know if a child can generate multiword utterances if the child's computer is preprogrammed with frequently used phrases? (1992, p. 4)

How, indeed? Clearly, strategies specifically aimed at language development need to be an integral part of every communication intervention. In the section that follows, we describe some of the most commonly used and/or promising methods for language development.

> Over the years, . . . [Adam] has added some of the structure, rules, and intricacies of language. He added these in the same way he adds to his vocabulary: when he wants and needs them to communicate, when he's given the words with which to do them, and when it isn't too much trouble to use them! Come to think of it, that's just about the way my daughter developed her language, and she doesn't use AAC. The only difference between the kids was that my daughter didn't have to wait for someone to give her a way to express those words. (The mother of Adam, a 9-year-old boy who uses a variety of AAC techniques, in Gregory & McNaughton, 1993, p. 22)

INTERVENTIONS TO SUPPORT LANGUAGE LEARNING AND DEVELOPMENT

Symbols and Language

One of the challenges in representing any language system for persons who use AAC and do not (yet) know how to read involves how to "translate" spoken language into a visual form without losing specificity and flexibility. There is wide variability in the extent to which current AAC symbol sets enable individuals to communicate precisely when using closely related (but linguistically distinct) words and concepts such as *eat, ate,* and *eating; mouse* and *mice; small* and *smaller;* and *boy, boys, boy's,* and *boys'.* Do certain symbol approaches facilitate language development (or certain aspects thereof) more than others?

The answer depends on whom you ask! For example, proponents of Blissymbolics have stated for many years that the use of this pseudolinguistic system allows people who use it to learn about the rules of morphology, syntax, and message construction (Soto, 1996):

> Blissymbolics is a language with a wide vocabulary, a grammar which allows for sentences in past, future and present tenses, and markers for possession, plurality, questions and commands. . . .It is a totally generative system with each new symbol interpretable by the receiver through analysing the component parts. (Retrieved from http://www.blissymbols.org/ on May 19, 2004)

Similarly, DynaSyms®, a symbol set used on some dynamic display SGDs, includes grammatical markers and symbols that allow representation of tense, plurals, possessives, and other grammatical forms. Manual coded language systems such as Signing Exact English also use modified and supplemented American Sign Language signs to give a clear and complete visual presentation of spoken English. Other symbol sets, such as the popular Picture Communication Symbols (Mayer-Johnson, Inc.), incorporate a few specific symbols that can be used to indicate past and future tense or relative size (e.g., big, bigger, biggest) but do not provide many other indicators (e.g., plural or possessive indicators).

Some researchers have also argued that iconic encoding (e.g., Minspeak) promotes language development because people who use it learn a certain set of words and icon sequences and then apply knowledge of that set to decode and spell new words and select new icon sequences (Erickson & Baker, 1996). Others have questioned its use entirely, especially for individuals who have not yet achieved a strong language base and for whom early language concepts are still developing (e.g., Jennische, 1993). Such critics question both the theoretical underpinnings of the technique and the practical implications of spending many hours teaching an individual to encode messages in a way that is quite different from the way spoken and written language is encoded.

In the end, it is clear that some individuals who use AAC symbols—regardless of the type—develop generative language while others do not (see Goldstein, 2002; Mirenda, 2003b; Soto & Toro-Zambrana, 1995; Williams & Krezman, 2000). However, aside from published case studies, little empirical evidence is available to suggest that any one symbol set is more facilitative of language development than any other. Thus, perhaps the best advice for now is to find ways to create links between whichever system a person uses for face-to-face communication and whichever system he or she uses for language and literacy instruction, so that he or she is not faced with the daunting task of learning completely separate systems for each of these domains (Pierce, Steelman, Koppenhaver, & Yoder, 1993).

The fact that we know very little about the development of language in young children with severe speech and physical impairments who require AAC is not surprising. At this point in time, we have many more questions than answers. . . . If we think of our knowledge in this area as a Tootsie Roll Pop, we have barely taken the first lick. The chocolate goodie in the center is still a long way off. (Bedrosian, 1997, p. 179)

Organizational Strategies

When an individual uses graphic symbols of any kind for AAC, the symbols must be organized in ways that promote maximally efficient and effective communication. This is particularly crucial when an individual has a large number of symbols in his or her system. Several organizational strategies are commonly used, some of which have the potential to encourage language learning. These strategies fall into two main categories: grid displays, in which the elements are typically individual symbols, text (words/phrases), or pictures that are arranged in various ways; and visual scene displays, in which the elements depicted are the events, persons, objects, and related actions that are inherent components of the scene (Blackstone, 2004). Symbols can also be organized on both grid and scene displays that appear together (i.e., a hybrid display). Both grid and scene displays will be discussed in the sections that follow.

Semantic-Syntactic Grid Displays

The first type of grid display organizes vocabulary items according to the parts of speech and their relationships within a syntactic framework (Brandenberg & Vanderheiden, 1988). By mapping the symbols according to spoken word order and/or usage, this strategy is intended to facilitate language learning, although there is no empirical evidence that this actually occurs. A commonly used semantic-syntactic display strategy is the Fitzgerald key or some modification thereof (McDonald & Schultz, 1973). The original form of the Fitzgerald key organized symbols from left to right into categories such as *who, doing, modifiers, what, where, when,* and so forth, with frequently used phrases and letters clustered along the top or bottom of the display. The order was intended to facilitate word-by-word sentence construction from left to right. Bruno (1989) described the design of a Minspeak display for a young child using a modified Fitzgerald key that involved a left-to-right clustering of symbols for people (nouns and pronouns), verbs, adjectives, prepositions, object nouns, time words, and place words. Goossens', Crain, and Elder (1994) standardized their published activity displays using a modified Fitzgerald key with the following categories: miscellaneous words (e.g., social words, *wh-* words, exclamations, negative words, pronouns), verbs, descriptors, prepositions, and nouns. Regardless of the categorization strategy used, symbols on semantic-syntactic displays are usually color coded to allow easier visual access.

Taxonomic Grid Displays

A second grid display strategy involves grouping symbols according to superordinate categories such as people, places, feelings, foods, drinks, and action words. Garrett, Beukelman, and Low-Morrow (1989) used this scheme to develop an AAC system for an older man with aphasia because he had retained substantial semantic knowledge despite a severe expressive language impairment. Mirenda, Malette, and McGregor (1994) described a similarly organized system for an adolescent with cognitive disabilities in which symbols were placed on pages (i.e., categories) for snack foods, lunch foods, transportation, after-school activities, weekend activities, personal care activities, friends, and family members. Research with typically developing children suggests that they do not find this type of organizational structure useful until sometime between ages 6 and 7 (Fallon, Light, & Achenbach, 2003). Thus, this strategy may not be appropriate for individuals who communicate through AAC and are developmentally younger than age 6.

Activity Grid Displays

Perhaps the most popular grid display strategy involves organizing vocabulary according to event schemes, routines, or activities; some researchers refer to these as "schematic grid layouts" (e.g., Drager, Light, Speltz, Fallon, & Jeffries, 2003; Fallon et al., 2003). Each display contains vocabulary items that are specific to an activity (e.g., Birthday Party) or to certain routines within an activity (e.g., Going to the Party, Eating Cake, Opening Presents, and Playing Games; Drager et al., 2003). Each display contains symbols for the people, places, objects, feelings, actions, descriptors, prepositions, and other vocabulary items that are relevant to the activity or routine. In so doing, activity displays provide a vehicle for participation while promoting language development and complex expressive output (e.g., multiword combinations). Typically, vocabulary items are organized on activity displays according to semantic categories—for example, all of the people words might be grouped together in one area, the action words might be grouped together in another, and so forth. Figure 12.1 provides an example of such an activity display that might be used by a child to play "Space Explorers." Burkhart (1994) suggested that activity-based displays are preferable to semantic-syntactic displays because the latter adds to the cognitive demands of the task for individuals who might not think in semantic categories.

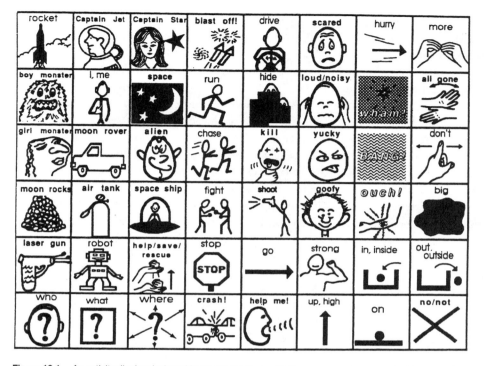

Figure 12.1. An activity display designed for a preschool-age child to encourage language development. (The Picture Communication Symbols © 1981–2004 by Mayer-Johnson LLC. All Rights Reserved Worldwide. Used with permission.)

Activity displays can be used in both low-tech and electronic (e.g., dynamic display) applications. Mirenda (1985) described a variety of strategies for designing and organizing low-tech activity displays in order to facilitate their usefulness. For example, AAC teams can place divider tabs in communication books to separate activity sections and facilitate easy access, or can provide core displays with supplemental border overlays for people who use lap-tray aids (Goossens' & Crain, 1986a). Such strategies are important in order to provide a wide selection of vocabulary items while allowing the person using the system to find a desired display quickly.

Participation is enhanced when multiple activity displays are available, perhaps in addition to a generic communication board or overlay that is used routinely. Several authors have discussed the construction of activity displays for children who use eye gazing, rotary scanners, communication books, dynamic display devices, and other display formats (Burkhart, 1994; Goossens', 1989; Goossens' & Crain, 1986a; Goossens', Crain, & Elder, 1992; Musselwhite & St. Louis, 1988). Low-tech activity displays can be mounted in specific locations, such as on the wall (e.g., in each room of the home at the child's height), on aquatic flotation devices (e.g., kickboards, inner tubes), or on the dashboard of a car. Activity displays can also be designed for use by individuals across the age range in community, school, and vocational settings (Elder & Goossens', 1994). The advantage of using this organizational strategy is that facilitators can construct new displays relatively quickly using only the vocabulary items appropriate to the activity or event. Low-tech displays for special events can be constructed and stored until the next occasion for their use (e.g., next Christmas, the next time Grandma visits). This strategy enhances the probability that specialized vocabulary items for specific contexts will be available when they are needed.

In addition to enhancing participation, activity displays also can promote the use of multiword linguistic structures and build a strong receptive language base. Unfortunately, many individuals who use AAC do not have access to vocabulary items that they can combine flexibly; instead, they have boards that contain only symbols that represent wants and needs, such as basic objects, people, places, and food items, plus a few verbs such as *eat*, *drink*, and the inevitable *go bathroom*. Thus, it is not surprising that their language development and use patterns often lag behind those of their peers who do not use AAC. Facilitators can provide relevant vocabulary items from a variety of semantic categories for specific activities with multiple low-tech activity displays. In addition, the natural branching capabilities of dynamic display devices can be used to promote sentence construction within specific activities. Burkhart (1994) suggested that, at first, partial sentence starters (e.g., *see*, *can't see*) should appear on the first page with a natural branch to a second page after any selection (see Figure 12.2a). Page 2 should have vocabulary items that might naturally come next as options (e.g., *big*, *quiet*, *good*), as depicted in Figure 12.2b. When an individual selects one of the second options, the display would naturally branch to a third page (see Figure 12.2c) with final-position words or phrases (e.g., animals, vehicles, people).

Visual Scene Displays

A relatively new addition to the menu of organizational options, visual scene displays are similar to activity displays in that they contain vocabulary words associated with specific activities or routines. However, the words in a scene display are organized schematically rather than semantically. This organizational strategy is most appropriate for use with speech-generating devices (SGDs) that have dynamic screen displays. For example, a scene display for Going to the Park might show a playground with swings, a slide, a teeter-totter, and a jungle gym. A number of children might be featured as well, along with dogs, trees, birds, adults, benches, and a variety of other pictures of items typically found in a park. When any of the individual pictures (i.e., symbols) in the scene are activated, an associated message is spoken.

Research suggests that scene displays are easier for young, typically developing children (as young as age 2.5 years) to learn and use than either activity displays or taxonomic displays (Drager, Light, Carlson, et al., 2004; Drager et al., 2003; Fallon et al., 2003). Because of this, scene display AAC technologies are likely to become increasingly common over the next decade. Scene displays can also be used in low-tech AAC systems, although with less efficiency than when they are used on SGDs.

Language is a powerful tool for communication, socialization, and thought. Clinicians strive to achieve a balance between language acquisition and acting on (and reacting to) immediate communication challenges facing the AAC user. (Sutton, Soto, & Blockberger, 2002, p. 201)

---

a.

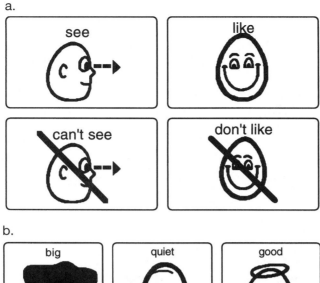

b.

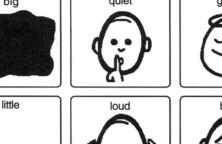
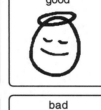

c.

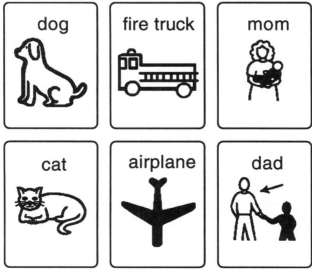

Figure 12.2. Dynamic displays for sentence construction. a) Partial sentence starters on page 1 of display; b) descriptors on page 2; c) final-position words on page 3. (Boardmaker and Picture Communication Symbols copyright © 1981–2004 by Mayer-Johnson LLC. All Right Reserved Worldwide. Used with permission.)

Message Units: From Sentences to Morphemes

Another issue that confronts AAC teams and undoubtedly affects language development has to do with the size of the message units made available to individuals who communicate through AAC. Message units can range in length from 1 symbol = 1 paragraph (e.g., a symbol for HAMBURGER accompanied by the printed message HELLO. I WOULD LIKE A HAMBURGER WITH TOMATO AND LETTUCE, NO MUSTARD, NO KETCHUP, AND EXTRA ONIONS. THANK YOU.) to 1 symbol = 1 morpheme marker (e.g., an arrow pointing to the left that means *past tense* or an arrow pointing to the right that means *future tense*). In between these two extremes are symbols for sentences (e.g., a single symbol that means *leave me alone*), phrases (e.g., I WANT or I DON'T WANT), and single words. The issue here is "How does use of different message unit lengths affect both long- and short-term language development?"

The short answer is: We really don't know. In order to answer this question, we would need to have access to the results of a large-scale, longitudinal study involving several carefully matched groups of young children who use AAC and are exposed to only one type of message unit for a long period of time (e.g., 3–5 years). We would then be able to compare the language abilities of children in the different message unit groups to see if some show evidence of more advanced language development than others. Of course, conducting such a study would be impossible. In fact, there is almost no research examining this issue; rather, decisions regarding the appropriate types of message units to provide to individual learners are made through a combination of theoretical knowledge derived from typical language development and clinical experiences with children who use AAC.

Of course, good rationales exist for the selection of both longer (e.g., paragraph and sentence length) message units and shorter ones (i.e., phrase-, word-, and morpheme-length units). Longer message units speed up the communication process, which is usually both slow and cumbersome, especially for individuals who access their AAC systems through scanning (Blockberger & Sutton, 2003; Paul, 1997). In addition to functionality, longer message units require fewer cognitive/linguistic resources and thus may be advantageous for individuals who fatigue easily, are minimally motivated to communicate, and/or are just learning to use AAC techniques (i.e., beginning communicators). Finally, longer message units permit the person to produce messages that actually exceed his or her productive language ability (Light, 1997), such as occurs when Jason, a beginning communicator, selects his own photograph to activate the spoken message, MY NAME IS JASON, WHAT'S YOUR NAME? on his SGD.

On the other hand, longer message units may also impede communication accuracy, as illustrated in the following anecdote:

> Tim vocalized to get his mother's attention, then looked at his mom, looked at his dinner, looked back at his mom, frowned, then selected the line drawing of the dog from his computer-based AAC system (thus retrieving the preprogrammed message *My dog's name is Skippy*). After numerous attempts, Tim's mother eventually determined that Tim intended to communicate the intrinsic message "dog," not the extrinsic message produced by the speech synthesizer, and that he was trying to tell her to give his dinner to his dog because he didn't like it. (Light, 1997, p. 165)

For Tim, having only a single sentence associated with the symbol for DOG actually slowed down his communication and forced his mother to play "20 questions" in order to understand what he meant. Clearly, the ability to communicate more flexibly is one of the advantages of shorter message units such as words and morpheme markers. Having opportunities to manipulate word- and morpheme-length units is also likely to enhance language development because the ability to break down and analyze message components is directly under the control of the individual who uses AAC (Blockberger & Sutton, 2003). Hence, correct language structures can be reinforced and expanded (e.g., Child: WANT BALL (points); Father: "Oh, you WANT the BIG ball; here you are!"), and incorrect structures can be corrected through modeling (e.g., Child: HAT ME (shows hat); Teacher: "What a nice hat you have! Try saying it this way: MY HAT"). Finally, the provision of shorter message units reduces the need for the individual to have to "translate" the language he or she hears (input modality) into the language he or she is able to use (output modality; Smith & Grove, 1999, 2003).

Given the clear advantages and disadvantages of these contrasting approaches to message unit size, perhaps the best solution at the present time is the compromise suggested by Blockberger and Sutton (2003):

> The possible benefits of more grammatically complete and correct output must be carefully weighed against the cost in terms of the longer time it will take to produce that utterance . . . The answer may lie in continuing to provide . . . phrases or sentences for certain functional situations [while] ensuring that the individual has the opportunity and AAC tools to segment and construct the linguistic forms in other situations. (p. 97)

Clearly, research is needed to clarify the questions related to this issue and to clarify the long-term impact of the various options. In the meantime, AAC teams must consider the pros and cons of providing symbols to represent both short and long message units for each individual and context and then rely on clinical judgment to make decisions that seem optimal.

Instructional Approaches

In order to use symbols effectively, individuals who use AAC must learn both their meanings, alone and in combination (receptive language), and how to produce them in communicative contexts (expressive language). Some instructional approaches treat receptive and expressive language as separate instructional entities, whereas others take a more holistic perspective. In Chapter 11, we introduced naturalistic teaching and general-case instructional procedures (see Tables 11.3 and 11.4) for teaching functional communication skills such as requesting, rejecting, and yes/no. We also introduced the adapted Strategic Instruction Model (A-SIM), structured practice, conversational coaching, and graduated prompting techniques for teaching conversation skills. In the sections that follow, we describe additional approaches that are designed to focus on specific aspects of receptive and/or expressive language development. In Chapter 13, we discuss instructional approaches related to literacy (including phonological skills).

Structured Approaches

Structured teaching is grounded in the traditions of both experimental (e.g., Remington & Clarke, 1993a, 1993b) and applied behavior analysis (e.g., Reichle, York, & Sigafoos, 1991). It is characterized by adult- or computer-delivered discrete trials that are usually conducted with one learner at a time. Typically, each trial consists of a stimulus (e.g., the facilitator holds up a cookie and asks "What's this?"), a prompt (e.g., from an array of two photographs, a cookie and a shoe, the facilitator gestures toward the symbol for cookie), a response by the learner (e.g., he or she points to the cookie photo), and a reinforcer (e.g., the facilitator says "good work!"). The trials are repeated several times with a pause between each, and the prompt is faded gradually until the learner can produce the correct response independently.

This type of instruction is often used to teach expressive labeling, as in the above example. It can also be used to teach receptive labeling; in this case, the facilitator might say "Show me the cookie" while holding up a photograph of a cookie, and then prompt the learner to select the correct object from a cookie–shoe array. When the goal is to teach labeling, the facilitator provides reinforcement that is *unrelated* to the target word; for example, if the learner correctly points to the symbol for cookie when asked "What's this?" he or she might be provided with verbal praise or a brief period of time with a favorite activity. This is done in order to distinguish labeling from requesting, which *should* result in a related reinforcer (Reichle, Rogers, & Barrett, 1984).

It is important to note that the use of a structured teaching approach to teach labeling may have some advantages over other instructional approaches, especially when applied in natural contexts (see Remington, 1994). For example, some individuals may require a large number of trials to learn a basic core of signs or symbols (e.g., Hodges & Schwethelm, 1984; Romski, Sevcik, & Pate, 1988). If this is the case, physical prompting or guidance techniques may be more efficient than less intrusive modeling procedures (Iacono & Parsons, 1986). Also, when an individual frequently communicates manual signs or symbols inaccurately, a structured approach may be preferable. If the individual requires corrective feedback on a regular basis during communication interactions, he or she may come to view communication as a negative experience. In such situations, the facilitator may use some structured teaching sessions to build a repertoire of accurate sign or symbol productions and may restrict corrections of inaccuracies to these times only. Carr and Kologinsky (1983) recommended such a "two-pronged approach" for teaching manual signs, with structured discrete trial techniques to teach language forms and incidental instructional paradigms to teach the use of the forms. Similarly, Reichle, Sigafoos, and their colleagues have recommended and used a complementary blend of more and less structured techniques to teach a variety of pragmatic functions (e.g., requesting, rejecting, commenting) using manual signs or pictorial symbols (e.g., Reichle & Brown, 1986; Reichle et al., 1984; Reichle, Sigafoos, & Piché, 1989; Sigafoos & Couzens, 1995; Sigafoos & Reichle, 1992; Sigafoos & Roberts-Pennell, 1999).

Structured approaches have been used to teach receptive labeling in the context of the fast-mapping phenomenon discussed previously. Wilkinson and her colleagues described both concurrent and successive introduction procedures that can be used in this regard; both are depicted in Figure 12.3. In the concurrent introduction procedure, each of two new symbols being taught—in this case, chair and shoe—appear in separate learning trials where they are contrasted with already-known symbols like dog, banana, and tree (top left and top right of Figure 12.3). The first time the learner sees the two novel symbols together is during a test for learning outcomes (middle of Figure 12.3). In contrast, the successive introduction procedure requires the learner to contrast the two novel

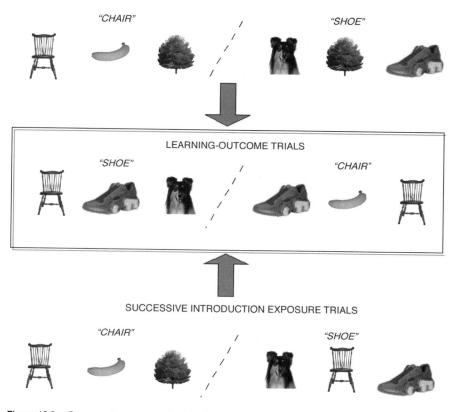

Figure 12.3. Concurrent and successive introduction procedures for teaching new vocabulary words.

symbols right from the beginning of instruction. First, one of the new symbols (in this case, CHAIR) is contrasted with well-known items like BANANA or TREE, as in the concurrent procedure (bottom left of Figure 12.3). Then, the second new symbol (SHOE) is contrasted with a well-known item like DOG and the now somewhat-familiar first new symbol, CHAIR (bottom right of Figure 12.3). Thus, the successive introduction procedure requires participants to mark the difference between the two new words even during initial training. Testing for learning after successive introduction is identical to testing after concurrent introduction. It appears that, although some learners seem to acquire new words more efficiently with concurrent presentation, simultaneous presentation usually results in better outcomes (Wilkinson, 2005; Wilkinson & Albert, 2001; Wilkinson & Green, 1998).

Structured approaches can also be used to teach morphemic and syntactic language forms using AAC techniques (e.g., Harris, Doyle, & Haaf, 1996; Iacono, Mirenda, & Beukelman, 1993; Remington, Watson, & Light, 1990; Romski & Ruder, 1984). For example, Lund and Light (2003) used a direct instruction strategy to teach four grammatical forms, including possessive pronouns (e.g., That computer is *theirs*) and correct word order in adjective phrases (e.g., I can't find my *blue sweater*), to two adults with cerebral palsy who used SGDs. Instruction consisted of 1) an explanation of the relevant grammatical rule, 2) identification of both correct and incorrect forms in sentences, and 3) practice correcting incorrect forms. The facilitator provided prompts following incorrect responses and praise following correct responses. Although both adults learned the target grammatical forms, one required additional instruction to maintain the gains over time, and generalization was not measured. Nonetheless, this study and that of Iacono et al. (1993) demonstrate that structured approaches can be used to teach language forms beyond labeling to both children and adults who do not acquire them naturally.

Children learn language in dyads involving people with whom they have meaningful relationships. (Wetherby, 1989, p. 25)

Interactive Model

As noted in Chapter 10, interventionists have established numerous training programs situated within an interactive model of language development that are designed to teach parents to provide rich language input, respond to their child's communicative attempts, and encourage the use of a variety of language forms and functions. These include the *Hanen Early Language Parent Program* (Pepper & Weitzman, 2004) and associated offshoots such as *More than Words* (Sussman, 1999) and *Allow Me!* (Ruiter, 2000); the Communicating Partners approach (MacDonald, 2004); and Prelinguistic Milieu Teaching (Yoder & Warren, 1998, 2001, 2002). Although these parent training programs are all based on current research about how to promote early speech and language development in typically developing children, there is no reason to suspect that they are not equally effective for children who communicate through AAC, because the principles on which they are based are universal (Blockberger & Sutton, 2003). Readers are referred to Chapter 10 for more detailed information about these programs.

If a facilitator with competent communication skills cannot effectively communicate by using [a communication display], then we cannot reasonably expect the augmented speaker to develop communication competency with that [display]. (Elder & Goossens', 1994, p. 164)

Aided Language Stimulation and the System for Augmenting Language (SAL)

Aided language stimulation (Elder & Goossens', 1994; Goossens' & Crain, 1986a; Goossens', Crain, & Elder, 1992) and the SAL (Romski & Sevcik, 1992, 1993, 1996) were both designed specifically for AAC applications, and both use total-immersion approaches to teaching individuals to understand and use graphic symbols. Their purpose is to provide individuals with rich contextual models for combining symbols in a flexible manner and opportunities to do so. They are based on the premise that, by observing graphic symbols being used extensively by others in natural interactions, "the [learner] can begin to establish a mental template of how symbols can be combined and recombined generatively to mediate communication during the activity" (Goossens' et al., 1992, p. 101). Because both techniques mimic the way natural speakers learn to comprehend language, they are intended to teach language in a very natural way that eliminates the need for more structured training interventions.

Aided Language Stimulation   In aided language stimulation, a facilitator "highlights symbols on the user's communication display as he or she interacts and communicates verbally with the user" (Goossens' et al., 1992, p. 101). In this way, it is similar to the "total communication" approach used to teach manual signs to individuals with hearing or other impairments (Karlan, 1990). For example, the facilitator might say, "It's time to put the cookie mix in the bowl," while pointing to the symbols PUT, COOKIE, IN, and BOWL on an eye-gaze vest or board, SGD, or activity display. Obviously, in order for this type of communication to occur, displays must be accessible to the facilitator, who should ensure in advance that they contain the necessary key vocabulary items for each activity in the learner's day. The facilitator should also provide numerous opportunities for interaction in the context of natural routines and activities. Table 12.1 details the steps of selecting vocabulary for aided language stimulation displays. See Figures 12.4 and 12.5 for examples of aided language communication displays that could be used in a preschool setting and a community setting, respectively.

Integral to aided language stimulation are a variety of unique instructional techniques that are used both to augment input (i.e., receptively) and to encourage the use of the communication display. The facilitator augments input by pointing to or highlighting symbols while he or she is talking, as described previously. Goossens' et al. (1992) noted that facilitators can accomplish this in several ways: 1) index finger pointing, 2) index finger pointing with a small squeaker concealed in the palm of the hand to draw attention to the display, 3) pointing to each symbol with a small flashlight or squeeze light (this is called *shadow light cuing* in descriptions of aided language stimulation), and 4) using a "helping doll" with an elongated pointer (e.g., a small dowel) taped to one hand of the

Table 12.1.   Aided language stimulation vocabulary selection

Example: Doll play

1. *Choose* an augmentative modality that incorporates pictorial symbols: This could be eye gaze, a communication board, or a voice-output device, for example.
2. *Delineate* a variety of doll play activity themes (e.g., cooking, doctor, kitchen, baby care).
3. *Delineate* subthemes associated with the activities (e.g., baby care—changing diapers, mealtime, dressing/undressing, grooming, bedtime).
4. *Select* vocabulary to reflect the interactions that can occur within each subtheme (e.g., baby care—changing diapers: stinky, wet, dry, change, pin, cry, no way, yucky, put on, take off, baby, mommy, wipe, bottom, powder, diaper, finished).
5. *Include* vocabulary commonly used across subthemes (e.g., more, yes, no, help).
6. *Develop* pictorial symbol displays for each subtheme, and post in the relevant activity area for easy access (e.g., in the doll play area of the classroom).
7. *Use* the pictorial symbols during interactions with the child, much as key word manual signing would be used. Encourage and support the child in attempts to use the symbols as one component of a multimodal communication system that might include speech/vocalizations or gestures, for example.

Source: Goossens', 1989, and Goossens' and Crain, 1986a, 1986b.

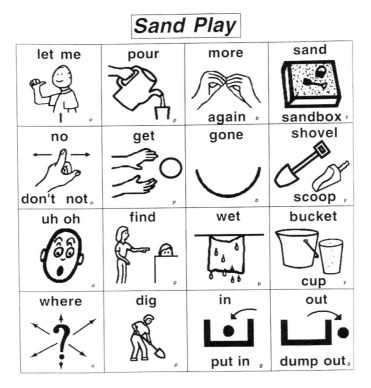

Figure 12.4. Aided language stimulation display for a young child to use during a sand play activity. (From Goossens', C., Crain, S., & Elder, P. [1994]. *Communication displays for engineered preschool environments: Books 1 and 2* [p. 128]. Solana Beach, CA: The Picture Communication Symbols © 1981–2004 by Mayer-Johnson LLC. All Rights Reserved Worldwide. Used with permission.)

doll. Regardless of the technique used, the aim is to provide speech and symbol input during activities, in much the same way total communication is used to combine speech and manual signs.

Aided language stimulation also incorporates a variety of techniques for eliciting communication using symbols and other AAC modes. *Nonverbal juncture cues* are "nonverbal signals (achieved via facial expression, gesture, body posture) performed by the facilitator that precede the highlighting of a symbol on the communication display" (Goossens' et al., 1992, p. 111). The cues serve two functions: They code the target symbol in nonverbal form, and they help the individual to anticipate symbol selection by providing a brief time delay during which the individual might jump ahead of the facilitator and select the symbol spontaneously. For example, the facilitator might blow a bubble during a bubble game and then point to it in an exaggerated manner with wide eyes before pointing to the symbol BIG. Related to these are a series of *verbal and light cues* that are used to encourage use of the symbols. These are delivered in a least-to-most prompt hierarchy, as illustrated in the following script.

Martha (M) is the facilitator, and George (G) is an adolescent with autism who uses a PCS display. They are baking cookies together. Martha points to each capitalized symbol on George's display while talking.

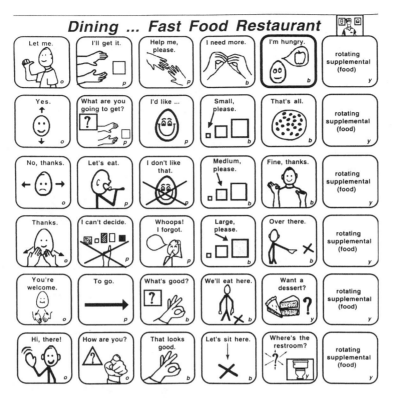

Figure 12.5. Aided language stimulation display for an adolescent or adult to use in a fast food restaurant. (From Elder, P., & Goossens', C. [1996]. *Communication overlays for engineering training environments: Overlays for adolescents and adults who are moderately/severely developmentally delayed* [p. 195]. Solana Beach, CA: The Picture Communication Symbols © 1981–2004 by Mayer-Johnson LLC. All Rights Reserved Worldwide. Used with permission.)

M: Let's get the cookie mix and the bowl. I'll put the cookie mix in the bowl. [uses a *sabotage routine* by putting the box in the bowl without opening it, thus providing a *contextual cue* to elicit George's use of the symbol open]

G: [laughs but does not point to open]

M: Uh-oh! I guess I did something wrong here! I wonder what the problem is? [pauses for 5 seconds to give George time to point to the open symbol (*indirect verbal cue*)]

G: [vocalizes agreement that something is wrong but does not point to the symbol]

M: [uses a *search light cue* by scanning her small flashlight across all of the symbols on George's display, and then pauses for another 5 seconds]

G: [watches but does not respond]

M: I forgot to do something with the cookie mix box. [*direct verbal cue* and 5-second pause]

G: [still does not point to the open symbol]

M: [provides a *momentary light cue* by flashing her light directly on the open symbol for 2–3 seconds]

G: [still does not respond]

M: [provides a *constant or flashing light cue* by shining her light directly on the OPEN symbol until George points to it]

G: [points to the OPEN symbol]

M: Oh! Right! I need to OPEN the COOKIE MIX before I PUT it IN the BOWL! Thank you, George! [opens box]

Of course, the prompt hierarchy would only be used in the above interaction up to the point at which George points to the target symbol.

Because aided language stimulation requires that, as much as possible, communication displays be available for each activity in the person's school and/or home setting, this intervention can be very labor intensive. Mayer-Johnson Inc., however, offers books of communication displays for 100 activities in preschool classrooms (e.g., snacktime, bubble play, Mr. Potato Head; Goossens', Crain, & Elder, 1994) and 63 activities for adolescents and adults in community settings (Elder & Goossens', 1996).

Numerous case studies and anecdotal reports have documented the effectiveness of interventions incorporating aided language stimulation (e.g., Basil & Soro-Camats, 1996; Cafiero, 1998, 2001; Goossens', 1989; Heine, Wilkerson, & Kennedy, 1996). In addition, two research studies examined aided language stimulation systematically. The first involved three preschoolers with moderate cognitive disabilities (e.g., Down syndrome) and little functional speech (Harris & Reichle, 2004). Aided language stimulation was used in scripted routines for preferred play activities; each child was exposed to 12 PCSs representing objects, four times each per routine, over approximately 35 play sessions. All three children learned to recognize and use the symbols and showed evidence of fast mapping in doing so. The second study involved nine learners (ages 4–18) who attended a week-long AAC summer camp in the United States (Bruno & Trembath, 2004). They used color-coded low-tech and dynamic displays with symbols depicting people; actions; adjectives; objects; morpheme markers such as *-ing* and *-s;* the auxiliary *is;* and function words such as *the* and *a.* Aided language stimulation was provided using the displays, in the context of a daily arts and crafts activity. Results indicated that three children whose language performance was highest during a pre-test made the greatest gains in syntactic performance, but all nine participants made gains in their ability to use the displays communicatively. Although this study was hampered by a weaker research design than that used by Harris and Reichle, the results are promising, especially because the intervention occurred over a very short period of time.

The System for Augmenting Language (SAL)   The SAL approach (also known as augmented communication input; Romski & Sevcik, 2003) is similar to aided language stimulation, with two notable exceptions: the use of an SGD is a critical component of the intervention (Romski & Sevcik, 1992, 1993, 1996), and SAL techniques are much simpler than the elaborate procedures for elicitation used in aided language stimulation. In SAL, communication displays using graphic symbols with a printed word gloss are constructed for the learner's SGD, and communication partners learn to activate symbols on the device to augment their speech input in naturally occurring communication interactions. For example, a teacher might say, "Johnny, let's go outside and play," while pointing to the symbols OUTSIDE and PLAY on his SGD. Thus, Johnny would see the teacher model the use of the symbols OUTSIDE and PLAY at the same time that he heard both the teacher and the SGD say the words. Aside from this, "communicative use of the device [is] not taught in the traditional sense. . . .Loosely structured naturalistic communicative experiences [are] provided to encourage, but not require, the children to use symbols when natural communicative opportunities [arise]" (Romski & Sevcik, 1992, p. 119). Because the SAL, like aided language stimulation, relies heavily on partners' cooperation and use of the technique on an ongoing basis, a variety of strategies are also included in the SAL to ensure that partners' perceptions and experiences with the technique remain positive.

Romski and Sevcik (1996) described the outcomes of a 2-year longitudinal investigation of the use of SAL with 13 ambulatory students with severe expressive communication impairments (i.e., 10 or fewer spoken words) who lived in Atlanta, Georgia (Romski & Sevcik, 1996). All of the students had intellectual impairments requiring limited or extensive supports and were in primary or secondary school classrooms. Experimenters provided each of them with portable SGDs in integrated home and school settings. Words were represented on devices with arbitrary symbols (i.e., lexigrams) accompanied by their printed English equivalents. Communication partners learned to operate the devices and to use them in accordance with the basic principles of SAL, as described previously.

The results of the SAL project are quite impressive. All of the students learned to use arbitrary symbols in combination with gestures and vocalizations to request items, assistance, and information; to make comments; and to answer questions, among other functions. In addition, meaningful and functional symbol combinations spontaneously emerged in the repertoires of 10 of the 13 participants (Wilkinson, Romski, & Sevcik, 1994). These included, for example, symbol combinations for verb + noun (e.g., WANT + JUICE) as well as those for descriptor + noun (e.g., HOT DOG + GOOD, MORE + BASEBALL) and noun + social regulator (e.g., JUICE + PLEASE). In addition, some of the participants learned to recognize, at minimum, 60% of the printed words displayed on their communication devices, even though they received no direct instruction related to either symbol–word or referent–word associations. Another important outcome was a general increase in the quantity and quality of some of the participants' intelligible spoken word productions (Romski & Sevcik, 1996). Finally, and perhaps most important, all of the participants showed evidence of generalized use of their communication devices with both familiar and unfamiliar adults as well as with peers without disabilities in a variety of environments.

In a follow-up study, Romski, Sevcik, and Adamson (1999a) compared the 13 participants' communication performance during structured interactions with and without their SGDs. With 5 years of SAL experience, the youth were able to convey more conversationally appropriate, clearer (i.e., less ambiguous), and more specific information to an unfamiliar adult partner with their devices than without them in this structured communicative interaction. Romski, Sevcik, Adamson, and Bakeman (2005) also compared the 13 participants with comparable youth who were able to talk and with youth without either speech or SAL experience. In general, the persons who rely on SAL fell in the middle of the range, communicating better than the nonspeaking, non-SAL participants yet not quite as well as the natural speakers. These follow-up studies serve to support the distinct contributions the SAL experience made to the participants' communicative interactions long term. Because of the many similarities between SAL and aided language stimulation, the outcome data for SAL are likely to have at least some application to aided language stimulation interventions (Romski & Sevcik, 2003).

Romski and Sevcik have continued to implement the SAL concept with school-aged youth with moderate to profound cognitive disabilities through Project FACTT (Facilitating Augmentative Communication Through Technology; Sevcik & Romski, in press). They have also extended their work to apply SAL to toddlers (e.g., Romski, Sevcik, & Adamson, 1999b; Sevcik, Romski, & Adamson, 2005). Currently, Romski, Sevcik, Adamson, and Cheslock (2002) are assessing the relative effects of three early communication intervention strategies—augmented communication input (based on SAL), augmented communication output, and communication interaction with no augmentation—in an on-going, randomized, longitudinal study that involves 60 toddlers and their primary caregivers. Through this study, the authors hope to be able to articulate the relative effects of augmented communication input and other intervention approaches for young children with severe developmental and communication disabilities. Additional research such as this is sorely needed to identify the critical intervention factors that enhance language learning and development in individuals who communicate through AAC.

CHAPTER 13

LITERACY DEVELOPMENT OF CHILDREN WHO USE AAC

WITH JANET STURM

Literacy is the ability to read and write in a desired language. It includes having knowledge about the use of reading and writing in everyday life. Literacy requires active and independent engagement with print and includes both sending and receiving orthographic messages. (Harris & Hodges, 1995)

Reading is the process of constructing meaning from written texts. It is a complex skill requiring the coordination of interrelated sources of information (Anderson, Hiebert, Scott, & Wilkinson, 1985, p. 6). Reading, defined as silent reading comprehension, "is the ability to read a text for a personally or externally imposed purpose and gain an understanding from it" (Mirenda & Erickson, 2000, p. 351).

Writing is a holistic and authentic communication process that is generated through the meaningful construction of . . . text. Writing is best understood as a set of distinctive thinking processes which writers orchestrate during the act of composing (Flower & Hayes, 1981). It is the "written composition or the translation of words into written text" (Mirenda & Erickson, 2000, p. 351).

Most individuals consider reading and writing skills to be a valued component for successful participation in society. These skills allow them to use literacy as a tool for communication, critical thinking, and the attainment of social and cultural power (Bishop, Rankin, & Mirenda, 1994). For people who rely on AAC, literacy skills facilitate successful participation at multiple levels across a variety of environments—home, work, school, and social settings. At a communication level, literacy skills improve their ability to participate successfully in face-to-face interactions by providing them with access to language (Koppenhaver, Coleman, Kalman, & Yoder, 1991). Literacy skills for these individuals are not only about the ability to read books and write text; they are also about access to a means of self-expression to communicate thoughts and opinions and to foster personal independence (DeCoste, 1997b). Literacy skills provide access to a range of so-phisticated AAC systems that allow them to express their thoughts through a combina-tion of symbols and orthography. Finally, literacy skills provide access to educational and vocational opportunities (Light & McNaughton, 1993). For people who rely on AAC, the development of reading and writing skills fosters self-expression by supporting the acquisition of knowledge about the world. The acquisition of literacy skills also cultivates independence by providing access to the outside world (Sturm, 2003).

There is no question that learning to read and write is a complex process that has been particularly challenging for people who rely on AAC. The process of learning is made more difficult as a result of their cognitive, language, sensory, and motor needs. People with severe speech and physical impairments (SSPIs) not only have motor needs that limit their access to books and writing tools, but also they may have language and cognitive limitations that may further complicate the literacy learning process. People with developmental disabilities such as autism also have cognitive and linguistic needs that make the acquisition of literacy skills especially challenging (Mirenda, 2003b).

In recent years, we have made considerable gains in understanding the literacy learn-ing process for people who rely on AAC. We have greater knowledge about how to iden-tify the literacy learning skills of these individuals and make choices about best practices of instruction. Unfortunately, comprehensive literacy assessment tools and programs for instruction for these individuals are not yet available in published formats. We also lack a substantial body of research that can guide AAC teams to set up literacy programs that support individual learning needs. Limited research is available to describe the literacy learning process and the best instructional strategies for these students. There is much work to do yet in the field of AAC and literacy, and we still have a lot to learn!

The purpose of this chapter is to start AAC teams on the path toward AAC compe-tence and expertise in the area of literacy. Because there are no comprehensive literacy assessment or practice guidelines available, we write about what we know today and pro-vide current information about the development of emergent and conventional literacy skills in people who use AAC. In this chapter, we review literacy development from pre-school through the school years as well as instructional and technical considerations based on current knowledge.

Many individuals require AAC to support the development of reading and writing. These people typically have language, cognitive, or motor limitations that inhibit their ability to fully participate in literacy learning. The goals of these AAC supports are to fa-cilitate ease of access to reading and writing and to assist individuals to develop language and communication in literacy. The following section will describe the populations of in-dividuals who may benefit from AAC supports in literacy and discuss instructional con-siderations.

WHO REQUIRES AAC SUPPORT FOR LITERACY?

Our definition of AAC support for literacy is broad and includes the use of high- and low-tech AAC communication systems (e.g., communication boards, dedicated devices), assistive literacy software (e.g., word prediction, concept mapping programs), desktop and laptop computers, handicap access features (e.g., Sticky Keys), input technologies that support access to reading and writing (e.g., alternate keyboards, joysticks), high- and low-tech tools that support access to books (e.g., screen readers, page turners, book holders), and fine motor supports (e.g., hand splints, adapted pencils). Most important, AAC support also includes communication partner scaffolds in the form of models as well as various types of visual and verbal input.

Primary Motor Impairments and Severe Speech and Physical Impairments (SSPIs)

A large number of individuals experience complex communication needs as a result of primary motor impairments that limit their ability to speak and write. These include people with congenital impairments such as cerebral palsy and arthrogryposis, as well as those with acquired impairments (e.g., spinal cord injuries). Typically, individuals with primary motor impairments do not experience significant primary cognitive or learning problems that contribute to their communication difficulties. At a minimum, they must be provided with appropriate alternative access to literacy curricula.

Children with SSPIs, especially those with cerebral palsy, have clearly documented difficulties with learning to read and write. Most children who use AAC are not literate even at the most basic levels (Koppenhaver & Yoder, 1992a). A review of the research showed that more than 50% and as many as 90% cannot read at all or read well below age-level expectations (Koppenhaver & Yoder, 1992a). Even children with cerebral palsy who have measured IQs in the average range demonstrate reading skills that are significantly below grade level (Berninger & Gans, 1986; Koppenhaver & Yoder, 1992a). Physical limitations have a significant impact on the writing production of people who use AAC. These individuals tend to compose very slowly (i.e., at an average 1.5 words per minute) and do so with great difficulty (Koke & Neilson, 1987; Smith, Thurston, Light, Parnes, & O'Keefe, 1989). The literacy learning process for children with SSPI is also influenced by visual and auditory perceptual difficulties that impact both reading and writing (Smith, 1992). For example, Erickson (2003) noted that the strategic eye movements used to read text are particularly challenging for people who use AAC. When writing, they also experience difficulty with semantics, morphology, grammar, syntax, and spelling that inhibit clear communication of their intended message (Sturm & Clendon, 2004).

While these factors present great challenges when providing literacy instruction for children who use AAC, the greatest barrier to literacy learning may be reduced opportunities to engage in authentic reading and writing opportunities and erroneous beliefs that individuals with SSPIs are not capable of learning to read and write (Erickson & Koppenhaver, 1995; Light & McNaughton, 1993). The reading and writing opportunities of these children are known to be restricted in amount of time and in the number, range, and quality of experiences (Coleman, 1991; Koppenhaver & Yoder, 1993; Mike, 1995). Lack of knowledge about literacy curricula and supports to literacy learning has been one of the critical challenges in supporting the literacy learning of students who use AAC (Sturm et al., in press).

Fine Motor Impairments

It's not like I could read it and nobody else could; not even the creator could control it! (Kent, a 12-year-old boy with fine motor needs who was describing his illegible handwriting)

Some students have fine motor problems that inhibit the mechanics of actually producing words on paper. This difficulty with handwriting, often referred to as dysgraphia, may be related to underlying fine motor control or eye–hand coordination problems, visuo-spatial impairments, or attention deficits (Lerner, 1988). These difficulties in producing legible handwriting and fluent text limit writing effectiveness and enjoyment for many individuals. Students who struggle with handwriting typically produce considerably shorter written products than their peers. Some simply complain when they have reached their physical limits, whereas others stop writing entirely (or refuse to write at all), regardless of whether they have completed assigned tasks. Students whose progress with handwriting development (e.g., very slow or illegible handwriting) has fallen behind their ability to express their thoughts in writing may benefit from access to standard keyboards, alternate keyboards, and assistive writing software that supports rate enhancement.

Cognitive Impairments

So is he ready for me to get out some books? (A response made by a skeptical parent of a 3-year-old child with moderate cognitive impairments who was told by the classroom teacher that her son really enjoyed looking at picture books)

Individuals with cognitive impairments are people whose intellectual abilities lag behind their same-age peers. The severity of their impairments may vary widely and is usually established in terms of scores on both norm-referenced intelligence tests and adaptive behavior scales (Luckasson et al., 2002). (Chapter 9 provides more extensive information about intellectual disabilities and unique AAC issues.)

Because of these individuals' cognitive limitations, educators may not consider literacy learning as an educational goal. As a result, individuals with cognitive impairments are at risk of experiencing both reduced expectations and lack of exposure to literacy materials, both at home and at school. We know that many children with cognitive impairments can develop both emergent and conventional literacy skills and should receive access to the same instructional opportunities as typically developing children. When decisions are made about literacy instruction for individuals with cognitive impairments, educators must consider not only the intellectual disability but also any additional learning needs that might be present. For example, many individuals may experience difficulty

understanding and expressing language, maintaining attention, and interpreting perceptual patterns. Thus, they may require additional scaffolding or educational adaptations to
achieve success. With the appropriate instructional support, many individuals with cognitive impairments can experience the same rewards from literacy experiences (e.g., composing personal letters to a friend or relative) as their classmates without disabilities.

A full account of literacy development must consider not only the child's cognitive processes for acquiring literacy skills, but also the support systems provided by the family and social community for learning these skills. (Blackstone,
1989c, p. 1)

Autism Spectrum Disorders

The symptoms and characteristics of autism can present themselves in a wide
variety of combinations, from mild to severe. Although autism is defined by a
certain set of behaviors, children and adults can exhibit *any combination* of the
behaviors in *any degree of severity*. Two children, both with the same diagnosis,
can act very differently from one another and have varying skills. (Autism Society
of America, 2004)

Children with one of the disorders on the autism spectrum (ASD) usually have identified
needs in areas such as language, cognition, nonverbal communication, understanding abstract terms, and social relations (American Psychiatric Association, 1994), all of which
can have an impact on the development of reading and writing. As many as 20%–60% of
children with ASD do not use speech as their primary mode of communication (Owens,
2004). The implementation and use of multimodal communication strategies, both aided
and unaided, is essential to this population of children (Mirenda & Erickson, 2000). Research exploring the literacy skills of children with autism suggests that some of these individuals have significant strengths in word recognition (e.g., hyperlexia) and relative
deficits in comprehension that are evidenced across language and literacy (Mirenda &
Erickson, 2000).

Because many children with ASD are identified as having significant impairments
across many areas, educators may not consider literacy learning as an education goal for
these children and they are also at risk of being held to reduced expectations and opportunities, both at home and at school (Mirenda, 2003b). Children with ASD can benefit
greatly from AAC strategies and assistive literacy software that supports them to process
and use language in meaningful ways while reading and writing. It is essential that AAC
strategies also support the development of language and text comprehension so that children with ASD have opportunities to engage in meaningful, text-based interactions with
teachers, peers, and caregivers.

Visual Impairments

The term visual impairment (VI) is used generically to refer to a wide range of visual problems (Scholl, 1986). These visual problems can be placed on a continuum that ranges from mild interferences in the visual system to total blindness (see Chapter 7). A number of children, especially those with multiple disabilities, have VIs that interfere with their ability to read and write, although the vast majority are not totally blind. Children with low vision can use their vision as a learning channel for reading and for many other school activities; however, some may need to use tactile materials, such as braille, to supplement printed text or other visual materials (Barraga, 2001).

Approximately 50%–60% of school-age individuals with VI have additional impairments, with physical and/or intellectual abilities occurring most often (Gates, 1985; Sadowsky, 1985). Approximately 40% of people with cerebral palsy have concurrent visual problems and loss of visual acuity (Miranda & Mathy-Laikko, 1989). In addition, research has suggested that as many as 75%–90% of individuals with severe or profound intellectual disabilities also have visual impairments (Cress et al., 1981). Given the high incidence of visual impairments with special needs populations, access to reading and writing should consider the degree and type of visual problem. Educational adaptations for this population should consider use of enlarged text, enlarged keyboards, screen magnifiers, speech-output text readers, or braille (Nelson, Bahr, & Van Meter, 2004).

> The typical American child enjoys many hundreds of hours of storybook reading and several thousand hours of overall literacy support during her or his preschool years. (Adams, 1990, p. 336)

LITERACY EXPERIENCES OF CHILDREN WHO USE AAC

Across both home and school environments, the literacy experiences of children who use AAC are distinctly different from those of typical children. We review the research in both areas in the sections that follow.

Home Literacy Experiences

When compared with parents of typical children, parents of children with SSPIs read aloud to their children fewer times per week, ask for fewer labels during reading (e.g., "What's this?"), and make fewer requests for the child to point to pictures (e.g., "Where's the [object]?") (Light & Kelford Smith, 1993). Communication exchanges during storybook reading are also unbalanced. Parents of children with SSPIs tend to dominate communication exchanges and, as a result, their children who use AAC give up many communicative turns (Light, Binger, & Kelford Smith, 1994). Preschoolers with disabilities also seem to have much less access to writing and drawing materials and writing opportunities than do preschoolers without disabilities (Light & Kelford Smith, 1993). This evidence suggests that children with SSPIs receive reduced opportunities to engage in repeated readings, to actively participate in early literacy interactions with parents, and to explore emergent writing through a range of composing materials.

One explanation for these differences appears to be related to parents' perspectives of the importance of literacy in their children's lives. Many parents of children who use AAC report that they primarily focus their priorities on communication and on meeting the children's physical needs (Light & Kelford Smith, 1993). In contrast, parents of typically developing children place the highest priorities on communication, making friends, and literacy activities. Of course, all parents of children with disabilities do not share this perspective. Four parents described by Coleman (1991), for example, had high expectations for their children, provided a print-rich environment, and offered a broad range of literacy learning experiences. Three of the four teachers of these children, however, had limited expectations for literacy learning.

Martine Smith (1992) described two children with severe speech impairments due to cerebral palsy who had reading abilities within the typical range. She suggested that important factors contributing to their success in reading were relative strength in language competence, support for reading at home, physical independence, and motivation for reading.

Pierce and McWilliam (1993) summarized a number of factors that influence literacy development in preschool children with severe communication impairments. These children often have difficulty manipulating and playing with literacy materials (e.g., selecting books, turning pages of books, playing with pencils and crayons) because of their motor impairments. In addition, parent modeling of literacy opportunities may be less frequent when the children are less mobile. Positioning and seating difficulties, paired with vision impairments, may make it difficult for these children to see the illustrations while their parents and teachers read to them; this, in turn, influences the quality of the interactions during storybook reading activities. Finally, language and cognitive factors may affect the development of play skills related to literacy (e.g., pretending to read). Overall, the nature and quality of interactions during literacy activities changes, as parents dominate to compensate for the children's inability to participate. The result is that the children are often unable to ask questions or make comments and, without access to messages on an AAC system, are also restricted in their ability to respond to parent questions. Finally, the children may also be unable to provide their parents with feedback related to their level of understanding as well as their preferences.

The substantial differences in the communicative and hands-on literacy learning experiences between children who do and do not have disabilities provide the former with a limited foundation for literacy learning. The unintended result is that children with disabilities often enter school with restricted understanding about text and are likely to be perceived as incapable of learning to write. We know that the knowledge, attitudes, and beliefs of both parents and teachers have a significant impact on the literacy learning opportunities of children with SSPIs. We also know that physical constraints these children usually face make it challenging to set up ideal literacy learning environments for them. Nonetheless, it is imperative that children with SSPI and other developmental disabilities be provided with active engagement in language, communication, and literacy opportunities that build core understanding about text prior to entering school.

The single most important activity for building the knowledge required for eventual success in reading is reading aloud to children. (Anderson et al., 1985, p. 23)

School Literacy Experiences

Classroom literacy learning experiences have also been found to be substantially different for school-age students who use AAC compared with their typically developing peers. Instruction differs not only in quantity but also in quality and amount of time spent engaged in literacy tasks. For example, late elementary and middle-school boys with SSPI had less than 2% of their total instructional time devoted to literacy tasks, and only 55%–63% of the total school time was allocated for actual teaching (Koppenhaver & Yoder, 1993). The majority of their literacy instruction focused on reading or writing words and sentences in isolation, completing fill-in-the-blank exercises, and performing spelling drills. Similarly, adolescents with cerebral palsy received direct instruction in reading for an average of 30 minutes per day, the majority of their instruction was conducted through seatwork, and they seldom interacted with one another (Mike, 1995). Factors that promoted literacy learning were also identified in their classroom, including the provision of a text-rich environment, opportunities for students to make decisions about their literate behavior, opportunities for daily story reading, and the use of computers.

In a related study, Wasson and Keeler (cited in Koppenhaver & Yoder, 1993) conducted an observation of the daily instruction provided to a set of 6-year-old twin girls. One twin had severe disabilities and was placed in a special education classroom; the other did not have disabilities and was placed in a general education classroom. Both girls demonstrated typical IQ scores and had similar home experiences. Shortly after starting first grade, the twin with severe disabilities began to fall behind her sister in literacy learning. In fact, the child with severe disabilities received 30 minutes of instruction for every 60 that her sister received. In addition, the twin with disabilities received one fifth the number of opportunities to communicate (i.e., to ask and answer questions and to make comments). This occurred despite the fact that this child had the benefit of a more favorable student-to-teacher ratio (8:3) than did her sister. Koppenhaver and Yoder (1992b) identified similar conditions in two additional classroom studies of individuals who used AAC systems. They also noted that, in a follow-up intervention for the twin with severe disabilities, her AAC team made numerous educational adaptations such as cutting up workbook activities and placing the response choices in quadrants, and facilitating eye pointing during practice activities. Her communication response opportunities more than tripled as a result of these adaptations. This is a good example of the importance of assessing and manipulating contextual variables as part of an overall literacy intervention.

Together, these studies provide insight into the type and amount of participation students with SSPIs typically have for literacy instruction. The challenges described are not meant to depress or discourage—rather, they are meant to inspire us to act in support of increased literacy instruction for people who use AAC, regardless of age and ability! The good news is that it is now possible to better understand the literacy abilities and needs of children with SSPIs. We have made gains in our knowledge about instructional practices, and the technology to support literacy learning has made great advances over the past few years. In the remainder of this chapter, we describe the language and literacy relationship, discuss literacy assessments for children with disabilities, and describe instructional and technical supports for these students.

THE RELATIONSHIP BETWEEN LANGUAGE AND LITERACY LEARNING

Language is central to the development of reading, writing, listening, and speaking. A solid foundation in each of these interconnected yet independent language skills is essential to classroom success. If individuals with AAC systems are to be successful in school, their language knowledge and skill base must be well-developed by the time they enter the elementary grades. However, the reality is that many of these children struggle to acquire even basic language and communication skills. They demonstrate significant difficulties across language domains, including vocabulary delays, a predominance of one- to two-word utterances, poor syntax, morphological difficulties, impaired pragmatic skills, and restricted speech acts (Sturm & Clendon, 2004).

Integrating Language and Literacy

As discussed in Chapter 12, the language learning of young children with complex communication needs must be accomplished using AAC approaches. Language and literacy should be an integral part of their lives from infancy. Development of literacy skills will be enhanced when these children have rich background knowledge, access to a broad range of vocabulary to express that knowledge, and the communication competence needed to convey their background knowledge using a range of AAC systems (Sturm, 2003). If children who use AAC are to be academically competitive or active, it is essential that they master considerable language knowledge before entering the elementary grades. The development of conventional literacy skills is inextricably linked to the potential of their language and communication systems. If AAC systems are acquired in the school years, it is important to recognize that these children are building language skills across multiple domains. They are simultaneously developing receptive language skills, learning to express themselves through the language code of their AAC system, and being asked to learn to compose text using an orthographic system that draws upon their receptive language skills (Sturm & Clendon, 2004). The role of symbolization on literacy learning remains unclear; however, it is important to explore the contribution of symbols in the process of literacy acquisition. We discuss this issue further in the following sections.

Graphic Symbols and Language Development

Most young children who cannot speak are also unable to read and spell in order to prepare their messages. Obviously, young children who use AAC must have some means to interact conversationally, and they cannot wait until they are able to spell in order to do so. Therefore, interventionists must teach them to use some type of AAC symbol system that may itself have significant learning requirements. For example, a child must have systematic instruction and experience in order to learn to use Picture Communication Symbols (PCS), DynaSyms, the Blissymbolics system, or iconic encoding (e.g., Minspeak). At the same time, many children are attempting to learn the orthographic form of their language while they are enrolled in general education elementary school classrooms. The combination of these tasks places considerable, competing demands on students' learning time.

There is no simple solution to this dilemma. AAC specialists face the important task of learning how to assist children who use AAC to achieve communicative competence while allowing them to participate successfully as students. Because many of these children must focus on the simultaneous acquisition of three modes of communication—speech, graphic symbols, and orthography—it is important that instructors consider overlapping features of the three modalities and utilize instructional time as a means to foster integration of concepts across modes (Erickson & Baker, 1996).

The mother of Justin and Jason, six-year-old twin boys with cerebral palsy who communicate through AAC, described the struggle to balance language and literacy development: "In the midst of this spurt of literacy interest and development, we have seen a DECREASE in use of Justin's AAC device for communication! Go figure! Instead of a complete sentence, we are getting a key word and a lot more of the invented sign language. When very frustrated at the grown-ups' inability to translate, Jason and Justin will resort to the AAC device, but not nearly with the language forms we were seeing. I am wondering if the finite amount of focused mental energy available is simply being redirected toward these new skills, while communication (at least at home) is being rerouted to the old standby signs they have used in conversation since the beginning of communication with us. I am very excited to see this self-imposed drive towards literacy, but I am unsure what to do about the decrease in communication attempts on the device. My gut instinct says 'let them tell us things in the easiest possible way right now, so they can focus on learning new skills.' I am at a loss to know where to find a middle ground that acknowledges their need to communicate multimodally, and yet encourages the skills they need to communicate with those who don't know their signs, and often don't even see that a communication attempt is being made! In addition, I am afraid that continued pressure to use limited resources to communicate sentences on the device right now will result in a decrease in the literacy development that we are beginning to see in such a wonderful, child-driven way!"

Symbolization and Literacy Learning

Both language development and literacy development in young children are greatly influenced by early learning experiences. Just imagine how many words a typical child hears and sees before saying (or reading) that precious first word! For that matter, think about how many manual signs the deaf child of deaf parents sees before making that first sign! Now think about young children who use AAC who communicate using symbols: How many of those symbols do they see others using before they are expected to use them to send messages, read, spell, and write? Did you say "Zero?" Often, sadly, that is the case— we expect young children with disabilities to use AAC symbols with almost no experience seeing others do so! This is but one example of the potential impact graphic symbols have on the language and literacy learning processes.

Researchers agree that good readers use their knowledge of spoken language and its sound segments (e.g., syllables, phonemes) to decode and interpret text (Adams, 1990). They also consider this knowledge of grapheme–phoneme correspondence to be critical to skilled reading. Because graphic symbols map spoken language at a morphemic or word level, their use may encourage the development of some of the basic skills and processes that individuals use when engaging in meaningful reading and writing (Bishop et al., 1994). When researchers have considered phonemic (i.e., print-to-speech) mapping, they have asked the following question: "Can graphic symbols and word labels support the acquisition of skilled reading and writing?"

In order to provide some insight into this relationship, Bishop et al. (1994) reviewed the literature relative to the development of early reading acquisition. They used Strickland and Cullinan's (1990) six concepts about print as a basis for interpretation. Through exposure to print, children learn: 1) that print conveys meaning; 2) that there is directionality to the way we read; 3) a basic understanding of the concepts of words, letters, and sounds; 4) that the words we speak are mapped onto print and there are certain patterns in speech-to-print correspondence; 5) that each letter has a shape and a name; and 6) that letters can represent sounds. Bishop et al. (1994) speculated that exposure to graphic symbols with word labels potentially facilitates acquisition of the first three of these skills. Table 13.1 summarizes the hypothesized contributions of graphic symbols on literacy learning.

In addition, it is important to recognize that children who use AAC and who have had limited early language experiences may have language difficulties that severely restrict their ability to comprehend text. Rankin, Harwood, and Mirenda (1994) described several important skills related to the influence of language abilities on reading comprehension. These critical variables include 1) phonologic processing skills, 2) word recognition abilities, 3) problem-solving skills, 4) lexical processing abilities, 5) syntactic awareness,

Table 13.1.   The contributions of graphic symbols to literacy learning

- When learning AAC symbols, children develop the knowledge that symbols convey meaning, and they may be able to transfer this concept to understand that print also conveys meaning.
- When communication displays support left-to-right progressions, children may also learn the concept of print directionality.
- When symbols are paired with traditional orthography, children who use AAC are exposed to the concept of words.
- When facilitators draw attention to the concept of letters, and communication displays utilize sound–symbol mapping rules, knowledge of words, letters, and sounds may be fostered.
- Because symbols are presented at the whole-word level, the ability to recognize words out of context, and the ability to discriminate individual letters through paired associative learning (i.e., letter–phoneme associations and speech-to-print matching) is not facilitated.
- Because symbols are not orthographic in nature, they are unlikely to teach children who use AAC that letters have shapes and names and that letters can represent sounds.

From Bishop, K., Rankin, J., & Mirenda, P. (1994). Impact of graphic symbol use on reading acquisition. *Augmentative and Alternative Education, 10,* 113–125; reprinted by permission of Taylor & Francis Ltd, http://www.tandf.co.uk/journals.

Table 13.2.   The relationship between graphic symbols and reading comprehension

- When considered as a feature of reading comprehension, phonological awareness skills in students who use AAC also play a role in facilitating word recognition and thus support their ability to understand text.
- For students who use AAC, word knowledge relates directly to the availability of symbols to communicate. The more symbols the student has, the more vocabulary words he or she can manipulate and use.
- Graphic symbols play a role in supporting syntactic awareness and competence if facilitators or teachers teach the student who uses AAC to integrate symbols into sentence sequences.
- Pragmatic awareness is the ability to recognize relationships between groups of sentences, to create an overall representation of the sentences, and to use prior knowledge to gain the full meaning of a passage. Because this skill develops through experience with written paragraphs, the influence of graphic symbols on comprehension at this level is unclear.

From Rankin, J.L., Harwood, K., & Mirenda, P. (1994). Influence of graphic symbol use on reading comprehension. *Augmentative and Alternative Communication, 10,* 269–281; reprinted by permission of Taylor & Francis Ltd, http://www.tandf.co.uk/journals.

6) semantic knowledge, and 7) narrative discourse processing skills. Difficulty with any one of these skills may have an impact on the individual's ability to comprehend text. Table 13.2 provides a summary of the phonologic, semantic, syntactic, and pragmatic skills related to reading comprehension, as outlined by Rankin et al. (1994).

In summary, it appears that frequent exposure to graphic symbols and orthography may not automatically give students who rely on AAC an "upper hand" in the early stages of literacy. Graphic symbols appear to influence emergent literacy primarily because they facilitate the development of linguistic and metalinguistic skills. The extent to which graphic symbols promote the development of basic reading skills appears to depend on how students are taught the spoken-to-written symbol relationship. The primary power of graphic symbols may lie in their power to increase communication with others (Bishop et al., 1994). Those who are interested may refer to several published articles that provide a more thorough review of symbolization and its relationship to reading acquisition and comprehension (e.g., Bishop et al., 1994; Blischak, 1994; Foley, 1993; McNaughton, 1993; McNaughton & Lindsay, 1995; Nelson, 1992; Rankin et al., 1994).

All children engage in a similar set of print-specific cognitive processes in learning and using print. (Erickson & Koppenhaver, 2000)

LITERACY ASSESSMENT AND CHILDREN WHO USE AAC

For children who use AAC, reading and writing instruction must take into account multiple factors, including the identification of literacy abilities; the recognition of individual learning needs; the selection of appropriate materials, teaching strategies, and tools; the school literacy curriculum; and the integration of AAC systems. Conducting literacy assessments that identify the child's literacy learning capabilities and needs will help school teams make decisions related to materials, strategies, and tools in relation to the literacy curriculum. Literacy assessments also serve a secondary purpose by assisting AAC teams to determine whether AAC strategies that include orthographic features at the word, phrase, or spelling/letter level are appropriate. Unfortunately, commercially available reading and writing assessment tools that enable a valid and reliable understanding of the literacy abilities of children who use AAC are only now being developed. Chapter 6 describes these efforts as well as specific instruments that can be used or adapted for literacy assessment. In this section, we briefly describe the primary assessment areas that should be targeted.

Emergent Literacy

Emergent literacy assessments assist in understanding the foundation skills of reading and writing such as concepts about print (e.g., book orientation), phonemic awareness (e.g., rhyming), and letter identification (e.g., show me "t"). Table 13.3 provides a summary of six components of an emergent literacy observation process first described by Clay (1993). In addition, Erickson (2000) described ways in which assessment methods can be adapted to examine the emergent literacy skills of children with disabilities (see Table 13.3). Results of the emergent literacy assessment can assist in gaining insights into a child's level of literacy skills and understandings about text. The results are used to make placement decisions, but rather to identify areas of strength and weakness in print awareness.

In addition, writing to dictation (Clay, 1993), also referred to as hearing and recording sounds in words (Clay, 2002), can be used to examine a child's ability to hear the sounds

Table 13.3. The six components of Clay's assessment process and possible adaptations

Original task	Possible adaptations
Running record: Child reads a short text aloud while the adult records the words read correctly and incorrectly.	Use graded passages from informal reading inventories in conjunction with the oral reading to support observations about comprehension. There are currently no viable alternatives for children with significant communication impairments.
Letter identification: Child labels first uppercase and then lowercase letters of the alphabet presented in random order.	Present three or more uppercase and lowercase letters at a time, in random order, and ask the child to point to a letter named by the adult.
Concepts about print: Child reads a text that has been manipulated (Sand and Stones) to assess the developing understandings of book, picture, and print orientation, directionality, and other print conventions.	Create your own manipulated text using an off-the-shelf children's book on a topic that is meaningful and interesting for the child. Follow the format of the original manipulated texts.
Word tests: Child reads words in a list from a curriculum-based sample of words (the child should have encountered them in instruction) that have not been taught directly.	Present words three or more at a time and ask the child to point to a word named by the adult. Select nouns from the list that can be clearly represented by pictures. Show three or more of the pictures and the target word printed on an index card. Ask the child to point to the picture that matches the word.
Writing: Child writes any known words for 10 minutes. The adult prompts with possible words when the child requires assistance (e.g., child's name, animals, little words). In addition to the word generation task, collect independently produced writing samples.	Use a word processor and keyboard, alternative keyboard, scanning array, or communication device to complete both tasks. In the word generation task, disable word prediction and any features other than letter-by-letter spelling (e.g., word prediction, pre-stored messages) in the overall analysis of change over time.
Dictation: Child writes a sentence the adult dictates word-by-word. The adult does not elongate individual phonemes.	Complete the dictation with the technologies listed in writing above. Compare child's performance completing the task with letter-be-letter spelling both alone and in combination with other strategies.

Source: Clay, 1993.

(phonemes) he or she would like to write (graphemes). In this task, the adult dictates a sentence aloud and the child is asked to "write the sounds you hear" (see Table 13.3); the child receives credit for every correct phoneme. A child who struggles to understand sound-to-letter correspondence can benefit from instruction in phonemic awareness.

Word-Level Knowledge

Reading assessments have also been conducted with children who use AAC using informal reading inventories that contain a series of graded word lists (e.g., preprimer, grade 1, grade 2) and graded passages. Reading assessments examine word-level knowledge such as automatic word recognition (e.g., naming or identifying graded words) and decoding (e.g., identifying words that begin with "f" or end with "ack"). Table 13.3 provides an adapted format for examining word-level knowledge in children who use AAC. Results of word level assessments assist in understanding whether instructional emphasis should be placed on development of automatic word recognition skills or decoding skills (Cunningham, 1993).

Listening Comprehension and Silent Reading

Reading assessments also examine listening comprehension (e.g., a graded passage is read aloud to the child and he or she is then asked comprehension questions) and silent reading comprehension (e.g., the child reads a graded passage and is then asked comprehension questions). Results of listening comprehension tasks can be compared with those of silent reading tasks to understand whether the child has difficulties with knowledge of text structures and language comprehension (listening task) and/or with print processing (silent reading task), which includes factors such as inner voice (processing text by holding words in working memory) and eye movements (strategic left-to-right eye movement with stops to fixate on text) (Cunningham, 1993). The standard format for asking comprehension questions in an informal reading inventory is to have the child respond verbally. In the adapted format, a child who uses AAC is asked to respond to the question by pointing to the answer among a multiple choice set. Although these reading assessment procedures provide our best estimate of the literacy abilities of children who use AAC, it is important to know that the task adaptations may influence the constructs being examined. For example, automatic word recognition is typically assessed by quickly flashing a word and asking the child to name that word aloud. In the adapted procedure, the child is shown a word and asked to identify the target word out of a choice of three to four multiple choice options. The obvious problem with this adaptation is the potential inflation of the child's score with respect to word level knowledge.

Collaborators at the Center for Literacy and Disability Studies at the University of North Carolina at Chapel Hill have contributed greatly to the advancement of literacy assessment and instructional practices for individuals who use AAC. Readers interested in the activities of the Center are referred to their Web site, listed in the Resources section.

Writing Assessment

Writing assessments focus on understanding both the child's writing processes and his or her writing products. Writing processes include planning, revising, composing, editing, and publishing. Interviews and observations can be conducted to examine a child's ability to be successful while engaged in these processes. A writing products assessment includes an examination of both spelling skills and writing samples. One method that can be used to examine how a child approaches the task of spelling is a vocabulary writing task in which the child is asked to write any known words for a period of 10 minutes (see Table 13.3). A child's spelling level can also be examined using a developmental spelling test such as the one described in Table 13.4 (Ferroli & Shanahan, 1987; Koppenhaver & Yoder, 1988). In this task, the child is asked to spell each of the words. The words are then compared with word pattern examples and assigned a developmental level (e.g., phonetic cue, transitional, and conventional). If a child demonstrates delayed spelling development on either the vocabulary writing task or the developmental spelling test, instructional components designed to strengthen his or her knowledge of spelling patterns in reading and writing would be recommended. These spelling tests may also assist in understanding whether alphabetic cueing is a viable strategy for both children and adults. A writing sample assessment can also be used to assist the AAC team to understand which features of print—such as letter knowledge, left to right sequencing, letter formation, and letter order—students have mastered and which they have not (Clay, 2002). Writing sample assessments might also target examination of the best type of "pencil" used for text input (e.g., standard keyboard, alternate keyboard, on-screen keyboard). To get the most accurate assessment of writing processes and products, it is important that the child's method of text input be the easiest and most efficient mode.

If possible, it is also important to examine the student's writing processes and products when composing narratives or expositions. To obtain the most representative sample, the student should be asked to compose a self-selected topic and should be provided with an input method that addresses any access constraints (e.g., alternate keyboard). The assessor can then observe the child while writing to understand his or her planning, com-

Table 13.4.   Developmental spelling test

Print has meaning	Visual cue	Phonetic cue	Transitional	Conventional
RE		BET BEC	BAK	BACK
E		SE SEK	SINCK	SINK
3	A	MM MOL MAL	MAEL	MAIL
	S	DN JS GAS	DRES	DRESS
AH	E	L LAE LAK	LACE	LAKE
TTT		PF PT PECT	PEKED	PEEKED
IEIX	I	LSIE LAT LIT	LIET	LIGHT
ATJA	O	JK GAN DAGN	DRAGIN	DRAGON
F	I	S STC SEK	STIK	STICK
TC		ST CI SID	CIDE	SIDE
8V	T	F FT	FET	FEET
ABT		TS TST TAST	TEEST	TEST

From Ferroli, L., & Shanahan, T. (1987). Kindergarten spelling: Explaining its relationship to first grade reading. In J.E. Readence & R.S. Baldwin (Eds.), *Research in literacy: Merging perspectives* (36th Yearbook of the National Reading Conference). Rochester, NY: National Reading Conference; reprinted by permission.

posing, and revising processes. For example, the student may pause for extended periods and become frustrated after 10 minutes, terminating the task prematurely. The student's writing products should also be examined to understand his or her abilities and needs and to identify instructional areas that require emphasis (e.g., difficulty choosing topics or generating ideas). Sturm, Rankin, Beukelman, and Schutz-Meuhling (1997) and Nelson et al. (2004) provide overviews of additional methods that can be used to examine students' writing, as well as guidance in identifying instructional areas and assistive literacy software supports.

Below is an example of the writing produced by Chris, an 8-year-old boy with SSPI who received limited literacy instruction in early elementary school and obtained his first AAC device in the second grade. This sample took him an extensive amount of time (30 minutes) and physical effort to compose. Whereas grammar and syntax were relative strengths, spelling and writing fluency were identified as areas of need.

Kraz Anems
I like kraz anems. My favoert anem is a meke. I like to wach thm sweg.
(Translation: *Crazy Animals*
I like crazy animals. My favorite animal is a monkey. I like to watch them swing.)

EMERGENT LITERACY

Emergent literacy addresses the earliest phase of literacy development and includes the period between birth and when the child begins to read and write conventionally (Sulzby & Teale, 1996). This perspective about literacy learning seeks to understand changes over time in how the child thinks and uses strategies to comprehend or produce text (Teale, 1995). This continuing development is acknowledged through the recognition of early literate behaviors such as scribbling and reenactments of books.

An emergent literacy viewpoint contrasts with a reading readiness perspective, which espouses that children should be taught a series of prerequisite skills prior to reading and that writing should be delayed until children are reading conventionally (Yaden, Rowe, & MacGillivray, 2000). Unfortunately, for children who use AAC, the reading readiness perspective often influences their literacy learning opportunities more than an emergent perspective. This belief is especially true for those children with developmental disabilities that include cognitive impairments. Often, literacy is not considered to be an appropriate educational goal for these children, who struggle to master skills deemed to be prerequisites to learning to read (see Kliewer & Biklen, 2001; Mirenda, 2003b). Reduced expectations and lack of exposure to literacy materials, both at home and at school, often create conditions that make it difficult for these children to acquire literacy skills. In contrast, when educated in environments that embrace an emergent literacy perspective, these same children are often able to demonstrate varying degrees of literacy learning success (e.g., Erickson & Koppenhaver, 1995; Erickson, Koppenhaver, & Yoder, 2002; Fossett, Smith, & Mirenda, 2003; Koppenhaver & Erickson, 2003). The following sections address the importance of an emergent literacy perspective with all children, especially those with the most complex communication needs.

Emergent Literacy at Home

Research in the area of emergent literacy has shown that exposure to a wide array of literacy experiences in the home provides children with a solid foundation for successful literacy learning at school (Adams, 1990; Sulzby & Teale, 1996). At home, adults can provide models, facilitate interactions, and guide children in a variety of experiences with reading and writing materials. For example, during home literacy experiences children can:

- Actively read stories aloud with their parents

- Engage in multiple readings of favorite stories

- Examine and talk about print through encouragement by their parents

- Connect ideas in the book with the world around them

- Play with reading and writing materials in literacy rich environments

- Watch adults use written materials (e.g., reading newspapers)

- Enjoy books and talk about the content and structure of stories

- Develop literacy tools and a sense of story structure (Adams, 1990; Pierce & McWilliam, 1993)

Through repeated exposure to favorite books, children also learn a host of literacy concepts, including story schema, plot structure, anticipation of events, and how story language is used to create emotions such as surprise and humor (Clay, 1991). For example, in one home literacy program, girls with Rett syndrome gained emergent reading skills and improved their interactions with storybooks when provided repeated opportunities to engage in storybook reading experiences together with their parents (Koppenhaver et al., 2001; Skotko, Koppenhaver, & Erickson, 2004). In addition, as they watch adults read newspapers, magazines, Web sites, books, emails, grocery lists, letters, and other printed materials, children also learn that print occurs in a variety of forms, holds information, and can be produced by anyone (Adams, 1990). Clearly, early literacy experiences in the home lay the foundation for literacy learning in school.

> Literacy learning, like language learning, begins at birth, and perhaps most importantly, speech production is not a prerequisite to literacy learning. (Erickson et al., 2002, p. 5)

Emergent Literacy Instruction at School

Literacy instruction in early childhood classrooms that draws upon an emergent literacy perspective supports students by actively engaging children in reading and writing from the first day of school (Teale, 1995). A small body of evidence contributes to our understanding of early childhood learning environments that foster emergent literacy learning in children with SSPIs and other developmental disabilities (e.g., Katims, 1991; Erickson & Koppenhaver, 1995; Koppenhaver & Erickson, 2003). Some of the key instructional practices in such environments include

- Creation of a well-stocked, accessible library that includes both familiar books (i.e., those read aloud by an adult) and predictable books (i.e., those that include repeated themes or language)

- Daily storybook readings in which children choose the book to be read aloud to the group

- Opportunities for children to write about functional and meaningful events several times a week

- Provision of a wide variety of reading and writing tools as well as time to explore the use of those tools

- Adult scaffolding during storybook reading that draws attention to the forms, content, and use of written language

- Routine integration of text into classroom routines (e.g., song lyrics on charts, labels on activity centers)

- Individual and small group instruction that exposes children to new reading and writing activities. Such instruction includes oral interpretations of what the children draw and scribble as well as adult models of alternative ways to use literacy materials and tools during parallel play activities (Katims, 1991; Koppenhaver & Erickson, 2003)

In addition to the above instructional components, young children develop emergent literacy skills by engaging in "pretend readings" of books that have been read aloud by an adult; responding to literature that has been shared (e.g., through discussions or writing); and actively participating in phonemic awareness, letter, and letter-sound activities (Teale, 1995). To participate in pretend readings, children who use AAC need access to communication tools that support them to retell stories. For example, an alternative keyboard might be provided with symbols that support the retelling of the children's storybook, *Brown Bear, Brown Bear, What Do You See?* (see Figure 13.1 for a sample story overlay). Responses to literature can be supported by assisting children who use AAC to offer their opinions about books by using either low-tech or electronic "multiple choice" communication displays with symbols representing options (e.g., "I thought the book was [silly/funny/sad]"). Finally, phonemic awareness and letter knowledge development can be encouraged by providing children who use AAC with opportunities to hear and manipulate sounds and letters that make up the English language (see Gillon et al., 2004). Providing auditory feedback in literacy experiences may have a positive impact on the reading skills of children who use AAC (Dahlgren Sandberg, 2001; Foley, 1993; Vandervelden & Siegel, 1999). Reading and talking about books (and the words and letters therein), playing with language, and using nursery rhymes and poems are excellent ways to foster these skills. A variety of adapted access methods can be used to assist students to actively engage in these activities (see the Barkley AAC Center's Web site for examples).

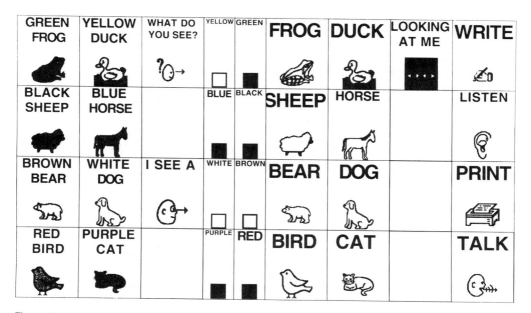

Figure 13.1. A sample story overlay based on the book *Brown Bear, Brown Bear, What Do You See?* (Martin, 1967). Courtesy of Denise Bilyeu (1995). Created with the Discover Create program from Don Johnston, Inc.

> What the child who is least ready for systematic reading instruction needs most is ample experience with oral and printed language, and early opportunities to begin to write. (Anderson et al., 1985, p. 29)

Storybook Reading

Blackstone (1989c) summarized a number of strategies that family members, teachers, and others can use to encourage the development of reading skills. For example, parents and teachers should read age-appropriate stories aloud frequently and repeatedly because young children enjoy hearing the same story over and over. Such repetitive readings help children to learn that the language of stories is different from the language of speech. During story reading, children who use AAC should be positioned on the lap of or next to the person who is reading, so that they can see the pictures and words on a page. As children become familiar with a story, the reader can encourage them to indicate key pictures, fill in the blanks of a refrain vocally, or participate in other ways that help "tell" the story. Similarly, talking switches (e.g., the BIGmack) that activate single repetitive phrases (e.g., "No more monkeys jumping on the bed!") can be used to assist children to participate actively in book reading (see Chapter 10). Once children are interested in this aspect of reading, it is important to indicate key words to them by pointing to the words or using other cuing techniques. Many children also enjoy learning the meaning of logos for places or activities and learn to read the names of fast food restaurants and cereals long before they enter kindergarten!

The speech-language pathologists in a preschool program for children with complex communication needs provided parents with a list of book titles as well as communication overlays that their children could use at home prior to the start of each theme-based unit. One mother purchased a book before a reading unit started and read the book aloud at home with her son. When she arrived at the preschool that week, she noted that her son did not seem to enjoy the book very much at all. However, after watching a preschool story reading session, this mother obtained ideas about how to adapt the text and provide interactive activities. She then used these literacy techniques at home with her son, and the book became one of his favorites. In fact, his name happened to be the same as the boy featured in the story, and he took great delight each time he heard his name read aloud! (from West, Bilyeu, & Brune, 1996)

Additional ways to encourage literacy development include visiting the public library with the child to borrow books from an early age, and involving the child in story time activities sponsored by many libraries (Koppenhaver, Evans, & Yoder, 1991). It is also important to remind relatives and friends to purchase books and other printed materials for young children with disabilities as birthday or holiday gifts; otherwise, they may forget that, without such early stimulation, it will be difficult for the children to develop a later interest in literacy. Seventy-one percent of literate adults who used AAC and participated in a survey by Koppenhaver et al. (1991) reported that people read to them as children at least two to three times per week, and an even greater number reported receiving books as gifts for their personal libraries.

Caroline Musselwhite and Pati King-DeBaun wrote a book entitled *Emerging Literacy Success: Merging Whole Language and Technology for Students with Disabilities* (1997) that is available from Creative Communicating. The book contains hundreds of illustrations and mini case examples to illustrate activities designed to support emerging literacy in students of all ages who have disabilities.

Children who use AAC also need integrated communication and literacy activities that allow them to engage in active, meaningful interactions about texts. One useful strategy in this regard involves the use of thematic curricula in which all activities center around a central topic that can also relate to literacy activities (e.g., the topic of bears, with stories such as *Goldilocks and the Three Bears* and *Brown Bear, Brown Bear, What Do You See?* [Martin, 1967]). Access to integrated literacy experiences requires creativity and planning on the part of the support staff and parents as they select relevant vocabulary words for discussing book content, making comments, predicting events, making inferences, and playing with the sounds of language. They will also need to create communication boards to address book reading in general or to target specific books. Many resources are available to assist parents, educators, and support staff in this regard (see the Barkley AAC Center's Web site for a list of resources).

Joey, age 5, who was getting ready to start kindergarten, enjoyed playing with the letters on the alphabet overlay on his AAC system. One day his mother, who was in another room, heard his AAC device saying "Mom." Without formal instruction, Joey was playing with his knowledge of letters and sounds and managed to spell the name of an important person in his life. As you can imagine, his mother was thrilled to hear her name and to realize that he had spelled it independently!

Emergent Writing

Children also need opportunities to learn writing, drawing, and other composition skills that involve the use of various output tools. Many children with SSPIs and other disabilities are highly motivated to try to manipulate crayons, paint brushes, and other drawing and writing aids that they see their peers use, and they should have opportunities to do so whenever possible. Occupational therapists or other motor specialists may recommend adaptations to standard drawing or writing tools. Children should be encouraged to compose and produce drawn and written materials such as art projects (to be posted on the refrigerator at home or on school bulletin boards, of course!) and letters to Santa Claus, so that they learn to enjoy artistic and written expression.

Children who use AAC also need home and school environments that offer multiple opportunities each week to engage in emergent writing experiences. For example, beginning writers learning to make meaning through text can use invented spellings to generate important words in their environment (e.g., family names), make grocery or other lists, label pictures (e.g., This is . . .), and offer their opinions (e.g., I like . . .) (Cali & Sturm, 2003; Clendon, Sturm, & Cali, 2003). Many children who use AAC need access to computer-based writing tools on desktop computers, laptop computers, or dedicated AAC devices that support them in these writing experiences. Additional information about supportive environments for beginning writers will be addressed later in this chapter.

To relax and wait for "maturation" when it is experience that is lacking would appear to be deliberately depriving the child of opportunities to learn. (Clay, 1991, p. 22)

Assistive Literacy Software for Emergent Readers and Writers

As noted previously, limited access to both reading and writing has been a substantial barrier to the development of literacy skills in many children who use AAC. While reading, these individuals often have difficulty selecting books, turning pages, and reading aloud. While writing, many are unable to use pencils or other instruments to compose text. However, thanks to an increased awareness of the potential of computer technology, access to emergent literacy software for children who use AAC has increased dramatically over the past decade.

A number of emergent literacy software programs for young children are available to support emergent reading and writing concepts targeted at home and school. Early reading software programs such as *All My Words* (Crick Software) and *Balanced Literacy* (IntelliTools, Inc.) provide children who use AAC with access to storybook reading and to activities that foster phonemic awareness, letter identification, letter sounds, phonics, word recognition, and spelling. Emergent writing software tools such as *Writing with Symbols 2000* (distributed by Don Johnston, Inc.), *Kid Pix Studio* (The Learning Company), and *Clicker 4* (Crick Software) offer access to drawing and picture selection, word processing, word banks, publishing features, and communication symbol use for writing.

The potential positive effects of literacy software on the development of emergent literacy skills are especially promising for children who are at risk of developing literacy problems due to motor limitations. Because computer keyboards or other alternative access methods may become primary vehicles for text composition for these students in the primary grades, software programs used in preschools should allow them to develop mouse control skills and a basic understanding of computer operations (e.g., opening a file, saving, shutting down). It is important to remember that technologically supported activities should not replace the emergent literacy activities described previously; rather, they should support and enhance literacy learning in early childhood.

> Language, literacy, communication and assistive technology use can be integrated for learners of any age or ability. It's never too late to start, and no one is "too disabled" to reap the benefits. (Erickson et al., 2002, p. 5)

CONVENTIONAL LITERACY

There is no doubt that the field of AAC has focused heavily on emergent literacy instruction for children with SSPIs and other disabilities over the past few years. As a result, we have a relatively strong understanding of how to support emergent literacy learning. However, it is important to view emergent literacy as a place to start and not as an end goal (Koppenhaver, 2000). Individuals who rely on AAC will realize the full power that literacy offers only through the development of conventional literacy skills. In this section, we describe approaches to formal reading and writing instruction and offer examples of instructional adaptations and technical supports.

> *Conventional literacy* refers to reading and writing that adhere to accepted conventions of form, content, and use. It includes such behaviors and understandings as using written syntax that others can understand, spelling words as they appear in a dictionary, understanding the main ideas of texts written by others, and being able to communicate in print with people we have never met before. (Koppenhaver, 2000, pp. 271–272)

The field of education in general is beginning to reach a consensus about what constitutes good literacy instruction. One vehicle for achieving this consensus has been through examination of the literacy teaching practices that teachers rate as "exemplary." Such practices draw on a balanced model of instruction that includes both skill-based as well as literature and language-rich practices (Baumann, Hoffman, Duffy-Hester, & Moon Ro, 2000; Baumann, Hoffman, Moon Ro, & Duffy-Hester, 1998). Within a balanced approach to literacy, teachers maximize instructional time in the classroom through the sheer density of literacy activities. They also balance instruction across the core skills needed for successful literacy learning, including decoding, automatic word recognition, reading comprehension, independent reading, and writing. They use extensive scaffolding to support beginning reading and focus on developing the ability of students to self-regulate during the learning process (Pressley et al., 1996). In a balanced literacy approach, reading and writing experiences are multifaceted and authentic, and they allow students to have repeated opportunities to internalize concepts. Balanced literacy instruction in general education classrooms serves as a useful guidepost for the instruction of students who use AAC (Sturm et al., in press).

Reading Instruction for Children Who Use AAC

Increasingly, educators and researchers working with children who use AAC incorporate balanced literacy practices in both curricula and instruction, with positive results. For example, published case studies of Thomas and Jordan, two boys with cerebral palsy and associated multiple disabilities, provide evidence that an early focus on language development, paired with a focus on balanced literacy in the school years, can result in the acquisition of conventional literacy skills (Blischak, 1995; Erickson, Koppenhaver, Yoder, & Nance, 1997). The literacy curricula for both boys included instruction in word recognition, decoding, reading comprehension, and writing. Their AAC systems allowed them to participate actively in literacy activities and to communicate with teacher and peers. Similarly, a balanced literacy program that blended traditional skills-based instruction with literature and language-rich instruction resulted in measurable reading and writing gains with elementary students with mental retardation (Hedrick, Katims, & Carr, 1999). These studies can be used as reference points to develop literacy programs across a number of related areas for students who use AAC.

Automatic Word Recognition

Automatic word recognition involves the ability to pronounce words quickly and without effort, and it is essential to reading fluently with comprehension (Cunningham, 1993, 1999). Word recognition instruction targets the development of the ability to recognize words rapidly in meaningful contexts. When providing instruction that facilitates automatic word recognition in students who use AAC, it is important that their experiences with words be both repeated and meaningful. In the early grades, students can be engaged in numerous opportunities to read predictable text, engage in repeated readings of books, and participate in activities that target recognition of high-frequency words (Sturm et al., in press). By the later grades, most students independently develop automatic word recognition skills by reading easy texts, so word recognition instruction can receive less direct emphasis. However, it is essential that students who use AAC be provided with high-quality word recognition instruction in the early grades, in order for such automaticity to develop.

Participation in activities that target recognition of high-frequency words can be facilitated by having those words programmed into speech-generating devices (SGDs) or available on low-tech communication displays. For example, "Word Walls" consisting of words that children use every day for reading and writing are used in many classrooms to build reading, spelling, and decoding skills (Cunningham, Hall, & Sigmon, 1999). New words are added to the wall over time (e.g., 5 words per week) for students to use while reading and writing. During instruction, teachers may use the word wall to ask students to chant word spellings aloud, find words that match a series of clues (e.g., "It's a four letter word, it starts with *b*, and you use it to play sports"), and compose dictated sentences. Students who use AAC can access the same words on communication displays or as core vocabulary words programmed into their SGDs.

I was in Justin's class for the holiday party and he began practicing his letters on his AAC device as the other children were putting on their coats. The teacher looked at me as if to say, "See, he's doing it again. He can't use his device." What he was practicing was one of the most recent letters the class had been focusing on, and also the first letter of his aide's last name [the teacher and aide chose to go by the first letters of their surnames because one of their surnames was difficult to pronounce]. When I commented that Justin was working on one of the letters they had just talked about in class, the teacher seemed to have a "light bulb" moment. I think it hadn't ever occurred to her that the only way the boys can practice their letters is to say them on their device, and that it is perfectly acceptable to do so during odd moments in the day. (Justin and Jason's mother)

Decoding

Decoding is the process of analyzing and identifying unknown words. There are many different ways that students can employ knowledge of phonics as well as other word analysis strategies (e.g., patterns and analogies) to identify unfamiliar words (Ehri, 1992; Foorman & Torgesen, 2001; Goswami & Mead, 1992; Moustafa, 1995; Treiman, 1985; Tunmer & Nesdale, 1985; Wylie & Durrell, 1970). Like word recognition instruction, instruction that focuses on the development of decoding skills is also at its peak in the first and second grade when students are encountering a large number of unknown words while reading. Students in first grade, for example, typically engage in activities at least twice each week that target manipulation of word sounds, onset-rime patterns, reading and reciting nursery rhymes, word sorting, recognizing word chunks, and counting sounds in words (Sturm et al., in press). In the upper grades, instruction in decoding decreases as students require fewer new strategies in this area. Across the grades, skill in decoding unfamiliar words in text leads to efficient development of a growing automatic word recognition bank.

It is essential that reading instruction for students who use AAC supports frequent and active participation in the broad range of decoding instructional activities that typically occur in classrooms. Teachers should draw attention to the concept of letters, letter–sound correspondence, word onsets (e.g., *b* and *ch*), and syllable chunks (e.g., *at* and *ack*). Communication displays should support students to use and manipulate letters, sounds, rhymes, and word patterns. The word wall example described previously as a strategy to build automatic word recognition can also be used to teach decoding skills. For example, one activity might require students to name all of the words on the wall that start like *ball* or that rhyme with *bat*. Students who use AAC can use communication displays and/or SGDs to name these words and then spell them letter by letter. Because learning to decode is not age dependent, decoding instruction should not be arbitrarily discontinued at a particular grade level; rather, it should continue until the student no longer struggles to decode new words in text.

We have also seen some "spelling" of words at home: trk for truck, and prsnt for present. How exciting! The *speak display* feature [on the boys' SGDs] has been fun and a great learning tool. When they type things and hit *speak display,* the boys hear some very unusual noises from their device at times! They enjoy repeating the consonant blends on the device and hearing how they are pronounced. (Justin and Jason's mother)

Reading Comprehension

The ability to read with comprehension is considered the most important aspect of reading—without comprehension, true reading cannot be said to occur! Reading comprehension is the most demanding aspect of reading because it requires the integration of all skills (automatic word recognition, language comprehension, and print processing) to construct meaning from text (Cunningham, 1993). Reading comprehension instruction in the early grades includes teacher models and scaffolds to support students to approach text with strategies that promote understanding (e.g., decoding unknown words or finding the gist of the story). Such instruction also helps students to self-regulate the reading process and understand when to draw on a range of tools that allow them to integrate their background knowledge with the text being read, make predictions, read new words, synthesize the text content with other curricular content, and offer their thoughts and opinions about the text content. By the upper grades, the instructional emphasis shifts to include a greater amount of content area reading; thus, it is important that students who use AAC be taught strategies for comprehending longer, more sophisticated expository texts from early on.

Self-regulation is a form of metacognitive awareness where the reader knows when reading makes sense by monitoring and controlling one's own comprehension (Harris & Hodges, 1995).

When supporting students who use AAC to participate actively in reading comprehension instruction, it is important to select texts that are at the student's instructional level (i.e., texts in which the student is able to read 90%–95% of words automatically). When in doubt, it is better to err on the side of selecting text that is too easy rather than too difficult. Students who use AAC should have repeated opportunities to use each of the reading comprehension strategies taught to their classmates, with extensive verbal modeling and scaffolding by the teacher, at least initially. These students should also have access to communication messages that support them to interact with both teachers and peers regarding the text being read. Examples of these messages, for both beginning and strategic communicators who use AAC, are provided at the end of this chapter.

Independent Reading

In general education classrooms, independent reading is also known by many names, including *Sustained Silent Reading* (SSR) and *Drop Everything and Read* (DEAR). During independent reading time, which occurs daily in a balanced literacy curriculum, both teachers and students stop all other classroom activities and read silently for a sustained period of time. Students are allowed to choose books that are of interest to them and are generally easy for them to read. Independent reading shows students the high value placed on reading and allows them to both enjoy the reading process and build their general world knowledge. Repeated exposures to interesting texts also provides essential opportunities for students to use decoding and reading comprehension strategies while expanding their automatic word recognition bank. Independent reading helps students become more fluent and confident readers.

Many students who use AAC have text read aloud to them frequently by others in order to access grade-level content, but they have limited opportunities to read independently. Of course, it is important to provide access to curricular content and to support its use as part of a student's literacy curriculum across all grade levels. However, because the central educational goals of independent reading are to foster gains in word recognition and silent reading comprehension, it is also important to provide sufficient time for them to engage in this activity. When supporting students who use AAC in independent reading activities, the following factors should be considered:

- The classroom should contain a broad range of books (or other accessible text formats) at the student's independent reading level.

- The book selection should offer choices that reflect the student's interest and age. For example, an adolescent who reads at a first-grade level needs access to texts that are of interest to teenagers, yet written at the first-grade level. Each day, the student should be allowed to self-select a book for independent reading.

- Given the print processing (i.e., strategic eye movement) difficulties experienced by some students who use AAC, adaptations to the text format may be necessary, including: 1) increased font size, 2) double spacing between lines, and/or 3) fewer words or sentences per page.

- Students should have independent access to the text through adaptations such as book holders, page turners, or electronic formats that allow them to maneuver through text independently.

- Students should also have access to communication tools that allow them to share their thoughts and opinions about the texts they are reading.

Ethan, a boy with cerebral palsy, was in fourth grade and communicated using eye gaze, gestures, and an SGD. Assessment of Ethan's reading skills revealed that he performed at grade level in the areas of phonemic awareness, letter and letter sound identification, and listening comprehension skills. His needs were in the areas of reading comprehension (pre-primer level), automatic word recognition and decoding (first-grade level), and independent writing (pre-primer level). Each day, Ethan spent time reading 1) books that were at his independent reading level of pre-primer to primer, where he could read at least 95% of words automatically; 2) challenging books that were written at his instructional level of primer to first grade, where he was able to read approximately 90% of words automatically, and 3) books for listening comprehension at the fourth grade level. For independent reading, it was important that Ethan have choices that were interesting to him. Eye-gaze and/or partner-assisted auditory scanning were used to enable him to choose the book he wanted to read each day. The text was available to Ethan in a computer-based format that allowed him to use a single switch to "turn pages" independently. The text was enlarged using a 36-point font, with no more than three to four words per line and double spaces between each line. Initially, he only read for brief periods but he was eventually able to read for 15 minutes at a time. Assisted by a peer, Ethan kept a record on the computer of the books he read, including indicators of whether he liked each of them. His teacher assessed reading comprehension by offering a variety of opinion messages that were spoken aloud, written on a dry-erase board, or written on an eye-gaze frame.

Writing Instruction for Students Who Use AAC

Written language is a powerful vehicle for learning, and, for students who use AAC, it is also a powerful vehicle for communicating. Calkins reminded us that "writers live their lives differently because they write" (1994, p. 7). In order to learn to write well, students need regular and frequent time for writing and opportunities to write about topics that are meaningful to them (Atwell, 1987; Calkins, 1994; Graves, 1994; Reif, 1992). When they are learning to write, students need to know that writing involves composing a message using their own words to communicate with other people. They also need the freedom and flexibility to express their thoughts without being constrained by requirements for correct spelling, "neat" handwriting, or appropriate grammar. The teacher's role is to help students write and to keep them writing by providing models, strategies, support, tools, and conditions that are conducive to writing (Graves, 1994).

For many children who use AAC, composing is a slow and laborious process, even with the aid of adaptive equipment. Nonetheless, it is essential that they have ample opportunities to compose continuous written text, and not merely to write single words in isolation as part of workbook exercises (Koppenhaver & Yoder, 1990). Allowing these students to get their thoughts down on paper is much more important than emphasizing correct grammar, spelling, and punctuation, at least initially. Consistent with the balanced literacy approach, young children who use AAC should have frequent opportunities to "create literacy events by dictating stories; labeling; creating charts or bulletin boards; writing journals, stories, and poems; and by producing their own books" (Chaney, 1990, p. 245).

In addition, the commonly used "process writing" model views writing as a process in which students engage in planning, composing, and revising prewriting (planning), writing (composing a draft), and rewriting (editing and revising) activities (Pressley & McCormick, 1995). The principles of process writing focus on student responsibility for learning and place a strong emphasis on informal methods for learning (e.g., Atwell, 1987; Calkins, 1994; Graves, 1994; Reif, 1992). Students with learning difficulties who lack strategies for approaching all phases of the writing process may require additional supports of a more formal nature because the minimal guidance that teachers provide in process writing approaches may not be sufficient to help students with disabilities to acquire the skills they need to write successfully (Graham & Harris, 1997).

Students who struggle with process writing need a balanced approach that allows for frequent writing time, collaboration, individual student learning, and explicit skill instruction. These students often have difficulty with both low-level (e.g., conventions and mechanics) and high-level aspects of the composition process (e.g., organization and generation of content). Students who use AAC, who usually have extremely slow writing rates, may have restricted ability to monitor these complex cognitive demands, and the form of their written language may be affected (Blackstone, 1989c).

A method of explicit skill instruction known as "strategy instruction" can be used to aid struggling writers to develop problem-solving skills for approaching academic writing tasks (Harris & Graham, 1996; Pressley & Woloshyn, 1995). Educators have used strategy instruction successfully to teach a range of writing skills to students with learning disabilities (Graham & Harris, 1989, 1993, 2005; Graham, MacArthur, Schwartz, & Page-Voth, 1992; MacArthur, Harris, & Graham, 1994) but, at least in principle, it can also be applied to students who use AAC. Strategy instruction should not be approached in isolation but should be embedded in the process writing approach described previously. This type of writing instruction involves goal setting, self-regulation, and performance evaluation. Students who participate in strategy instruction interventions in which teachers convey information about and model good writing appear to gain greater awareness of the writing task, learn strategies for approaching writing, and are able to generalize these skills to other writing tasks (Seidenberg, 1988).

In the sections that follow, we describe instructional considerations for beginning and skilled writers who use AAC. Writing development, cognitive models of the writing process, and principles of good instruction are used as points of reference throughout.

One of the most important advances for children who are nonspeaking is the ability to produce their own words by spelling them. . . . Given enough time, a literate person using a letter board can produce any possible message. (Nelson, 1992, p. 11)

Beginning Writers

Beginning writers are students who are in the emergent to early conventional stage of writing development. During the initial stages of writing development, beginning writers focus their energy on producing ideas and generating text (Bereiter, 1980; Berninger, 2000). Because the principle obstacle to idea generation for beginning writers is knowledge of topical material, students need to have opportunities to write daily about authentic, self-selected topics about which they are quite familiar (Calkins, 1994; Graves, 1994). The habit of daily writing supports children to rehearse topics and ideas regularly and to have an elaborate bank of ideas on hand at any time (Graves, 1994).

Beginning writers typically use drawings to rehearse their topics before they begin to write (Dyson, 1986). Thus, both drawing and writing are important aspects of early elementary classrooms. Typical first-grade children produce an average of 85 writing samples per school year and create over 100 drawings (Sturm et al., in press). These repeated experiences allow them to gain an understanding of how to produce text that can be understood and appreciated by others and provides a critical foundation for sophisticated conventional writing. Nonconventional spelling (also known as inventive spelling) is also valued and respected in many kindergarten and first-grade classrooms. For example, a typically developing kindergartener produced the following sample: IA MRIDMIKIK WHI MIS (I am riding a bike with my sister) (Cali & Sturm, 2003). Her writing accompanied an elaborate picture of two girls on their bicycles as well as a verbal report to the teacher about what she had written. For this girl and her classmates, drawings and the oral language communicated during the writing process help to ensure a joint reference between the creator and the receiver and assist the receiver to understand the text created using inventive spelling (Sturm, 2003).

In contrast, consider the limited writing and drawing opportunities available to most children with SSPIs and other disabilities that require AAC support. Koppenhaver and Yoder (1992b) noted that, even when literacy instruction for children with disabilities places great emphasis on reading, it almost always excludes writing. In our work with children who use AAC, the frequency of writing experiences for these children is often limited to worksheet completion; writing topics are often chosen for them; they rarely have access to personal drawings, pictures, or ways to communicate about what they have written; and inventive spelling is often seen as evidence of their "lack of writing readiness." Thus, students who rely on AAC are at a distinct disadvantage with regard to writing, compared with their typically developing peers.

How can this be remediated? First, beginning writers who use AAC and have motor impairments that interfere with their ability to draw need access to pictures related to personally relevant topics that can facilitate self-selection of writing topics. Clinical evidence suggests that, when children with SSPIs are presented with photographs and content-specific vocabulary choices that are linked to preferred topics, they are able to use a wider variety of vocabulary and compose more fluently. Second, as children who use AAC engage in beginning writing experiences, they need assistance to utilize a broad range of writing forms. These should include the typical narratives and journals as well as writing forms such as text labels, written opinions, and story retellings (Cali & Sturm, 2003). Students who use AAC also need numerous opportunities to engage in this range of self-selected topics and writing forms. They can learn about text structures through reading and writing models in the classroom (e.g., peer writing, books read aloud by the teacher, and books read independently by classmates).

Third, beginning writers should be encouraged to make improvements to their writing by "saying more," without the implication that editing for grammatical and spelling errors is necessary. It is important to remember that the primary goal for beginning writers is to focus on the fluent expression of ideas in words. In order to share ideas through writing, students who use AAC need rich life experiences, a solid language base, and extensive experiences with literacy. Finally, it is important to remember that people who use AAC can be beginning writers at any age. Understanding the principles behind writing development and the cognitive processes involved in writing are essential to providing appropriate and meaningful writing opportunities for these individuals.

Colin, a fully included first-grade student with cerebral palsy, uses an SGD as well as gestures and facial expressions to communicate. He can recognize numbers 1–50, most colors, and all of the letters of the alphabet, and can identify rhyme in words. His teacher uses a "Writers' Workshop" model of instruction in which students choose their own topics; share and discuss ideas with teachers and peers before, during, and after writing; and publish writing projects of their choice. Colin's teacher provides writing instruction through a series of short mini-lessons that help students pay attention to different aspects of the writing process. During a typical large group lesson, his teacher provides a model for writing by thinking aloud about her own writing process. For example, she may talk aloud about how she generates and chooses a writing topic. Following the lesson, Colin and his classmates are asked to create a folder that contains a list of possible topics for their daily writing. Colin and his parents take and choose photographs that reflect important events in his life, to be included in his folder. He then uses these photographs to choose topics that are important to him. To participate in classroom writing sessions, Colin has access to vocabulary on his SGD that allows him to communicate with his peers and teacher. For example, he may ask a peer, "Hey, let me see what you picked," to ask about a writing topic. Colin also uses several other AAC tools to compose text, including an eye-gaze frame, an alternate keyboard, and an alternate mouse system. He uses a word processing program that enables him to compose text at a faster rate, as well as word banks that allow him to choose among words that set him up for different types of emergent text forms. For example, he can choose "I like . . . " to compose a text reflecting his opinions. He also composes fewer writing products each week so that he can produce writing forms that are of the same quality as his peers. Once each week, Colin's teacher uses Author's Chair, a Writers' Workshop activity that features student sharing of writing products and includes a follow-up large-group peer discussion. When it is Colin's day to share, he introduces himself using his SGD and tells the class about his writing topic. He then releases the written text that he and his parents have stored in his SGD, one line at time. Colin also has access to publishing software that allows him to print and share his work. (adapted from Sturm, 2003)

Skilled Writers

By second grade, typical students make many changes in their approach to writing. They shift from using pictures to begin writing to writing first and then drawing to illustrate their text (Newkirk, 1989). They begin to juggle the multiple aspects of the writing process by moving recursively among the planning, composing, editing, and revising aspects of writing (Flower & Hayes, 1981). They also begin to write multiple drafts as well as changing, reorganizing, and adding to ideas before finishing a piece of writing. By the end of second grade, most students are able to clearly communicate text messages through more conventional spelling, manipulate word choices to convey their messages, compose longer documents, and use a broader range of writing forms to inform their readers (e.g., topic-based reports). These increasingly sophisticated writing forms also require students to integrate information from personal knowledge, the classroom curricula, and outside text resources.

By late elementary and middle school, students are able to compose multiple types of writing and are expected to communicate what they know through text. Skilled writers approach writing tasks strategically (e.g., setting goals), spending an extensive amount of time planning, generating ideas, and deciding how to say what they want in ways that are both organized and coherent. Skilled writers are able to manage these multiple constraints by quickly moving among these factors while in the writing process (Flower & Hayes, 1981).

What do these increased writing demands mean for students who use AAC? As these students are supported in general education environments, it is critical that they have access to instruction and technologies that allow them to participate in all writing processes, including planning, composing, revising, and editing. Because language development, especially vocabulary and syntactic complexity, continues to grow in the upper grades through extensive reading, it is also important that these students have access to curricular content through classroom discussions, textbooks, and other text resources. In our work with adolescents who use AAC and are considered conventional writers, we often observe two related problems in this regard. First, their literacy curriculum often contains writing assignments but does not include explicit instruction in writing. The implication is that these students can attain more sophisticated writing skills simply by writing *more*. Second, drafts of writing products are often deemed sufficient by their teachers, without the usual editing, revising, and other processes required of their classmates. Thus, students who use AAC are not held to the same high expectations for writing that are applied to their classmates, nor do they receive the systematic instruction that might assist them to improve their writing over time. As a solution, the process writing approach, paired with the principles of strategy instruction, would be an ideal instructional combination for skilled writers who use AAC but still require writing instruction. This combined approach would provide repeated practice while supporting them to become strategic writers who can self-regulate the writing process and produce a broad range of sophisticated writing products for any community of readers.

I received an e-mail from the [Justin and Jason's] teacher asking how to implement writing in the classroom for the boys. She seemed worried about using all of the technology. She wanted to know if they should begin trying to teach the boys to write with a pencil, or use letter stamps to construct words, or use the aide to write things down. The boys don't have the motor skills to form letters with a pencil. The OT says that maybe by age eight they'll be able to print their names. I don't know what to say about the letter stamps. It seems like an awful lot of motor work when we are trying to teach a new cognitive skill. How do I reassure these folks the technology really isn't that hard? I am tempted to invite the entire school team over to our house to see that it takes two seconds to hook up the computer to the AAC device, and also to show how independent the boys can be with the technology that releases them from battling with their motor skills. (Justin and Jason's mother)

ALTERNATIVE ACCESS TO LITERACY

Most children without disabilities enter elementary school with the ability to hold and manipulate pencils and other writing implements. Educators then take responsibility for developing the motor and language skills the children need for writing. When students who use AAC enter school without any way to handle and compose texts, they cannot gain access to most literacy experiences. Thus, they need to enter school with alternative ways to read and write independently so that they can benefit from typical classroom instruction and avoid the need for personalized literacy curricula.

Adaptations for Access to Reading and Writing

Rosenthal and Rosenthal (1989) suggested that school personnel utilize a "backwards elimination" approach to determine the writing adaptations needed by an individual student. Using this approach, the teacher simply works backward from the standard materials and procedures used by students without disabilities. Initial adaptations might involve modifications of worksheets or textbooks. For example, the teacher might standardize workbook pages by changing fill-in-the-blank questions to those that require multiple-choice or matching responses. Then, the teacher can code answer options with a letter or number so that the student can respond by writing, typing, or pointing to a single character. In some cases, simply enlarging a worksheet by photocopying may be sufficient to allow a student with a motor disability to use a pencil to write in answers. Alternatively, shortening the length of assignments or modifying the overall workload may be appropriate strategies that allow the teacher to evaluate the quality of a student's work without lowering academic standards. If simple solutions to participation prove ineffective, the backward elimination approach requires that the teacher then try low-tech adaptive equipment or materials as solutions. For example, headsticks; splints with pencil attachments; modified pencil holders; or large pencils, crayons, and markers may be useful. Figure 13.2 illustrates examples of these adaptations.

Many students with motor impairments use handwriting for short writing tasks but find that it is not functional, efficient, or accurate for longer text production. It may be useful to identify primary and secondary "pencils" for such students, to allow them to re-

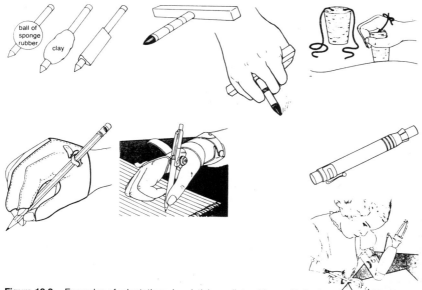

Figure 13.2. Examples of adaptations: headsticks; splints with pencil attachments; modified pencil holders; or large pencils, crayons, and markers. (From Best, Sherwood J.; Heller, Kathleen W.; Bigge, June L., *Teaching Individuals With Physical Or Multiple Disabilities, 5th Edition,* © 2005, pp. 445, 446. Reprinted by permission of Pearson Education, Inc., Upper Saddle River, NJ.)

main academically competitive or active. It is essential that these students, whose easiest method of text generation is usually computer-based, are identified as they enter the school system and provided with access to appropriate alternative access computer tools. To enhance the rate of their writing, many of these students also require rate enhancement techniques such as encoding or linguistic prediction (see Chapter 3 for a discussion of this issue). AAC teams should document in students' educational plans which tasks will be completed through handwriting (e.g., signing one's name and completing short fill-in-the-blank worksheets) and which tasks will require a word processor or other alternative access format. Of course, some students with SSPIs will require computer-based formats to produce all written work. Table 13.5 provides a list of writing input tools and alternative mouse access options.

Table 13.5. Writing input tools and alternative mouse access

Keyboard input	Input tools and mouse access
Standard keyboard	Keyboard modifications
Enlarged keyboard (depressable)	Cursor enlargers
Alternate keyboard (membrane)	Mouse emulator
Assisted keyboard	Optical pointer
Onscreen keyboard	Eye pointer
Dedicated AAC device	Touch window
Voice recognition	Mouse pad
Joystick	
Trackball	
Microswitch	

Sources: Glennen and DeCoste, 1997, and Nelson, Bahr, and Van Meter, 2004.

Specialized reading techniques will also be needed by many students with visual impairments (i.e., low vision or blindness). Such techniques may include large-print text, braille text, low-vision devices, computers, optical character recognition devices, speech systems, or some combination of these. The expressive communication and writing systems used by these individuals may include braille, typewriting, handwriting, audio recordings, and computers. Individual preferences for particular techniques generally depend on a variety of factors, including the person's visual status and functional needs as well as the subject matter.

A valuable reference to help with making decisions about literacy access for students with visual impairments is entitled *Learning Media Assessment of Students with Visual Impairments: A Resource Guide for Teachers,* by Alan Koenig and Cay Holbrook (1995). It provides a process and rationale for conducting learning media assessments, and has a variety of forms for gathering objective data. This text also reveals the characteristics of students who might be likely candidates for a print or a braille reading program.

Assistive Literacy Software

A multitude of assistive literacy software tools are also available to foster the development of literacy skills. For example, many tools offer access to or support the process of writing. Students can use 1) images and organizational features to plan writing, 2) word supports to assist them with vocabulary and idea generation when composing, 3) spelling- and grammar-checking features to assist with editing, 4) text reading features to monitor all phases of writing, and 5) publishing features to share their writing in official formats. Table 13.6 provides an overview of assistive writing features currently available and the potential function of these tools for students who use AAC. For additional information, Nelson et al. (2004) and Sturm et al. (1997) offer a comprehensive discussion of the use of these assistive writing software tools with a range of students.

Numerous reading software programs are also available to enable students who use AAC to read, review, highlight, obtain definitions, manipulate, and copy text sources in a computer-based environment. Such computer applications, along with alternative access and screen reader options (via speech synthesis), allow students to choose and load text, display it on a computer monitor, and advance through the text independently. Students can also use speech synthesizers to read words, lines, or entire screens of text. Screen readers may also provide additional supports to students who use AAC through visual and auditory exposure to text information. Many talking word processors (and communication software products) highlight text as the device speaks it aloud. Students who use AAC can also use talking word processors as tools that allow them to "read aloud" when participating in oral reports with their classmates. Table 13.7 provides a summary of these features and their primary functions for students who use AAC.

When choosing assistive literacy software tools for individual students, it is important that AAC teams base their decisions on students' abilities and needs, their purposes

Table 13.6. Assistive writing software

Writing tools	Functions of the tools
Planning	
• Pictures and photographs	• Pictures and photographs can provide access to drawings and pictures to support text.
• Locked text	• Locked text can be inserted into a word processing file and used to provide self-regulatory question prompts to guide the student (e.g., Who are your characters?).
• Mapping and webbing	• Mapping can be used to assist with organization of content and text structure.
• Outlining	• Outlining can also be used to assist with organization of content & text structure.
Composing	
• Symbol writing	• Symbol writing software can be used to support students in composing using picture communication symbols.
• Word banks	• Word banks can be used to support a fixed set of vocabulary choices.
• Word prediction	• Word prediction can be used to support a broad range of vocabulary choices.
• Frozen text	• Frozen text can be used to provide question prompts to guide the student.
• Talking word processors	• Talking word processors can provide regulatory feedback to the student.
Editing and revising	
• Spell checker	• Spell checkers can identify misspellings. Some tools also offer alternative word choices, definitions, and text readers.
• Grammar checker	• Grammar checkers can identify a broad range of sophisticated grammatical errors.
• Talking word processors	• Talking word processors can read text aloud for the student when reviewing text to be revised and edited.
Publishing and sharing	
• Publishing features	• Tools that offer publishing features can offer students a variety of formats to publish their writing (e.g., newspapers and books).
• Talking word processors	• Talking word processors support students in listening to their final product and sharing their writing with others.

for writing, and the specific curricula to which they are exposed. Many software tools that are used in schools were not designed for use by students with SSPIs. Thus, they may be too motorically or visually demanding (e.g., those that feature a large number of small buttons on each screen) and/or may require complex mouse operations that are beyond students' capabilities (Sturm, Erickson, & Yoder, 2003). It is also important to consider the extent to which specialized software tools are necessary for developing literacy skills (e.g., those that allow students to compose text using picture symbols), or whether a student might do equally well with repeated opportunities to compose text using traditional orthography. Some questions to ask when selecting software tools for students who use AAC include:

• Is this software tool in alignment with the student's literacy abilities?

• Does this tool provide a range of authentic and meaningful literacy learning experiences?

• Does the tool allow for independent access (or support independent access through assistive hardware and software)?

Table 13.7 Assistive reading software

Reading tools	Functions of the tools
Drill and practice/learning game software	Supports the literacy curriculum and provides alternative access to repeated engagement with literacy concepts such as letter identification, phonemic awareness, decoding, word identification, spelling, and guided reading.
Optical character recognition software	Allows books and educational materials such as worksheets to be scanned and entered into an electronic format. Provides student with access to electronic texts for reading and researching for informative writing. Some tools provide exact representations of text, including pictures.
Screen readers/talking software	Reads text aloud for students.
Web sites and CD-ROM texts	Provides student with access to electronic texts for reading and researching for informative writing.
Text enlargers	Allows student to enlarge text and add additional spacing with minimal mouse operations. This feature is especially helpful to students with motor or visual impairments.
Text highlighters	Allows student to highlight text being reviewed. The student is also able to move highlighted text to a word processor.
Definition features	While reading, allows the student to highlight words and get a definition for that word.

- Does the tool provide ease of access to the activity or reading and writing process?

- Does the tool support the general education literacy curriculum and is it a good match with the teacher's philosophy about reading and writing?

- Does the tool allow for continued use as the student's literacy abilities grow and develop?

Of course, any assistive literacy software tools selected for students who use AAC should be reviewed annually to ensure that they are an appropriate fit with the student's changing abilities and needs and the literacy curriculum.

COMMUNICATING IN READING AND WRITING

It is important to emphasize that the development of literacy skills is highly dependent on the ability of the child who uses AAC to communicate effectively with teachers and peers while engaged in all aspects of the literacy learning process. It is important that AAC teams examine the communication used by all students in the classroom and ensure that the student who uses AAC has access to appropriate messages at appropriate times. For example, students participating in the Writers' Workshop communicate frequently in the context of very specific writing events such as peer conferencing (e.g., where ideas are exchanged and feedback given) and Author's Chair (e.g., where students share their writing and peers offer praise and make suggestions). Figures 13.3 and 13.4 provide examples of communication displays that have been created to support students using AAC while they are engaged in such writing processes. In addition, communication displays with generic messages linked to specific reading and writing events can be developed to

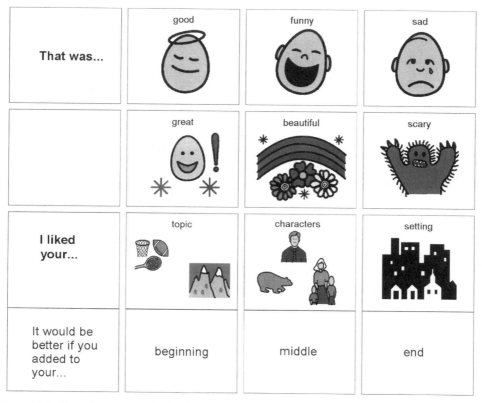

Figure 13.3. Examples of communication displays that have been created to support students using AAC while engaged in the writing process. (The Picture Communication Symbols © 1981–2004 by Mayer-Johnson LLC. All Rights Reserved Worldwide. Used with permission.)

Table 13.8.   Adapted response techniques

Open-ended written or spoken responses can be adapted into yes/no responses or multiple choice responses through:
- Dry-erase boards
- Charts
- Chalkboard
- Eye-gaze board (ETRAN)
- Eye-gaze frames

Response modes for the child might include:
- The student directly selecting the message
- Using partner assisted scanning where the communication partner slowly reads each choice aloud two times. During the second pass, the adult pauses to allow the student to make a choice.
- Coding answer options with a single letter or number so that the student can respond by writing, typing, or pointing to a single character

allow students using AAC to communicate across types of texts. These displays are meant to serve as a point of reference and will need to be individualized for specific students.

> Ethan, the fourth grader featured previously in this chapter, uses two large, side-by-side dry-erase boards to manage the communication demands of the classroom. At the beginning of each lesson, his teacher writes down four possible brief answers on each board and reads them aloud to Ethan, one board at a time. When she asks him a question, Ethan uses eye gaze to indicate whether the answer is on the right or the left board. His teacher then reads the four choices on the board he selected and he makes a choice by producing a "yes" gesture with his eyes. The eight choices can be used to obtain multiple answers from Ethan during the lesson.

Adapting communication events to support active participation in content-specific interactions (e.g., a classroom discussion about the Civil War) may also be achieved by changing open-ended written or spoken responses into yes/no or multiple-choice responses. Both generic message systems and adapted response techniques serve as options for increasing the frequency of participation and the depth of responses of children who use AAC. To be successful, many students will need repeated opportunities to use these messages. At least initially, they will also require assistance, in the form of verbal or visual scaffolds, to know when and how to use the messages. Table 13.8 provides examples of ways in which message choices could be presented. Additional options are presented in Chapter 14.

> Anne, a 9-year old girl who uses AAC, received literacy and communication intervention that fostered her ability to independently compose narratives and later use them to communicate longer, more sophisticated messages across communication partners and classroom settings. The integration of personal

stories and communication in authentic contexts resulted in Anne becoming a more assertive and active communicator. (Waller, O'Mara, Tait, Booth, Brophy-Arnott, & Hood, 2001)

CONCLUSIONS

The possibility for greater numbers of individuals who use AAC to lead rich lives through the power of literacy is on the horizon. Today, we have a better understanding than we did even 5 years ago about how to identify the literacy needs and abilities of students who use AAC and make decisions about instruction that foster literacy learning. Research studies and case descriptions both show that good instruction can result in the development of emergent and conventional reading skills in students who use AAC. Research is currently being conducted that will allow AAC teams to understand the silent reading comprehension skills of individuals who use AAC. This assessment information will enable teams to make individualized instructional decisions that will support students in ongoing development of their reading skills. In addition, research is currently being conducted that will assist in understanding best practices of literacy instruction, including the use of technical and instructional supports, for individuals who use AAC. Future technological advances will also assist students who use AAC in ease of movement among reading, writing, and communication, as well as tools that support them in each stage of literacy development. It is an exciting time! It is essential that all students who use AAC have access and opportunities for literacy learning. The successful implementation of literacy programs for students who use AAC will require that AAC teams draw on current knowledge about literacy development, cognitive models of the literacy learning process, best practices of assessment and instruction, and assistive literacy technology to foster literacy learning.

As this book went to press, a new text titled *Literacy and Augmentative and Alternative Communication,* by Martine Smith of Trinity College, Ireland, became available from Elsevier. It investigates a range of research and application issues relating to AAC and literacy and provides a balanced view of both whole language as well as more analytic approaches to reading instruction.

CHAPTER 14

EDUCATIONAL INCLUSION OF STUDENTS WHO USE AAC

> Education is a specialized form of communication. Human beings have developed particular times and places in which the scripts of their cultures are to be communicated from one generation to the next. We have come to call the set of practices by which this communication of cultural scripts is accomplished "education." The communication that occurs in educational contexts happens in oral, written, verbal, and nonverbal modes . . . . [Our] role is to facilitate the communication, thus the education, that occurs in the classroom. (Hoskins, 1990, p. 29)

In North America and many other places around the world, the educational environments considered to be appropriate for children with significant disabilities have changed dramatically (Fisher & Ryndak, 2001). Whereas special schools and segregated special education classrooms were once the accepted norm, these students are increasingly educated in the same schools and classrooms as their chronological age peers without disabilities. *Inclusion* is the term most commonly applied to this practice, which includes "physical integration, social integration, and access to normalized educational, recreational, and social activities that occur in school" (Alper, 2003, p. 15).

Because participation in the general education classroom requires many types of communication, effective AAC systems that are age- and context-appropriate serve as critical tools for success for students with complex communication needs across the ability range. Unfortunately, it is not uncommon for such children to attend schools for several years without having access to the writing, drawing, reading, or conversational tools available to their fellow students. Students who cannot hold pencils or crayons may not have access to augmented writing systems. Students who cannot hold books, turn pages, or use their voices to sound out words and read may not be given adapted reading equipment or computers. Students who have difficulty answering questions in class and participating in social conversations may not be provided with AAC systems for interaction. Thus, it is not at all surprising that many of these students are unable to participate suc-

cessfully in general education classrooms because their communication skills and the resources with which they have been provided place them at a distinct disadvantage for both
academic and social learning. Sadly, when educational or social participation is not evident, these students are often deemed "failures" or "inappropriate for inclusion" and assigned to segregated classrooms, resource rooms, or other separate settings. In time, they
find themselves increasingly isolated from general education classrooms and placed with
typical students only during nonacademic classes such as music, art, or physical education.
As this chapter shows, parents and school personnel who support students who use AAC
must learn to collaborate in order to avoid this outcome. Instead, they need to work together to deliver inclusive communication and educational services within general education classrooms whenever possible.

FROM PRESCHOOL TO ELEMENTARY SCHOOL

When students with complex communication needs enter elementary school without
communication systems that permit them to participate in typical curricular activities,
their educational experiences are quite different from those of their peers. For example,
they are unable to write or speak in class at times when the teacher expects other students
to do so. Instead, they must either passively observe other students or communicate
through a paraprofessional. In addition, students with severe communication disorders
often spend months and even years engaging in assessment and instructional activities related to AAC system use. These activities may conflict with regular classroom activities,
causing them to fall further behind classmates because they must forfeit "academic time"
in favor of "communication time."

A clear solution to this dilemma is to begin providing AAC services to children with
complex communication needs during their preschool years (Judge & Parette, 1998;
Romski, Sevcik, & Forrest, 2001). Early AAC attention allows children to develop the linguistic, operational, and social competencies that are necessary to support participation
in elementary school. In the United States, the Individuals with Disabilities Education
Act Amendments of 1997 (PL 105-17) mandate publicly funded preschool education for
children with disabilities who are older than age 3 years and provide the legal basis for
early AAC interventions. AAC teams must design such interventions to meet the conversational and interactional needs of young children—communication for today—as well
as the academic and social needs of the general education classroom—communication for
tomorrow. It is important to ensure that by the time children who use AAC reach first
grade, they have the tools necessary for academic participation and instruction. These include augmented writing and reading supports (either electronic or nonelectronic), in addition to whichever communication system is appropriate to meet their needs for social
interaction (see Chapters 9–12). Children who use AAC are also likely to need a variety
of other tools to enable active participation in the educational activities of the general education classroom.

Ideally, the AAC team should begin planning for the child's elementary school (i.e.,
kindergarten) placement at least 1 year before the end of preschool so that the necessary
adaptations and arrangements can be put in place (Sainato & Morrison, 2001). One way

for interventionists to facilitate a smooth transition to kindergarten is to visit the target entry-level classroom well before the beginning of the school year in order to gather information about the participation patterns of typical children in that setting. Some kindergarten settings are quite structured and academically oriented, whereas others emphasize building concepts through play, exploration, and cooperative learning. The nature and expectations of the kindergarten environment greatly influence the interactive requirements placed on the child, which will, in turn, influence the direction of intervention planning during the preschool years. Regardless of the type of classroom, kindergarten teachers themselves have identified a number of critical work-related and social skills that they consider to be important for successful kindergarten entry. Examples of some of the most commonly cited kindergarten entry skills are listed in Table 14.1.

Pretransition visits also facilitate dialogue between the kindergarten teacher and the preschool AAC team concerning the child's needs and abilities as well as the supports necessary for accommodation. For example, the school may need to make architectural modifications to facilitate physical accessibility or may need to hire a part-time paraprofessional to assist the teacher to optimize the student's classroom participation. The speech-language pathologist and motor specialists in the new school may want to establish a plan for learning to use whatever communication equipment is in place or for sharing the day-to-day management of the communication program. Family involvement in the transition and planning process is also critical because family members are likely to be the only people with whom the child has regular contact until the transition is complete. Thus, family members often play a crucial role in the transfer of information about technology, interaction, and other components of the child's communication program.

Table 14.1. Examples of kindergarten entry skills

Type of skill	Skill
Social	Cooperates, takes turns, and shares with other children
	Has self-control and is able to interact without aggression
	Is curious about and interested in unfamiliar events, activities
	Is self-confident and eager to learn
	Attends and listens to the teacher
	Is able to play independently with other children
Communication	Is able to express feelings and needs (e.g., asks for help, communicates wants and needs)
	Asks peers for information or assistance
	Initiates and maintains appropriate peer interactions
	Answers questions
	Relates ideas and experiences to others
Work-related	Follows established classroom routines
	Uses playground and classroom equipment and materials appropriately
	Respects the property of others
	Works on activities for appropriate lengths of time with minimal supervision
	Follows group and individual directions
	Accepts positive and corrective verbal feedback and changes behavior accordingly, as needed

Sources: Chandler (1992); Foulks and Morrow (1989); Hains, Fowler, Schwartz, Kottwitz, and Rosenkoetter (1989); Harradine and Clifford (1996); Johnson, Meyer, and Taylor (1996); Knudsen-Lindauer and Harris (1989); and Piotrkowski, Botsko, and Matthews (2001).

We received a card announcing Maria's graduation from high school. It was her way of saying thanks and caused us to remember her as a preschool child with few ways to communicate. Because of her cerebral palsy, she could not speak, walk, or eat independently. She had very expressive eyes, an infectious laugh, and quite a temper!

In just a few years, she made the transition from a home-based early childhood program, to an inclusive preschool, to kindergarten, to first grade. She arrived in first grade with an electronic AAC system and a powered wheelchair. She had not mastered using either, but she had the tools. With the help of her school district personnel and parents, she was a competitive student who always performed at grade level and never needed to repeat a grade. Along the way, she participated in several summer sessions to enhance her reading, writing, and communication interaction skills. Would she have been this successful if she hadn't received her communication and mobility equipment until entering fourth grade? *What do you think?*

The specific transition planning process depends on the school district and the individuals involved and is likely to vary widely. However, a few general guidelines can be applied. First, during the first several months after transition, the educators and staff in the new school need to pay careful attention to the child's needs in order to avoid "reinventing the wheel" by providing redundant or unnecessary interventions. For example, the AAC team should not modify the child's existing AAC system unnecessarily during the first year of school. If a child has been prepared well for school, drastic changes to the communication system should not be necessary. If the AAC team makes substantive changes, the child is at risk for falling behind the other students academically while he or she learns to use the revised system. Of course, if AAC preparation prior to entry into elementary school has been inadequate, the elementary school AAC team faces a difficult problem and will need to intervene aggressively during the first few years, although this timing is not optimal.

Second, the elementary school AAC team needs to be "up to speed" with regard to the knowledge and skills required to facilitate the communication efforts of young children who use AAC. If team members must learn about an unfamiliar AAC system over the course of the school year, the student's ability to participate in the classroom will probably be affected adversely. We have found that one way to avoid this problem is for a paraprofessional to follow the student from preschool, to kindergarten, and then to elementary school, especially if his or her AAC system has sophisticated technical requirements. When this is not possible, providing facilitator training for the elementary school staff prior to the beginning of the academic year should be a priority component of transition planning.

FOUR COMPONENTS OF INCLUSION

Although inclusion has become more widespread over the past decade, various types and levels of participation still exist in inclusive classrooms for students both with and without

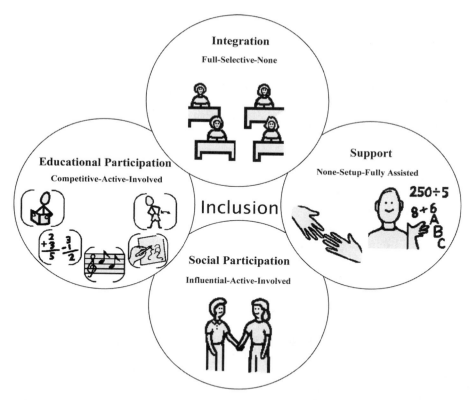

Figure 14.1.   Four components of inclusion.

disabilities. We propose four components of inclusion that interventionists can consider to achieve a participation pattern that is appropriate to meet the needs of an individual student. These include two levels of integration, three levels of educational participation, three levels of social participation, and three levels of support, as depicted in Figure 14.1.

Integration

The term *integration* refers to the amount of time each day a student is physically present in a general education classroom, "breathing the same air" as his or her same-age classmates without disabilities. Integration is a *necessary but not sufficient* component of inclusion. Integration can occur at two levels that are related to inclusion—full and selective. A third level, no integration, may also be available but is generally not recommended.

Full Integration

Students who are *fully integrated* are physically present in the same educational settings as their same-age peers during the entire school day (i.e., essentially 100% of the time). As a result, they have numerous opportunities to participate in the educational and social activities of the classroom, and—given the appropriate supports—are likely to be seen by both their classmates and teacher as full members of the class (McGregor & Vogelsberg, 1998; Schnorr, 1990, 1997). It is important to note that a student can be fully integrated and still spend part of his or her school day outside of the general education classroom, in environments such as the school library, gymnasium, music room, and so forth. In many school districts in North America, all high school students (both with and without disabilities) participate annually in community-based vocational "internships" and/or community volunteer experiences that are appropriate to their long-term goals. The issue here is not whether a student spends time outside of the general education classroom—rather, the issue is the extent to which his or her same-age classmates also do so at the same time. Full integration means doing what everyone else does, when and where everyone else does it.

Selective Integration

Students who are *selectively integrated* spend part of each day in learning environments *other than those* that are typical for their classmates, such as resource rooms, special education classrooms, and so forth. Selective integration may be an appropriate option in some situations for some students, depending on their academic or social needs. For example, we know several high school students (some of whom use AAC and some of whom are able to speak) who choose to spend one or two periods of each school day receiving remedial literacy instruction in a resource room environment rather than attending study hall, music, art, or other elective classes. Others receive speech-language, occupational, and/or physical therapy services in settings outside of their general education classrooms one or more times each week. However, these selectively integrated students participate in various ways in the general education curriculum for the remainder of their school day.

Of course, when students are selectively integrated, they may spend anywhere between 1% and 99% of their time in general education classrooms. Research suggests that the amount of time a student is integrated is likely to have a significant impact on the perceptions of both classmates and teachers (e.g., Schnorr, 1990, 1997). Thus, the student who is "mostly" in a special education classroom but who attends a few selected general education classes each week (typically, for electives such as art, music, and physical education) is likely to be considered by classmates to be a "visitor" rather than a true member of the class (Schnorr, 1990). Similarly, it is unlikely that a teacher will assume "ownership" of a student who "drops into" the general education classroom for a few activities each week but is otherwise educated separately. Thus, it is important to consider the potentially negative impact of such episodic integration and aim for a situation in which pull-out services are minimized rather than the norm.

No Integration

Finally, some students with AAC systems may experience *no integration* during 1 or more years of their school careers. As noted previously, a variety of social, legal, and educational mandates are rapidly reducing the availability of this option in many parts of the world. Special circumstances, however, may exist in which AAC and educational services provided in separate settings benefit the children involved. For example, Hunt Berg (in press) reported on the outcomes over a 15-year period for students with severe speech and physical impairments who attended the Bridge School in California. One of the primary goals of the Bridge School is to "ensure that . . . students achieve full participation in their own communities through the use of AAC technologies" (p. 3). Hunt Berg reported that, of 16 students who attended Bridge for an average of 4.5 years each, 10 eventually transitioned to fully integrated educational settings, 3 were selectively integrated, and 3 were placed in separate school settings. When professional expertise and the commitment to long-term educational and AAC gains are not available in inclusive settings, separate educational programming such as this may be a short-term solution.

Lindsey is a 10-year-old student with severe, multiple disabilities who is included in a general education classroom. Assistive technology along with the support of school personnel and classmates who view her as a full-fledged member of the class help her to participate actively during classroom activities such as the following:

- A classmate records the weekly spelling words on an audiotape, and on Fridays Lindsey activates the tape recorder to announce each word and a sentence that includes the word. After about 8 seconds, her Powerlink (AbleNet, Inc.) automatically turns off the tape until Lindsey activates the switch again to announce a subsequent word and sentence.
- In physical education class, also called "Sweating with Lindsey," the students must exercise as long as the music plays, and, of course, Lindsey controls the switch. At the end of the class, the students spontaneously line up and file by her wheelchair to give her "high fives" for a job well done.
- Lindsey uses a BookWorm (AbleNet, Inc.) to participate in "read aloud" activities during the daily reading period. The story is recorded into the BookWorm and Lindsey uses her switch to read a page when it is her turn to do so.
- Lindsey uses a digital AAC device to announce her choices during snack time and break time.
- When the teacher asks a question in class, Lindsey selects the student who is to respond. She activates a slide projector with a carousel containing two slides of each student, one with a serious and one with a silly pose. By changing the order of the slides occasionally, the students cannot predict when they will be called on to respond to a question. Also, anticipating the silly photo keeps the students attentive, as well as entertained (Locke & Piché, 1994).

Educational Participation

One of the primary reasons for including students who use AAC in general education classrooms is to expose them to the educational curriculum and learning culture designed for all students. Several negative consequences may result if this does not occur. First, when students are excluded from the general education curriculum, teachers (often special educators) must develop personalized educational plans to meet their needs. They deliver this instruction either in segregated settings (e.g., resource rooms, special education classrooms) or in general education classrooms during activities that are parallel to, but not the same as, those engaged in by other students. Although a personalized curriculum may not appear problematic in theory, the reality is that such a curriculum often lacks continuity because its content depends on the preferences and philosophies of individual educational staff. Thus, an individual's curriculum may change dramatically with the arrival of each new teacher, paraprofessional, or speech-language pathologist. Furthermore, inadequate longitudinal management of a totally personalized curriculum over the years usually results in a splintered educational program that is replete with gaps, redundancies, and oversights. In contrast, the general education curriculum provides an overall program structure for educational staff that, at a minimum, encourages a cohesive scope and sequence of instruction.

Second, failure to be involved in the general education curriculum reduces peer pressure and support for learning. For example, in the early elementary school years, there is considerable peer pressure related to learning to read and write. Children with disabilities in general education classrooms are subject to this pressure as much as their classmates without disabilities, and they often respond with the desire to learn what their peers are learning. Peer pressure also encourages children with disabilities to learn at a rate similar to that of other students so that they don't stand out from their peers. A personalized curriculum in which no other students participate eliminates such opportunities for peer pressure and support.

Third, failure to be involved in the general education curriculum diminishes opportunities for peer interaction and instruction. Even if a student with disabilities is physically present in a general education classroom, opportunities for social and academic involvement with other students are reduced if he or she has a personalized curriculum. In addition, a personalized curriculum eliminates almost all opportunities for peer instruction in either direction (i.e., a child with disabilities tutoring a peer without disability or vice versa).

Fourth, lack of participation in the general education curriculum may shape students' negative perceptions of themselves and may also foster negative impressions and low expectations in the eyes of classmates, teachers, and family members. If, however, students are able to participate successfully in the same curricular activities as their peers—with adaptations as needed—they learn to see themselves as academically able in the same arena as their peers.

We suggest three levels of educational participation to describe how students who use AAC can participate in the same general education activities as their peers: competitive, active, and involved. Of course, a fourth possibility—no educational participation—is not appropriate in an inclusive model, although we will discuss this option briefly.

Competitive Educational Participation

Competitive students participate in the same educational activities as their peers *and* are expected to meet the same educational/academic standards. However, they may not complete the same amount of work in the same amount of time with the same level of independence as their peers. For example, most competitive students with AAC systems cannot write as rapidly as their peers. Thus, their teachers may expect them to complete a reduced amount of written class work in order to save time, as long as they meet the same academic standards as their classmates. Similarly, competitive students who use AAC often require more time to take tests or complete assignments, and some may require increased levels of personal assistance in order to stay in the general education curriculum. Again, the issue here is not whether adaptations are required; the issue is whether the student is expected to learn the same curricular content as his or her peers. It is important to note that students may be competitive in one, several, or all areas of the curriculum. Thus, an elementary school student may be competitive in math, reading, music, and art, while performing at a different level in other areas.

Claudia: A Competitive Student in Science Class

Claudia is a student with muscular dystrophy who uses a wheelchair and a computer with word prediction and Morse code to write. She participates in a unit on "rock studies" in her Grade 6 science class. As a competitive student, she is responsible for meeting the same educational goals as her peers. These goals include 1) identifying the difference between rocks, crystals, and minerals; 2) demonstrating an understanding of the rock cycle and erosion; 3) identifying the three main types of rocks (igneous, sedimentary, metamorphic); and 4) explaining how to identify different types of rocks. She and her classmate Venesa work together on in-class activities that require manual dexterity and/or drawing skills, both of which are impossible for Claudia. Venesa acts as Claudia's "hands," but they are both responsible for the quality and content of each project. At the end of the rock unit, Claudia is given more time than her classmates to take a multiple choice test that covers the same content as their essay test. Like many of her classmates, Claudia gets a B+ for her performance in the rock unit.

Competitive educational participation requires that families, teachers, and specialists coordinate efforts so that the student can work with maximal efficiency. The expectations of competitive educational participation do not allow for a remedial curriculum that is different from that of the general education classroom and is taught by specialists. Rather, educational specialists who support competitive students act as consultants to general education teachers so that all school activities contribute to the student's overall educational goal. Educators should expect that competitive students will meet the same standards expected of the peers, with adaptations as needed.

Active Educational Participation

Educationally active students also participate in the same educational activities as their peers and learn content related to academic subject areas such as language arts, math, science, and so forth. However, the expected learning outcomes are not the same as those of their peers, and their progress is evaluated according to individualized goals or standards. Active students often perform at one or more grade levels below the grade in which they are placed and require more extensive curricular accommodations in order to participate. Active students may also receive supplementary instruction to develop skills in certain areas such as math or reading. Many students with AAC systems will be competitive in some subject areas and active in others. Maintaining these students as active participants in general education classrooms allows them to experience many of the benefits of inclusion, such as exposure to a structured educational sequence, peer social contact, and peer instruction. A number of authors have provided rich case studies documenting the progress of students with complex communication needs who were active students in general education classrooms (e.g., Downing, 2002; Erickson, Koppenhaver, Yoder, & Nance, 2001; Fossett, Smith, & Mirenda, 2003; Jorgensen, 1998; Nickels, 1996; Ryndak, Morrison, & Sommerstein, 1999; Sax, 2001; Sonnenmeier & McSheehan, in press).

Aaron: An Active Student in Science Class

Aaron is an active student with autism who uses a communication book with more than 150 picture symbols. His Grade 6 science class is also studying rocks, and Aaron participates in the same instructional activities as his classmates. Like Claudia, he is also learning basic information about the rock cycle and erosion, and about the three main types of rocks: those made from fire or heat (igneous); those made from bigger rocks (sedimentary), and those made from pressure (metamorphic). In addition, some of Aaron's learning goals are quite different from Claudia's. For example, he is learning various rock-related words and their corresponding picture symbols, including MOUNTAIN, BOULDER, ROCK, STONE, PEBBLE, SAND, DUST, and so forth. He is also learning to recognize the symbols for rock descriptors such as BIG, LITTLE, HEAVY, LIGHT, ROUGH, and SMOOTH. He works on all of his goals by participating in the same educational activities as his peers. At the end of the unit, Aaron takes a different test than this classmates, to assess how well he met his goals. Aaron's final B+ has a different meaning than Claudia's because some of the learning expectations for him were different.

Involved Educational Participation

Educationally involved students, like their competitive and active counterparts, also participate in the same educational activities as their peers. However, they are primarily expected to learn content in cross-curricular areas such as communication, social, and motor skills, rather than in academic subjects. As with active students, their expected learning outcomes are not the same as those of their classmates, and their progress is evaluated according to individualized goals or standards. Involved students may require extensive adaptations in order to participate in the same activities as their peers. Again, students who use AAC may be involved in some areas, active in others, and competitive in still others.

Nicole: An Involved Student in Science Class

Nicole is a student with multiple disabilities who communicates primarily through gestures, vocalizations, and eye gaze to objects. During the rock unit in her Grade 6 classroom, Nicole participates in most of the same activities as her peers, to work on motor and communication goals rather than academic ones. At the beginning of each class while the teacher explains various rock concepts, Nicole's paraprofessional wheels her up and down the aisles and provides assistance to help her put one small rock on the desk of each of her 30 classmates. At the end of the class, they reverse the process to pick up the rocks. Thus, each day, Nicole gets 60 practice trials of "fine motor grasp-and-release," a goal identified as important by both her family and her occupational therapist. Every day, Nicole also practices using a head switch to operate a Step-by-Step Communicator (AbleNet, Inc.) and make comments to her science group (e.g., COOL! CAN I SEE? EXCELLENT! CAN I HAVE A TURN?). This occurs during a daily activity in which the students use their small rocks for experiments or other projects. At the end of the unit, Nicole is evaluated on the amount of assistance she requires to pass out and collect the rocks and on the number of times she activates her head switch appropriately to make comments. Her grade of B+ reflects her progress with regard to these cross-curricular goals.

No Educational Participation

Unfortunately, there are two ways that students can be *educational nonparticipants* in general education classrooms. Some students are integrated (i.e., physically present) in general education classrooms during the same activities as their peers but are passive and uninvolved for the majority of the time. Others are integrated in general education classrooms but participate in substantially different educational activities than their peers and receive separate instruction delivered by paraprofessionals or therapists. For both types of nonparticipants, there are often either no explicit learning goals at all, or there are expected outcomes that are substantially different from those of their classmates; if progress is evaluated, individualized goals or standards are applied. Nonparticipation may occur for a number of reasons, often because the student does not have the AAC tools that are needed for involvement in the activities of the class. Even fully integrated students may be nonparticipants in one or more classroom activities. Clearly, this highly undesirable option requires prompt remediation.

Dharma and Rajinder: Nonparticipating Students in Science Class

Dharma is a student who has cerebral palsy and is learning to use an electronic AAC device to communicate in her sixth-grade classroom. During the rock unit, Dharma listens passively to the teacher for the first part of the class, and then watches as the other members of her science group complete their project. Occasionally, one of her classmates shows her what he is doing or makes a comment but, for the most part, she is uninvolved in the activity. Because she is not expected to learn anything from the rock unit, she is not assessed at the end of it and receives no grade. Periodically, her teacher asks the AAC team, "What is Dharma supposed to be doing in here?" They respond that "She is just there for the social experience of being around other kids."

Rajinder is a student with Down syndrome who uses manual signs to communicate. During the rock unit in his Grade 6 class, Raj sits in the back of the room with a paraprofessional and works on activities such as matching objects to pictures, counting from 1 to 10, and writing his name. He does this because, in the opinion of his AAC team, "there is nothing relevant for him to learn in the context of the rock unit." His progress is assessed with regard to his separate curricular goals, and he is assigned a grade that bears no relationship at all to the grades assigned to his classmates.

From this discussion and based on the examples provided, it should be clear that there are many *appropriate* ways in which students who use AAC, regardless of ability, can participate in the educational activities of typical education classrooms. In general, research suggests that several things are required in order for appropriate educational participation to occur. These include

- Administrative support for and commitment to inclusion of all learners (Soto, 1997)

- Availability of an AAC system with functions that are appropriate to meet individual student needs in general education classrooms (Kent-Walsh & Light, 2003)

- Attitudinal skills among AAC team members such as creativity, flexibility, open mindedness, a willingness to take risks and suspend judgment, mutual respect, patience, persistence, humility, and a strong commitment to inclusion (Soto, Müller, Hunt, & Goetz, 2001a, 2001b)

- Willingness of the general education teacher to develop the necessary skills related to both AAC and strategies for including students who use AAC in general education classroom activities (Kent-Walsh & Light, 2003; Soto, 1997)

- A team (including the general education teacher and parents) whose members have a working knowledge of the general education curriculum as well as knowledge of strategies for adapting/modifying the curriculum and assessing students' individual learning styles in order to plan instruction (Hunt, Soto, Maier, Müller, & Goetz, 2002; Mirenda & Calculator, 1993; Soto, 1997; Soto et al., 2001b)

- A team with specific expertise in assistive technology whose members know how to operate, maintain, and make use of the student's AAC system and other learning technologies (e.g., computer and appropriate software) across classroom activities, and provide the vocabulary needed in the classroom (Hunt et al., 2002; Mirenda & Calculator, 1993; Schlosser et al., 2000; Soto, 1997; Soto et al., 2001b)

- A team whose members know how to use inclusive instructional practices such as cooperative learning, team teaching, and small group instruction (Mirenda & Calculator, 1993; Soto et al., 2001b)

- A clear understanding of the roles and responsibilities of each AAC team member, combined with a willingness to be flexible around role boundaries (Soto et al., 2001b)

- Sufficient time for AAC team members to meet regularly, in collaboration with parents (Hunt et al., 2002; Kent-Walsh & Light, 2003; Soto et al., 2001b)

At first glance, this may seem to be a tall order, but the fact is that many of these requirements apply to the provision of meaningful educational programs for students who use AAC *regardless* of where they are educated. Given the many educational benefits available by including such students in general education settings, efforts in this regard are clearly warranted.

"Beyond Access" is a 4-year model demonstration project being conducted through the Institute on Disability, University of New Hampshire. The goal is to design, implement, and evaluate the effectiveness of the Beyond Access Model for students with the most significant disabilities who use AAC in general education classrooms (Sonnenmeier & McSheehan, in press). Information about the project is available at the Institute on Disability, University of New Hampshire Web site.

Social Participation

School involves more than just academic learning because all curricular and extracurricular activities occur within social contexts. Parents of typical students show their awareness of this aspect of school when they request that their children be assigned to the same classroom as their friends or that they be assigned to specific teachers who encourage social development. The inclusive participation patterns of students with disabilities can be described at three levels of social participation: influential, active, and involved. A fourth option, no social participation, will also be discussed briefly.

Influential Social Participation

Socially influential students have friends that include their classmates without disabilities and assume leadership roles in their peer social groups. They are intimately involved in the activities of the group and also exert direct influence over group decisions and social choices, both in school and after school. For example, a socially influential student might initiate activities such as birthday or slumber parties on occasion and, in turn, is invited to similar activities by other group members. A student who is socially influential typically plays, visits, "hangs out," or otherwise interacts with his or her classmates after school hours (e.g., weekends, evenings).

Active Social Participation

Many students (both with and without disabilities) are not socially influential but may be *socially active.* They have friends, make choices about, and are involved in the social activities of their peer group, although they may not exert much direct influence over the social climate of the group or its interaction patterns. Some socially active students are shy, artistic, or studious individuals who have small circles of like-minded friends. Generally, socially active students interact with classmates both inside and outside of school, although they may spend more time alone after school than do their socially influential counterparts.

Involved Social Participation

Students who are *socially involved* have smaller circles of friends without disabilities, exert less choice and influence in social situations, and are often passive participants or observers in social activities. Typically, they do not maintain contact with their typical peers after school hours, and spend evenings and weekends engaged in activities primarily with family members or other peers with disabilities. Students may be socially involved by their own choice or because they require additional supports to be more active or influential. Often, socially involved students do not have adequate AAC systems to enable social participation with typical peers.

No Social Participation

Students who are *social nonparticipants* have limited or no access to peers without disability during school hours and thus have no opportunities to form friendships or make acquaintances with them. They are not real members of a classroom social group during either school or nonschool hours. As is the case with educational participation, social nonparticipation is generally undesirable and requires remediation.

Social participation patterns coexist with the patterns of integration and educational participation described previously. For example, when students with disabilities are at least selectively integrated in general education classrooms for the majority of the school day, they have opportunities for social participation at some level, regardless of whether they are educationally competitive, active, or involved. In order for social opportunities to be realized, AAC team members must know how to facilitate social interactions between students who use AAC and their peers unobtrusively, cultivate natural supports, and teach peers to be good communication partners (Hunt et al., 2002; Mirenda & Calculator, 1993; Soto et al., 2001b).

"Yes, but what about students with problem behaviors?" This is perhaps the most frequently asked question encountered in any discussion of social participation in inclusive classrooms. Unfortunately, problem behavior and related strategies are not the focus of this book. However, readers are referred to the Web sites of the Rehabilitation Research and Training Center on Positive Behavior Support, the Center for Effective Collaboration and Practice, the Online Academy of Positive Behavioral Support, and the Center for Evidence-Based Practice: Young Children with Challenging Behavior for more state-of-the-art information about this important topic.

AAC team members must also know how to set social interaction goals and plan associated interventions that are appropriate for a wide variety of social contexts and communication partners. One way to accomplish this is through use of the "Social Networks" process and inventory discussed in Chapter 10 (Blackstone & Hunt Berg, 2003a, 2003b). This process was designed specifically for individuals with AAC who live, work, and go to school in inclusive environments. It begins by assisting AAC team members to identify individuals with whom the person using AAC interacts regularly, across five "Circles of Communication Partners": lifelong partners such as family members, close friends and relatives, acquaintances, paid workers such as teachers and other professionals, and unfamiliar communication partners (see Figure 14.2). Next, a structured inventory is used to compile information regarding the individual's current modes of expression, representational strategies, selection techniques, strategies used to support interaction, and topics of conversation. In addition, the types of communication used with partners in each Circle are identified along a continuum. This information is then summarized and used to plan unique intervention goals and strategies that apply to each Circle. The Social Networks approach combines the concepts of person-centered planning and inclusion to AAC and can be used with individuals across the range of age and ability.

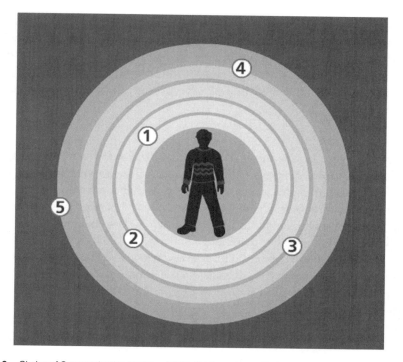

Figure 14.2.   Circles of Communication Partners (CCP). 1) Life partners; 2) close friends/relatives; 3) acquaintances; 4) paid workers; 5) unfamiliar communication partners. (From Blackstone, S., & Hunt Berg, M. [2003]. *Social networks: A communication inventory for individuals with complex communication needs and their communication partners— Inventory booklet* [p. 30]. Monterey, CA: Augmentative Communication, Inc.; reprinted by permission.)

The Social Networks video/DVD presents interviews with AAC experts and consumers and shows how individuals with complex communication needs can broaden their social networks of friends, acquaintances, and people in the community. The DVD includes expanded interviews. Both are available from the Attainment Company and from Augmentative Communication, Inc., along with the Social Networks manual and inventory booklets.

Support

In order for students who use AAC to participate in meaningful ways in the educational and social activities available to their peers, they will most likely require additional support. Support can occur at three different levels, depending on the activity and the student: none, setup, and full assistance. Support can be provided by either adults or peers.

No Support

Some students who use AAC require *no support* in some activities—that is, they are able to position themselves appropriately, equip themselves with the necessary tools for participation, and engage in the activity independently. For example, Aaron, the educationally active student we met previously, ambulates independently to move around his Grade 6 classroom and uses his communication book to interact with peers and adults without assistance. Similarly, Claudia uses a power wheelchair to move around her classroom and school and is able to turn on her computer, boot the necessary software, and complete in-class writing assignments independently using technology that has been individualized to enable her to do so.

Setup Assistance

Most students who use AAC require, at a minimum, *setup assistance* at the outset of an activity to change position or organize their work area in the classroom. Once these setup activities are completed, many students can function independently. For example, even though Aaron can interact socially without assistance (as described previously), he needs a paraprofessional to set him up for most of his schoolwork by making sure he has the appropriate writing tools and other materials. Similarly, Jaqui is an educationally involved high school student with multiple disabilities whose peers wheel her from class to class and help to position her appropriately so that she can use her eye-gaze system to communicate.

Full Assistance

Some students require *full assistance* in order to participate in general education classrooms. This may include help manipulating writing instruments, using a computer, reading, counting, or engaging in other ways in the activities of the classroom. Jermaine, a deaf-blind kindergartener, is one such student who has a full-time paraprofessional to provide support. Of course, teachers and paraprofessionals are not the only available sources of such human assistance; in fact, classmates should be utilized in this regard as much as possible, in ways that do not adversely affect their own participation or learning. For example, Ethelyn, an adolescent with acquired brain injury, needs full assistance in many activities and receives this from a combination of peers and paid adults.

Ideally, all students who use AAC systems should have opportunities to function independently (either with or without setup assistance) during at least some parts of each school day. For example, in the early grades, AAC teams can often facilitate such independence during language arts activities in which students tend to work in small reading groups with other students at a similar academic level. It is important that students who use AAC participate independently at least some of the time because it communicates to the students themselves and to their classmates that they are capable of functioning autonomously in both educational and social areas. Independence also requires well-coordinated support efforts from the AAC team. For example, if a student is unable to participate independently in a subject area for several days, it is often a sign that the AAC team is not fulfilling its responsibilities by keeping the vocabulary current or by maintaining the AAC device. What is critical to remember is that support need not be provided on an "all-or-none, one-to-one" basis by an adult. Peers can—and often do—provide intermittent support to students who use AAC in ways that are more socially normative and useful than when it is provided by adults. Furthermore, we cannot emphasize enough that neither independence nor the ability to be educationally competitive is an appropriate prerequisite to general classroom inclusion.

THE PARTICIPATION MODEL FOR INCLUSION

We use the general idea of the Participation Model (see Figure 6.1) as a framework for making decisions associated with including students who use AAC in general educational programs. This requires several sequential steps that are linked together: constructing a student profile, developing an IEP, planning lessons that include all students, developing a goal/context matrix, and identifying individualized adaptations for participation. The process begins by identifying a student's current and desired participation and support patterns.

Identify Current and Desired Participation and Support Patterns

The foregoing discussion related to the four components of inclusion can be used by the AAC team as both a conceptual and a practical tool. First, the team (including the student who uses AAC, his or her family, and appropriate professionals) should consider the student's current levels of integration, educational and social participation, and support. How much is the student currently integrated? At what level does the student currently participate in the educational activities of the rest of the class in each subject area (e.g., language arts, math, science, social studies, music, art)? How can the student's current social participation best be characterized? What level of support does the student currently receive in each subject area, and who are the sources of support? Figure 14.3 provides an "inclusion map" that the team can use to summarize the current situation. This form is adapted from tools developed through two projects conducted in Ontario, Canada, from 1999 to 2003 (Blackstien-Adler, 2003; Schlosser et al., 2000).

Next, the team should discuss the integration, participation, and support goals for the next school year. Is there a need to increase the amount of integration and if so, what is the appropriate goal? Should there be increased emphasis on improving the level of educational and/or social participation and if so, what are the goals in this regard? Is there a need to adjust the amount of assistance provided, or to explore ways to enlist assistance from different sources; again, what are the goals? This approach contrasts with a less systematic approach to inclusion that involves placing the student in a general education classroom and then "seeing what happens." We have found that, for most students with AAC needs, the latter approach almost guarantees confusion, frustration, and often failure. Again, Figure 14.3 can be used to document goals across the four components.

Figure 14.4 provides an example of an inclusion map completed for a student with autism named Mitchell at the end of his Grade 9 year. As can be seen in this example, Mitch was selectively integrated into a Grade 9 general education classroom for approximately 75% of each day. He received special education services for language arts and physical education and participated in the activities of the Grade 9 classroom, both educationally and socially, as an involved student. He required full support from a paraprofessional for all educational activities. For his Grade 10 year, his team's goal was that Mitchell should be fully integrated and more active in the general education curriculum rather than simply involved. They also wanted to see if they could reduce the amount of educational support he required in two of his classes (drama and applied skills), from full

Current Level of Integration

(circle most appropriate)

Full: in the same general education environments as typical peers for the entire school day

Selective: in the same general education environments as typical peers for parts of the school day

% integrated: _____   % not integrated: _____

None: in different general education environments than typical peers for the entire school day

Desired Level of Integration

Classes to target for integration during the upcoming school year:

1.

2.

3.

4.

Educational Participation and Level of Support

Key: Comp = competitive; Act = active; Inv = involved; None = no participation; N/A = not applicable (new class this year or not on schedule next year)

Support codes: NS = no support; SA = setup assistance; FS = full support

Subject	Current					Desired				
	Comp	Act	Inv	None	N/A	Comp	Act	Inv	None	N/A

Social Participation and Level of Support

Key: Infl = influential; Act = active; Inv = involved; None = no participation; N/A = not applicable (new class this year or not on schedule next year)

Support codes: NS = no support; SA = setup assistance; FS = full support

Subject	Current					Desired				
	Infl	Act	Inv	None	N/A	Infl	Act	Inv	None	N/A

In *Augmentative and Alternative Communication: Supporting Children and Adults with Complex Communication Needs, Third Edition,* by David R. Beukelman and Pat Mirenda. Copyright © 2005 Paul H. Brookes Publishing Co., Inc. All rights reserved.

Figure 14.3. Current and desired inclusion map for individualized planning. (Blackstien-Adler, S. [2003]. *Training school teams to use the Participation Model: Evaluation of a train-the-trainer model.* Unpublished master's thesis, Ontario Institute for the Study of Education, University of Toronto; adapted by permission.)

Current Level of Integration
(circle most appropriate)
- Full: in the same general education environments as typical peers for the entire school day
- Selective: in the same general education environments as typical peers for parts of the school day
  % integrated: __75%__   % not integrated: __25%__
- None: in different general education environments than typical peers for the entire school day

Desired Level of Integration
Classes to target for integration during the upcoming school year:

1. English (reading, writing) (now in special ed room)
2. Physical Education (PE) (now in adapted PE)
3. Drama (new class)
4. Applied Skills (new class)

Educational Participation and Level of Support

Key: Comp = competitive; Act = active; Inv = involved; None = no participation; N/A = not applicable (new class this year or not on schedule next year)

Support codes: NS = no support; SA = setup assistance; FS = full support

Subject	Current					Desired				
	Comp	Act	Inv	None	N/A	Comp	Act	Inv	None	N/A
English				FS			FS			
Math			FS				FS			
Science			FS				FS			
Socials			FS				FS			
PE				FS			FS			
Drama			FS				SA			
Applied skills			FS				SA			

Social Participation and Level of Support

Key: Infl = influential; Act = active; Inv = involved; None = no participation; N/A = not applicable (new class this year or not on schedule next year)

Support codes: NS = no support; SA = setup assistance; FS = full support

Subject	Current					Desired				
	Infl	Act	Inv	None	N/A	Infl	Act	Inv	None	N/A
English				FS				FS		
Math			FS					SA		
Science			FS					SA		
Socials			FS					SA		
PE				FS				FS		
Drama			FS					SA		
Applied skills			FS					SA		

Figure 14.4.   Inclusion map completed for a student with autism at the end of Grade 9, to plan for Grade 10.(Blackstien-Adler, S. [2003]. *Training school teams to use the Participation Model: Evaluation of a train-the-trainer model.* Unpublished master's thesis, Ontario Institute for the Study of Education, University of Toronto; adapted by permission.)

support to setup assistance only. With regard to social participation, the team, which included his family, believed that Mitch was doing well as an involved student and that his social needs were being met. However, they believed he had the skills to communicate with his peers with setup assistance only, so their goal was to encourage him to become more socially independent in all classes except English and physical education, where they believed full support would still be needed. We will continue to follow Mitchell as we discuss the other components of the Participation Model for inclusion.

It is wise to choose a school that your neighborhood friends attend. I was no surprise to the majority of my classmates; they had known me and how I did things for many years before I became a fellow classmate. They also were able to explain about me to any new students who had never met me or had any exposure to a person with disabilities. (Victor Valentic, a man with cerebral palsy who uses AAC, in Valentic, 1991, p. 9)

Develop a Student Profile

Especially when the general education teacher and/or key members of the AAC team change regularly, it is important to develop an annual strengths-based student profile that can be used to guide decision making and goal setting. This profile can be developed through informal interviews with family members and others who know the student well; through more formal, facilitated group processes such as MAPs, PATH, or person-centered planning (see Chapter 10); or through the use of an inventory such as the Social Networks inventory mentioned previously. Whatever process is used, some of the key questions to be answered include:

- Who is this student, as a person? What are his or her preferences and/or affinities? What are his or her strengths and gifts?

- Who is this student, as a learner? How does he or she learn best? In what contexts is he or she challenged to learn?

- What are the student's current literacy (i.e., reading, writing, spelling) abilities? Numeracy and math abilities? Social/emotional and behavioral abilities? Language and communication abilities? Daily living and personal hygiene skills?

- What are the student's challenges and needs?

Table 14.2 summarizes the personal profile developed for Mitchell. It should be evident from this profile that Mitch was a unique learner who had a unique set of preferences, strengths, and challenges and was not performing at the academic level of his Grade 10 classmates.

Develop Appropriate Individualized Education Programs

It is important for the AAC team to determine priority goals for each student at least at the beginning of each school year, so that meaningful educational programs can be de-

Table 14.2. A personal profile for Mitchell

Who is Mitchell?	Current literacy and numeracy skills?	Current personal hygiene skills?
• Age 13, entering Grade 10 • Diagnosed with autism • Lives at home with parents, brother • Attends his neighborhood school • Selectively integrated in Grade 9 • Involved student in Grade 9	• Reads at a Grade 1 level • Can count to 100 and add and subtract simple numbers • Knows basic concepts such as color, size, and so forth. • Can match anything to anything!	• Is ambulatory • Eats and uses toilet appropriately • Needs help with dressing and fasteners • Needs prompts to wash/dry hands • No meal prep skills

Preferences, strengths, gifts?	Current social/emotional skills?	How does he learn best?
• Likes music, karaoke, watching videos, looking at pictures in books • Likes being with other kids as "one of the gang" • Good at singing, running, matching • Fun to be around (happy) most of the time; good sense of humor	• Tries hard to please • Tries to control behavior when confused or frustrated but has "meltdowns" 2–3 times per week • Likes to watch for a while before trying new things	• Verbal instructions are supported visually (pictures, printed words) • He is offered choices, even small ones • He is praised frequently for effort as well as success • He is given short breaks when he asks for them • He is encouraged to be independent and monitored from a distance

Dislikes and needs?	Current language/communication skills?	How is he challenged to learn?
• Dislikes unpredictability, sudden changes in routine, not understanding expectations • Needs supports to become more independent and interact with peers on an ongoing basis • Needs to improve literacy skills	• Spanish is his first language; can say a few words and understand basic phrases and sentences in Spanish • Follows 1- to 2-step directions in Spanish and English; understands more than people assume!! • Can answer simple yes/no questions with head shakes, nods • Started using a TuffTalker with Speaking Dynamically Pro last year	• Directions are too complex • No visual supports are provided • He is not given enough time to process information • He is told to do something over and over again (tunes out) • Adults pay attention to little problem behaviors (they will escalate to big ones!)

signed and implemented. Such individualized education programs (IEPs) should include academic, social, and cross-curricular goals (e.g., in areas such as communication, daily living, and motor skills) as appropriate for each student, along with instructional strategies and criteria for determining whether each goal has been met. Unfortunately, a comprehensive discussion of how to identify appropriate goals and develop meaningful education plans is beyond the scope of this book. However, Table 14.3 describes a number of appropriate resources that can be used in this regard. Although none was developed specifically for students who use AAC, several were designed for students with moderate to severe disabilities who are included in general education classrooms.

It is important to emphasize that team members need to "think outside of the box" and adopt what Donnellan (1984) referred to as the "principle of the least dangerous as-

Table 14.3.   Tools for developing individual education programs for students in inclusive classrooms

Tool	Designed for	Available from
Adapting Curriculum and Instruction in Inclusive Classrooms (Cole et al., 2000)	Students who require intermittent or limited supports in inclusive settings	National Professional Resources, Inc.
Choosing Options and Accommodations for Children, Second Edition (COACH-2) (Giangreco, Cloninger, & Iverson, 1998)	Students who require limited or extensive supports in inclusive settings	Paul H. Brookes Publishing Co.
Curriculum and Instruction for Students with Significant Disabilities in Inclusive Settings (Ryndak & Alper, 2003)	Students who require intermittent, extensive, or pervasive supports in inclusive settings	Allyn & Bacon

sumption" when making decisions about educational goals that are appropriate for individual students. This principle states that, in the absence of conclusive data about a student's abilities, assuming competence has less dangerous consequences for the student than assuming incompetence, should the assumption ever be proven wrong. Failure to adhere to this principle often results in goals that are set too low and that limit both teacher expectations and student progress. Taking the risk of setting educational goals that are "too high," in the end, is less likely to negatively affect student progress than setting them too low. Table 14.4 displays some of the key IEP goals that were identified for Mitchell by his educational team, based on the least dangerous assumption.

Use the Principles of Universal Design to Design Lessons That Include All Students

Universal design principles were originally developed with regard to physical accessibility for people with disabilities, based on the concept that it is less expensive and more efficient to build physical accessibility features into blueprints and community designs from the outset than to do so as an afterthought (Rose & Meyer, 2002). Thus, when new buildings are constructed following this principle, they automatically include features such as ramps, accessible washrooms, braille legends in elevators, and tactile stairs. When new communities are universally designed, they automatically include sidewalks with curb cuts, street intersections with both visual and audio signals, and so forth.

When applied to general education classrooms, the principles of universal design for learning (UDL) encourage teachers to set lesson goals and to design related activities that are inclusive from the outset (Bauer & Matusek, 2001; Kame'enui & Simmons, 1999; Rose & Meyer, 2002). Three basic principles are involved:

1. To support recognition learning, teachers should provide *multiple, flexible methods of presentation*

2. To support strategic learning, teachers should provide *multiple, flexible methods of expression and apprenticeship*

3. To support affective learning, teachers should provide *multiple, flexible options for engagement*

Table 14.4. Example educational goals for Mitchell, Grade 10

Goal: Mitchell will read and write simple texts
- Mitchell will read age-appropriate texts adapted to his current reading level
- Mitchell will use a computer with PixWriter software to write short stories, poems, and adapted tests

Goal: Mitchell will attend to classroom activities, discussions, and presentations
- Mitchell will use follow-along materials and strategies (e.g., circle the number of the question being discussed)
- Mitchell will pay attention when requested to do so

Goal: Mitchell will participate in classroom activities, presentations, and discussions
- Mitchell will respond without protest to simple directives given by the teacher or a peer (e.g., take out a book, transition from one activity to the next, direct attention to specific items when asked)
- Mitchell will use his TuffTalker to respond to two questions asked by the teacher during <u>each classroom activity</u> (e.g., "What is the answer to the flashcard problem?" "What is in the picture?" "What is this word?")
- Mitchell will present a report on at least one concept from each unit, using visual materials and his TuffTalker
- Mitchell will demonstrate mastery of at least three concepts from each unit
- Mitchell will manage his materials in an appropriate manner (e.g., keep his locker neat, arrange materials neatly in/on his desk, bring supplies to class)

Goal: Mitchell will participate in social activities in the classroom
- Mitchell will initiate conversation and interactions with peers with his TuffTalker
- Mitchell will converse at appropriate times in the classroom with his TuffTalker
- Mitchell will demonstrate appropriate turn taking and sharing
- Mitchell will greet unfamiliar adults appropriately by shaking hands or saying *hi*
- Mitchell will participate in extracurricular activities with peers in his social network at least twice each week

When teachers set lesson goals that are "fuzzy" and open-ended, all students—including but not limited to those who use AAC—are likely to benefit (Rose & Meyer, 2002). For example, consider a language arts lesson related to *Romeo and Juliet* that was taught in Mitchell's Grade 10 classroom by Mrs. Johnson. Mrs. Johnson's original goal for the lesson was that "Students will read the play *Romeo and Juliet* and write a 10-page essay describing the key plot elements and character motivations"—a goal that made it virtually impossible for Mitchell to participate in any meaningful way. However, when Mrs. Johnson applied the principles of UDL to her lesson planning, she considered three types of learning outcomes: what *all* students will learn, what *most but not all* students will learn, and what *some* students will learn (Schumm, Vaughn, & Leavell, 1994). Her revised goal for all students (including Mitchell) was "Students will act out an abbreviated version of the play *Romeo and Juliet* and will be able to identify the setting, main characters, main plot elements, problem, and solution." Note that this goal does not specify *how* students will demonstrate their knowledge, only what the content should be. In addition, Mrs. Johnson's goal for most but not all students was that "Students will demonstrate an understanding of the motivations underlying the decisions made by the main characters." Again, note that the mode of demonstration is left open-ended. Finally, her goal for some students (e.g., those who wanted to complete extra-credit work out of special interest) was "Students will be able to to analyze the political and sociological contexts in which the play is situated." For Mitchell, only the first goal applied, whereas for other students, the second and perhaps the third applied as well.

A number of Web sites serve as excellent resources for information about and resources related to Universal Design for Learning. These include the Web sites of the Center for Applied Special Technology (CAST), Association for Supervision and Curriculum Development (ASCD), National Center to Improve the Tools of Educators (NCITE), and Closing the Gap.

Once the goals are identified, the teacher can proceed to design the lesson using UDL principles as well. For example, Mrs. Johnson assigned roles from *Romeo and Juliet* to each student in the class, including Mitchell. This meant that the AAC team had to ensure that his lines were programmed into his TuffTalker (Words+, Inc.) so that he could practice them in class. Mrs. Johnson also added a new component of instruction because she knew that Mitch, like many students with autism, was a visual learner. Thus, before they read each scene, she had the class watch that scene in the Hollywood movie version of the play. For Mitchell's sake, she also had students work in cooperative learning groups to practice their parts, which had not occurred in the past. As is typically the case when the principles of universal design are utilized creatively, the changes Mrs. Johnson made were of benefit to *all* of the Grade 10 students, not just Mitchell—so much so that she continued to teach the lesson the "new way" in subsequent school years, even after Mitch was no longer in her class.

Develop a Goal/Context Matrix

Once the goals for the student who uses AAC and those for all students have both been identified, the two can be combined in a goal/context matrix. The matrix is a planning map that identifies when and where each of the student's goals will be taught in the context of the general education activities of the classroom. As depicted in Mitchell's matrix (see Table 14.5), the goals are listed in the left-hand column and the general education contexts are listed across the top. In consultation with the classroom teacher, goal–context intersections are then identified and marked. The matrix provides the teacher and other members of the AAC team with a "blueprint" that indicates which goals will be targeted for instruction in which subject areas or environments.

We can, whenever and wherever we choose, successfully teach all children whose schooling is of interest to us. We already know more than we need in order to do this. Whether we do it must finally depend on how we feel about the fact that we haven't done it so far. (Edmonds, 1979, p. 29)

Identify Individualized Adaptations Needed for Participation

Even when teachers use UDL principles to plan lessons inclusively, students who use AAC often require additional adaptations as well. Researchers have identified seven main ways that teachers can adapt curricula so that students with disabilities can participate in the

Table 14.5. Goal/context matrix

Mitchell will	English	Math	Science	Social studies	Lunch	PE	Drama	Applied skills
Read age-appropriate texts adapted to his current reading level	X		X	X				X
Use a computer with PixWriter software to write short stories, poems, and adapted tests	X	X	X	X			X	X
Use follow-along materials and strategies	X	X	X	X		X	X	X
Pay attention when requested to do so	X	X	X	X		X	X	X
Respond without protest to simple directives given by the teacher or a peer	X	X	X	X	X	X	X	X
Use his TuffTalker to respond to two questions asked by the teacher during each classroom activity	X	X	X	X	X	X	X	X
Present a report on at least one concept from each unit, using visual materials and his TuffTalker	X	X	X	X			X	X
Demonstrate mastery of at least three concepts from each unit	X	X	X	X				
Manage his materials in an appropriate manner	X	X	X	X	X	X	X	X
Initiate conversation and interactions with peers with his TuffTalker	X	X	X	X	X	X	X	X
Converse at appropriate times in the classroom with his TuffTalker	X	X	X	X	X	X	X	X
Demonstrate appropriate turn taking and sharing	X	X	X	X	X	X	X	X
Greet unfamiliar adults appropriately by shaking hands or saying *hi*	X	X	X	X	X	X	X	X
Participate in extracurricular activities with peers in his social network at least twice each week	X	X	X	X	X	X	X	X

same activities as their classmates (Cole et al., 2000). The seven ways can be used singly or in combination, depending on both the needs and abilities of the student and the lesson itself. The seven types of adaptations are summarized in Table 14.6, with examples of each. As can be seen from Table 14.6, Mitchell required a few individualized adaptations in order to participate in the *Romeo and Juliet* unit. Note that the adaptations designed for Mitchell are well-articulated with several of the IEP goals identified for him in Table 14.4

Table 14.6.   Types and examples of adaptations and modifications

Type	Definition	Examples
Size	Adjust the number of items a student is expected to learn or complete	• Seamus is a competitive student who types using sip and puff Morse code. To accommodate his relatively slow rate of text entry, his math test consists of 5 problems rather than 10. • Mitchell is expected to write two sentences in his daily journal rather than the page expected of his classmates.
Time	Adjust the amount of time allotted for learning, task completion, or testing	• Stacy is an active high school student who uses an optical pointer and a speech-generating device (SGD). Her history teacher asks her a question at the end of each class period. She prepares her answer each evening at home and stores it in her SGD. The next day, Stacy "calls up" the answer in class when asked to do so. This arrangement enables her to answer questions without spending time in class preparing her response. • Mitchell is given additional time to complete a science project on endangered species.
Level of support	Adjust the amount of personal assistance or technology use	• Jamie and his friends work together to complete a map on Africa for a social studies project, using Intellipics Studio 3 software. • During the *Romeo and Juliet* lesson, Mitchell's educational assistant programs his character's lines into the TuffTalker and helps him to practice activating related symbols to speak them out loud. He plays the part of the Apothecary who sells poison to Romeo.
Input	Adjust how instruction is delivered	• When giving instructions for a science project, Mr. Marsh uses an overhead projector to list the key steps, using words and hand-drawn pictures. • Mrs. Johnson, Mitchell's teacher, uses the NASA website to help Mitchell understand about the planets, rockets, and space travel.
Output	Adjust how the student is expected to demonstrate learning	• In Foods class, Terry cuts out magazine pictures of the four food groups to show what he has learned, rather than taking a test. • Mitchell uses PCSs to complete a story map to show what he has learned about *Romeo and Juliet*.
Difficulty	Adjust the skill level, problem type, or rules about how the learner approaches an activity.	• Ramona combines adjectives and nouns using shape grid to guide her selections. • Mitchell reads a simplified version of *Romeo and Juliet* that his educational assistant created using Writing with Symbols 2000.
Participation	Adjust how the learner is actively involved in the activity	• Todd uses a Big Red switch and All-Turn-It Spinner (AbleNet, Inc.) to select multiplication problems for his classmates to complete. • When his classmates rehearse scenes from *Romeo and Juliet* that do not include his character, Mitchell is responsible for placing the appropriate props on the stage.

Source: Cole, S., Horvath, B., Chapman, C., Deschenes, C., Ebeling, D., & Sprague, J. (2000). *Adapting curriculum and instruction in inclusive classrooms* (2nd ed.). Port Chester, NY: National Professional Resources.

(e.g., reading age-appropriate texts adapted to his current reading level, writing using a computer with PixWriter software, demonstrating mastery of at least three concepts from each unit). This is at the heart of inclusive education—providing opportunities for meaningful instruction in priority goal areas while participating in the same curricular activities as the rest of the class.

In addition to the seven basic types of adaptations depicted in Table 14.6, there are several more that are unique to students who use AAC and deserve specific emphasis because of the dramatic impact they can have on students' learning, both today and tomorrow. These adaptations fall into several categories, including those related to adapting the educational environment, managing the academic workload, and assisting students to manage time constraints.

Adapt the Educational Environment

Teachers may need to adapt the physical environment in order to enhance access in a classroom. For example, it is not uncommon for teachers to position students who use wheelchairs off to the side or at the back of a room because their chairs make it difficult for others to get around them. Creating wider aisles between student desks and classroom furnishings is a preferable solution to this problem because this allows students who use AAC to stay with the group instead of being physically marginalized. Wider doors adapted with special pull handles or electric eyes allow easy entrance into the classroom and other areas of the building, such as the music room, gymnasium, and cafeteria. Teachers should position student working surfaces (ideally, adjustable desks and tables) at appropriate heights for comfort and efficiency. Cutout desktops may be necessary so that students have a suitable distance between their wheelchairs and their working surfaces. Chalkboards placed at lower-than-usual levels and extended slightly out from the wall allow students in wheelchairs to position themselves appropriately for writing activities. Teachers can also lower other items such as pencil sharpeners, coat racks, and light switches to heights accessible to all students. Finally, classroom assignments should be made after taking into consideration the mobility needs of students, because some classrooms are more accessible than others.

It should be emphasized that saying it can be done is not the same as saying it will be easy. (Stainback & Stainback, 1990, p. 7)

Managing the Academic Workload

Another adaptation has to do with helping students who use AAC to manage the academic workload. For example, Jason, a middle school student who requires AAC, received some resource room assistance to increase his literacy skills. He was learning to use a computer with a standard word processing program and Co:Writer 4000 (Don Johnston, Inc.), a writing program with rate enhancement features. Early in his augmented writing program, Jason's resource room teacher gave him writing assignments without considering the many written assignments that his general education teachers required. It soon became apparent that Jason, who wrote very slowly, was being asked to manage a workload that was far beyond his capabilities. Through collaborative efforts, the general and special education teachers began to adapt their assignments and expectations so that Jason had sufficient writing practice and was still able to complete his general classroom assignments. For example, his English teacher agreed to accept the letters and stories that Jason wrote in the resource room as fulfilling his language arts requirements. In addition, the resource room teacher agreed to design assignments to relate to the subject matter covered in the general education classes.

Assist Students to Manage Time Constraints

Students with severe communication and motor impairments often find it difficult to keep up with the pace of a general classroom because they have difficulty manipulating educational materials such as books and worksheets. Without adaptations to deal with these difficulties, students may experience academic failure because they cannot complete their work, although they have mastered the content. Educators often use one of several approaches to accommodate the time constraints of students with disabilities.

Advance Preparation   It may be necessary for AAC teams to work with general education staff to preview upcoming assignments, topic areas, and class projects, so that they have ample time to create related adaptations. For example, if the AAC support team knows that upcoming science units will include planets, rocks, and dinosaurs over the next 2 months, they can begin to construct related communication displays or plan how to program the needed vocabulary words into an electronic AAC device in advance.

In addition, teachers can encourage students who use AAC to prepare questions in advance or compose their answers to assigned questions at home in order to compensate for their reduced communication rates. For example, in her Teen Living class (a health and personal responsibility class), Ginger was involved in a unit on sex education. Although she was not able to grasp all of the class material, she clearly understood at least some of the discussion related to dating etiquette. She managed to convey to her paraprofessional that she had some questions about this subject. Prior to class, the paraprofessional recorded a series of questions into Ginger's Step-by-Step Communicator. Ginger's classmates also used this technique when Ginger was assigned class reports in a cooperative learning group. Ginger worked with her classmates after school to prepare the report, and they recorded it in segments into her Step-by-Step Communicator. Ginger was then responsible for playing the report the next day in class, when cued to do so by her classmates. Such advance preparation strategies allow students with AAC systems to participate actively in general classes without requiring teachers and peers to wait while they compose messages or questions.

Use of Peer Instruction and Support   The use of cooperative learning groups and peer instruction is increasing in general education classrooms. Applying these approaches to students who use AAC systems can be very effective in helping them meet classroom time demands. In addition, when teachers include students with disabilities in small cooperative learning or informal peer-instruction groups, they are often able to participate more effectively than they can in large classroom situations.

In junior high, senior high, and college or university classes, educators can also enlist peer students to take notes in class for students with disabilities. They can insert carbon paper between pages of their notebooks so that a copy is made automatically, or the notes can be photocopied. However, regardless of grade level, students with AAC systems should be encouraged to at least outline their class notes whenever possible, in order to stay mentally involved in the subject matter of the class. Alternatively, many students prefer to tape classroom lectures and use the tapes to clarify information from the peer notes. Some tape recorders have a feature that allows the operator to press a button to mark specific sections while recording. Then, as they review the tapes with the notes, they can fast forward to the marked sections rather quickly. This reduces their listening time and encourages students to stay involved in the class so that they can mark important segments on the tape.

Selective Retention   In the United States, children with disabilities are eligible to remain as public school students past the age of 18 when most of their peers graduate. This extra time for students who use AAC systems means that rather than rushing through an educational program at the same pace as their peers without disabilities, they and their families may opt for retention at a grade level in order to meet specific academic goals. Such retentions tend to occur at four different times. First, some students may not have the AAC equipment that they need to enter first grade. Their parents may choose to retain them in preschool or kindergarten for an additional year so that the AAC team has time to develop the appropriate communication supports. Second, we know of a number of parents who have elected to retain their children in the third or fourth grade. In particular, this option has been chosen by parents who had children with literacy skills not developed sufficiently to allow learning to occur. The additional work in reading and writing that these students completed was often sufficient to narrow the gap in this area. Third, some students may participate in junior high school for an additional year. In schools in the United States, much of the junior high school curriculum consists of an enhanced version and review of the concepts and processes taught in earlier years to ensure that students are fluent in this material before they enter high school. Students who do not master this material in elementary school may benefit from an extra year in junior high for academic reasons. Finally, students may choose to extend the length of their high school programs in order to complete academic requirements.

Retention should only be considered if both the student and his or her parents consent to it. Of course, in many cases the detrimental social impact of retention may outweigh any potentially positive academic benefits. In fact, it is primarily the social implications of selective, voluntary retention that make this such a controversial topic. In addition, many general educators and administrators believe that retaining even typical students serves no constructive purpose, which may or may not be true. Regardless, applying the same logic to students with disabilities and rejecting selective retention for philosophical reasons only appears to be equally nonconstructive. To our knowledge, there is simply no reason not to consider this type of adaptation for competitive or active students who experience academic difficulties because of their reduced communication efficiency.

Early in his elementary years, we discussed with Grant's parents the possibility of academic retention. For several years, Grant performed at grade level. However, by the end of sixth grade, he had begun to struggle with writing, spelling, and math. Grant enrolled in a 2-year junior high program. By the end of eighth grade, his academic difficulties remained, so his parents and teachers decided to retain him in junior high for an additional year. In 1998, he graduated from high school. He took 5 years to complete a 4-year program and plans to enroll in junior college the fall following his graduation.

SUPPORTING STUDENTS WHO USE AAC IN GENERAL EDUCATION CLASSROOMS

Once decisions have been made with regard to the appropriate educational goals, instructional contexts, lessons, and adaptations for a student who uses AAC, we can turn our attention to classroom-wide strategies for providing ongoing instructional support. In general education classrooms, students typically encounter a range of instructional arrangements over the course of the day, each of which has specific support implications. In this section, we describe what we know about these instructional arrangements and their implications for students who use AAC, suggest classroom-wide strategies for providing appropriate language input and vocabulary support, and suggest a variety of strategies that can be used to plan for today and tomorrow.

Identify Typical Instructional and Interaction Patterns of the General Education Classroom

The ultimate goal of inclusive education for students who use AAC is that they are able to be engaged in meaningful ways, both academically and socially, in general education classroom environments. In order to accomplish this, such students must have appropriate access to educational and social vocabulary items in their AAC systems. However, it is often a real challenge to keep vocabulary in the AAC system current because the communication content in general education classrooms changes so rapidly. This leads to a tendency to provide AAC students with communication systems that are solely designed to address wants/needs and social interaction functions rather than the information-sharing functions that are integral to classroom participation. If this happens, people who rely on AAC are often forced to be passive learners: They cannot ask or answer questions in class, deliver topical reports, or otherwise participate in subject-oriented discussions because they do not have the vocabularies to do so. However, the AAC team can take advantage of the fact that most teachers are able to predict ahead to upcoming units or lessons and, if asked to do so, identify core vocabulary words that are essential for each unit. It is critical that the AAC support team aggressively attempt to translate the curriculum into communication units that will allow students who use AAC to participate in these classroom interactions. This is particularly crucial during the early elementary years before students are able to spell well enough to compose their own messages.

It is essential for the AAC team to identify the naturally occurring instructional strategies used by teachers in the classroom or classrooms in which the student who uses AAC is included. This should be assessed for each subject area individually (e.g., language arts, math, science, music, art, physical education), because most teachers tend to use different strategies across subject areas. Of course, as students get older, there is also the likelihood that each subject area will be taught by a different teacher in a different classroom, making such subject-by-subject assessment even more essential.

In the sections that follow, we review the four areas that require assessment—instructional arrangements, interaction patterns, supports for language comprehension, and vocabulary and response supports. Table 14.7 summarizes these areas in a format that can be used for initial assessment and to identify adaptations that are needed. This form can be used while observing the classroom teacher as she or he teaches a class of typical students in each subject area.

Instructional Arrangements

Teachers use a variety of instructional arrangements in classrooms, each of which has different implications for educational and social participation by students who use AAC. The most commonly used arrangements are described below.

Teacher-Led Large-Group Instruction   Teacher-led large-group instruction tends to predominate in most classrooms (Katz, Mirenda, & Auerbach, 2002). In a study of communication patterns in first-, third-, and fifth-grade general education classrooms, Sturm and Nelson (1997) identified 10 unofficial "rules" that guide most teacher-led large-group instructional activities:

1. Teachers mostly talk and students mostly listen, except when the teacher grants permission to talk.

2. Teachers give cues about when to listen closely.

3. Teachers convey primarily subject-related content and procedures about how to complete related activities.

4. Teacher talk gets more complex in the upper grades.

5. Teachers ask questions and expect specific responses.

6. Teachers give hints about what is correct and what is important to them.

7. Student talk should be brief and to the point.

8. Students should ask few questions and keep them short.

9. Students are expected to talk to teachers, not to other students.

10. Students can make a limited number of spontaneous comments, but only about the process or content of the lesson.

Together, these 10 unofficial rules have implications for students who use AAC to participate in teacher-led group instructional activities. First, teachers expect students to be brief and provide relevant information. Second, teachers tend to ask questions only about information that they think is important. Third, teachers of large groups control most interactions and already have an established agenda about the information that they expect students to know. This often means that teachers can be very effective informants regarding key AAC vocabulary that is required.

Table 14.7. Assessment of classroom and teacher variables and required adaptations for students who use AAC

Natural instructional arrangements	How students are expected to interact/participate	Natural supports provided for language comprehension	Natural vocabulary and response supports available
1) Teacher-led, large group	1) Bid for response/question opportunities (e.g., raise hand)	1) Tangible items	1) Tangible items
2) Teacher-led, small group	2) Answer questions individually	2) Photographs, pictures, maps, illustrations	2) Photographs, pictures, maps, illustrations
3) Teacher led, sharing time	3) Answer questions in group	3) Videotapes	3) Writing/drawing on overhead transparencies
4) Student-led, cooperative learning groups	4) Ask questions	4) Slides	4) Writing/drawing on flipchart, blackboard, word wall
5) Learning centers or stations	5) Ask for help, clarification, or feedback as needed	5) Writing/drawing on overhead transparencies	5) Graphic organizers
6) Adult–student 1:1 instruction	6) Make comments	6) Writing/drawing on flipchart, blackboard	6) Visual schedules
7) Peer–peer 1:1 instruction	7) Offer ideas, suggestions, etc.	7) Graphic organizers	7) Teacher asks multiple choice questions
8) Group or paired seat work	8) Tell story/give oral report	8) Visual schedules	8) Teacher asks yes/no or true/false questions
9) Independent seat work	9) Lead/coordinate group project	9) Computer software	9) Teacher uses nonverbal response modes
10) Independent test taking	10) Take notes/act as recorder	10) Internet	10) Other: _____
11) Other: _____	11) Role play/act	11) Role playing	
	12) Listen as the teacher lectures	12) Other: _____	
	13) Follow instructions and engage in activities as directed		
	14) Work quietly and independently (no interaction)		
	15) Other: _____		

Adaptations required

1) More large group instruction
2) More small group instruction
3) More cooperative learning groups
4) More group or paired seat work
5) Increase adult support
6) Increase peer support
7) Adapt how independent seat work is completed
8) Adapt test or mode of learning assessment
9) Other: _____

Adaptations required

1) Provide switch + buzzer/light for response bids
2) Provide yes/no device for answering
3) Provide vocabulary displays with key words for questions, comments, idea generation
4) Pre-record oral reports, stories, show-and-tell
5) Use visual displays for oral reports, stories, show-and-tell
6) Record notes on audiotape
7) Use more role playing/acting
8) Other: _____

Adaptations required

1) Make tangible items available
2) Make photographs, pictures, maps, illustrations available
3) Increase use of videotapes
4) Increase use of slides
5) Write/draw on overhead transparencies
6) Write/draw on flipchart, blackboard, word wall
7) Use more graphic organizers
8) Use more visual schedules
9) Increase use of computer software
10) Increase use of Internet
11) Increase use of role playing
12) Other: _____

Adaptations required

1) Keep tangible items available
2) Keep photographs, pictures, maps, illustrations available
3) Keep writing/drawing on overhead transparencies available
4) Keep writing/drawing on flipchart, blackboard, word wall available
5) Keep graphic organizers available
6) Keep visual schedules available
7) Provide vocabulary displays with key words
8) Adapt teacher question format (multiple choice, yes/no, true/false)
9) Increase group responding with nonverbal signals
10) Other: _____

Augmentative and Alternative Communication: Supporting Children and Adults with Complex Communication Needs, Third Edition, by David R. Beukelman and Pat Mirenda.
Copyright © 2005 Paul H. Brookes Publishing Co., Inc. All rights reserved.

Teacher-Led Small-Group Instruction   Usually, the purpose of small-group instruction is to develop language, literacy, problem-solving, and critical thinking skills, with an emphasis on comprehension of text material and verbal expression. Small-group interactions tend to be topical but conversationally based, with an emphasis on teacher-initiated questions and student responses. Individual students may interact by competing for turns or by being called on either randomly or sequentially; at times, the teacher may encourage whole-group discussion as well. Katz et al. (2002) found that students with developmental disabilities in inclusive classrooms were more likely to be actively engaged when they were involved in small group instruction (both teacher- and student-led) than when they were involved in any other grouping arrangement, including one-to-one instruction. Thus, small-group instruction appears to have advantages with regard to student participation. In addition, because the teacher tends to control both the topics discussed and the questions asked in small-group instruction, he or she can often act as an informant to guide the advance preparation of AAC communication displays for students who need them.

Teacher-Led Sharing Time   Teachers often employ a "sharing" format for current event presentations, reports, and show-and-tell activities. According to Duchan (1995), people use language sharing contexts primarily to describe events in a logical and temporal sequence, usually in the past tense (e.g., "Last weekend, we went to visit my grandmother. We drove there in a car. We stopped for lunch at Perkins. When we got there . . . . "). Often, the teacher will comment following the completion of a student's narration and perhaps ask questions to expand or clarify the content. At times, the teacher encourages other students to ask questions. Thus, sharing interactions are very much like the storytelling contexts described in Chapter 2, and AAC teams can design messages as described in that chapter.

Student-Led Cooperative Learning Groups and Learning Stations/Centers
Putnam (1998) described several approaches to cooperative learning that vary considerably with regard to how groups and learning activities are structured. However, they all have a number of elements in common: 1) they involve a common task or learning activity that is suitable for small group work, 2) they emphasize cooperative behavior and positive interdependence, and 3) they include structures related to individual accountability. Learning stations or centers are often used in the context of cooperative learning. In this type of instructional arrangement, students are usually expected to move around the classroom from station-to-station and to engage in different cooperative learning activities related to an overall lesson theme at each.

A few studies have demonstrated that educators can use small, cooperative learning groups successfully as contexts for instruction of students with significant disabilities (Dugan et al., 1995; Hunt, Staub, Alwell, & Goetz, 1994; Katz et al., 2002). The communication patterns among students in such groups tend to more closely resemble those that occur in peer conversational interactions than those that occur during teacher-led group instruction (Katz et al., 2002), so the vocabulary requirements may be less predictable. In addition, for students who use AAC, mobility and increased task variability may become challenges when learning stations are employed. Nonetheless, many current texts on inclusive education promote the use of cooperative learning groups for students across the range of age and ability because they are conducive to both active engagement and social participation (e.g., Downing, 2002; Jorgensen, 1998; Kluth, 2003; Putnam, 1998; Ryndak & Alper, 2003).

Seth was unable to speak and communicated with an AAC system. He was assigned to a cooperative learning group to prepare a class report on tornadoes. Each member of the group was responsible for a different aspect of the report. With the help of his paraprofessional, he entered the report in his AAC system. He gave the presentation, releasing the report one sentence at a time, and participated in a panel discussion by asking questions of the other members in his group. He was also able to answer some questions from his classmates.

One-to-One Instruction   Simpson (1996) videotaped a series of students who used AAC systems in general classrooms and observed that communication patterns varied considerably from one student to another. Some of the students communicated primarily with their teacher; others distributed their interactions quite equally among the teacher, the paraprofessional, and their peers; and still others interacted almost exclusively with their paraprofessionals in one-to-one teaching contexts (Simpson, Beukelman, & Sharpe, 2000). Of course, one-to-one instruction can be delivered by both adults and by peers (e.g., peer tutoring). Regardless, question-and-answer interactions tended to predominate, with fairly predictable words and phrases needed by the student using AAC.

Seat Work   In most classrooms, students spend some portion of instructional time each day completing work sheets or exercises, taking tests, writing in daily journals, and engaging in other types of seat work activities. During these activities, they may be expected to work in small groups, student–student pairs, or individually; regardless, interaction is usually neither required nor encouraged. For many students who use AAC, seat work activities may need to be adapted so that they can be completed using adapted writing software or other alternative response modes such as pictures. Often, students who use AAC have an easier time participating in meaningful ways in classrooms in which seat work is used minimally rather than regularly, because it is often quite time consuming for the teacher or paraprofessional to adapt seat work so the student can complete it. When adaptations are not in place, students run the risk of either not participating at all or of being assigned to activities separate from the rest of the class.

Expected Student Interaction Patterns

A second component of classroom instruction has to do with how teachers expect students to interact and participate in lessons or activities. In some classrooms, "silence is golden" is the rule; in others, students are encouraged to "speak up and speak out" regularly. Some teachers place a lot of emphasis on relatively predictable question-and-answer interactions over which they have control, whereas others prefer discussion-type interactions that are less structured and more student directed. Some teachers encourage students to read or respond individually, whereas others use whole-class response formats in which all students are expected to read or answer questions as a group. Classrooms also vary widely with respect to requirements related to sharing, story telling, and reporting; participating in discussions; recording/note taking; following instructions; listening during teacher lectures; and so forth.

Instructional arrangements and expected interaction patterns often occur independent of one another, so both need to be assessed. For example, consider the difference between a typical physical education class (PE) and a typical social studies class, both of which are conducted predominantly through teacher-led large group instruction. In the PE class, students are expected to participate by simply listening to the teacher's instructions (e.g., related to a new game) and following them. They are expected to ask the teacher for help, clarification, or feedback as needed, but no other types of interaction are required. Students are likely to interact with one another as they play the games or engage in other activities. In the social studies class, on the other hand, the teacher first asks students to discuss the chapter they read as homework (expectation: students will make comments), then engages in a question-and-answer session about the main ideas (expectation: students will answer questions in a group and individually), and finally presents a lecture about the information in the next chapter (expectation: students will listen quietly and ask for clarification as needed). Students are not encouraged to interact socially with one another; in fact, they are discouraged from doing so. Thus, these two teacher-led large group lessons have very different interaction requirements, with very different implications for students who use AAC! Table 14.7 can be used by the AAC team to identify the typical interaction and participation requirements expected of students in each subject area.

ChalkTalk: Augmentative Communication in the Classroom (Culp & Effinger, 1996) describes a process that gives school teams a place to start when developing communication programs for students who use AAC systems. This manual provides observational protocols that help a team profile the communication patterns and needs of students in school settings. Additional activities guide the development of action plans that include the actions to be taken, the person or people responsible, the target date of completion, and the procedures to be used.

Natural Supports Provided for Language Comprehension

As teachers present concepts, information, or instructions, they often supplement their speech with additional audiovisual media. For example, Mr. Zaidman uses illustrations; manipulables; and model squares, rectangles, and triangles when he teaches geometry concepts to his Grade 5 class. He does this for two primary reasons: 1) to enhance students' attentiveness and thus decrease off-task and other problem behaviors, and 2) to enhance the likelihood that students will understand the target concepts, information, or instructions (i.e., to enhance language comprehension). For students who use AAC, especially those with significant language delays or deficits, teachers' use of various types of instructional media may be critically important to their ability to learn even basic information in a lesson. If teachers do not use such media regularly or in sufficient quantities, the AAC team may need to provide input and suggestions about how to include them, emphasizing that this is likely to enhance learning for all students, not just those who use AAC.

There are two main types of supports in this regard: those used to augment comprehension and those used to map language (Wood, Lasker, Siegel-Causey, Beukelman, & Ball, 1998). Teachers often augment the meanings of instructional events by using real objects, maps, drawings, photographs, slides, videotapes, and other media to augment spoken language, especially when they teach new information or unfamiliar concepts. In addition, almost all teachers visually map new language forms as they teach. For example, as they provide verbal information to students, they may write key words or even entire texts on the blackboard, an overhead transparency, or a flipchart. Table 14.7 lists the media that are most commonly used in classrooms to support language comprehension.

Natural Vocabulary and Response Supports

Teachers also vary widely with regard to the supports they provide for a student responding during instructional interactions. As noted previously, some teachers augment comprehension or map language regularly with real objects, photos, or illustrations, or provide written word or messages on flipcharts, blackboards, word walls, and so forth. These same teachers will often pool potential response options by leaving the tangible items or words on display so that students can use them as memory aids or point to them in response to teachers' questions. Such teachers often find it rather easy to include students who use AAC when asking questions during large- and small-group instruction because these strategies apply to them as well. However, other teachers tend to remove tangible items or erase words once a lesson is completed, and then require students to demonstrate what they have learned through writing or speech only. These teachers may need help to learn to use more effective response pools that do not require AAC students to rely almost entirely on their memories and on the vocabulary items available in their AAC systems.

Many teachers also use verbal strategies to pool responses, especially during question-and-answer activities. For example, a teacher might use a multiple choice format to ask questions such as, "Marco Polo's book gave Europeans their first information about what? Here are your choices: Canada, Russia, and the Far East." This same teacher might then provide alternatives to the traditional verbal answer format by saying, for example, "If you think the correct answer is Canada, look at me; otherwise look at the ceiling," and so forth with the remaining options. Another teacher might use a yes/no or true/false format such as, "True or False? 8 times 12 equals 86," followed by the instruction "If you think the answer is True, put your head down," and so forth. Such strategies allow the teacher to check the understanding of *all* students, *including* those who use AAC systems. Of course, questions and answers structured in this way can also be used to determine the knowledge of individual learners. In either case, from the perspective of the student using AAC, such strategies are vastly preferable to the more traditional "raise your hand if you know the answer" option that primarily rewards students who can move quickly and efficiently and speak well. Furthermore, they make it easy for students who use AAC to respond and participate without the need to have the answers on their personalized communication displays. The AAC team can use Table 14.7 to identify the vocabulary and response supports that are naturally available during instruction in each subject area.

Identify Instructional and Interaction Adaptations that Are Required

Once the natural instructional and interaction arrangements, expectations, and supports have been identified for each subject area, the AAC team can use Table 14.7 to determine the need for adaptations or changes. Which natural instructional arrangements already enhance educational and social participation for the student who uses AAC? Which ones interfere with participation and need to be adapted or replaced? Which natural interaction and participation expectations are already achievable by the student, and which require adaptation? Which natural language comprehension supports are appropriate for the student, and which require enhancement? Similarly, which vocabulary and response supports are appropriate, and which require enhancement? The AAC team should encourage the teacher to continue to use existing strategies that are appropriate and provide assurance that they are likely to be as successful with the AAC student as they are with his or her typical students. On the other hand, if specific strategies appear to be incompatible with the AAC student's sensory, motor, linguistic, or other abilities, the team may need to coach the teacher to modify or expand his or her repertoire to meet the student's needs.

In this regard, the team should again encourage the teacher to apply the principles of UDL—in this case, to "engineer the classroom" and provide the types of supports needed by the student who uses AAC to *all students in the class* (Goossens' & Crain, 1992). For example, teachers vary considerably in the ways they expect their students to bid for response opportunities and provide answers in the classroom. Some teachers may call on specific students to respond, one at a time. Others may expect students who know an answer to bid for a turn by raising their hands; the teacher then selects one student to respond. As noted previously, teachers who find it rather easy to include AAC students tend to develop ways for the entire class to bid and provide answers without being disruptive. Alternatively, a student may be provided with an adapted way of "raising her hand," such as a switch-activated buzzer, light, or call button. Some of the most commonly used adapted response options are listed in Table 14.7 under "How Students are Expected to Interact/Participate," along with adaptations in other areas.

It is important to create a socially supportive environment for students with severe disabilities who are included in general classrooms. Hunt, Alwell, Farron-Davis, and Goetz (1996) provided a detailed discussion of their efforts to include students with multiple disabilities. They summarized their experiences with the "focus students" as follows:

1. **Information provision and friendship programs:** Ongoing information on the ways in which the focus students communicated and the adaptive equipment they used was provided to schoolmates in the context of interactions between the student and a classmate. Further information was provided to schoolmates through participation in "clubs": a "support circle" for Isaac, a "sign club" for Todd, and a "recess club" for Daniel.

2. **Identification and utilization of a variety of media for interactive exchanges:** The various interactive media utilized fell into three categories:

1) multimodal communication systems; 2) interactive computer activities; and 3) toys, games, and cooperative educational activities.

3. **Third-party facilitation through buddy systems, arrangement of interactive activities, and prompting to promote interactions:** A buddy system was established in which each focus student had a peer partner for the day who sat by him in class and accompanied him to recess, the cafeteria, and other school activities. Paraprofessionals received information during training meetings and feedback periods on facilitation strategies that included 1) arranging classroom and other school contexts to ensure that the focus student was involved in an activity and that a peer partner, communication devices, and adaptive equipment were available, 2) prompting interactions between the focus student and classmates, 3) prompting the focus student to use a variety of communicative means, and 4) interpreting the communicative behaviors of the focus student for classmates (Hunt et al., 1996, p. 58).

Implement Instruction and Evaluate Outcomes

By this point, the AAC team has completed all of the necessary planning. They have determined current and desired inclusion parameters, completed a personal profile of the student who uses AAC, and identified relevant goals. They have worked with the teacher to help him or her learn to design lessons based on the principles of UDL and have also identified additional adaptations that may be required for the individual student. Finally, they have identified typical instructional and interaction patterns of the general education classroom and made suggestions about how these can be continued and/or enhanced. Finally—it is time to implement instruction and evaluate the student's progress!

Within the Participation Model as it applies to inclusive educational environments, two main questions should be assessed for each lesson or activity: 1) Was the student able to actively participate in a meaningful way in the activities of the general education classroom? 2) Was the student able to meet his or her learning goals? These two questions are certainly related but can also be separated—for example, a student might be able to participate actively in a lesson or activity but fail to learn anything relevant to his or her individual educational goals. Thus, both aspects should be examined.

Let's revisit Mitchell's Grade 10 English class as an example of how this can be accomplished. His class has successfully completed the *Romeo and Juliet* unit. With regard to participation, the primary lesson activities were 1) reading the play and discussing it in class; and 2) participating in key scenes from the play. How did Mitchell participate? Along with his classmates, he watched scenes from the Hollywood movie version of the play before reading and acting out each scene. As summarized in sections of Table 14.6, his version of the play was adapted by his paraprofessional, based on *Shakespeare for Children: The Story of Romeo and Juliet* (Foster, 1989) and *The Sixty-Minute Shakespeare: Romeo and Juliet* (Foster, Shakespeare, & Howey, 2000). Using his TuffTalker (Words+, Inc.), he recited his character's lines (he played the Apothecary who sold poison to Romeo); when he was not in a scene, he was one of two "propmasters" who were responsible for making sure that the appropriate props were available on the "stage." Did he participate in meaningful ways? Clearly, yes!

The second issue to assess is: Did Mitchell meet his learning goals? As displayed in Table 14.5, several of Mitchell's goals were identified as appropriate for English class, including "Mitchell will read age-appropriate texts adapted to his current reading level," "Mitchell will use his TuffTalker to respond to two questions asked by the teacher during each classroom activity," and "Mitchell will demonstrate mastery of at least three concepts from each unit." The latter goal overlaps considerably with the classroom-wide goal Mrs. Johnson identified *for all students:* "Students will act out an abbreviated version of the play *Romeo and Juliet* and will be able to identify the setting, main characters, main plot elements, problem, and solution." As noted previously, Mitchell read an adapted version of the play. He also used his TuffTalker to answer questions during the discussion that occurred in every class (e.g., "What was Romeo's mother's name?" "How did Romeo die?"). Finally, he completed an adapted story map using printed words and drawings to demonstrate his ability to meet both the classroom-wide goal and his mastery of at least three key concepts (see Figure 14.5). Did Mitchell meet his learning goals? Yes, again!

The assessment process illustrated by Mitchell's story can be used to answer the two key outcome questions for students who use AAC in general. If the answer to either question is "No," the team should identify interfering factors and incorporate potential solutions into future lesson plans and activities, either for the entire class or for the individual student. Our experience is that, once this plan-implement-evaluate-revise cycle has occurred several times, the amount of time and effort required for each step decreases

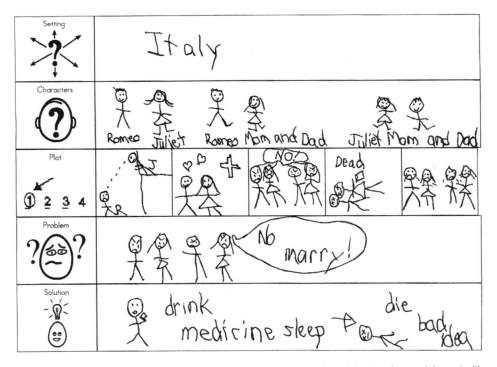

Figure 14.5.   Adapted *Romeo and Juliet* story map completed with words and drawings by an adolescent with autism. (From Diane Lea Ryndak & Sandra Alper [Eds.], *Curriculum and instruction for students with significant disabilities in inclusive settings* [2nd ed.; p. 200]. Published by Allyn & Bacon, Boston, MA; Copyright © 2003 by Pearson Education. Reprinted by permission of the publisher.)

dramatically. As teams develop fluency around this process, both students who use AAC and team members themselves are increasingly able to use UDL principles and other strategies to develop meaningful, inclusive lessons that benefit all learners.

Felipe is an educationally involved student with multiple physical and sensory impairments who attended a junior high biology class that was considerably beyond his academic ability level. Nevertheless, he was involved in various plant experiments with his peer group, enjoyed learning to use a microscope to examine cells, participated in a presentation about ecology by helping his classmates collect examples of recyclable materials, and listened to recorded portions of the textbook using a tape recorder and a single switch. He benefited both academically and socially from involvement in this class.

A Final Note

It is important to emphasize that inclusion *does not mean* placing students in general education classes in which they are passive nonparticipants nor in classes from which they cannot benefit. For example, placing Felipe, the student described in the vignette above, in a junior high math class would probably have been quite pointless because he was not interested in or able to learn the material at all, and the teacher was not open to making changes to accommodate him. However, Felipe was fully integrated into biology, English, Earth science, music, drama, and home economics classes and stayed awake and alert in those classes for the entire school day for the first time in his school career. He learned to use a low-tech communication display with photographs and remnants (see Chapter 11), and he was actively involved in classroom activities where he worked primarily on communication, social, and motor goals. At the completion of eighth grade, he attended his class school graduation dance and had a great time wheelchair-dancing with his friends. If you asked Felipe, his family, or the members of his school team, "Was it worth all the hard work and time? Did inclusion *really* make a difference for Felipe?" there is no doubt that they would say "YES!" For Felipe, Mitchell, and many other students at all academic levels who use AAC, inclusive education is not only here to stay—it is changing their lives.

PART III

AUGMENTATIVE & ALTERNATIVE COMMUNICATION INTERVENTIONS FOR INDIVIDUALS WITH ACQUIRED DISABILITIES

CHAPTER 15

ADULTS WITH
ACQUIRED PHYSICAL DISABILITIES

WITH LAURA J. BALL

Madonna survived amyotrophic lateral sclerosis (ALS) for 7 years. She first noticed leg weakness while enjoying her favorite pastime, golfing. When the weakness began to affect her arms, she decided to see a neurologist and was diagnosed with ALS. After about 4 years, her speech began to slow. A speech-language pathologist from the ALS clinic urged her to complete an AAC assessment even though her speech was still intelligible, so that she would have time to acquire and learn to operate an AAC system before her speech deteriorated further. At that time, Madonna's speaking rate in sentences was about 120 words per minute (compared with 190 words per minute by typical adult speakers). Within a month after her AAC assessment, she began to notice that listeners were straining to understand her in noisy situations. After that, her speech began to deteriorate very rapidly and she was no longer understandable at all within 3 more months. Because an AAC assessment had been completed in a timely manner, her AAC technology arrived and she had the time to learn how to operate it before she became unable to speak. With a head switch, she controlled a computer-based speech-generating device (SGD) using alphabet scanning, word prediction, and message retrieval. In addition, she maintained an active social life over the Internet. Although she was no longer able to work as an accountant, she used her computer system to "keep the books" for a volunteer organization. In addition to her high-tech AAC system, Madonna used an eye link low-tech system when she was not in her wheelchair or in a specially equipped chair at her dining room table. About 1 month prior to her death, she became too weak to use her computer system, so she used eye-linking alone to communicate with her caregivers, close family, and friends.

The mechanics of spoken communication are so automatic for natural speakers that the content of interactions, not the speaking processes involved in them, is the primary focus of most communicative exchanges. It is almost impossible for those who have learned to speak as children and continue to speak without difficulty to imagine what it would be like to be unable to speak due to an acquired disability. This chapter briefly summarizes assessment and intervention approaches to a number of such disabilities, including ALS, multiple sclerosis (MS), Guillain-Barré syndrome, Parkinson's disease (PD), brain-stem stroke, and others. Subsequent chapters discuss information related to the acquired disabilities of traumatic brain injury (TBI), aphasia, and dementia secondary to stroke.

The Barkley AAC Center's Web site contains links to many excellent sites that provide a range of information on the neurological conditions and syndromes discussed in this chapter.

A MODEL FOR INTERVENTION

Augmentative and alternative communication (AAC) teams have employed a somewhat streamlined version of the Participation Model (see Figure 6.1) with adults who have severe acquired communication disorders. This model involves three simultaneous types of assessment, all of which are represented in Figure 6.1: 1) an identification of participation and communication needs, 2) assessment of capabilities to determine available and appropriate communication options, and 3) assessment of constraints. In addition, strategies for evaluating the effectiveness of AAC interventions are important to this model. (See Chapters 6 and 7 for a detailed discussion of assessment.)

Identify Participation Patterns and Communication Needs

Individuals who experience acquired physical disabilities that affect their ability to communicate usually experience other dramatic changes in their lives as well. Depending on the progression of the specific condition or disease, these changes may occur gradually (as with a degenerative disease) or more abruptly (as with trauma or stroke). Individuals' physical disabilities as well as their personal lifestyle preferences determine their communication needs and their participation roles and contexts. For example, some people with severe degenerative disabilities, such as ALS, prefer to center their lives within their home environment; Madonna was an example of such an individual. These individuals find that it is more efficient and less demanding on their families to establish their homes as their primary work, social, and care setting, rather than to continue to participate extensively in the larger community. Thus, they may work at home if they are active vocationally. Friends and family visit them at home, and they travel only for special events. Some use the Internet to maintain contact with their social and support networks. Eventually, they may go through numerous transitions involving their living situation (e.g., private home, assisted living, nursing home, hospice), which will have an impact on the available funding for AAC, as well as necessitate changes to their AAC systems (Ball, 2003).

Although Madonna did not work when she was diagnosed with ALS, continued employment plays an important role in the lives of some individuals with this disorder (McNaughton, Light, & Groszyk, 2001). Interventions for people with ALS who wish to continue to work should include both computer literacy and Internet training so they have the option of furthering their employment and can access a range of support networks. Expanded electronic communication options such as e-mail, the Internet, electronic conferencing, and cellular technology have resulted in expanded opportunities for employment, volunteerism, distance learning, financial transactions, and commercial activity. Participation in virtual activity is of little interest to some people who use AAC technology; however, others participate regularly, both socially and vocationally, using the Internet.

Other individuals adopt a different participation strategy and attempt to stay active in the community as long as they possibly can. These individuals may continue to work outside the home, travel, and attend recreational activities, religious services, and social events with friends and family. For example, Tom and his family maintained a very externally focused lifestyle even after he was diagnosed with ALS. During the first 18 months following his diagnosis, Tom and his wife traveled extensively, at times with their children, at times with Tom's siblings, and often with friends. When he began to rely on a wheelchair and eventually on AAC technology, they scheduled "Time with Tom" at a local restaurant every Monday during the dinner hour. Friends, former colleagues, members of their church, neighbors, and relatives all stopped by at their convenience. Tom also continued to attend athletic events and concerts and hosted lunches with friends in his home regularly. He also continued to phone family and friends to celebrate birthdays and anniversaries. Needless to say, Tom developed extensive AAC skills in order to participate in these extensive social interactions.

Decisions about patterns of participation substantially affect an individual's communication needs and corresponding AAC strategies. For example, an individual who communicates primarily at home may need an AAC system that can be moved to various rooms on a cart or on a computer stand with wheels, rather than an AAC device that attaches directly to a wheelchair. Individuals who participate actively in the community need communication systems that are self-contained, compact, and fully portable. Some require efficient internet access via their AAC technology whereas others do not. Most require a means to use the telephone. During assessment and intervention, it is important to consider the individual opinions and preferences of adults with acquired disabilities regarding participation and lifestyle patterns.

Consensus Building

It is also important to develop consensus between the person who uses AAC and the individuals who support him or her when developing a communication needs and participation profile. One way to build consensus is to identify potential communication needs and assign each a level of importance. A review of the information provided previously about Madonna and Tom reveals that many of their communication needs were similar; however, their lifestyle choices dictated unique communication solutions.

A detailed needs assessment has advantages for both the person with the disability and the members of his or her family and support networks. For example, it is not uncommon for adults with acquired communication disorders to insist that their AAC systems return (or maintain) all of the functions of natural communication to them. This is quite natural because many people struggle to accept their disabilities and are often frustrated by their inability to communicate in the same way that was possible with natural speech. In the process of completing a communication needs inventory, these individuals are forced to go beyond the generic expectation of "being able to do everything that I could do before this happened," in order to identify *specific* communication needs and assign them priorities. In a study examining the purposes of AAC device use for people with ALS as reported by their caregivers, Fried-Oken, Rau, Fox, Tulman, and Hindal (2004) found that the two most frequent and highly valued purposes involved regulating the behavior of others (basic wants and needs) and staying connected (social closeness).

In addition, it is not uncommon for family members and friends who surround a person with an acquired physical disability to have differences in opinions regarding the person's communication needs as well as the use of assistive technology as a solution. There is no way to predict what these differences will be, but it is important to try to achieve some degree of consensus among these people about the individual's communication needs or, if that is impossible, to at least clarify their differences of opinion. We discuss this issue with regard to specific disorders in subsequent sections of this chapter.

Assess Specific Capabilities

As we discussed in Chapter 6, AAC teams usually conduct assessments of cognitive, motor, language, and sensory capabilities with people who have acquired physical disabilities. One particularly important aspect of the assessment process for these individuals involves predicting the natural course of various capabilities. People with degenerative diseases will gradually lose some capabilities while other capabilities remain stable. People in stable condition following a brain-stem stroke or SCI may regain certain capabilities either naturally or with therapeutic intervention. Subsequent sections of this chapter address these issues in more detail with regard to specific disabilities.

Assess Constraints

A variety of external constraints may affect the AAC decisions in general, and some of these constraints are especially common for people with acquired communication disorders. As noted previously, the attitudes of family members and friends about the communication disorder in general and the acceptance of AAC technology in particular may influence decisions. For example, families of some older adults appear to have difficulty accepting the use of electronic communication techniques for a spouse or parent because they struggle with accepting their loved one's loss of speech or writing ability. Families of teenagers or young adults may resist low-tech options, even if these are the most appropriate techniques for the time being, because they believe that their child "deserves the very best" and mistakenly equate sophisticated equipment with the best intervention choice.

Another constraint involves the availability of facilitators to learn about the operation and use of an electronic AAC system in order to assist the person who relies on AAC to learn and maintain it. In some locations, facilitators may not be able to obtain adequate support for certain types of communication options. Another important external constraint involves the availability of funding for equipment and instruction. Funding patterns for AAC systems vary dramatically in different parts of the world. Some countries, provinces, or states fund AAC systems for children who participate in educational programs but provide little financial support for adults. In the United States, Medicare, Medicaid, Tricare, and many insurance plans now fund AAC technology and instruction. It is impossible to outline such funding constraints in detail in this book, because funding policies change frequently. The Web site maintained by the Rehabilitation Engineering and Research Center in Communication Enhancement provides current AAC funding information for the United States. As is the case with children, successful AAC interventions require that the AAC team assess constraints and focus on the remediation of these limitations as vigorously as they focus on the individual's communication needs and capabilities.

Evaluate Intervention Outcomes

There are three primary reasons for measuring the outcomes of interventions with adults who have acquired physical disabilities. The first is to identify the communication needs that have and have not been met. When an intervention approach succeeds in meeting certain communication needs, the AAC team should document these for the sake of the individual and his or her family. If an initial intervention does not meet certain communication needs, the team should refine the approach and intervene accordingly. The second reason for measuring intervention effectiveness is to document the effectiveness of the AAC agency providing service. Agencies that provide funding for AAC interventions with adults usually demand this documentation for continued funding. The third reason for measuring intervention effectiveness is to document the overall AAC efforts of a particular center or agency, which may result in increased administrative support for AAC efforts over time.

The following sections of this chapter discuss AAC approaches that apply to specific impairments and syndromes. We cannot provide complete clinical descriptions of these conditions here, so we highlight only those aspects of the disease process that most directly influence AAC interventions.

AMYOTROPHIC LATERAL SCLEROSIS

ALS is a progressive degenerative disease of unknown etiology involving the motor neurons of the brain and spinal cord. Because between 75% (Saunders, Walsh, & Smith, 1981) and 95% (Ball, Beukelman, & Pattee, 2003) of people with ALS are unable to speak by the time of their deaths, these individuals need AAC services. Emery and Holloway (1982) defined the mean age of onset for ALS as 56 years. The most common early symptom is weakness, with approximately one third of those affected reporting initial upper extremity (arm and hand) weakness, one third reporting leg weakness, and one quarter presenting with bulbar (brain-stem) weakness manifested by dysarthria and dysphagia. Extraocular muscle movements are usually spared, as is sphincter control. As the disease progresses, motor weakness may become pervasive, leaving the individual dependent on others for personal care, mobility, and feeding. Of individuals with ALS, 14%–39% survive for 5 years, about 10% live for up to 10 years, and a few may live for 20 years after onset. Individuals with primarily bulbar symptoms tend to have a more rapid course, with a median survival of 2.2 years after the appearance of initial symptoms (Yorkston, Miller, & Strand, 2004).

Communication Symptoms

Dysarthria, a motor speech disorder, results from the weakness and spasticity inherent in ALS. Dysarthria of the mixed flaccid-spastic type is almost universally present at some point (Darley, Aronson, & Brown, 1975; Dworkin, Aronson, & Mulder, 1980; Yorkston, Beukelman, Strand, & Bell, 1999). People with predominantly bulbar (brain-stem) involvement experience this speech disorder early in the disease process, and their speech and swallowing functions may deteriorate rapidly. Such individuals may be able to walk and even drive, although they are unable to speak. Individuals with predominantly spinal involvement, however, may retain normal or mildly dysarthric speech for a considerable period of time, even as they experience extensive motor impairments in their extremities.

Ball, Beukelman, and Pattee (2001, 2002) monitored the speaking rate and speech intelligibility of more than 100 individuals with ALS from the time of diagnosis until they were no longer able to speak. The timing of speech deterioration cannot be predicted accurately based on ALS type and months post-diagnosis alone. However, regardless of the ALS type (bulbar, mixed, or spinal), speaking rate has been shown to be a relatively good predictor of the approaching decrease in speech intelligibility (see Figure 15.1). Generally, speaking rate slows but intelligibility remains above 90% during the early stages of the disease. After speaking rate decreases to about 120 words per minute, an increasing number of individuals achieve speech intelligibility scores below 90%. When speaking rate decreases to 100–120 words per minute, most speakers, regardless of the type of ALS, have speech intelligibility scores below 90% (Ball et al., 2002).

Although the progression of speech symptoms may differ from individual to individual, most people with ALS experience a severe communication disorder during the last months or years of their lives. In an older retrospective study of 100 hospice patients with ALS, 28% were anarthric (unable to speak) and 47% were severely dysarthric at the time of their deaths. Only 25% could speak understandably during the terminal stage of the illness (Saunders et al., 1981). Twenty years later, Ball and colleagues developed the Nebraska ALS Database in which they recorded data from consecutive participants in an ALS clinic sponsored by the Muscular Dystrophy Association. At the time this book was written, data had been collected every 3 months from more than 200 people with ALS. Of that group, only 6% communicated using natural speech at the time of their deaths and 94% required AAC strategies (Beukelman, Ball, & Pattee, 2004).

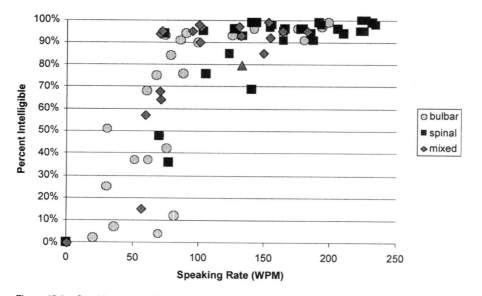

Figure 15.1. Speaking rate and intelligibility decline for people with ALS.

Identify Participation Patterns and Communication Needs

As noted previously, individuals with ALS tend to adopt a range of lifestyle patterns. Some, such as Stephen Hawking, the Nobel Prize–winning physicist, continue to participate actively outside the home in work and community affairs. Tom, whom we introduced earlier in this chapter, maintained a very active social schedule outside of his home. Others, like Madonna, transform their homes into social centers and work, socialize, and conduct their affairs within this stable and customized environment. For home-centered individuals, either movable (i.e., mounted on a table or cart) or portable AAC systems may meet their communication needs. These individuals may also use AAC systems that require extensive facilitator support (e.g., eye pointing, lipreading, residual speech) because they rarely need to function as independently as do their counterparts who participate actively in the community.

Assess Specific Capabilities

In this section, we describe the primary cognitive/linguistic and motor capabilities that require assessment prior to AAC intervention.

Cognitive/Linguistic Skills

Individuals usually retain their cognitive and linguistic functions as ALS progresses. The incidence of depression in people with ALS does not differ from that in other individuals with ongoing illnesses, nor is the suicide rate unusually high (Yorkston et al., 2004). Thus, most people with ALS are able to understand and relate to the world around them and formulate messages much like other adults.

On the other hand, AAC interventionists need to be aware that cognitive changes in ALS do occur. Recent research indicates that between 40% and 50% of people with ALS experience some degree of dementia (Lomen-Hoerth et al., 2003; Yorkston et al., 2004). Yorkston et al. (2004) estimated that approximately 25%–35% of individuals with ALS without overt dementia exhibit subtle changes in cognitive function, especially in the areas of executive functioning, reasoning, response generation, initiation, abstraction, planning and organization, new learning, verbal fluency, and picture recall. Measures of cognitive functioning, along with some evidence from brain imaging, suggest a mild frontal dysfunction (Kiernan & Hudson, 1994; Lloyd, Richardson, Brooks, Al-Chalabi, & Leigh, 2000). Cognitive deficits tend to be more pronounced in individuals with dysarthria (bulbar involvement) and pseudobulbar palsy. Together, these deficits are likely to affect an individual's acceptance of and ability to learn to use AAC systems.

In addition, Montgomery and Erickson (1987) suggested that overt dementia (i.e., frontotemporal dementia [FTD/ALS]) occurs in 1%–2% percent of individuals with ALS. The prevalence of dementia in familial ALS may be somewhat higher (Hudson, 1981). FTD/ALS is characterized by profound personality changes and breakdowns in social conduct. Most patients fail on tests of executive function and exhibit poor abstraction, planning, and organizational skills. Neurological signs are usually absent in the early stages. FTD/ALS is relatively rare. Frequently, the onset of dementia precedes other physical symptoms (Rakowicz & Hodges, 1998). It is unclear whether FTD/ALS constitutes the extreme end or range of this disease or represents a separate disease entity entirely.

Finally, there is growing evidence that aphasia can be associated with ALS (Bak & Hodges, 2001; Mitsuyama, Kogoh, & Ata, 1985; Tscuchiya et al., 2000). In a few rare cases, primary progressive aphasia appears to evolve to ALS. For example, Caselli et al. (1993) reported on seven patients in whom articulatory and language impairment preceded to rapidly progressive ALS. Recent research also describes a frontotemporal lobar dementia syndrome (FTLD) that has three categories: FTD (involving primarily personality changes), semantic dementia (e.g., fluent aphasia), and primary progressive aphasia (e.g., nonfluent aphasia with loss of word meaning; Lomen-Hoerth, 2004; Lomen-Hoerth et al., 2003). FTLD has been reported to be more common among people with ALS who have bulbar symptoms, are somewhat older ($M = 65$ years), and have decreased functional vital capacity ($M = 66\%$ predicted).

Motor Skills

Individual patterns of motor control capability greatly affect the selection of an AAC system for people with ALS. These capabilities generally differ markedly depending on whether the person first experiences bulbar or spinal symptoms.

Bulbar (Brain-Stem) ALS   For some time, people with predominantly bulbar symptoms are usually able to control AAC devices that they can operate via direct selection using their hands or fingers. For example, Yorkston (1989) described an individual with ALS who pointed to letters on an alphabet board in order to communicate messages and supplement her distorted natural speech. During the initial stages of the disease, she was able to write longer messages as well. Because she did not consider telephone communication to be a pressing need, this individual decided to defer the decision to use an SGD until her disease progressed. Another man with ALS communicated with an alphabet board and a small portable typewriter. As his disease progressed, he continued to type using a single finger and moved his arm and hand with the assistance of a mobile arm support (Beukelman, Yorkston, & Dowden, 1985).

Spinal ALS   People with ALS who exhibit predominantly spinal symptoms usually experience extensive trunk- and limb-related motor impairments by the time they are unable to meet their communication needs through speech. For these individuals, the need for an augmented writing system often precedes the need for a conversational system.

Individuals with severe impairments related to limb control usually require a scanning communication system of some type. For example, Beukelman, Yorkston, et al. (1985) described a man who was unable to move his upper or lower limbs and for whom using an optical pointer, even for very brief periods of time, was too fatiguing. However, he demonstrated the ability to activate, release, and reactivate a switch that was mounted on a pillow beside his head when he was seated in a large easy chair. Because he had the head rotation capability needed for this and because he could generate accurate as well as nonfatiguing switch control movements, until his death he used this motor pattern to operate a scanning AAC device.

The motor control site for alternative access may need to be changed several times during the progression of the individual's disease. For example, one woman controlled her system initially with a single switch operated by either hand. In time, her AAC team modified the switch so that she could control it with minimal movement of a single finger. Finally, her team mounted a P-switch on her forehead, as depicted in Figure 15.2. She operated this switch by wrinkling her forehead slightly as she raised her eyebrows.

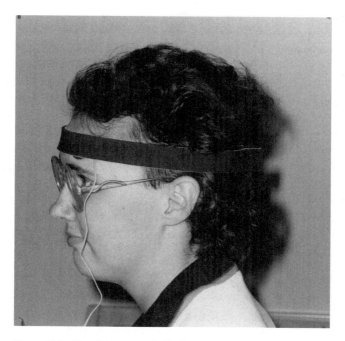

Figure 15.2.   P-switch worn on the forehead.

Assess Constraints

Although not specifically mentioned in the Participation Model (see Figure 6.1), certain constraints that are discussed in the following sections apply to people with ALS and their support systems.

Acceptance of AAC by People with ALS and Their Families

Usually, people with ALS demonstrate relatively high acceptance of AAC technology. As AAC technology improves and is more common in society, acceptance rates continue to increase. Mathy, Yorkston, and Gutmann (2000) reviewed AAC use by people with ALS (PALS) from numerous sources. They referred to data by Gutmann and Gryfe (1996), who evaluated trends in the use of AAC systems for 126 PALS seen at an assistive technology clinic in Toronto, Canada. Among these participants, 27% elected not to pursue AAC interventions. Gutmann and Gryfe (1996) developed a critical path strategy for service provision that identified early intervention, frequent intervention, and early introduction to AAC as key components to increasing AAC acceptance. Gutmann (1999), analyzing the same data, reported that "women preferred voice output systems twice as often as men (49% for women, 26% for men)" (p. 211). In addition, "almost an equivalent number of men (27.8%) and women (26%) did not wish any AAC intervention . . . " (p. 211).

In 2004, Ball and colleagues reported on the AAC acceptance patterns of 50 individuals who were referred consecutively to an ALS clinic. Ninety-six percent of the PALS in this study accepted AAC technology either immediately (90%) or after some delay (6%). Only 4% (i.e., two individuals) rejected AAC technology completely. None of the PALS discontinued use of their AAC technology more than 2 months before their deaths. Analysis of interviews with PALS and their family members revealed that family member resistance occurred most often because 1) they believed they could understand their loved one's communication sufficiently to meet his or her needs and 2) they believed they were providing adequate care without assistive technology. Two family members who initially resisted AAC expressed concern that the quality of their ability to provide care was being questioned; however, in both cases, they eventually accepted AAC technology as their family member's speech continued to deteriorate and they realized that they could not provide "good care" without communicating effectively. One PALS and his family reported physician resistance. According to their report, the physician viewed speech deterioration as an inevitable part of the disease progression and counseled the family to accept it rather than turn to technology. Three PALS resisted AAC because they denied that their speech was difficult to understand or that they would ever need AAC technology. In time, each of these individuals accepted AAC, often with the strong encouragement of their family. The three individuals who rejected AAC technology entirely were subsequently diagnosed with FTD.

Operational Competence

People with ALS, like most people who use AAC, require time and instruction in order to gain communicative competence with their AAC systems. Because ALS is predictably degenerative, these individuals are in the unique position of being able to select their AAC systems and learn to operate them while they can still use natural speech to meet at least their most basic communication needs. In fact, if an AAC system is selected and implemented after an individual is no longer able to speak, the AAC experience often becomes extremely frustrating for all involved.

Although rapid decline of speech function in ALS is certainly not inevitable, it occurs frequently enough so that sound clinical management dictates early preparedness. In our experience, exploration of AAC options should begin when speech has slowed to between 100 and 120 words per minute and/or intelligibility is inconsistent in adverse listening situations.

Facilitator Support

People with ALS require ongoing support from facilitators in order to use their AAC systems. This support may include instruction in technical or other skills that enable individuals to operate the devices efficiently and accurately. They may also need facilitator support to select and modify messages stored in their systems. In addition, as an individual's capabilities change with progression of the disease, facilitators may need to change the motor control options and the positioning of the system. Facilitators may also have to provide instruction in the social use of the AAC system.

Intervention Staging

Once an individual has received a probable or definitive diagnosis of ALS, the process of education, assessment, and intervention should begin in order to meet their changing needs. We organize our efforts in the communication area by using a staging system (Yorkston et al., 1999) that allows people with ALS, the members of their social networks, and their care teams to understand the intervention process.

Stage 1: No Detectable Speech Disorder

In this early stage of the disease, assessors can detect no (or minimal) changes in speech. This stage may be very short for people with primarily bulbar symptoms and may be extended for people with primarily spinal symptoms. The purpose of intervention at this stage is to monitor speech performance and present information to people with ALS and their decision makers, so that they will be ready to make intervention decisions in a timely manner. Early in a degenerative disease, individuals and their families require some time to accept the diagnosis and grieve their loss. Then, families often go through an educational phase in which they attempt to learn as much as possible about the disease and its impact on the individual and family. During this phase, individuals with ALS and their families usually welcome general information about communication impairment and AAC as well as information about the AAC service options that are available. AAC teams and medical personnel should take care at this stage not to be too graphic or detailed about the later communication difficulties that individuals may experience.

During Stage 1, we typically monitor speech performance, especially with regard to speaking rate. As noted previously, a gradual reduction in speaking rate usually precedes a decline in speech intelligibility. By systematically measuring speaking rate, we can prepare people with ALS and their supporters for the potential need for an AAC assessment and intervention.

Stage 2: Obvious Speech Disorder with Intelligible Speech

In the second stage of the disease, changes in speech are noticed by unfamiliar listeners, especially when the speaker is fatigued. Intervention at this stage should focus on learning to minimize environmental interference by muting the sound on the television, arranging conversations in quiet settings, choosing quiet restaurants, finding quiet places to talk with friends at social events, and so forth. It is often helpful at this stage to develop guidelines regarding when family members and friends should act as communication facilitators and interpreters if unfamiliar listeners cannot understand the speaker.

During this stage, most people with ALS experience a reduction in their speaking rates. Sentence reading tasks such as the Sentence Intelligibility Test (Yorkston, Beukelman, & Tice, 1996) or paragraph reading tasks such as Pacer/Tally (Yorkston et al., 1997) can be used to monitor speaking rate. When the speaking rate has slowed to 50% of what is typical (i.e., approximately 100–120 words per minute on a sentence reading task), AAC teams should initiate assessment and training with regard to AAC systems. Interventionists should also encourage frequent listeners to have their hearing checked, if there is any possibility of hearing impairment. Speakers with ALS at this stage should be taught strategies for establishing conversational topics, confirming that their listeners are aware of the topics, and coping with conversation in groups (e.g., learning to use and accept voice amplification).

Stage 3: Reduction in Speech Intelligibility

At the third stage, speakers with reduced speech intelligibility will find that listeners ask them to repeat messages with increasing frequency. If they have not already slowed their speaking rate to compensate for reduced speech intelligibility, the speech-language pathologist should encourage them to do so at this time. They also need to learn to reduce their breath group length (i.e., the number of words spoken on a single breath) in order to conserve energy. If speakers are leaking considerable air through their nasal cavities during speech and their speech articulation is still quite precise, they may be fitted with a palatal lift to position their weak soft palate more appropriately (Yorkston et al., 1999). They should also learn breakdown resolution strategies, such as rephrasing messages before repeating them. Finally, the AAC assessment and training that was started in Stage 2 should be completed early in this stage so that the individuals have AAC systems available to resolve communication breakdowns when needed.

During Stage 3, it is often helpful to provide people with ALS and their caregivers with information about how other people with the disease have used their AAC systems. For example, Mathy et al. (2000) reported on AAC use by 31 people with ALS. All of these individuals used multimodal AAC strategies, including both low-tech and electronic options. They used electronic AAC devices to talk on the telephone; write messages and letters; convey detailed, complicated messages; and communicate with strangers. They used low-tech or unaided communication options to provide brief instruction and to participate in face-to-face conversations with family members and familiar caregivers. Recent research (Fried-Oken et al., 2004) suggests that for some individuals, as AAC devices become more complex, the frequency with which they are used to discuss important issues, converse about work, and give instructions may decline. However, as in all areas of clinical practice, individuals with ALS vary considerably with regard to their preferences in this regard. By making such information available, families can be protected somewhat from having unrealistic expectations of either the person who relies on AAC or the technological supports that are available.

> Efficiency of communication becomes more critical as the amount of energy for John to respond increases and his endurance fades. His will to live depends on his ability to communicate. Communication is the last great love of his life available to him. (C. Brahne and V. Hall, writing about a man with ALS, in Brahne & Hall, 1995, p. 10)

Stage 4: Residual Natural Speech and AAC

During the fourth stage, AAC shifts from being a secondary to a primary communication system for most individuals with ALS. For a time, they may use alphabet supplementation (Beukelman & Yorkston, 1977), during which they point to the first letter of a word simultaneously as they speak the word using their residual natural speech. Of course, facilitators will need to help the individuals change their communication modes for various communication situations. For example, individuals will probably need an electronic communication system for speaking on the telephone, writing, and conversing with strangers.

Stage 5: Loss of Useful Speech

During the fifth stage, individuals lose functional natural speech and must rely on AAC entirely. It is important that people with ALS and their caregivers develop adequate yes/no communication systems to use during meals, in bed, and during emergencies. Eye-pointing or eye-linking systems are also helpful at this stage as an alternative to electronic communication systems in some contexts. During this phase, some individuals will choose ventilator support to compensate for their respiratory problems. If this occurs, special communication training to deal with ventilator care will also be required. Because most individuals also experience eating and swallowing difficulties during this stage, special communication messages and strategies will also be required so that they can communicate accurately and efficiently about eating- and drinking-related needs and supports.

> For a time, the only way I could communicate was to spell out words letter by letter, by raising my eyebrows when someone pointed to the right letter on a spelling card. It is pretty difficult to carry on a conversation like that, let alone write a scientific paper. However, a computer expert in California . . . heard of my plight. He sent me a computer program he had written . . . . This allowed me to select words from a series of menus on the screen, by pressing a switch in my hand . . . . When I have built up what I want to say, I can send it to a speech synthesizer . . . I can manage up to 15 words a minute . . . . Using this system, I have written a book and many scientific papers. I have also given many scientific and popular talks. (Stephen Hawking, describing the communication system he uses as a result of ALS, in Hawking, 1995)

MULTIPLE SCLEROSIS

MS is an acquired inflammatory disease of the white matter of the central nervous system. The lesions of MS result in multiple plaques that cause destruction of the myelin sheath.

In the northern part of the United States, the prevalence of MS is about 1 in 1,000; in the southern states, the prevalence is about one third to one half of this figure. Approximately 95% of all cases begin between the ages of 10 and 50 years, with a median onset age of 27 years. Although MS is considered to be a disease of young people, it is not uncommon for an initial diagnosis to occur between 50 and 60 years of age. The female-to-male ratio of occurrence is 3:2 (Yorkston et al., 2004). Racially, people with MS are more likely to be white than African American and more likely to be African American than Asian.

The natural course of MS differs greatly from person to person. The clinical course of MS is usually divided into five classes (Yorkston et al., 2004).

1. **Relapsing and remitting:** About 70% of young people with MS fall into this category. They experience virtually full recovery from the neurological signs and symptoms after each episode of relapse.

2. **Chronic progressive:** This is most commonly present in individuals who are older adults at the onset of the disease. The motor and neurological symptoms gradually worsen over time, with no intermittent remissions.

3. **Combined relapsing/remitting with chronic progression:** The majority of individuals reach this stage of the disease, which results in a gradual deterioration of capabilities over time, although individuals experience periods of relative remission.

4. **Benign:** About 20% of all individuals with MS have a typical life span with relatively typical functioning and little or no progression of the disease.

5. **Malignant:** A small percentage (5%–10%) of (predominantly) young people with MS show rapid and extensive involvement of cognitive, cerebellar, and pyramidal systems, which leads to death in a relatively short time.

The average life expectancy of young males with MS is about 35 years following the onset of the disease. The prognosis is worse 1) in males than in females; 2) if the age at onset is greater than 35 years; 3) if a chronic, progressive pattern appears at onset; or 4) if cerebellar symptoms occur at initial presentation (Poser, 1984).

Communication Symptoms

Dysarthria is the most common communication problem associated with MS, but the study of large groups of individuals with MS has shown that dysarthria is not a universal characteristic of this disease. In a study of 144 individuals with MS, Ivers and Goldstein

(1963) reported that dysarthria was present in 19% of the participants. Darley, Brown, and Goldstein (1972) reported that 41% of their MS sample demonstrated overall speech performance that was not "essentially normal" in terms of its impact on listeners. Nevertheless, when researchers utilized a self-reporting technique, only 23% of these individuals reported a "speech and/or communication disorder"; thus, a large percentage of this sample appeared to be unaware of the severity of their speech problems. Overall, a survey of studies related to the prevalence of dysarthria in MS revealed a range of occurrence of 19%–41%, depending on who made the assessment and how they sampled the population.

Although a number of individuals with MS demonstrate speech impairments, most do not require AAC systems. Beukelman, Kraft, and Freal (1985) reported that 4% of 656 survey respondents with MS indicated that their communication was so severely impaired that strangers were unable to understand them.

One evening . . . I had gone to the bathroom for a shower . . . . All was well as I entered the bathroom and showered. Then I began to wheel myself to the bedroom after I had finished. I tried to say something to my wife as I neared the door, but the words would not come and all I could manage was a babbling as I tried to express myself. My wife said to me, "What did you do, flush your voice down the drain?" Now this is not a real funny line. However, under those circumstances, it sounded hilarious. We both burst into laughter . . . . My voice control did not return for a few days . . . [but it] did return. (A man with MS, in Michael, 1981, p. 27)

Identify Participation Patterns and Communication Needs

Because the onset of MS occurs relatively early in life, individuals with MS are usually in educational programs or employed when they first experience symptoms. The intermittent and gradual onset of symptoms usually does not require people with MS to modify their lifestyles immediately, although some people with visual problems, which are quite common in MS, may require technological assistance to read computer screens or detailed printed materials. In time, however, impairments that are unrelated to verbal communication often prevent these individuals from attending school or working. For example, Kraft (1981) reported that arm and leg spasticity is an important reason why many people with MS drop out of the employment market. Loss of balance, loss of normal bladder control, and fatigue also interfere. In addition, a combination of weakness, spasticity, ataxia, and tremor may interfere with walking and necessitate the use of a wheelchair for mobility.

Because most people with MS whose speech is so impaired that they require AAC systems are no longer able to attend school or work, they rarely have communication needs related to these domains. Furthermore, some individuals with severe speech impairments require personal care assistance beyond what their families can offer; and they may live in residential or nursing centers, which may limit their communication needs even further. Thus, the primary communication needs of many people with MS are conversational, although individuals may require assistance with writing as well.

Assess Specific Capabilities

In this section, we describe the primary cognitive, language, sensory/perceptual and motor capabilities that require assessment prior to AAC intervention.

Cognitive Skills

The cognitive limitations of individuals with MS have been poorly documented, but more than half of these individuals seem to display definite evidence of cognitive impairment (Rao, 1995). There is general consensus that cognitive changes are specific rather than global and can be described as a subcortical dementia with 1) the absence of aphasia; 2) memory retrieval failure in the presence of relatively intact encoding and storage capability; 3) impaired conceptual reasoning in the context of near-normal intellect; 4) slowed information-processing time; and 5) personality disturbances including apathy, depression, or euphoria (Rao, 1995).

Language Skills

Although dysarthria is the most common communication problem associated with MS, aphasia has occasionally been reported. Several large studies of individuals with MS have noted no occurrence of aphasia (Olmos-Lau, Ginsberg, & Geller, 1977). However, Beukelman, Kraft, et al. (1985) noted that other researchers reported the incidence of aphasia as ranging from 1% to 3% of people with MS. Recently, Yorkston, Klasner, and Swanson (2001) indicated that people with MS commonly report difficulty with word-finding and changes in verbal or written organization. Murdock and Lethlean (2000) evaluated 60 people with MS and reported four potential subgroups: 1) those with pervasive language impairment (2%), 2) those with moderate to severe language impairment (13%), 3) those with mild to moderate language impairment (32%), and 4) those with essentially typical language abilities (53%).

Sensory/Perceptual Skills

Vision limitations are common in MS; in fact, 35% of people with MS experience optic neuritis, the acute or subacute loss of central vision in one eye with peripheral vision spared, as their first symptom (Wikstrom, Poser, & Ritter, 1980). Optic neuritis is often manifested initially by an inability to see text on a computer screen or to read small print in general. The visual limitations of MS cause particular problems in the context of AAC interventions because many of AAC techniques require extensive visual capabilities. Many individuals with MS cannot use visual scanning arrays; instead, they may require auditory scanning systems such as the one described in a subsequent section of this chapter. Large-print text is a common requirement of people with MS, as is synthetic speech feedback that echoes the letters and words selected in typing or from a communication display. For example, an AAC system designed for a 30-year-old woman with MS consisted of an expanded keyboard with 1-inch square keys and speech feedback (Honsinger, 1989).

[Here] is my list of lists: Long-term projects and obligations . . . daily tasks, projects, and obligations; spring cleaning tasks; items to be taken on overnight outings and trips, . . . personal care schedule; phone numbers; books on loan from the National Library Service for the Blind and Physically Handicapped and from

Recordings for the Blind, Inc.; two lists of physical therapy exercises; names and phone numbers of friends and former clients; names and addresses of out-often friends and family; calendar; medical and surgical supplies that must be stocked; and fears and questions I have concerning life with a progressive disease. Some of my lists are on large sheets of braille paper, others are in a looseleaf binder. All are on cassette tapes. (Denise Karuth, a young woman who is blind as a result of MS, describing the lists she keeps as memory aids, in Karuth, 1985, p. 27)

Motor Skills

An individual's motor control capabilities in MS vary considerably; therefore, careful motor assessment is an important aspect of all AAC interventions. According to Feys and colleagues (2001), intention tremor in the upper limb, which occurs during or is exaggerated by voluntary movement, is encountered in approximately one third of the MS population. The tremor often disrupts an individual's attempts to access assistive technology interfaces such as keyboards, computer mice, or switches. AAC teams can sometimes identify a way to stabilize the body part involved in access sufficiently so that the individual can make voluntary movements without excessive tremor. At other times, AAC teams may need to attach a switch to an individual's limb or hand so that the switch can move with the body part during tremor but still remain in position to be activated by a finger. Finally, specialized applications providing motion-filtering software that support multiple interfaces have also been developed (Feys et al., 2001).

Often, the motor control problems and visual impairments of MS combine to limit AAC options severely. For example, Porter (1989) described an AAC intervention that occurred near the end of a person's life. The individual's visual and motor control limitations were quite extensive, but he learned to control a simple call buzzer and auditory scanning system using a pressure switch that attached to a pillow beside his head.

Assess Constraints

Several characteristics of MS complicate many AAC interventions. First, symptom patterns vary considerably among individuals. Although the clinical course of MS follows five general patterns of progression, individual manifestations can be complex and vary over time. Obviously, changes in an AAC system may be needed to accommodate this variability. Second, as noted previously, visual impairments are quite common in MS and can make AAC interventions particularly challenging. Third, AAC interventions usually occur in conjunction with other efforts to compensate for the multiple impairments experienced by people with MS. Therefore, AAC teams must coordinate their interventions with other interventions in the context of changing symptom patterns.

Intervention Staging

As with ALS, interventions for MS can be described using a five-stage model.

Stage 1: No Detectable Speech Disorder

Early in the disease process, no (or minimal) changes in speech can be detected. In fact, many people with MS may not experience speech symptoms for an extended period of time. After confirmation of the diagnosis, people with MS and their families often engage in an educational phase in which they attempt to learn as much as possible about the disease and its impact. Individuals and their families often request general information about communication impairment and MS. Service providers should take care to explain the variable patterns of motor speech disturbance.

Stage 2: Detectable Speech Disorder

At the second stage, unfamiliar listeners notice changes in speech. Speech symptoms worsen and lessen slightly during exacerbations and remissions of the MS. Although phonation may be unstable, individuals usually do not experience reductions in speech loudness, but they may have difficulty maintaining appropriate volume levels in restaurants and at public meetings. AAC teams usually do not recommend speech intervention in this stage.

Stage 3: Obvious Speech Disturbances with Intelligible Speech

At the third stage, speakers with MS experience dysarthria that is severe enough to be apparent to anyone who speaks with them. Even at this stage, many may not receive intervention for speech, depending on how limited their participation patterns are due to other impairments (e.g., problems with fatigue, mobility, balance). Facilitators should teach breakdown resolution strategies at this stage, such as rephrasing messages before repeating them.

Stage 4: Reduction in Speech Intelligibility

During the fourth stage, speakers with MS will experience reductions in speech intelligibility. By taking care to establish the topic they are discussing and speaking in optimal listening conditions, their speech is likely to remain comprehensible to familiar listeners. Toward the end of this stage, some choose to use alphabet supplementation (Beukelman & Yorkston, 1977), in which they point to the first letter of a word as they speak in order to remain comprehensible. They often use the alphabet board to resolve communication breakdowns as well.

Stage 5: Loss of Most Useful Speech

During the fifth stage, individuals have very limited functional natural speech and must rely on AAC. It is important that people with MS and their caregivers develop adequate yes/no communication systems to use during meals, in bed, and during emergencies. Some people with MS have sufficient visual-motor ability to operate an electronic communication system. Individuals with severe visual impairments must rely on auditory scanning. A relatively small percentage of individuals with MS require a multipurpose AAC system. Given the range of motor control, visual, sensory, and cognitive impairments experienced in MS, interventions need to be very individualized.

GUILLAIN-BARRÉ SYNDROME

Guillain-Barré syndrome (GBS) results from the progressive destruction and regeneration of the myelin sheath of peripheral nerve axons. Paralysis progresses from the lower extremities upward, and maximal paralysis usually occurs within 1–3 weeks of onset. As the myelin sheath slowly regenerates, nerve function and associated muscle strength gradually return. Typically, motor recovery begins with the structures of the head and face and progresses inferiorly. About 80% of people with GBS recover completely with no residual impairments (Guillain-Barré Syndrome Fact Sheet, National Institute of Neurological Disorders and Stroke Web site [1997]).

Guillain-Barré syndrome occurs in about 1.7 cases per 100,000 people (or about 3,500 cases per year in North America) and is among the most common neurologic causes of admission to the ICU. [It is] characterized by the acute onset of a symmetrical descending paralysis that extends from the legs to the trunk, arms, and cranial nerves. Treatment includes ventilation in about one third of all cases. If respiratory failure occurs, the average period on a ventilator is 50 days, with a 108-day period of hospitalization. (Fried-Oken, Howard, & Stewart, 1991, pp. 45–46)

Communication Disorders

The weakness associated with GBS causes flaccid dysarthria and in many cases anarthria (complete loss of speech). In addition, severe weakness often requires ventilator support through oral intubation or tracheotomy. Language and cognition are usually unaffected.

Intervention Stages

The stages of progression of GBS require different types of AAC support, as described in the following sections.

Stage 1: Deterioration Phase

As noted previously, people with GBS experience maximal paralysis within 1–3 weeks of onset. Because weakness progresses upward from the lower extremities, the diagnosis usually is made before speech becomes impaired. Little time usually passes, however, between diagnosis and onset of severe speech impairment. Typically, individuals with GBS are hospitalized following their diagnosis so that medical personnel can monitor their symptom progression and provide appropriate supports and intervention. As part of this effort, medical teams should monitor these individuals' communication impairment so that AAC intervention can be provided at an appropriate time.

Stage 2: Loss of Speech

During this stage, the progress of symptoms stabilizes. Those people who require AAC intervention are usually unable to speak by this stage and receive respiratory support from a ventilator. Initially, AAC intervention consists of low-tech options, with emphasis on the establishment of a reliable yes/no system, followed by the development of an eye-pointing or eye-linking technique. AAC teams should develop communication boards that will support the individual's needs through dependent (i.e., partner-assisted) visual and auditory scanning, yes/no responses, and eye pointing. Usually, these communication boards will include social messages, health-related messages, and letters and numbers for message construction.

Stage 3: Prolonged Speechlessness

The period of time during which people with GBS are unable to speak varies from individual to individual. Some people may experience weeks or months of dependence on AAC systems to communicate with family, friends, and health care staff. Typically, these individuals continue to use the low-tech strategies introduced in Stage 2; however, electronic options may also be appropriate to allow greater independence and less need to rely on knowledgeable, well-trained listeners. Usually, the extensive motor impairments of these individuals require them to use scanning AAC systems, often with a switch controlled by eyelid or head movement. Given the temporary nature of these individuals' AAC use, most learn to communicate with letter-by-letter spelling and retrieval of a limited number of alphabetically encoded messages. Typically, these people do not use systems that require them to memorize extensive codes.

Stage 4: Spontaneous Recovery of Speech

During the fourth phase, the individual with GBS makes the transition from speechlessness back to normal speech. Often, this transition takes several weeks or months. As muscle strength returns to the oral mechanism, the individual may still depend on a ventilator and a tracheostomy tube. Some speakers find an oral-type electrolarynx (see Chapter 18) very helpful at this point. By controlling the sound sources of the electrolarynx with a head switch, the sound can be turned on when the person wishes to speak and turned off when she or he wishes to listen or rest. While the muscles of the oral cavity are still weak, the individual may have imprecise articulation and reduced speech intelligibility. Some individuals find it helpful to first establish the communicative topic or context with their AAC system, then attempt to use their residual speech, and finally resolve communication breakdowns with their AAC system. As recovery progresses, medical personnel will remove ventilator support and the individual will again be able to speak independently. Usually, the individual requires no ongoing natural speech interventions.

Stage 5: Long-Term Residual Motor Speech Disorder

As mentioned previously, 85% of people with GBS experience complete recovery of motor control; the remaining 15% experience residual weakness. Of this residual group, only a few experience long-term motor speech disorders (i.e., dysarthria). For them, speech interventions to maximize the effectiveness of their natural speech are appropriate. We do not know of any individual with GBS who required long-term AAC support.

Botulism [a form of food poisoning] clinically resembles Guillain-Barré syndrome . . . . [It] is an infection of the nervous system caused by the organism *Clostridium botulinum,* which when ingested produces widespread muscle weakness. The disease often occurs when someone eats uncooked canned food that has not been sterilized properly. (Fried-Oken et al., 1991, p. 46)

PARKINSON'S DISEASE

Parkinson's disease (PD) is a syndrome composed of a cluster of motor symptoms that include tremor at rest, rigidity, paucity (i.e., reduction in movement), and impaired postural reflexes. PD results from a loss of dopaminergic neurons in the basal ganglia (especially the substantia nigra) and the brain stem. The onset is typically insidious; in retrospect, many individuals recall stiffness and muscle aches, which they first attributed to normal aging. The symptom that often initiates the first visit to a physician is tremor in a resting position.

Medical treatment since the 1970s has greatly altered the natural course of PD. Prior to the availability of current medications, about one fourth of all individuals with PD died within the first 5 years following diagnosis, and 80% died after 10–14 years (Yorkston et al., 1999). Although the changes in mortality rate due to levodopamine (L-dopa) and other medications are not yet clear, these treatments have certainly altered dramatically the lifestyles of people with PD. Individuals with PD are able to move much more freely and manage their lives much more independently with medication than without it. Surgical treatments have come back into favor for selected people with PD, as has deep brain stimulation. For a more detailed discussion of medical and surgical interventions, see Yorkston et al. (2004).

> The average annual incidence of parkinsonism (excluding drug-induced cases) is 18.2 cases per 100,000 people. The prevalence is estimated to be between 66 and 187 cases per 100,000. There is no significant difference of incidence between males and females. The incidence increases sharply above age 64, and peak incidence is between 75 and 84 years of age. There is a trend toward increased age at the time of diagnosis (Yorkston et al., 1999).

Although pharmacological treatment dramatically improves the performance of many people with PD, some side effects of the medication can interfere with the use of AAC approaches. Individual fluctuations in motor responses (also known as an on–off response) may occur, probably due to differences in medication absorption and dopamine receptor responsiveness. With long-term therapy, some people also experience involuntary movements that interfere with functional activities. These involuntary movements may cause emotional distress as well.

Communication Symptoms

Dysarthria is common in Parkinson's disease. Recently, Hartelius and Svensson (1994) surveyed 230 people with Parkinson's disease, and noted that 70% of these individuals reported that speech and voice were worse than prior to disease onset. The speech symptoms of people with PD are described in detail by Yorkston and colleagues (2004). Typically, symptoms include reduced pitch variability, reduced overall loudness, and decreased use of all vocal parameters for achieving stress and emphasis. Articulation is imprecise and is produced at variable rates. Voice quality is often harsh and sometimes breathy.

Speech disorders among people with PD are not uniform. Some speakers are difficult to understand, primarily because they speak excessively fast. Their speaking rates may exceed those of typical speakers or exceed those that are optimal for people with motor control disorders. Other speakers are difficult to understand because they speak with reduced intensity or loudness. Still others speak with such limited movement of their articulators that they have difficulty producing precise speech sounds. As PD progresses, many speakers demonstrate combinations of these speech disorders.

Researchers have not documented the natural course of symptoms in people with PD who have communication disorders. Clinical observations reveal a gradual process, with speech becoming increasingly difficult to understand. Most people with PD communicate with natural speech to a greater or lesser extent. Therefore, when they use AAC techniques, the techniques make up part of a multimodal communication system that includes natural speech.

> My ability to form thoughts and ideas into words and sentences is not impaired; the problem is translating those words and sentences into articulate speech. My lips, tongue, and jaw muscles simply won't cooperate. What words I do smuggle through the blockade can be heard, though not always comprehended. Try as I might, I can't inflect my speech to reflect my state of mind. And it's not like I can liven up my halting monotone with a raised eyebrow; my face, utterly expressionless, simply won't respond. Like Emmett Kelly, but without the greasepaint, I often appear sad on the outside while actually smiling, or at least smirking, on the inside. (Michael J. Fox, describing his PD symptoms in *Lucky Man* [2002])

Identify Participation Patterns and Communication Needs

The communication needs of people with PD depend on two primary factors. Many people with PD are older adults, and most are retired. Therefore, their communication needs reflect, first of all, the social environments of their retirement. In addition, the range of physical impairments in PD varies greatly from person to person. Some people have such severe physical limitations that they require extensive physical assistance from attendants or family members. The level of dependence greatly influences each individual's communication needs.

Assess Specific Capabilities

In this section, we describe the primary cognitive/linguistic, sensory/perceptual, and motor capabilities that require assessment prior to AAC intervention.

Cognitive/Linguistic Skills

People with PD acquire their disability late in life, so they usually have developed typical language skills. Therefore, they can spell and read at levels necessary to support most

AAC interventions. Controversy exists as to whether dementia is a feature of PD (Bayles et al., 1996). During tests, examiners have found that some individuals have specific memory impairments, and some individuals complain of slowness in problem solving. The AAC team must consider whether such cognitive limitations are likely to interfere with AAC interventions. The team may provide additional instruction and practice in order to help the person compensate for learning or memory difficulties.

Sensory/Perceptual Skills

Disturbances in sensory function usually do not interfere with AAC interventions for people with PD.

Motor Skills

Clinical reports describe people who have successfully used direct selection AAC techniques such as alphabet boards, as discussed previously. Because researchers have reported few AAC interventions with speakers who have PD, the motor control problems that may influence such AAC interventions are not well documented. Thus, AAC teams may need to consider several motor control problems. Many individuals have reduced range and speed of movement due to the rigidity associated with PD. The AAC team will need to reduce the size of the selection display (e.g., on an alphabet board) for these individuals. Other individuals experience extensive tremors that are usually worse when they are at rest. Many can dampen the tremors if they can stabilize their hands on the surface of a communication board or device. A keyguard is often helpful with devices that have keyboards. Some people experience hyperkinesia (excessive movement) as a side effect of the medication that controls their parkinsonian symptoms. These excessive movements may interfere with the fine motor control required for some AAC options.

> Micrographia is precisely what it sounds like—tiny writing . . . . Without drugs, my own penmanship becomes . . . microscopic. Combined with the stubborn refusal of my "off" arm to move in a smooth, lateral, left-to-right direction, the result is a fractured column of miniature scribbles. (Michael J. Fox, describing his PD symptoms in *Lucky Man* [2002])

Assess Constraints

Two types of constraints are usually associated with AAC interventions for people with PD. First, because most people with PD are able to speak to some extent, they may display some resistance toward the need for an AAC intervention. Some will blame their listeners for their communication failures, even if this is not the case. Communication partners need to actively encourage these individuals to use AAC techniques. Second, many people with PD are older adults and have spouses and friends in the same age group. Therefore, the hearing limitations of their listeners may act as a significant barrier to effective communication.

Intervention Stages

Again, we use a five-stage model of support to describe potential AAC interventions for individuals with PD. For a detailed discussion of speech intervention for people with PD, readers are referred to Yorkston and colleagues (2004).

Stage 1: No Detectable Speech Disorder

Early in the disease, people with PD have received a diagnosis but do not yet exhibit speech symptoms. As with other degenerative diseases, individuals and their families often engage in an educational phase after a time of acceptance and grief. During this phase, they will often ask about communication disorders. During Stage 1, intervention involves the confirmation that speech is now normal and the provision of information about the types of available supports, should the individual need and desire them.

Stage 2: Obvious Speech Disorder

Usually, the presenting symptom that signals the beginning of the second stage is a reduction in speech loudness (Logemann, Fisher, Boshes, & Blonsky, 1978). Speech intervention is recommended during this stage and usually follows the guidelines provided by Ramig, Pawlas, and Countryman (1995) that include intensive instruction and practice to speak with increased loudness, respiratory support, effort, and flexibility. It is beyond the scope of this book to discuss this intervention program. However, research strongly supports the implementation of such a speech intervention program early in the disease when speech symptoms begin to appear so that speech intelligibility disorders can be delayed or prevented (Ramig, Sapir, Countryman, et al., 2001; Ramig, Sapir, Fox, et al., 2001).

Because many people with PD speak with reduced voice loudness, portable speech amplification systems may improve communication interactions effectively during this stage (see the Barkley AAC Web site for links to voice amplification products). Small, portable voice amplifiers are most effective when speakers produce consistent phonation (i.e., voicing) during speech, although voice loudness may be severely reduced. In addition, many telephone adaptations are available to people with PD and other disorders who have difficulty using the telephone because of communication impairments (see Blackstone, 1991). If the individual whispers, however, amplification usually does not improve intelligibility.

Stage 3: Reduction in Speech Intelligibility

During the third stage, reduction in speech intelligibility becomes apparent due to imprecise consonant sound production, reduced speech loudness, and voice breathiness. For some speakers with PD, alterations in the speaking rate also occur; these may include rushes of excessively rapid speech, difficulty initiating speech, and excessive overall speaking rates. Intervention includes speaking rate control and/or voice amplification, depending on the speaker.

Individuals who speak too rapidly often benefit considerably from interventions designed to slow their speech rate. Several AAC techniques may help slow the speech rate, thereby often helping to increase speech intelligibility. Beukelman and Yorkston (1978) introduced alphabet board supplementation, which was among the first of such interventions documented in the literature. This procedure requires the speaker to point to the first letter of each word on an alphabet board or other type of AAC device as he or she utters the word. This not only forces speakers to slow their speaking rates but also provides their communication partners with extra information in the form of the first letters of words. For some speakers, the slowed speaking rate alone appears to be the major factor contributing to improved intelligibility. For others, the communication partner's knowledge of the first letter of the spoken word also contributes to more effective communication. In addition, when communication breakdowns do occur, speakers can use their alphabet boards to spell messages. For a more complete discussion of speech supplementation, readers are referred to Yorkston et al. (1999).

Mary's family complained that they were no longer able to understand her. She had difficulty initiating speech, as she seemed to freeze on the first word of some utterances. Once started, she spoke with bursts of excessive speech rates. Due to a lack of movement related to her PD, Mary showed no facial expression. Thus, during speech, her articulators barely moved. Mary learned to use a small alphabet board and pointed to the first letter of each word as she spoke. With this technique, she reduced her overall speaking rate to about 35–40 words per minute and eliminated the rushes of excessive speech rates. Her speech was quite understandable even when her listeners did not observe the communication board to determine the first letter of each word. When people had difficulties understanding her, she spelled her message with her board. Although Mary had success with this approach, she was reluctant to use it. She felt that it looked strange. It also required more effort than speaking her messages. However, with encouragement from her family, she used the alphabet supplementation approach for several years. Toward the end of Mary's life, her motor control deteriorated to the point at which she was unable to point efficiently. Her facilitators abandoned the alphabet board and helped her use a dependent scanning approach until her death.

The intelligibility of poorly articulated speech usually improves considerably when the communication partner is aware of the topic of conversation. Thus, people with PD may be encouraged to provide their listeners with the topic of a message or a conversation before beginning to speak. At times, the individual can communicate the topic successfully through natural speech, but he or she may also need to identify the topic using an AAC device such as a topic display. Topic displays often appear on the same communication boards used for alphabet supplementation of rate-reduced speech. Figure 15.3 illustrates this combination.

It is important that people with PD and their frequent communication partners act as informants and identify relevant topics to be included on the board. Some people with PD may also find it useful to employ a "remnant book," as described in Chapter 11. Individuals may use remnants such as theater tickets, napkins from restaurants, traffic tickets, bank statements, programs from plays, church bulletins, and racing forms to communicate topics as well as to clarify the details of an experience.

Small Talk	Sports	Shopping	Weather
Family	Food	Church	Computers
Personal Care	A B C D E F G H I J K L	Yes No	Please repeat each word I say, so I know you understand.
Transportation	M N O P Q R S T U V W X	Maybe I don't know.	You misunderstood! Start over.
Trips	Y Z	Forget it. I have something to say.	This is important! Wait a minute!
Appointments	I will spell the word. I will say the word.		

Figure 15.3.   Alphabet-topic board.

Stage 4: Natural Speech Supplemented with AAC

In the fourth stage of PD, the individual does not have functional natural speech. AAC interventions may include the use of pace-setting boards or alphabet supplementation to control speaking rate and increase the comprehensibility of residual natural speech. Some individuals prefer to use portable typing systems to prepare written messages because their handwriting is illegible.

Stage 5: Loss of Useful Speech

A very small percentage of people with PD lose all functional speech during the fifth stage of the disease. Clearly, when an individual has such a severe speech disorder, he or she requires AAC intervention. Given the overall motor control impairment and relatively frequent cognitive impairments late in the disease, AAC interventions are often difficult to institute and are very individualized.

BRAIN-STEM STROKE

Strokes (i.e., cerebrovascular accidents) that disrupt the circulation serving the lower brain stem often cause severe dysarthria or anarthria (i.e., an inability to produce speech). Because the brain stem contains the nuclei of all the cranial nerves that activate the muscles of the face, mouth, and larynx, damage to this area of the brain may result in an inability or a reduced ability to control these muscles voluntarily or reflexively. The nerve tracts that activate the trunk and limbs via the spinal nerves also pass through the brain stem. Therefore, severe damage to the brain stem may impair motor control of the limbs as well as motor control of the face and mouth.

Communication Symptoms

Communication symptoms associated with brain-stem stroke vary considerably with the level and extent of damage to the brain stem. Some people with dysarthria can communicate partial or complete messages through speech. These individuals usually experience dysarthria of the predominantly flaccid type due to damage to the nerve nuclei of the cranial nerves. Other individuals may display a marked spastic component in addition to flaccidity. Many people with brain-stem stroke are unable to speak because of the severity of their impairments.

Identify Participation Patterns and Communication Needs

Medical and lifestyle issues influence the communication needs of people who experience brain-stem stroke, as does the extent of their communication disorders. Following brain-stem stroke, an individual may require extensive personal and medical care, depending on the severity of the stroke and subsequent health conditions. People who survive a brain-stem stroke are usually unable to work. Some can be cared for at home, whereas others may live in settings that range from independent living to nursing care centers. Individuals who experience brain-stem strokes are usually aware of the world around them and are able to exchange information and achieve social closeness through their message formulations. Thus, they may have extensive communication needs.

Ruby was 44 years old when a severe brain-stem stroke left her unable to speak or swallow. When we first met her on the rehabilitation unit, she was able to communicate by answering yes/no questions and by using a dependent scanning approach. She communicated no by closing her eyes and yes by leaving them open and raising her eyebrows slightly. The dependent scanning approach included a small chalkboard with the letters of the alphabet positioned vertically on the left and right sides. To communicate a message, Ruby's communication partner pointed to each column of letters (A–L on the left side and M–Z on the right side). Ruby raised her eyebrows to signal the desired column of letters. Then her partner scanned down the column until Ruby signaled the preferred letter. In order to remember the letters that had already been chosen, the partner wrote each letter on the chalkboard. Ruby's partners were encouraged to guess the remainder of a word or message when enough of a message had been communicated. With proper positioning and head support, Ruby was able to move her head voluntarily to some degree, and she began to practice controlling a headlight pointer that was mounted on a headband and positioned over her right ear. In time, she was able to point to the letters on the chalkboard; with this technique, her communication rate was three times faster than with dependent scanning. Finally, Ruby learned to access an electronic AAC device using an optical head-pointing strategy. In time, the AAC device was mounted on her wheelchair and could also be transferred to her bed when needed. Ruby used this system for about 8 years (Beukelman, Yorkston, et al., 1985).

Assess Specific Capabilities

In this section, we describe the primary cognitive, language, sensory/perceptual, and motor capabilities that require assessment prior to AAC intervention.

Cognitive Skills

No accompanying cognitive limitations are expected if the stroke involves only the brain stem. If the stroke extends higher into the brain or is associated with a more extensive medical episode that interfered with the supply of oxygen to the brain, a wide variety of cognitive impairments may exist. These need to be assessed on an individual basis.

Language Skills

If brain-stem stroke does not affect the cortical or subcortical structures associated with language functioning, language skills should not be impaired. Thus, the skills of people with brain-stem stroke usually reflect their prestroke linguistic performances.

Sensory/Perceptual Skills

A high brain-stem stroke may affect the cranial nerve nuclei that control muscles for eye and eyelid movement, whereas a middle or low brain-stem stroke probably will not impair these muscles. Thus, visual functioning may or may not be impaired. In either case, brain-stem stroke generally leaves hearing unimpaired but often damages tactile and position senses.

Motor Skills

People with severe dysarthria or anarthria following a brain-stem stroke usually experience motor control problems of their limbs as well as control of their speech mechanisms. AAC specialists have reported interventions that employ eye or head pointing as the alternative access mode for these individuals who experience motor control problems. For example, Beukelman et al. (1985) reported case studies of two people with brain-stem strokes who successfully used electronic AAC systems via optical pointers mounted on their eyeglasses. Both individuals were required to spend much time in bed for medical reasons and learned to operate their AAC systems while in their wheelchairs and also while lying supine. AAC teams designed special mounting systems to support their devices in bed.

Intervention Stages

Throughout the years, a number of individuals with severe brain-stem strokes have received AAC services. The pattern of these interventions is quite similar and is outlined in the following sections.

Stage 1: No Useful Speech

The initial goal during Stage 1 is to provide an early communication system so that those people who are unable to speak due to brain-stem stroke can respond to yes/no questions. These individuals frequently report that they were well aware of their situation and were able to comprehend spoken information long before those around them realized it. Given the severe impairment of motor control that accompanies brain-stem stroke, yes/no responses usually involve slight head or eye movements. It is usually confusing if such an individual learns to signal "yes" but simply stares at the communication partner to signal "no." Early in recovery, it is usually easy for people with brain-stem stroke to signal "yes" by looking upward toward the ceiling and to signal "no" by looking downward toward the floor. Once an AAC team has identified a response mode for the individual, the team will often need to train communication partners to formulate communication interactions in a yes/no format.

According to his medical records, Merle sustained a thrombosis of the basilar artery that resulted in a severe brain-stem stroke. At the time of his admission to a rehabilitation center 1 month later, he was quadriplegic and ventilator dependent. Reports from his family indicated that an upward eye movement for "yes" and a downward eye movement for "no" had been his first and only volitional movements since the stroke. Merle demonstrated 100% accurate responses to concrete and biographical questions using this method. Eye-linking was introduced to Merle and his support team. A series of single-word, full-message, and alphabet boards were developed. Full word and message boards were used for messages that needed to be communicated quickly and easily regarding basic needs, as well as some messages that facilitated social closeness. Alphabet boards were used to spell out word-level responses initially. Two weeks after admission to the rehabilitation facility, Merle was spelling novel, one- to two-word messages using this process. Subsequent intervention efforts focused on the use of head movement to point to choices on communication boards. Utilizing the safe laser access system, a low-tech head-pointing system was implemented. The safe laser was mounted on the bow of Merle's glasses, and a 9 × 14-inch laser-sensing surface was positioned in front of him on an adjustable table. When it was not directed toward the laser-sensing surface, the laser operated at reduced output power, greatly improving eye safety for passers-by. However, when the laser was directed toward the laser-sensing surface, the laser output power increased to provide an easily visible, continuous beam. After 8 days of training, Merle began to demonstrate a limited amount of horizontal head rotation with the safe laser access system such that he could access an alphabet board requiring horizontal as well as lateral movements. During the following weeks, a variety of communication boards were developed with help from Merle's family and care staff, including a nursing page, family page, question page, visitor page, pain page, and emotion page. Merle indicated a strong preference for the alphabet page by choosing to use it during all communicative interactions. Thirty months after his stroke, Merle relies on the safe laser access system to communicate most of his messages. In the low-tech mode, he spells messages by directing the laser toward an alphabet board on the laser-sensing service. His communication partner composes messages based on the letters to which Merle points. In the high-tech mode, he composes messages using the safe laser on a laptop computer. These messages are spoken both word by word and sentence by sentence. Merle still does not speak.

For those individuals who stabilize at Stage 1 and never regain functional speech, AAC teams usually implement a three-phase intervention sequence.

Phase 1: Initial Choice Making   Those who are unable to recover natural speech after brain-stem stroke will need to develop progressively more complex AAC systems. In time, some of these individuals may be able to respond to visual and/or auditory dependent scanning techniques to support the formulation of messages. Once AAC teams have developed a yes/no response strategy, communication intervention usually focuses on choice-making responses signaled with the eyes. Teams use two strategies most often: eye pointing and eye linking. Eye pointing (see Chapter 4) involves teaching the individual to look directly at the item of choice. During eye linking, the choices are displayed on a transparent board; however, in this case, the augmented communicator is instructed to look at the item of choice while the partner looks at the user's eyes. The communication partner then moves the transparent board until their eyes "link" (i.e., meet) across the symbol of choice. This strategy is preferable when the eye gaze of the person using AAC is difficult to "read." When an individual's eye movements are limited to the vertical dimension, as is common in locked-in syndrome, eye-linking charts need to be organized vertically.

Phase 2: Pointing   In time, some individuals with brain-stem stroke are able to move their heads sufficiently to direct a light beam (e.g., a safe laser) at items of choice (e.g., letters, symbols). Depending on the recovery of motor control, some individuals may also be able to point to messages with their fingers or hands.

Phase 3: Use of a Multipurpose Electronic AAC Device   After progressing through Phases 1 and 2, some people with brain-stem stroke are able to learn to control a high-tech AAC device. Usually, the individual manages alternative access by head pointing (with either a light, laser, or sonar pointer); however, due to lack of motor control or to fatigue, some individuals require a scanning system all or some of the time (Culp & Ladtkow, 1992; Fager, Beukelman, & Jakobs, 2002; Soderholm, Meinander, & Alaranta, 2001).

Stage 2: Reestablish Subsystem Control for Speech

During this stage, people unable to speak because of brain-stem stroke work systematically to develop voluntary control of their respiratory, phonatory (vocal), velopharyngeal, and articulatory subsystems while they continue to use their AAC systems for communication interactions. Because weakness is such a predominant symptom of brain-stem stroke, intervention at this stage involves strengthening the muscles of the subsystem and coordinating actions of the subsystems during speech-like and speech behaviors. Early in this stage, the AAC system will support the majority of communication interactions; however, late in this stage individuals will convey an increasing percentage of messages through natural speech. (For a complete description of these intervention strategies, see Yorkston et al., 1999.)

Stage 3: Independent Use of Natural Speech

During this stage, speech intervention focuses on speech intelligibility, with the goal of meeting all communication needs through natural speech. We have worked with several speakers who used alphabet supplementation early in this stage. In time, they used AAC only to resolve communication breakdowns, and finally, AAC became unnecessary for communication interaction, although writing was still difficult or required the use of AAC.

Stage 4: Maximizing Speech Naturalness and Efficiency

By this stage, the person with brain-stem stroke will no longer need to use an AAC system. The goal is for the individual to speak as naturally as possible by learning to use appropriate breath groups and stress patterns.

Stage 5: No Detectable Speech Disorder

Few individuals who have sustained a brain-stem stroke achieve typical speech patterns.

Locked-in Syndrome

Closely related to brain-stem stroke is locked-in syndrome (LIS, also known as ventral pontine syndrome), which results in a conscious quadriplegic state that limits the individual's voluntary movement to vertical eye movements and perhaps eye blinks. The usual cause is a basilar artery stroke (occlusion or hemorrhage), a tumor, or trauma that results in damage to the upper pons or occasionally the midbrain. In a follow-up study of 29 people with LIS, Katz, Haig, Clark, and Dipaola (1992) reported an 85% survival rate for 5 years, with survival ranging from 2 to 18 years. None of these individuals regained the ability to speak in full sentences, although one was able to utter single words consistently and four could produce single words occasionally. Low- and high-tech AAC strategies were used.

In another follow-up study, Culp and Ladtkow (1992) followed 16 people with LIS for at least 1 year. Fifteen of these individuals experienced LIS following stroke, and one experienced LIS following a blow to the occipital region. All remained nonambulatory, and nearly half experienced sufficient visual difficulties to interfere with their AAC interventions. Eight eventually developed adequate vision and motor skills for direct selection AAC access, and nine relied on scanning access. Thirteen of the 16 individuals chose high-tech AAC systems.

Finally, Soderholm and colleagues (2001) followed the AAC use of 17 people with LIS. On average, these individuals were involved in rehabilitation for 3–4 months, during which they received computer-based AAC systems. Switch access sites included the head, mouth, fingers, and hands. AAC technology was used for communication, Internet access, email, writing, telephone, games, and vocational duties. Through the years, AAC intervention evolved as these individuals' capabilities, living situations, and personal roles changed. Eventually, 2 of the 17 individuals regained speech as their primary communication method.

In 1997, Jean-Dominique Bauby, a French man with LIS, completed a book entitled *Le Scaphandre et le Papillon [The Diving Bell and the Butterfly]*. After a stroke in 1995, Bauby required ventilator assistance to breathe and was fed via a gastric tube; he was unable to move, except for blinking his eyes. He wrote the book with the help of an assistant, who repeatedly recited the alphabet arranged according to the frequency of letter use in the French language. Bauby used eye blinks to indicate to his assistant which letters to use to spell out words. At the end of the book, Bauby asked, "Is there a key out in the cosmos that can unlock my bubble? A currency valuable enough to buy my freedom? I have to look elsewhere. I'm going there." Bauby died less than 72 hours later.

CONCLUSIONS

Numerous factors influence AAC interventions for people with severe communication disabilities due to acquired physical impairments. First, the diseases, conditions, and syndromes associated with the physical impairments usually require close medical monitoring. Therefore, frequent, detailed, and accurate communication with medical personnel is necessary.

Second, the medical and physical status of individuals with acquired physical impairments can affect their capability levels. Because fatigue is common for these individuals, interventionists should take care to provide them with AAC systems that they can control even when tired. In addition, these individuals' responses to medication can vary. For example, people with PD may experience a range of physical abilities, depending on their medication regimens. Those with physical impairments may be susceptible to health problems such as infections and respiratory disorders, both of which limit physical endurance.

Third, people with severe communication disabilities due to acquired physical impairments often experience additional disabilities in areas such as mobility, object manipulation, eating, and swallowing. Their communication needs are usually influenced by the nature and severity of these associated disabilities. In order to obtain appropriate services, they must request assistance, instruct caregivers and attendants, and interact with professional personnel regarding the range of their disabilities. Thus, AAC teams must plan their interventions to accommodate other assistive technologies, such as powered wheelchairs, electronically controlled beds, and respiratory support equipment.

Electronic communication options, such as email, Internet chat rooms, closed Listservs, and Web sites, provide people who use high-tech AAC systems important additional communication options. Several characteristics make these electronic communication options quite comfortable for people who communicate using AAC. For example, off-line preparation of messages allows people with slow message preparation rates to take as much time as they need during the process. Also, individuals can access electronic communication options according to their personal schedules.

CHAPTER 16

ADULTS WITH SEVERE APHASIA

Kathryn L. Garrett and Joanne P. Lasker

Aphasia is an impairment of the ability to interpret and formulate language that results from brain injury. In aphasia, the sequence of neurological steps required to communicate may be interrupted at any point—when comprehending what others say, creating ideas, retrieving words and sentence structures, or executing the motor movements to speak. Some people with aphasia may have a profound expressive and receptive communication impairment because of overwhelming breakdowns in this chain of events. Other individuals may communicate some information verbally but demonstrate intermittent difficulties with comprehension, language formulation, and/or speech production. Typically, people with aphasia have relatively preserved intellectual ability. However, there may be reductions in processing speed, attention, memory, or problem solving that cannot be completely explained by the loss of language (McNeil, 1983).

Most individuals acquire aphasia as a result of a cerebral vascular accident (CVA), commonly known as a stroke. Other etiologies for aphasia include brain injury related to accidents, tumors, or neurologic illnesses such as meningitis or epilepsy. In the large majority of individuals, the injury is in the left hemisphere of the brain. Most people acquire aphasia after the age of 60–70 years and a lifetime of communicating normally. However, a substantial number of children and younger adults can also develop aphasia while in the prime of their school-age or working years.

Each year, 400,000 individuals experience a stroke, and 80,000 of these cases result in aphasia. Approximately 1 million people, or 1 out of every 275 adults in the United States, have aphasia. The incidence of aphasia is equal for males and females; people of all races and educational and socioeconomic backgrounds experience aphasia. Despite speech-language therapy, 72% of all individuals with aphasia who responded to a 1988 National Aphasia Association survey could not return to work. Approximately 70% of those surveyed believed that people avoided contact with them because of difficulty with communication. (National Aphasia Association, 1988)

The experience of having aphasia differs for each individual, depending on the extent and location of the brain injury, the person's pre-morbid language and intellectual abilities, and the availability of therapeutic and social-emotional support. In the early stages of recovery, some individuals rapidly recover their speech and language capabilities. Most never communicate as efficiently or effectively as before their stroke or other injury. Up to 40% of people with aphasia have chronic, severe language impairments across modalities and are thus continuously challenged by their reduced ability to comprehend, speak, read, and write (Collins, 1986; Helm-Estabrooks, 1984).

Aphasia can have a profound impact on the lives of individuals with the disorder as well as their significant others and family members, who often share the burden of caregiving and communication for many years. One of the unique challenges of aphasia is that it is a less tangible impairment than some physical disabilities. Sometimes, family members, physicians, and health care providers assume that people with aphasia can understand everything but are unable to express themselves through speech. At other times, they may perceive the individual as having an intellectual impairment and, therefore, treat the individual as having less competence than is truly the case. In almost all scenarios, direct medical treatments are not effective at reducing the impairment because of the complexities of the neurolinguistic system. This can frustrate those affected by aphasia because progress seems slow and beyond the control of those participating in the rehabilitation process. Affected individuals must rely on external behavioral interventions to relearn language—language that once was swift, automatic, unconscious, and perfectly tuned to the dynamic challenges of communicating with others in a variety of situations.

Communication Disorders

In aphasia, individuals usually have reduced abilities in all language and communication modalities, including speaking, auditory comprehension, reading, writing, and gestural communication (Chapey & Hallowell, 2001). The degree of deficit in each modality is different across individuals, creating distinct patterns of impairment. People with injuries in the posterior region of the left hemisphere may experience an auditory comprehension deficit that is relatively severe when compared with their other language deficits. Often, these individuals also produce sentence-length utterances that are relatively unintelligible because of numerous sound substitutions, or jargon. This collection of symptoms is associated with an aphasia syndrome called *Wernicke's aphasia*. Individuals with damage to the frontal regions of the left hemisphere may have relatively good comprehension but poor expressive skills because of reduced sentence length, significant word retrieval difficulties, or reduced intelligibility as a result of groping or imprecise oral-motor movements (also known as apraxia of speech, or AOS). Many of these individuals also have limited or no use of their right arm, hand, and leg, a condition known as right hemiparesis. This aphasia syndrome is referred to as *Broca's aphasia*. Some people with *transcortical aphasia syndrome* have a relatively preserved ability to repeat what they hear. Although others may assume they are reasonably functional communicators, these individuals often have extreme difficulty generating their own utterances. People with *anomic aphasia* demonstrate mild or moderate language impairments that allow them to function quite well in familiar contexts but hinder their communication in unfamiliar contexts, particularly when they are naming or creating complex sentences. Finally, individuals with *global apha-*

sia have a profound communication impairment in all modalities. A detailed discussion of the various types of aphasia is beyond the scope of this text, and the reader is referred to Goodglass (1993) or Brookshire (2003) for more extensive descriptions of the classic aphasia taxonomy and neurologic aspects of the disorder.

AN ALTERNATE TREATMENT APPROACH

Traditional aphasia treatment focuses on improving the disability level of people with aphasia by, for example, assisting them to speak more effectively, comprehend more fully, or write with fewer errors. Many reports show that stimulation-type aphasia therapy works for many individuals—i.e., people with aphasia do indeed become better speakers or listeners as a result of such treatment (Holland, Fromm, DeRuyter, & Stein, 1996; Wertz et al., 1986). However, other reports suggest that some individuals with aphasia, in particular severe aphasia, never recover enough from their disabilities to become functional, competent communicators unless alternate intervention models are introduced (Fox & Fried-Oken, 1996; Holland, 1998; Lyon, 1992; Poeck, Huber, & Willmes, 1989).

The Participation Model (see Figure 6.1) may be a more effective framework for organizing interventions for people with severe aphasia than traditional therapy approaches. This model is based on the philosophy that interventions for individuals with communication disabilities should focus on enhancing their ability to participate actively in important life activities. In accordance with this approach, individuals with aphasia are encouraged to use both natural communication modalities, such as residual speech, gestures, and writing, and specific AAC techniques. Each of the components of the Participation Model will be incorporated into an assessment protocol for communicators with severe aphasia described later in this chapter.

Participation Patterns

People with aphasia live in a variety of different environments. Some continue to live in their own homes, either alone or with a spouse and possibly with children. They may have frequent opportunities to interact with neighbors, friends, and relatives. Other individuals are no longer able to live at home and may reside in retirement centers, assisted living facilities, nursing homes, or the homes of children or relatives. Many people with severe aphasia who were employed prior to their strokes have to retire because of residual impairments. Some individuals continue to participate quite actively in community activities, whereas others noticeably decrease the frequency of their contact with others. Thus, the participation patterns of individuals with aphasia are often quite different after a stroke than before. It is important to identify and customize AAC strategies to match post-stroke participation patterns, while simultaneously envisioning the activities that people with aphasia *could* participate in, if given access to AAC.

Functions of Communication

It is also important to analyze the purposes of communication prior to designing AAC interventions for people with aphasia. As mentioned in Chapter 1, Light (1988) suggested that communication interaction can be divided into four general functional categories:

expression of basic wants and needs, information transfer, social closeness, and social etiquette. With careful planning, these interaction functions can be incorporated into AAC strategies for adults with aphasia.

Wants and Needs

Before a severe stroke, many older people were able to care for their own wants and needs. They prepared their own food, managed their dressing and bathing, and transported themselves from place to place. They may have required occasional assistance with household chores and taking care of their property or finances, but, in general, they spent little of their energy on communicating wants and needs. Following a stroke, the proportion of time spent on communicating wants and needs may increase somewhat because these individuals must request items for comfort and environmental access more frequently from others. Communication of needs should be rapid and specific so communicators can get what they need in a timely manner. Therefore, communicators with aphasia must learn to referentially point, gesture, verbally produce key words, point to pre-stored messages on a communication board, or utilize speech-generating devices (SGDs) to request items that fulfill their wants and needs.

Social Closeness

Following a stroke or other injury, most people continue to strive for social closeness in their interactions. Before their strokes, they typically spent much time interacting with relatives, acquaintances, and friends, and, unless they are very elderly, they continue to expand this social network throughout their lives. Younger individuals with aphasia will want to maintain close connections to their school-age children or friends from work. Thus, for most people with aphasia, the ability to communicate for social closeness is a very important interaction function.

In contrast to the brief, precise communication needed for basic needs and wants, communication about social closeness can be lengthier and moderately specific but is generally less predictable. To illustrate, adults will predictably ask each other about the weather or inquire after others' family members, but the news that they share to maintain social connections will vary greatly depending on recent events (e.g., "Did you hear about Edith's surprise visitor yesterday?"). Many AAC strategies can provide a means for maintaining social closeness, both in the content of the messages as well as in the interactional structure of the strategy. For example, the written choice conversation strategy (see next section) automatically establishes social closeness because communication partners are continuously involved in the communication process. For independent communicators, social closeness messages must sometimes be purposefully included in the message set (e.g., "You look lovely today").

Information Transfer

The ability to share information remains important for people with aphasia in two primary ways. As participants in a consumer culture, they may need to provide *facts*—for example, they may need to answer questions about their disability, provide details about an item they want in a department store, or order food cooked to their specifications in a restaurant. In addition, as people enter their later decades of life, information transfer increasingly reflects their cultural roles as *storytellers*. In this role, they often reiterate the oral histories of their families, recount past events, and attempt to interpret present experiences in terms of past events (Fried-Oken, 1995; Stuart, Lasker, & Beukelman, 2000). Awareness of both of these information transfer issues is important in the design of AAC systems for communicators with aphasia. For example, AAC systems should facilitate retelling of rich narratives for individuals who enjoy this activity. AAC systems and message sets should also allow people to participate in favorite activities that require precise transmission of information, such as playing cards, teaching others about gardening with perennials, or conducting business at the bank.

Social Etiquette

Most individuals continue participating in the social etiquette routines of their cultures following a stroke or other injury. For example, they often appreciate being able to thank other individuals for assisting them. Fortunately, the awareness of what is proper and the ability to express "thank you" and "excuse me" through nonverbal modalities (e.g., gestures, intonation, facial expression) are usually retained in aphasia unless there is significant cognitive deterioration. Therefore, most AAC interventions for people with aphasia do not have to incorporate this vocabulary.

AAC INTERVENTIONS FOR APHASIA

People with aphasia may seem to be the most natural candidates for AAC systems. However, their history of competence as speakers and writers, the glaring gap between what they know and what they can say, and their clear desire to resume communication may tempt others to apply AAC strategies using a "more is better" motto. A classic scenario is a family member buying a new computer with the hope that it will automatically provide a means of communication for their nonspeaking family member with aphasia. Clinicians need a clear understanding of the competencies possessed by the communicator with aphasia and those required by specific AAC interventions, in order to achieve optimal improvement in communication.

Garrett and Beukelman (1992; Beukelman & Garrett, 1998) introduced a new classification system for severely aphasic individuals to aid in planning AAC interventions. We have revised the categories of this system to better assess differences in individuals' ability to communicate in *partner-supported* contexts versus *independently*. Within these two main groupings, the AAC classification varies depending on communicators' optimal participation levels, communication needs, or specific cognitive-linguistic competencies. Unlike in the other chapters in this book, we first describe various types of communicators with aphasia, along with appropriate interventions for each. We then follow this with a discussion of assessment strategies that can be used to determine an individual's AAC classification prior to initiating intervention.

Partner-Dependent Communicators

Some communicators with aphasia will always remain dependent on their conversational partners to manage informational demands and provide communication choices within highly familiar contexts (Kagan, 1998). These individuals can be termed "partner-dependent communicators." Three types of partner-dependent communicators are described in this section, in an ascending hierarchy of communicative competence, along with corresponding intervention goals and strategies.

Emerging Communicator

The emerging communicator (formerly called a basic choice communicator) has a profound cognitive-linguistic disorder across modalities as a result of extensive brain injury from one or more CVAs, trauma, or encephalopathy. Often, because of diminished arousal and comprehension skills, these individuals fail to respond appropriately to the physician's or speech-language pathologist's initial screening questions in an acute medical setting. Many of these individuals are subsequently discharged to long-term care facilities after minimal or no rehabilitation. Some of these individuals are capable of responding immediately if partners adopt slightly different ways of communicating and engaging their attention. Others may experience increased attentional capacities even months later, at which time additional therapy may be considered. A small proportion may eventually transition to more advanced levels of communication and develop some speech, functional gestures, or ability to use moderately complex AAC strategies.

Emerging communicators have extreme difficulties speaking, using symbols, and responding to conversational input. They seldom communicate purposefully; even fundamental nonverbal signals, such as pointing or nodding, are used infrequently. They are not readily able to associate photos or line drawings of common objects with their referents, which results in failure when clinicians provide picture symbol books to help them request wants and needs. They may not be able to participate in typical linguistic treatment programs used in aphasia rehabilitation; for example, when answering a series of unrelated "yes/no" questions in a stimulation-type therapy session, they may not respond or may answer with vague, imprecise head nods. Communicators who have such limited linguistic ability may initially benefit from contextual activities that elicit basic *referential* skills, such as pointing to request or looking in the direction of a mutually important item (e.g., out the window during a snowstorm), versus participating in highly linguistic question-and-answer tasks (Garrett, 2001).

Low-tech AAC strategies can be used to assist emerging communicators to both comprehend and control their personal environments by making basic choices, symbolized with real objects, within the context of familiar routines such as a morning dressing activity. For example, the therapist or caregiver can point to the calendar and discuss the season or weather, and then indicate several items of clothing. After ensuring that the emerging communicator has visually attended to the clothing items, the partner can then verbally present the choices at a slow pace, encouraging the individual to choose or show preference by nodding, vocalizing, reaching, or showing changes in facial expression.

To encourage participation in familiar social activities (such as selecting a gift for a family member), the therapist, caregiver, or family member can first show pictures of the individual for whom the gift is desired and can then discuss the occasion using props (e.g., for a birthday, present a calendar and birthday card). Then, prior to asking choice questions, the partner can encourage the person with severe aphasia to look at pictures of gift choices presented in a simplified catalog (i.e., pictures cut apart, pasted on blank paper and taped inside a real catalog) and to turn pages, if appropriate. After the person with aphasia chooses or shows preference for a gift, he or she can make other decisions regarding cost or color of the item, if appropriate. Emerging communicators should also be encouraged to "confirm" that a choice is desired as a preliminary step toward developing a linguistic response such as "yes" and "no."

Intervention Strategies   Treatment for the emerging communicator focuses on developing the following foundational communication skills: turn-taking, choice-making ability with tangible objects or photographs, referential skills, and clear signals for agreement and rejection (precursors to the linguistic "yes" and "no" signals). In addition, partners can benefit from instruction in how to provide choice-making opportunities throughout daily routines and reinforce the communicator's responses. Table 16.1 lists appropriate intervention goals and strategies for both emerging communicators and their communication partners.

Case Example and Therapy Outcomes

J.V., an individual with an aphasia quotient of 0.6 out of 100 on the Western Aphasia Battery (Kertesz, 1982), fit the profile of an emerging communicator. J.V. unexpectedly sustained a large hemorrhagic left CVA when he was 51 years of age (see Figure 16.1). He had experienced a lengthy hospitalization in an acute care facility, followed by several inpatient stays in rehabilitation facilities. Thanks to an attentive spouse and a generally sunny outlook on life, J.V. survived many bouts of pneumonia and other secondary ill-

Table 16.1.   Emerging communicator intervention goals and strategies

Communicator strategies	Partner strategies
Choose items to meet needs during daily routines by pointing or reaching.	Develop contextual routines, life activities, and opportunities in which the individual can utilize choice-making, turn-taking, referential, acceptance, and rejection skills (e.g., choosing nail polish to match outfit, selecting gifts for spouse from a catalog).
Reference familiar photographs in photo album by pointing OR demonstrating appropriate facial expression when participating in dyadic reminiscing activity	Create a simple scrapbook (1–2 pictures per page and key-word labels)
Choose pictured items in context of a functional activity (e.g., ordering garden seeds from a catalog)	Facilitate participation in simple, age-appropriate games (e.g., Tic-Tac-Toe, War)
Participate in turn-taking within context of familiar visual games (e.g., Tic-Tac-Toe, War)	Provide contingent feedback for communicator's referential, joint attention, affirmation, and rejection signals (e.g., "Oh, you're looking at the pink nail polish . . . so that's what you want!")
Consistently signal affirmation/agreement (head nod) during choice-making activities for preferred items	Utilize augmented input strategies: supplement person with aphasia's comprehension of auditory information by pointing to referents, gesturing, or drawing key conversational points.
Consistently signal rejection (pushing away, head shake) during choice-making activities for non-preferred items (e.g., dental floss, chewing tobacco)	
Demonstrate joint visual attention during interactions involving referential items (e.g., pictures, objects of interest)	

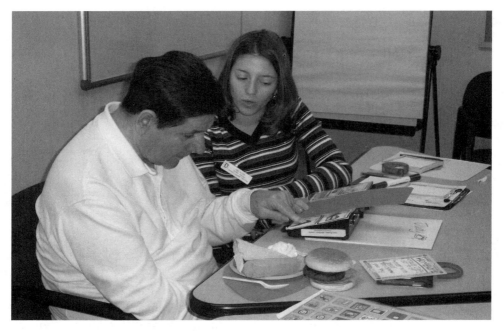

Figure 16.1. J.V., emerging communicator (left), learning to point to symbolized choices to choose favorite foods on a digitized VOCA. Copyright © 2004 K.L. Garrett and J.P. Lasker, with permission of J.V. and spouse, and student clinician.

nesses during the 10-year period prior to his evaluation at a university outpatient clinic. At that time, J.V.'s verbal expression consisted of a single stereotypy, "wah-wah-wah-wah," produced with a variety of intonation patterns and facial expressions. He did not typically point to items that he wanted. Profound limb apraxia interfered with any ability to produce symbolic gestures. J.V. had tremendous difficulty attending to communication partners, and he had no ability to recognize or use two-dimensional symbols as an alternate means of communication.

In the early phases of therapy, J.V. was encouraged to listen to the clinician, observe her gestural and referential communication, and inhibit his perseverative jargon. He also learned to visually attend to choices (initially objects, followed by photographs) that were presented within the context of a functional activity. Next, he was encouraged to select a choice by reaching or pointing to it during an interrupted routine. For example, when making coffee with J.V., the clinician completed one step of the activity (e.g., carrying the pot of coffee to the table), then stopped and offered J.V. a choice of a mug or a fork. When J.V. reached for an item, showed a preference for an item, or rejected an item, she provided contingent verbal feedback to increase his understanding that his communication effort conveyed meaning. J.V. eventually learned to choose his favorite activities (e.g., listening to Frank Sinatra music, playing cards or Bingo, and watching old movies) by pointing to photographs or line drawings, after which he participated in the actual activity for a few minutes. When symbols representing nonpreferred activities (e.g., flossing teeth, smoking) were added to the set of choices, J.V. quickly learned to scrutinize his choices before pointing. He then learned to shift his attention from objects and symbols to other communicators in group therapy and ask them a question by pointing to them.

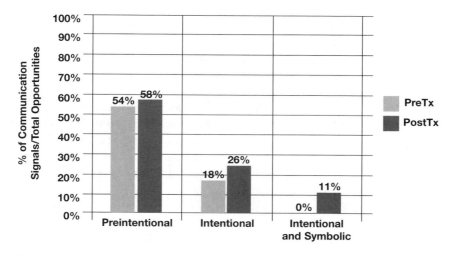

Figure 16.2. Pre- and post-therapy change in percentage of intentional communication behaviors based on a jury of five clinician ratings using the Communication Interview (modified from Schuler, Peck, Willard, & Theimer, 1989). This graph illustrates the change in percentage of preintentional, intentional, and intentional/symbolic communication behaviors from total rated behaviors (*n* = 14); total number of ratings = 159; 82% intrarater reliability. Copyright © 2004 K.L. Garrett and J.P. Lasker.

J.V. ultimately developed the consistent ability to demonstrate joint visual attention in individual and group activities, and to gain the attention of others and then point to props or drawings to indicate his focus of attention. He learned to purposefully inhibit his verbal jargon. He was approximately 80% accurate when making choices from a set of four items within a contextual activity, and even began to show his choices to other group members quite proudly. His wife was elated when J.V. took her by the arm one day, led her to the bathroom, and pointed to an overhead light bulb that needed to be replaced. Figure 16.2 represents J.V.'s gradual shift to more intentional and symbolic communication over a 1.5-year period during which emerging communicator strategies were implemented. J.V. eventually transitioned to the next category, contextual choice communicator, 10 years after the onset of aphasia.

Contextual Choice Communicator

Contextual choice communicators (formerly called controlled situation communicators) function more capably than emerging communicators. They can already indicate basic needs by spontaneously pointing to objects and items. They recognize visual symbols such as photographs, labels, written names, and signs. They are aware of daily routines and schedules. During conversations, they may demonstrate partial awareness of especially predictable topics, questions, and comments. However, contextual choice communicators do not have the linguistic ability to initiate or add to conversations on their own. Thus, these individuals may be quite isolated socially. With assistance, however, they can participate in topical conversations when communication partners provide written or pictorial choices on a turn-by-turn basis. Most of these individuals also benefit from augmented input techniques to supplement their comprehension of others' auditory messages. Many individuals with global, severe Broca's, transcortical motor, or severe Wernicke's aphasia may function as contextual choice communicators over either the short or long term.

Intervention Strategies   AAC interventions for contextual choice communicators are typically embedded within conversations about familiar topics. The primary expressive language goals involve teaching the communicator with aphasia to reference (i.e., point) to what he or she is talking about consistently, understand the meaning of graphic symbols, make choices to answer conversational questions, and begin to ask questions by pointing or using exaggerated intonation. Because these individuals participate more extensively in conversational exchanges than emerging communicators, partners can also help them to understand specific messages and ideas that are being presented by using "augmented input" techniques (Beukelman & Garrett, 1998; Wood, Lasker, Siegal-Causey, Beukelman, & Ball, 1998). Strategies to support both expression and comprehension are listed in Table 16.2.

Written Choice Conversation   A primary communication technique used with contextual choice communicators is *written choice conversation* (Garrett & Beukelman, 1992, 1995). This technique requires the facilitator to generate written key-word choices pertinent to a conversational topic (see Figure 16.3). The person with severe aphasia participates by pointing to the choices, thereby making his or her opinions and preferences known. Responses can be quite general, particularly when partners ask basic social questions (e.g., "Who visited this weekend?"). They also can be highly specific, particularly if the questions pertain to personal memories, beloved hobbies, or detailed knowledge associated with a past career. When facilitators present a sequence of related questions, interactions lengthen and communicators can discuss topics with relative depth.

Communicators with minimal reading ability on formal tests demonstrated more than 90% accuracy when responding to conversational questions by pointing to written choices, as long as the choices were presented within the context of a conversation and

Table 16.2.   Contextual choice communicator intervention goals and strategies

Communicator strategies	Partner strategies
Person with aphasia (PWA) will point to one of the following to answer conversational wh-questions: • Written word choices • Points on a scale • Locations on a map	Implement written choice conversation strategy: • Identify interesting conversational topics • Learn to generate consecutive, meaningful, conversational questions • Learn to generate potential/possible answers in the form of written word choices, scales, or locations on a map.
Answer partner's tagged "yes/no" questions with reliable gestures, head nods, or verbal responses.	Utilize "tagged" yes/no question format. Example: "Do you like Grace Kelly, the actress . . . yes (nod head up-and-down) or no (shake head side-to-side)?"
When cued, learn to ask questions by pointing, gesturing, and/or using rising intonation ("uh . . . [point]?")	Utilize "augmented comprehension" strategies when PWA does not appear to understand incoming auditory messages: • Write/draw key words, new topics, maps, family trees • Gesture (e.g., hand over back to indicate past) • Point to (e.g., reference) item being discussed
Visually attend to partner's presentation of augmented input; confirm whether message was understood via head nods, yes/no responses, or vocalizations.	Respond to all modes of communication and interpret PWA's communication attempts

Friend: Can you give me advice on what to make for the school bake sale tomorrow?

Person with aphasia (PWA):   [nods *yes*]

Friend: Should I take an angel food cake, brownies, or cookies? [writes choices vertically in notebook]
- ANGEL FOOD CAKE
- BROWNIES
- COOKIES

PWA: [points to brownies]

Friend: Yes, those always sell fast [circles BROWNIES]. Should I make them from scratch or get a box mix? [writes choices]
- SCRATCH
- BOX MIX

PWA: [laughs and points to BOX MIX]

Friend: [laughs and circles BOX MIX] Yeah, it's hard to make them as good as Betty Crocker!

Figure 16.3.   Sample written choice conversation. Copyright © 2004 K.L. Garrett and J.P. Lasker.

spoken aloud by the partner while he or she wrote them (Garrett, 1993). This implies that reading comprehension scores from formal tests may not be good predictors of success with this technique. Lasker, Hux, Garrett, Moncrief, and Eischeid (1997) also determined that some individuals can respond to written choices that are not supplemented with the partner's spoken output, whereas others can answer verbal choice questions without the accompanying written words. Thus, the presentation of a pool of choices seems to be the critical requirement for contextual choice communicators, but the optimal method of responding may be communicator specific.

Variants of the written choice conversation approach include presenting choices in the form of points on a rating scale or locations on a map. These graphic options are particularly useful when communicators want to answer opinion questions (e.g., "How do you think the election's going . . . good . . . so-so . . . or bad?"), quantitative questions (e.g., "How much should we spend on your birthday present . . . a lot . . . some . . . or a little?"), or questions about locations (e.g., "Where did your sister move . . . to New York . . . Texas . . . or Florida?") (see Figures 16.4 and 16.5).

The clinician's role is to introduce communicators to the written choice conversation strategy. Communicators can be encouraged to attend to the partner's questions, scan and

Friend: [Pause] what do you think about the kids' elementary school? Do you think they're getting a good education or a so-so one? [writes a rating scale on the page]

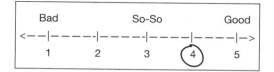

PWA: [hesitates, points to "4"]

Friend: [circles "4"] Yeah, we're pretty happy with the school district. Too bad the classes are so big, though!

PWA: [nods *yes*]

Figure 16.4.   Sample written choice conversation illustrating a person with aphasia's (PWA's) response on a rating scale. Copyright © 2004 K.L. Garrett and J.P. Lasker.

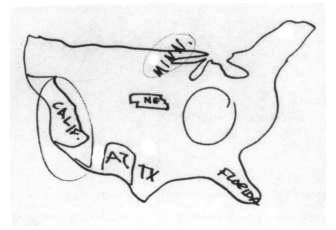

Figure 16.5. Map choices to answer question "Where do you go on vacation?" Copyright © 2004 K.L. Garrett and J.P. Lasker.

comprehend the choices, then respond thoughtfully by pointing. The clinician should also teach identified facilitators to use the strategy and then assist them to prepare simple notebooks to use in the supported interactions. An instruction card (see Figure 16.6) can be placed on the cover of the notebook to explain the procedure to unfamiliar communication partners.

Yes/No Responses to a Partner's Tagged Questions   Communicators with severe aphasia often have difficulty answering yes/no questions in a clear and unambiguous manner. Because of apraxia, they may have trouble coordinating their head movements to signify *yes* and *no*. Or, they may not know how to answer the question because the grammatical structure of questions does not explicitly tell them to answer with yes/no versus a more specific word or phrase. Other times, communicators simply do not understand the question. The simple strategy of "tagging" the question can bypass the first two problems. Partners add the phrase "yes . . . or . . . no?" to the ends of their yes/no questions. They simultaneously model the head movements. This effectively provides the communicator with a narrow pool of choices for how to respond within the context of a conversation. Figure 16.7 provides an example.

Asking Questions   Contextual choice communicators can become skilled conversational respondents when choices are pooled and presented in a contextual format. However, they may need additional intervention to initiate communication. One of the first strategies that can be implemented with contextual choice communicators is to encourage them to point or gesture toward conversational partners to ask questions. In treatment, individuals may initially benefit from hand-over-hand assistance to point; later, a model may suffice. To prompt generalized use of this gestural strategy in conversations, it may be beneficial to remind the communicator that a question would be appropriate ("So . . . don't you want to know about my weekend?"). Figure 16.8 provides an example.

Augmented Comprehension (Input) Techniques   Often, contextual choice communicators have accompanying auditory processing difficulties that interfere with their

I HAVE HAD A STROKE. I WOULD LIKE TO TALK TO YOU, BUT I CANNOT SPEAK.

WE *CAN* CONVERSE IF YOU ASK ME A QUESTION AND OFFER ME WRITTEN CHOICES TO POINT TO. HERE'S HOW:

1. THINK OF A QUESTION YOU WOULD HAVE ASKED ME BEFORE MY STROKE. TRY TO FIND OUT MY OPINION, GET MY ADVICE, OR FIND OUT MY PREFERENCE.

    Example:

    "What crops have you gotten out of your garden so far?"
    "Who's going to win the football game Saturday?"
    "What do you think of the new tax law?"

2. ONCE YOU'VE ASKED THE QUESTION, THINK OF POSSIBLE ANSWERS OR CHOICES. WRITE THEM IN THIS NOTEBOOK. USE A DARK PEN OR MARKER. USE LARGE CAPITAL LETTERS. PUT A DOT IN FRONT OF EACH CHOICE. USE A SCALE FOR "HOW MUCH" QUESTIONS.

    Example:

    *   (TOMATOES)
    *   CUCUMBERS
    *   BEANS

    _____

    *   NEBRASKA
    *   (PENN STATE)

    _____

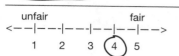

       unfair   fair
    <— —|— —-|— —-|— —|— —|— —>
        1   2   3 (4) 5

3. ENCOURAGE ME TO POINT. CIRCLE MY ANSWER. ASK PLENTY OF FOLLOW-UP QUESTIONS—I ENJOY CONVERSING!

Figure 16.6. Written choice communication notebook cover card. Copyright © 2004 K.L. Garrett and J.P. Lasker.

ability to understand language, especially language that is complex or that shifts the conversational topic. These individuals will nod their heads to indicate that they understand, but in fact may be "holding their place" in the conversation instead of signaling true comprehension. Thus, they often experience significant confusion and communication breakdowns as a conversation progresses. At other times, these people withdraw completely from complex discussions.

To avoid communication breakdowns, communication partners can supplement their spoken language by gesturing, writing key words, or drawing. This set of strategies, called *augmented input* or *augmented comprehension* strategies (Beukelman & Garrett, 1998; Garrett & Beukelman, 1992; Sevcik, Romski, & Wilkinson, 1991; Wood et al., 1998), can be implemented whenever the communicator with aphasia is having difficulty comprehending conversational questions, comments, or instructions. To provide augmented input, the communication partner first identifies that the communicator has misunderstood or is confused, after carefully observing the person's blank facial expression, ambiguous head nods, or incorrect responses. The partner then reiterates the message, while simultaneously

Partner: Richard, do you like omelettes . . . yes . . . or no? (nods head up-and-down while saying *yes* and shakes head side-to-side while saying *no*)

R.C.:   (tries to gesture thumbs up, then points down, then nods head *yes* after pausing to work out the movement sequence)

Partner: Yes?

R.C.:   Confirms *yes* by nodding his head up-and-down

Figure 16.7. Sample interaction with tagged yes/no question strategy. Copyright © 2004 K.L. Garrett and J.P. Lasker.

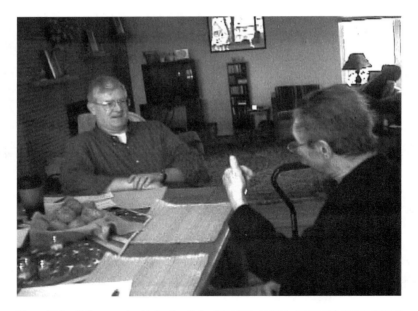

Figure 16.8.   R.C. answering his brother-in-law's tagged yes/no question with a "thumbs up" signal. Copyright © 2004 K.L. Garrett and J.P. Lasker.

pointing to the item being discussed; gesturing symbolically (e.g., throwing a hand over the shoulder to indicate past tense); pantomiming an event; showing photographs, drawings, or other diagrams; or writing key words and topics. Individuals with receptive aphasia can then use these visual representations to help them understand the conversational information. Individuals with aphasia can also point to these same visual representations to identify aspects of the interaction that they have not understood or about which they want additional information.

Augmented comprehension strategies are often used in conjunction with the written choice conversation technique described earlier. The technique of augmented input is similar in that it is completely partner dependent, which means that communication partners must learn to resolve communication breakdowns by initiating its use. The clinician can assist with this process by demonstrating the technique, providing a notebook with instructions on the cover to partners (see Figure 16.9), and teaching the person with aphasia to signal he or she is experiencing comprehension difficulties. Although a variety of individuals with severe aphasia may benefit from augmented comprehension tech-

Partner:	And so we went to the arboretum to see which trees grow best around here, and then we went to the nursery to pick out some varieties. . . .
Charles:	[raises hand to stop interaction, shakes head *no*]
Partner:	Oh, I'm sorry—I was going too fast again. Here [writes *arboretum,* draws a picture of a tree]. We went to the arboretum [points to word and pauses to check for comprehension]. . .then we went to the nursery to get some plants [writes *nursery* and draws arrow from previous message] and then we took them home to plant them [sketches house with plants by sidewalk]. Did I make sense?
Charles:	[nods *yes*]

Figure 16.9.   Example of conversation in which augmented input strategies are used. Copyright © 2004 K.L. Garrett and J.P. Lasker, with permission of R.C., spouse, and T.R.

niques at some point in their recovery, people with Wernicke's aphasia often require permanently augmented input. Other individuals with aphasia who demonstrate intermittent auditory processing problems may also benefit from this technique.

Case Example and Therapy Outcomes

R.C. was a 61-year-old, college-educated logistics engineer who sustained a sudden-onset, thrombolytic left CVA in the region of the middle cerebral artery shortly after retiring. He participated in 1 month of inpatient rehabilitation, after which he returned home with his wife. He also attended five outpatient therapy sessions 2 months after onset. At that time, he was not stimulable for speech because of profound AOS. An electronic AAC system was introduced, but R.C. was unable to use it. Eight months after his stroke, he was reevaluated at a university outpatient clinic. He achieved an aphasia quotient of 9.2 out of a 100, which corresponded with an impairment profile of global aphasia. However, his awareness of routines and his response to the clinician's humorous comments indicated hidden communication competencies. Within two treatment sessions, he learned to point to written choices to answer conversational questions about his teapot collection, political preferences, children's travel adventures, and attempts to learn to play the bass guitar. He also gradually learned to answer conversational yes/no questions by nodding his head or using a "thumbs up/down" signal. He was much more accurate when his partner used the tagged yes/no question format; because of apraxia, however, he also required tactile cues and a model for approximately 2 months until responses stabilized. Because of intermittent auditory comprehension breakdowns, R.C.'s clinician frequently supplemented her spoken questions by writing or drawing key concepts. R.C. then began participating in group therapy in addition to individual treatment sessions. Although he required initial hand-over-hand assistance to look at other participants and point at them to ask questions, he ultimately learned to initiate this simple request with only occasional cues. Interestingly, he also began to show other people his written choice responses in lieu of being able to announce them aloud, and he used this strategy frequently to participate in group interactions.

R.C.'s wife confirmed that his written choices and yes/no responses were accurate approximately 90% of the time after 1 month of biweekly therapy sessions. During the next year, R.C. became more attentive, initiated more requests by gesturing symbolically and pointing, and learned to tease others. His reading comprehension also increased, and he began to participate in traditional stimulation and motor speech therapy, through which he developed an imitative spoken repertoire of more than 200 words. However, he was not yet able to use speech in a communicative manner. Therefore, his sons and wife were trained in partner-supported strategies, including written choice conversation, tagged yes/no question presentation, and augmented input. In future treatment, clinical emphasis shifted to teaching R.C. to access stored message communication systems as well as to produce a limited repertoire of spoken language in response to partner questions.

Supported Conversation for Adults with Aphasia (SCA) is an approach developed at the Aphasia Institute in Toronto, Canada. SCA incorporates many of the techniques described for contextual choice communicators in this chapter, including using gestures, writing key words, drawing, and using pictures to ensure that people with aphasia understand what is being communicated and have opportunities to express themselves in conversations with others. The results of a recent randomized control study indicated that communication between facilitators and their partners with aphasia improved significantly after the facilitators were trained in SCA (Kagan, Black, Duchan, Simmons-Mackie, & Square, 2001). Training and support materials related to SCA are available through the Aphasia Institute.

Transitional Communicators

Transitional communicators are beginning to fully appreciate that external symbols and strategies can help them communicate. They increase their efforts to search for ways to convey their messages when unable to speak. They gesture or speak to start an interaction with a communication partner, and they may begin to search through their notebooks for written choices from prior conversations to find something relevant for the present discussion. They increasingly know the answers to questions before their partners even present written choices. Communicators may, by this time, have communication notebooks or SGDs containing message sets for common situations, such as telling about themselves or requesting snacks in the cafeteria. Some individuals will even spell in combination with locating stored messages. In therapy, they may locate these messages easily and use them communicatively in structured interactions. However, the hallmark of this category of communicators is that they cannot think of *how* to communicate the answer in spontaneous communication contexts *without cues*. Therefore, this category represents a transitional step between those communicators who need partner support to compose messages (i.e., emerging and contextual choice communicators) and those who locate or generate messages on their own in everyday contexts (i.e., stored message and generative communicators).

Intervention Strategies   Intervention goals focus on teaching transitional communicators to initiate conversations with as little cueing as possible (see Table 16.3). Strategies provide the communicator with a means of conveying significant content without taxing cognitive skills. For example, transitional communicators can learn to introduce themselves using a prepared card or message on an SGD (e.g., "I have aphasia following a stroke. Therefore I have difficulty thinking of words and saying them. I communicate by . . . . "). They may learn to initiate conversations by presenting remnants (i.e., tangible representations) of events they consider to be noteworthy (e.g., movie ticket stubs or newspaper headlines; Garrett & Huth, 2002; Ho, Weiss, Garrett, & Lloyd, in press). If clinicians have not yet assembled messages related to familiar topics (e.g., autobiographical information), it is appropriate to begin embedding these pages into notebooks or SGDs for these individuals' levels (see Figure 16.10).

Storytelling is another content-rich communication activity that matches the cognitive abilities of the transitional communicator. When consecutive segments of a story are pre-stored in a communication book or SGD (typically, in a left-to-right sequence if English is the primary language), the communicator simply has to point to the message square in the correct sequence to tell the story (see Figure 16.11). Visual scene display technology allows "hot spots" or key visual elements within a digitally stored picture to be programmed with appropriate messages on an SGD. Pilot work is underway to deter-

Table 16.3.   Transitional communicator intervention goals and strategies

Communicator strategies	Partner strategies
Call for assistance/signal a communication partner that he or she wishes to converse	Provide suggestions, hints, or direct instructions to encourage PWA to use strategies in appropriate contextual situations
Introduce self with low- or high-tech AAC strategy (card, wallet, SGD)	Pause and expect communication
Search for previous written choice responses to answer similar conversational questions	Provide opportunities for communication of specific information within contextual, familiar conversations and routines. Example: "Tell me about your vacation."
Search for biographical info in a simple reminiscing book/scrapbook to answer similar conversational questions	Assist PWA to develop a scrapbook or communication wallet
Answer predictable questions (e.g., autobiographical, topical) by searching for, selecting, and pointing to pre-stored messages on a simple SGD	Assist PWA to store autobiographical or topical messages on an SGD prior to conversing
Hand a potential communication partner a tangible topic setter or remnant to initiate a conversation	Assist PWA to identify, collect, and present tangible topic setters or remnants (e.g., travel brochures) to potential communication partners
Tell simple stories on an SGD by activating sequential messages	Assist PWA to identify favorite stories, then select and program the messages on an SGD

mine whether adult communicators can utilize this new means of representation to augment their storytelling or conversational skills (Beukelman et al., 2003). Regardless of storage method, clinical experience suggests that some transitional communicators learn to use AAC systems primarily because they are motivated to tell amusing or sentimental anecdotes.

Because of their history of relying on instructions and cues, transitional communicators often benefit from practicing their strategies in structured role plays (e.g., introduc-

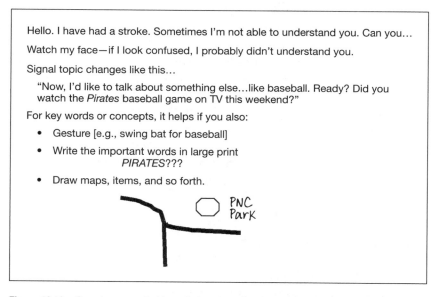

Figure 16.10.   Sample augmented input instruction card. Copyright © 2004 K.L. Garrett and J.P. Lasker.

Guess what! We went gambling and I won $500! $$$	It's spent already— on a necklace for my wife and a lobster dinner for me.	I'm such a great guy! #1

Figure 16.11. Sample storytelling page for a digitized VOCA. Copyright © 2004 K.L. Garrett and J.P. Lasker.

ing themselves to a bank teller, telling their life stories to a student clinician). Clinicians can set up an expectancy for communication by repeating the role play and then pausing for the communicator to introduce him- or herself or answer the question using the target AAC strategies. Sometimes, it is helpful to embed the target strategies into a written script that the communicator can refer to during the role play. For transitional communicators, therapists and conversational partners must learn to wait to cue the individual until it is clear they cannot think how to communicate without further instruction.

Independent Communicators

The individuals described in the preceding section require the assistance of a communication partner to maximally participate in conversations and important life activities. In contrast, a number of people with severe aphasia have enough cognitive and linguistic competence to converse independently. These individuals comprehend most of what is said to them even when little contextual support is available. They can intentionally share their own ideas using a variety of strategies and modalities that they select themselves. These people can be termed *independent communicators*.

It is important to note that, without focused clinical intervention and implementation of AAC strategies, independent communicators may experience frequent communication breakdowns. The connecting threads of conversation can easily dissolve when they try to communicate specific words (nouns, verbs, and/or functor words) in order to clarify locations, details, names, cause–effect relationships, or event chronologies. Fortunately, independent communicators can learn to utilize both natural communication strategies (e.g., speech, residual writing or drawing) and augmented strategies (e.g., pointing to elements of a picture to elaborate on a topic, finding messages stored in a multilevel SGD, spelling, drawing) to communicate effectively in multiple environments with a variety of communication partners. Many of these individuals have aphasia patterns that correspond most closely with the traditional syndromes of anomic, moderate Broca's, conduction, or transcortical motor aphasia.

Stored Message Communicators

Stored message communicators can independently locate messages that have been stored in advance in their AAC systems. For example, they may spontaneously activate an SGD to offer a toast at a celebration or to order their favorite kind of milkshake at an ice cream store. Or, they may utilize an SGD with messages programmed on multiple levels to alternate between greeting, exchanging small talk, and making predictions about the coming football season. In short, they are initiators who think to use their AAC systems to supplement or substitute for speech without prompting within familiar situations. With practice, they also may consciously intersperse some natural communication strategies (e.g., partially intelligible speech, symbolic gestures). However, they seldom can generate enough novel information to participate in a discussion about an unusual topic because their spelling, speech, and AAC skills are too limited to participate independently in free-form conversations.

Intervention Strategies   Stored message communicators should work with therapists and family members to create an inventory of messages and topics that they will need in specific situations where they must communicate specifically and efficiently. They can assist in storing these messages in their low-tech communication notebooks or wallets (see Figure 16.12), or they can help select locations and symbols for programming the messages into a multilevel SGD. Potential strategies for this group of communicators are listed in Table 16.4.

Clinicians may wish to conduct some intervention sessions with these individuals outside of the therapy room. For example, if an individual targets the post office as an en-

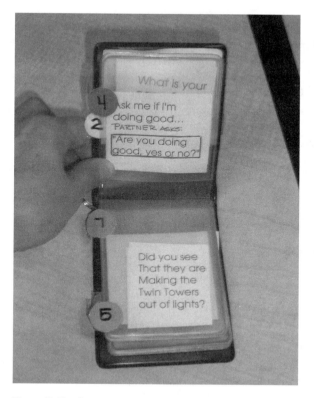

Figure 16.12.   Sequentially organized communication wallet with introductions, topic setters, and questions for conversational partners. Copyright © 2004 K.L. Garrett and J.P. Lasker.

Table 16.4.   Stored message communicator intervention goals and strategies

Communicator strategies
• Participate in identification of specific situations, stories, or communication routines (e.g., restaurant, vacation, family stories, bank, returning an item to a store, asking spouse out on a date)
• Participate in selection and storage of specific vocabulary for each situation
• Practice accessing vocabulary during structured, scripted role playing situations (in therapy)
• Practice communicating in real-life situations and evaluating:
• *Effectiveness*—did I get my message across?
• *Efficiency*—was the partner fidgeting or uncomfortable? How many communication breakdowns did I have?
• *Changes needed*—was there anything I could have done to make this interaction go better?
• Evaluate pros and cons of SGDs versus low-tech communication options, make an informed decision, and develop the final system with the clinician
• Gradually use the system in more demanding situations, such as returning an item to a store serviced by a clerk with no knowledge of aphasia

vironment for better communication, initial sessions might consist of identifying messages, storing them, and then practicing how to use both natural and AAC messages with a script (see Figure 16.13). Later sessions might take place with a novel communication partner, such as another clinician or secretary, in a simulated post office scenario. If it is possible to conduct community outings within one's facility, it would be beneficial to go to the actual environment and observe the communicator utilizing the strategies. Finally, the clinician and communicator should evaluate the effectiveness of the interaction and make changes in message content, sequence of delivery, or use of natural communication strategies if needed.

Case Example and Therapy Outcomes

The case of M.R., a 44-year-old man with moderate–severe receptive and expressive aphasia and AOS (Lasker & Bedrosian, 2001), is summarized to illustrate the category of stored message communicator. M.R. acquired aphasia as a result of a left CVA sustained 8 months before his evaluation. Prior to his stroke, he was employed as a mechanical press operator and was active in the community softball league and in a local church. He had

Clerk: Who's next?

PWA: (points to self)

Clerk: What do you need, sir?

PWA: (I WANT TO PICK UP MY PACKAGE.—VOCA)

Clerk: What is that thing?

PWA: (Goes to main level of VOCA—I HAD A STROKE. IT IS HARD FOR ME TO SPEAK. I USE THIS MACHINE TO COMMUNICATE.)

Clerk: OK, now what was that?

PWA: Patuj (returns to Post Office level on VOCA; reactivates I WANT TO PICK UP MY PACKAGE.)

Clerk: Your name?

PWA: Chim...no...no... (returns to Level 1 on VOCA—MY NAME IS JAMES GREEN)

Clerk: Jim Green...OK sir, I'll check. Just a minute.

Figure 16.13.   Sample script for post office scenario. Copyright © 2004 K.L. Garrett and J.P. Lasker.

completed 2 years of college and earned an associate degree. After his stroke, M.R. was unable to work due to his residual physical disabilities and communication limitations. He lived at home with his wife, teenage son, and 3-year-old granddaughter. However, he continued to drive and conduct errands in the community. He also had some parenting responsibilities at home while his wife was at work.

M.R.'s motor speech and language problems interfered with his ability to participate in daily communication activities. His verbal output was limited to "yes," "no," and automatic speech sequences, although he often attempted to repeat verbal models. After 7 months of traditional speech therapy with little improvement in speech production, M.R. acquired a dynamic display SGD through a combination of funds from vocational rehabilitation and private insurance. He was unable to formulate novel messages using words or letters; however, he used the device extensively as a model for speech practice. In collaboration with M.R. and his family, messages for various communication contexts were collected and stored on several levels of his electronic device. However, despite this individualized programming, M.R. was unwilling to utilize his SGD in public. He communicated that the device was "for the clinic" and "for practicing speech" but was not for "talking with friends . . . [or] strangers." When probed, M.R. admitted that he was ashamed of using the machine in public and was afraid that people in the community would think he wasn't "normal."

To address the issue of AAC system acceptance, M.R.'s subsequent intervention program focused on selecting or spelling appropriate messages, practicing with written scripts, rehearsing via role plays with the clinician, and finally utilizing the system in community locations. Luckily, when M.R. used his device for the first time in the post office, he received a favorable and interested response from the clerk. After his second experience communicating in public, M.R. offered suggestions for his next community communication experience and also assisted in developing the practice script. In addition, he requested that the clinician maintain greater physical distance from him during his interaction with the clerk so that he could "do it himself." During his staged intervention program, M.R. learned to access his stored message system in a variety of locations. His ability to participate independently in public encounters increased with each experience, and he ultimately demonstrated acceptance of his system.

Generative Message Communicators

Generative message communicators (formerly called comprehensive communicators) are speakers or writers with aphasia who can produce some novel information. Typically, they have maintained independent lifestyles and may wish to participate in various types of conversational exchanges that occur in many environments. In addition to limited speech, the comprehensive communicator's preserved skills may include drawing, gestures, pantomiming, first-letter-of-word spelling, word writing, and pointing to words or symbols. Because many of these modalities allow them to create unique messages, they do not have to rely solely on stored vocabulary or choices presented by partners. However, their generative communication skills are often too fragmented or inconsistent for effective communication to occur without some degree of conversational or AAC intervention. Breakdowns may occur in spoken communication and/or when writing. One individual we know with conduction aphasia and limited semantic specificity was an outstanding generative communicator. She was able to manage the social aspects of communication quite well using verbal communication, but she required extensive support when asked to communicate specific information to her friends, her lawyer, her doctor, and the bus driver. Another man with moderate anomic aphasia became a published writer with the assistance of augmentative writing software (King & Hux, 1995). General intervention strategies for generative speakers and writers are listed in Table 16.5.

Intervention Strategies   AAC interventions for generative communicators can be quite complex. In addition to identifying anticipated participation patterns, clarifying

Table 16.5.   Generative communicator intervention goals and strategies

Communicator strategies for generative speakers

- Initiate introduction of self and communication strategies
- Communicate specific semantic info about a variety of topics via AAC strategies and natural communication modalities (e.g., presidential elections, stories from childhood, events from past weekend, hobbies)
- Establish topics prior to communicating complex conversational information using tangible topic setters, topic cards (e.g., "I want to talk about . . . sports . . . family, etc."), and verbal skills
- Communicate in a variety of situations with familiar and unfamiliar communication partners (e.g., with family members and public places such as stores, banks, government offices, bars and social clubs, lectures).
- Locate stored messages relevant to the topic on "hidden" pages in a communication book or "hidden" electronic levels in an SGD
- Shift between accessing stored messages and creating novel messages to convey a complete idea
- Increase complexity of discourse by communicating relational semantic information via gestures, timelines, and some speech. Examples:
  - *Temporal:* past and present (motion backward for "ago")
  - *Spatial/locational:* point to map to indicate "down the road"
  - *Preferential:* saying "the best" while gesturing "thumbs up"
  - *Additive:* finding a message about baseball, saying "and," then finding a message about enjoying "Steelers – football"
  - *Actions:* Pantomiming doing the laundry, then saying "dryer"
- Combine symbols to convey novel meanings. Examples:
  - *Speech:* "Big one . . . " and "Washington" to mean "the President of the USA"
  - *AAC messages:* access [Pittsburgh] on SGD, then find "baseball" on hobbies page to communicate "Pirates baseball team"
  - *Combine writing and speech:* Write "2" then say "boys" to indicate size of family
- Ask questions of others by combining key words, enhanced intonation, and gesturing (e.g., "Vacation . . . you?" [point]). Point to symbolized question forms in communication notebook or SGD
- Utilize specific, metacommunicative communication strategies to resolve communication breakdowns in conversation. Examples:
  - Determine rule for number of times it is acceptable to repeat message (e.g., no more than twice—then you have to try something else)
  - Provide additional information/shift to new strategy during communication breakdowns
  - Signal partner that he or she has understood/not understood
  - Manage conversational dynamics and make decisions about whether to continue/quit
- Work with clinician to assemble components of multimodal system and learn the operational requirements of SGD.

Communication strategies for generative writers

- Spell/write partial or complete words/phrases to generate novel messages using a low-tech system (e.g., pocket-sized notepad).
- Learn to use word prediction or abbreviation/expansion computer-based to supplement spelling.
- Learn to use organizational templates (low-tech or computer-based) to generate written products such as letters, journal entries, summaries, and so forth.

communication needs, and identifying topics of interest, the AAC specialist must also teach the individual to manage a variety of AAC techniques. For example, Beukelman, Yorkston, and Dowden (1985) described a man with Broca's aphasia who used a series of AAC approaches as he progressed through various phases of recovery. Initially, he communicated with a simple communication book that contained photographs of familiar people, places, and activities; his family provided additional picture albums identifying family members, interests, and experiences. This man later learned to expand his conversations by showing portfolios of his work as an interior designer. The portfolio helped him to establish a topic and provided pictorial support for specific words and ideas. Eventually, a multimodal AAC system was developed for him that included an SGD, limited natural speech, gestures, a communication book, portfolios, books and blueprints on the walls of the design studio in his home, and a design assistant who also served as a facilitator.

An often overlooked but critical aspect of AAC interventions with generative message communicators is their need for substantial instruction and guided practice to teach them *when* to use the various AAC techniques provided. Garrett, Beukelman, and Low-Morrow (1989) described this process with M.J., whose low-tech AAC system contained many different components, including stored messages for specific environments, lists of family names and sports teams, a written autobiography, maps, rating scales, a pocket for remnants, and blank paper for writing and drawing. In addition, M.J. produced some partially intelligible key words and automatic phrases using speech, and gestured symbolically part of the time to convey specific ideas.

Three to four months were required to teach this man how to decide on a specific AAC technique and then implement it in conversations. His clinician then developed the instructional sequence summarized in Figure 16.14, which M.J. referred to when learning to choose the most effective communication strategy during intervention sessions. For example, M.J. would first attempt to say a message using his natural speech. If he experienced a communication breakdown, he would then attempt to gesture, write, or repeat the spo-

STEP 1

| GESTURE | WRITE | REPEAT |

STEP 2

| WORD NOTEBOOK | ALPHABET CARD (will work better for names) |

STEP 3

CLUES	DIRECTIONS
• Size	• Wait—don't guess.
• It looks like...	• You almost got it.
• Function	• Let's quit.

Figure 16.14. Modality instruction card for a generative communicator. Copyright © 2004 K.L. Garrett and J.P. Lasker.

ken message. If he was still unsuccessful, he would use the word notebook, alphabet card, or select a remnant to increase context for the communication partner. Finally, he would direct his listener to the clues or control phrases to manage the conversation from a metacognitive perspective if his initial communication attempts had failed. Following training, M.J. greatly reduced the amount of effort he spent on resolving communication breakdowns because he became a conscious and strategic multimodal communicator.

Unfortunately, the training phase that is so essential for generative message communicators may not receive enough attention in a multimodal intervention. Additional reasons that comprehensive communicators fail to use their AAC systems effectively include: 1) the vocabulary and content of the AAC materials provided are inappropriate, 2) important communication partners are not willing or are not encouraged to accept augmented modes of communication, and 3) teaching and training in naturalistic situations does not occur.

The role of technology with this group of communicators is still evolving (Koul & Harding, 1998). Many electronic AAC systems that have been developed for individuals with primarily physical impairments are simply not appropriate for communicators with aphasia. Their need for adapted access is often minimal, and some of the most common methods used to access messages (e.g., abbreviation expansion, iconic encoding, complex level changes) are too difficult for most people with aphasia to use functionally. However, a variety of emerging technologies show promise for selected generative message communicators who have the skills and the desire to use AAC. For example, some experimental software allows communicators to engage in small talk by accessing a category of communication messages stored by pragmatic function, such as "greetings" or "continuers" (Todman & Alm, 1997). Many dynamic screen SGDs can be programmed with messages that represent the continuum of speech acts needed to communicate in a given situation (i.e., from greetings to questions to responses). New methods of representing concepts visually using, for example, photos of significant events, nodes on a flowchart (e.g., a family tree), locations in a schematic layout, or points on a timeline are increasingly possible with off-the-shelf technology. However, the present challenge for many individuals, even those who fit the description of generative message communicators, continues to be remembering to use these messages, particularly when they are not immediately visible (Garrett & Kimelman, 2000; Kraat, 1990). Research is underway to develop a "smart access" electronic communication system, in which the communicator can locate words or phrases by beginning with and entering any association that comes to mind, such as the first letter, category, or situation related to a word or concept (Beukelman et al., 2003). Technologies that compensate for cognitive and linguistic limitations represent some of the potential future communication options for people with aphasia (Waller, Dennis, Brodie, & Cairns, 1998).

Case Example and Therapy Outcomes: Generative Message Communicator

R.M. was a retired airport manager with moderate expressive aphasia, AOS, and good comprehension (see Figure 16.15). He learned to use a portable dynamic screen SGD in combination with residual speech, partial word writing, and gestural communication (Fried-Oken et al., 2002). R.M. lived independently, drove a truck, and maintained his

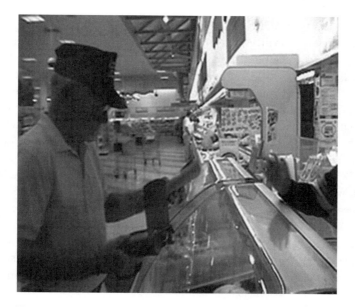

Figure 16.15.   R.M. ordering deli foods with his dynamic screen device, natural speech, and gestures. Copyright © 2004 J.P. Lasker and K.L. Garrett; used by permission of R.M.

own home. He was seen at a university clinic 7 years post-stroke for an AAC evaluation. At that time, he was already using a multimodal communication system consisting of residual speech, a small communication book, a notepad for word/letter writing, and various remnants. However, he required an SGD in order to participate more fully in all aspects of his life. He obtained a dynamic screen display device with Medicare funding support and then participated in several months of therapy to program his system with appropriate messages so that he could socialize and conduct business in the community. Many messages were stored holophrastically on multiple levels, but R.M. also demonstrated the ability to spell out single-word messages using the keyboard. He often typed in first letters of words to augment his speech attempts, help his communication partner guess a word, or access a number of pictured word prediction choices. He also learned to integrate natural communication modalities with AAC access. During role plays that gradually increased in difficulty, he learned to repair communication breakdowns by rephrasing, locating additional messages on his device, writing, or using conversational control messages such as "You're way off." At last report, he was using his system in the community independently on a daily basis whenever he believed it would enhance his communication effectiveness.

Case Example and Therapy
Outcomes: Generative Message Writer

Although writing may not be the first communication function that people with aphasia wish to target following a stroke, it can become an important focus for individuals who previously wrote extensively to communicate with others or to convey specific information at work. Some individuals with mild aphasia write for the first time to tell of their recovery from a devastating illness. Because many of the symptoms of aphasia are manifested in the written modality as well as in speaking and understanding, writers with aphasia are frequently frustrated by difficulties with word retrieval, spelling, and syntax formulation. King and Hux (1995) described the written output of an individual with mild aphasia who ultimately used AAC software to both select specific words and correct spelling errors as he wrote. This individual used a program called Co:Writer (Don Johnston, Inc.) to choose specific words from a list when he was not able to encode selected words into the correctly spelled form. He also learned to use standard spelling checker and grammar checker functions within word processing programs to write text accurately. We have also successfully assisted individuals with aphasia to use word prediction software that was built into their SGDs to generate written notes.

Alternatively, people with very severe aphasia cannot write independently. The composition, semantic, syntactic, and spelling demands of writing simply overwhelm their impaired linguistic systems. However, to address the specific need of writing personal letters, some individuals with severe aphasia and agraphia have used low-tech approaches that will be addressed in the next section on specific-need communicators.

Specific-Need Communicator

Some communicators with aphasia may not wish to use (and do not need to use) AAC as a primary communication method. However, they may describe specific communication situations that are problematic because of particular requirements for specificity, clarity, or efficiency. For example, an individual with aphasia might want to communicate on the phone, place bets at the racetrack, follow recipes, or record telephone messages. Any person with aphasia could have such well-defined, specific communication needs related to either speaking or writing. Individuals who live in settings that demand some independence generally require specific-need AAC techniques on an intermittent basis.

Intervention Strategies AAC interventions for specific-need communicators are usually limited in scope, because these individuals can often manage much of their communication through gestures and limited speech. When planning an intervention, it is first necessary to analyze the requirements of the specific communication task and to consider the person's current capabilities in light of the task. For example, an individual may need help setting up a system to allow verbal communication over the telephone. This might be managed through a simple tape recorder system in which a prerecorded message states, "Please ask me questions that can be answered 'yes' or 'no.'" Another common need is to communicate specific messages in a noisy place such as a cafeteria or bank. Often, a small communication card can be prepared with a restricted set of messages that are needed in the specific situation.

Another example of a specific need was tearfully expressed by one woman with mild expressive aphasia but severe agraphia, who was frustrated by her inability to recall the items she needed to purchase after arriving at the grocery store. Because she could not easily write the items she needed on a list before shopping, she had to rely on her memory and frequently forgot important items. A grocery list (see Figure 16.16) was created for her so she could simply circle items instead of writing them. Another individual was a speaker in most situations but was unable to order items by phone because of frequent

Date _____

We need to buy:

FOOD

Basic Foods
Bread
Cheese
Margarine
Ketchup
Mustard
Mayonnaise
Salt
Pepper
Lettuce
Potatoes
Rice
Macaroni
Spaghetti
• Sauce
• Noodles
• Mushrooms

Meats
Hamburger
Chicken breast
Bacon
Tuna
Rib eye
Delmonico steak

DRINKS
Milk
Coffee
Tea
Juice
• Orange
• Grapefruit
Pop
• Pepsi
• Coke
• 7Up

CLEANING SUPPLIES
Bath soap
Soft soap
Toilet paper
Ajax
Bleach
Scouring pads
Paper towels

COSMETICS
Shampoo
Deodorant
Band-Aids
Shaving cream
Razors

Figure 16.16.   Sample grocery list. Copyright © 2004 K.L. Garrett and J.P. Lasker.

semantic and phonemic paraphasias that interfered with saying the names of numbers. A list of the numbers 0 through 100 was printed for him. The number labels (e.g., FORTY) were written next to the number, which successfully cued him to state his credit card number or address correctly over the phone.

People with severe agraphia who wish to write letters may also benefit from a scaffolded letter-writing format (Garrett, Staab, & Agocs, 1996). In this augmented writing approach, individuals who have difficulty writing a letter without assistance can choose phrases from a list and copy them into partially completed sentences on a letter format (see Figures 16.17 and 16.18). One woman known to the authors wrote 50 letters in a 2-week period after initial instruction with the scaffolded letter format. Other individuals are able to progress from this approach to more independent letter generation with additional therapy. Scaffolded formats can also be useful in helping people with aphasia write email messages. The successful completion and mailing of a letter, the generation of a life story, or the sending of an email message to a friend or family member is another illustration of how the Participation Model, described earlier in Chapter 6, can be applied to all types of communication activities for people with aphasia.

Specific-need communicators may also benefit from situation training similar to that described previously. For example, if the person with aphasia needs to use a simple SGD for telephone communication, he or she may benefit from multiple opportunities to role play the situation. If a specific-need communicator is using a scaffolded letter-

1. __________ ______, 200__

Dear 2. ____________

3. ____________ ! How 4. ____________?

I am 5. ____________________. This month we

6. ____________________. We really

7. ____________________.

So, tell me about 8. ____________________.

I hope you are 9. ____________________.

Please 10. ____________________.

11. ____________________,

____

Figure 16.17. Blank letter format. Copyright © 2004 K.L. Garrett and J.P. Lasker.

writing format, it may be important to draft a few letters in a therapy session so the clinician can provide some initial cues before the individual completes the activity independently. Table 16.6 lists a few examples of goals for this group of communicators, for whom specific strategies are limited only by their needs and the creativity of their clinicians. Partners of specific-need communicators can contribute significantly by identifying situations at home or in the community that will require highly precise communica-

1.	Jan		Feb			March			April			May				June
	July		Aug			Sept			Oct			Nov				Dec
	1	2	3	4	5	6	7	8	9	10	11	12	13	14	15	16
	17	18	19	20	21	22	23	24	25	26	27	28	29	30	31	

2. (write in names of possible letter recipients here)
3. Hello! Hi! Howdy! Greetings!
4. . . . are you? . . . is it going? . . . is your family?
5. fine OK pretty good terrific a little tired
6. stayed at home visited the family worked around the yard vacationed in ____________ had the grandkids for a week
7. had a great time enjoyed ourselves were glad for Fall
8. your vacation your family school your job your friends
9. fine keeping busy taking it easy enjoying your grandkids
10. write soon call me sometime come visit take care
11. Sincerely, Fondly, With best wishes, Love,

Figure 16.18. Multiple choice letter format. Copyright © 2004 K.L. Garrett and J.P. Lasker.

Table 16.6. Specific-need communicator intervention goals and strategies

Communicator strategies (examples)
Utilize single-message SGDs to communicate information by telephone or in community situations (e.g., "I have aphasia—give me time to communicate") or to participate in rituals (e.g., prayers).
Present phrase cards to communicate specific needs in specific situations—e.g., to place bets at the race track, explain an upcoming bus stop, place bridge bets, ask grandchildren about school and sports, request a specific hairstyle at the salon.

tion on the part of the person with aphasia. Their continued participation in the message inventory process and role-playing activities is also very beneficial.

Case Example and Therapy Outcomes

J.K., a 53-year-old geography professor with aphasia, had been employed by a university for more than 20 years prior to onset of a left CVA. One year post-stroke, an evaluation revealed that her Aphasia Quotient of 79.1 of 100 on the Western Aphasia Battery (Kertesz, 1982) was most consistent with a diagnosis of anomic aphasia. She scored 80 of 100 on the reading subtest and 75 of 100 on the writing subtest. J.K. was determined to return to work as a college professor. She communicated in most daily situations using natural speech but required specific AAC supports to lecture on specific topics in her classes. J.K. obtained an SGD through a combination of vocational rehabilitation and university resources. She used her SGD to deliver class lectures on global hunger that she typed in advance, using software that allowed her to spell whole words or select whole words using word prediction. The software then allowed her to "speak" her lecture sentence-by-sentence through a speech synthesizer; she also learned to augment these prestored messages with natural telegraphic speech. Since she began to utilize this teaching approach to compensate for the challenges of acquired aphasia, her teaching evaluations have been excellent.

ASSESSMENT

In order to develop effective AAC interventions for people who have severe aphasia, clinicians need to evaluate communication needs as well as linguistic, cognitive, and communicative competencies. The guidelines and measurement tools in this section may assist clinicians in this process.

Assess Communication Needs in Real-Life Contexts

Prior to the onset of aphasia, adult communicators previously conveyed a wide variety of messages in myriad environments—messages that allowed them to greet others, share information, ask questions, see and provide solace, negotiate agreements, correct misunderstandings, and so on—all in a seamless sequence without much thought. Replacing this seemingly inexhaustible supply of internally generated language with a limited set of externally displayed messages is a tremendous task. Therefore, guidelines for developing the content of AAC systems generally start with a discussion of the individual's *needs*, by which we mean the environments and activities in which the person wishes to participate as well as the specific messages required to communicate in those contexts. Families and friends of people with severe aphasia often play a vital role in identifying these communication needs.

For clinicians who are conducting a formal evaluation with an individual who has severe aphasia, the following procedures may be helpful. First, during an *initial interview*, the clinician can simply ask the communicator, families, and significant others to list communication situations that are particularly challenging or difficult for the individual with aphasia. Next, ask interviewees *to imagine situations* in which they foresee opportunities for meaningful communication. Initially, families may often list situations in which physical needs are communicated (e.g., going to the doctor, getting dressed). Additional urging to think of situations in which the individual had an important life role prior to stroke may be necessary; providing the family with examples such as betting at the racetrack, saying the dinner prayer at Thanksgiving, attending sports events of grandchildren, and having coffee with a friend also may be helpful. Fox, Sohlberg, and Fried-Oken (2001) encouraged research participants with aphasia to sort topics into preferred and nonpreferred categories prior to engaging in conversational training. One of their three participants communicated much more extensively about topics that he had selected than those that had been chosen for him.

The *Communication Needs Assessment Form for Aphasia*, available through the Barkley AAC Center Web site, may assist clinicians to obtain this information in a systematic manner. For communicators who cannot verbally express the answers to these questions without supports, it may be useful to use the written choice conversation strategy described previously as well. Providing the communicator with written word choices representing potential communicative situations as well as scales for rating the relative importance of each situation can provide a window into his or her perceptions of important communication needs.

If it is not possible to conduct face-to-face interviews, clinicians can indirectly estimate communication needs by *assessing peer participation patterns*. Peers can be individuals of the same age or culture as the person with aphasia, or peers can have similar interests. For example, if a person with aphasia used to socialize at a Veterans' club in town, the clinician could observe or ask others about the types of messages or communication needs that typically arise in that situation. It might be helpful to ask the communicator to envision the sequence of communication events within each of these situations as well, so that a comprehensive message inventory also can be created.

Fox (personal communication, 2003) described how real-life communication needs were elicited from a group of people with aphasia and their significant others who attended a week-long "communication camp" experience. She asked these individuals to describe communication situations that had specifically challenged them and to share strategies that had been particularly effective in those situations. For example, one gentleman told about the difficulties he encountered when trying to order menu items in a fast-food restaurant. He developed an ingenious strategy—shining a red light from a laser pointer on the menu items posted behind the counter—to communicate his food order. Fox encouraged participants to develop and incorporate strategies such as the laser-light technique in their own "communication strategy toolbelt." Fox's "toolbelt" session is an excellent example of how clinicians can assist communicators with aphasia to identify important communication needs in a variety of life situations.

Assess Specific Capabilities

Traditional assessment procedures for aphasia typically identify the cognitive and linguistic deficiencies of an individual with aphasia; subsequent interventions then focus on remediating these deficits. Tests of impairment typically provide minimal extralinguistic context such as a topic, props, graphics, or functional routine. This traditional approach to assessment has been inadequate for individuals whose communication disorders are so severe that they cannot complete most test items. In addition, traditional tests do not assess an individual's residual abilities, a foundation upon which many AAC-oriented interventions are based. Therefore, it may be necessary to supplement standard aphasia tests with assessments of the person's language performance in functional settings and with familiar people. In the past few years, AAC clinicians have developed a variety of assessment procedures for creating profiles of competency and challenge. These are discussed in the following sections.

Linguistic Skills

Although people with aphasia may demonstrate extensive limitations in their linguistic systems, the words and structures with which they struggle are usually not lost or forgotten. Some individuals with aphasia use telegraphic speech to communicate because they have difficulty efficiently accessing the grammatical aspects of language. Other individuals may retain a conceptual awareness of grammar but have difficulty retrieving the specific words needed to communicate key ideas. Some people with aphasia, both fluent and nonfluent types, cannot always associate auditory language with meaning; therefore, they demonstrate some degree of comprehension difficulty. They may also make frequent sound-level errors when producing speech. These same individuals may comprehend or speak better when seeing the same information in printed form. Many people with aphasia who have poor reading scores on traditional tests have some ability to read when the written words are introduced in context. All of these observations of linguistic competence and challenge are compounded by the highly variable nature of aphasia (McNeil, 1983), which results in an intermittent pattern of performance on linguistic tests as well as in real-life communication.

Clinicians may find that an assessment battery that includes both traditional tests and contextual tasks will result in a more thorough understanding of linguistic skills. First, clinicians should assess expressive and receptive linguistic skills in a *conversational context*, both with and without AAC or contextual supports. Next, using a standard aphasia battery such as the Western Aphasia Battery (Kertesz, 1982), the Short Form of the Boston Diagnostic Aphasia Exam (Goodglass & Kaplan, 1983), or the Boston Assessment of Severe Aphasia (Helm-Estabrooks, Ramsberger, Morgan, & Nicholas, 1989), the clinician can measure the extent of the impairment when no external AAC strategies or partner support is available.

AAC-Related Skills

Several additional screening tools may assist the clinician in making AAC decisions for people with aphasia. Garrett and Beukelman's (1992) AAC Categorical Assessment for Communicators with Aphasia, recently revised by Garrett and Lasker (2004), provides the clinician with a means of checking off present or emerging communication competencies. This process may aid the clinician to make overall decisions about the nature of the primary AAC intervention based on the category the individual best fits at the time of the initial assessment. This form is available through the Barkley AAC Center Web site.

The second assessment tool, the Multimodal Communication Screening Task for Persons with Aphasia (Garrett & Lasker, 2004), reveals how a communicator answers situational questions (e.g., "How would you tell me you went to California in July?") by gesturing, spelling, pointing to locations on a map, or locating pictorial symbols throughout the eight-page booklet. It also provides information on the person's ability to categorize and to point referentially when telling a story. Pages include: 1) concrete concepts represented with pictures, photographs, and words (e.g., eat, lamp); 2) three categories represented with an incomplete series of visual symbols—the person with aphasia chooses from a row of six additional symbols to complete the categories; 3) graphic symbols representing descriptors (e.g., open, cold); 4) slightly more abstract concepts that can be combined with other items to represent complex meanings (e.g., grandchildren, money, monthly calendar); 5) two sets of written words and phrases, one for communicating in a pharmacy and another for conversing with grandchildren; 6) two sets of photographs representing different story sequences; 7) an outline map of the United States to represent locations of children's homes or favorite vacations; and 8) an alphabet board to communicate highly specific names (e.g., towns, restaurants) by spelling or pointing to the first letter. The picture stimulus book and administration manual for this descriptive tool are also available on the Barkley AAC Center's Web site.

Clinical experience suggests that this tool effectively distinguishes between communicators who will require partner support to indicate choices versus stored message communicators who can independently search through the booklet to locate symbols. It is also relatively easy to identify generative message communicators using the tool. Clinicians can ask the person with aphasia to communicate a complex message (e.g., "How would you communicate that your grandchildren are going to Disney World next month if their parents have enough money?"), and then observe if they can successfully communicate this idea by pointing to a logical sequence of pictures, words, letters, or map locations. In addition, observing this diagnostic activity may assist some family members to better understand why a clinician may suggest low-tech instead of electronic options for an individual with aphasia.

Nonverbal Communication Skills

Many individuals with severe aphasia retain a considerable repertoire of nonverbal communication skills, such as gestures, facial expressions, pantomimes, and vocalizations (Coehlo & Duffy, 1987; Kagan, 1995). Such skills allow some of them to communicate extensive information. Other individuals are impaired in their ability to produce nonverbal communication either consistently or efficiently. Instruction and practice are necessary for them to use these modes of communication. If nonverbal communication competencies do not show up during any of the preceding assessment activities, the clinician can specifically instruct the communicator to use gestures, drawing, or pantomimes while describing a recent event, such as losing a purse on the bus.

Motor Skills

Individuals with aphasia following a stroke usually retain the ability to control their limbs on at least one side of the body (usually the left). Therefore, they can typically gesture, turn pages, or point to communication choices in a direct selection mode. However, they may experience difficulties when asked to complete a complex sequence of motor movements (e.g., locating words on multiple pages of a book or SGD) because of limb apraxia or cognitive deficits. They may also have some difficulty physically carrying or manipulating heavy communication devices or the on/off buttons of those systems. Consultation with an occupational or physical therapist may be appropriate when deciding on a portable communication device or system.

Sensory Skills

The visual system may be spared entirely following a stroke. Frequently, however, there may be a visual field cut, usually on the right side. This means that the person is unable to see images with the right side of both eyes. Thus, AAC or other materials that are positioned in the right visual field are visually inaccessible. A person's ability to scan the visual field or the extent of field cut should be determined. In addition, it is important to assess the individual's residual visual capabilities and identify any visual deterioration that has occurred naturally with age, as well as any new deficits. A brief word cancellation/scanning task, in which the person with aphasia is asked to read line-by-line and circle a target word, may help to determine whether a functional visual field cut is present. An example test is available on the Barkley AAC Center Web site.

Perceptual Skills

People with aphasia often understand many of the visual images that are used to represent the world. For example, they recognize various "icons of geography" such as maps, and "icons of events" such as logos and signs. They also usually retain the ability to identify photographs and drawings that relate to people and places. Many people with aphasia retain knowledge about the relative relationships of size, shape, goodness, and importance among objects and experiences. For example, an aphasic individual may refer to another adult by gesturing to indicate his or her taller height as compared with a child. However, these skills should be probed. Asking an individual to tell about his or her family or childhood during a reminiscing conversation with a scrapbook will allow the clinician to observe these skills informally.

Some individuals with aphasia may also retain the ability to draw and can communicate messages through this modality (Lyon, 1995). Although these individuals may not have considered themselves artists prior to onset of aphasia, they can often depict ideas clearly enough through drawing that knowledgeable communication partners can understand their messages. Individuals with aphasia often retain knowledge of the chronology of events in their lives. For example, a person may indicate that a certain event, such as military service, occurred after high school but before her marriage. Or, an individual may refer to important events in terms of their proximity to the birth dates of his or her children. These skills can be assessed informally during reminiscing conversations.

Pragmatic Skills

Because most individuals with aphasia have communicated using natural speech and writing for most of their lives, they are quite familiar with how communication works. That is, they are aware of the turn-taking skills, speaker–listener roles, and topic coordination skills that are required in communication. They can also recognize and attempt to clarify ambiguous communicative messages. Thus, when compared with individuals who have had few or no normal communication experiences, individuals with aphasia are relatively aware of the structure and rules of conversational interaction. However, it may be important to assess pragmatic skills that are relevant for AAC communicators, including their ability to resolve communication breakdowns. For example, M.J., who was described earlier in this chapter, initially spent almost half of his communication effort on resolving breakdowns (Garrett et al., 1989). However, after he was instructed to shift to a different strategy (e.g., rewording or locating information in his communication notebook) instead of simply repeating words over and over, the proportion of his communication turns used to resolve communication breakdowns decreased from 46% to 11%.

Experiential Skills

Another skill area that is particularly relevant to people with aphasia involves the experiential skill base underlying communication. Most individuals with aphasia have lived for a considerable period of time and have experienced relatively normal, routine lifestyles, so their knowledge about the world is extensive. To gather "fuel" for upcoming AAC interactions, it may be helpful to informally assess interests, topics, and autobiographical information through interviews with family members prior to beginning an AAC intervention.

Cognitive Skills

Several aphasiologists have suggested recently that clinicians can gain predictive information regarding an individual's potential to communicate independently with AAC systems by administering specific cognitive assessment batteries. For example, the Cognitive Linguistic Quick Test (Helm-Estabrooks, 2001) contains several subtests that assess attention, memory, and reasoning without taxing linguistic ability. Nicholas, Sinotte, & Helm-Estabrooks (2003) suggested that several nonverbal reasoning tasks (e.g., trailmaking) may be useful for identifying individuals with adequate cognitive ability to use high-tech, symbol-based AAC systems. Research is underway to correlate subtest performance with each of the communicator categories described in this chapter.

Assess Constraints

As is the case with nonaphasic individuals who use AAC, constraints can originate in communication partners and the characteristics and demands of specific AAC strategies themselves.

Partner Skills

Because communication partners are so important in communication interactions with people who have severe aphasia, it is useful to assess their capabilities as well. This assessment usually cannot be conducted formally, so information about the communication skills of partners should be obtained from observing their interactions with the individual with aphasia. It is also important to determine whether the partner is able to learn or is interested in learning new ways of communicating with the person with severe aphasia. The clinician should also formally evaluate potential communication partners in basic skill areas that include speaking style and understandability, handwriting legibility, reading skills, hearing, and vision.

Demands of Potential AAC Strategies

Communication in general presents significant challenges to people with aphasia. They must learn how to map language onto ideas, even if that language is fragmented and difficult to retrieve and sequence. They must demonstrate the initiative and tenacity to convey a message to a partner despite frequent communication breakdowns. And, in some cases, they must also acknowledge that their efforts to communicate through speaking or writing are ineffective and then identify a more appropriate communication method.

Augmentative communication strategies and technologies may also add several cognitive and linguistic demands to this scenario (Garrett & Kimelman, 2000; Light & Lindsay, 1991). If a strategy requires writing, pointing, or access to digitally stored messages, the individual with aphasia must have competent alternative access, typically with the nondominant limb. Simply locating written or pictured messages in a book or electronic device requires the individual to translate symbols that are much more novel than natural speech. They must learn the meanings and internal representations of unfamiliar symbols such as line drawings or other symbols. When multiple symbols are used, people with aphasia must also learn to search one or more arrays or levels and possibly combine symbols to represent complex meanings. If a message encoding strategy is used, such as numeric encoding (e.g., N1 = "I need the bathroom"), the person with aphasia must recall these encoded representations. Even spelling, a more "natural" communication skill, is a type of encoding that requires sequential selection and sequencing of arbitrary symbols to represent sounds and meanings. Because successful spelling requires many repetitions of this procedure, it is often extremely difficult for people with aphasia. Therefore, providing people with aphasia with a typewriter or computer keyboard may be more frustrating than therapeutic.

People with aphasia who use AAC systems that store messages on one or more levels must also demonstrate sufficient working memory to complete the steps involved in accessing the messages before forgetting their intent or losing their partner's interest. In addition, if they are using technology, they may have to learn new operational skills such as turning the device on/off, comprehending synthesized or digitized speech, locating messages stored on invisible levels, using flowchart operational menus, keyboarding, and charging the device. Finally, individuals with aphasia must have the metacognitive skills to introduce their novel communication strategies to unfamiliar partners. They must know how to use their strategies in a dynamic manner—for example, a person might use speech and writing in certain contexts and then shift to an AAC strategy when communication breakdowns occur.

By definition, the disorder that is aphasia affects each of the levels of processing that AAC systems demand. For example, communicators with nonfluent aphasia typically exhibit difficulties with syntactic encoding. Therefore, strategies that require symbol combinations to communicate may frustrate them. Placing messages or symbols in leveled communication systems may impose significant processing challenges for many people with aphasia who demonstrate word retrieval or short-term recall problems. Complex visual displays may also affect people who have visual field cuts.

The purpose of this review of challenges inherent in the operation of AAC strategies and devices is not to warn clinicians away from trying to implement AAC with communicators who have aphasia. Instead, the message is that it is critical to match strategies to the individual's needs and skills.

Conduct Strategies Trials

To ensure that communication strategies match the skills and needs of the person with aphasia, it is useful to conduct trials in which the person with aphasia can try out the strategy in a simulated or real communication situation. Examples include planning a trip at a travel agency, returning an item to a store clerk, or talking about how aphasia affects one's life. For contextual choice and transitional communicators, it is important to see if they can successfully participate in several conversations, and whether their responses are accurate. For stored message and generative communicators, it is important to inventory vocabulary messages for a particular situation (e.g., beauty salon), represent and store the messages, model use of the system, and then see how well the person with aphasia communicates with the system in an actual role play of the interaction. It is only in the context of real-life communication trials that the individual can display his or her competencies and future training needs. A *Protocol for Implementing Strategies Trials* (Lasker & Garrett, 2004) is available on-line at the Barkley AAC Center's Web site.

INTERVENTION ISSUES

> The most difficult thing for us is actually thinking of when to use the [AAC system]—including it in our daily routines. (S.A.'s wife, B.A.)

Several issues may have an impact on the success of an AAC intervention. These include but are not limited to 1) the individual's or family's continued desire to work on speech alone, 2) difficulty with acceptance of AAC alternatives, 3) adherence to a medical model of treatment versus a participation model in available therapy centers, 4) premature discontinuation of treatment, 5) poor matching between AAC system features and communicators' capabilities, 6) limited availability of personalized messages, 7) lack of practice in contextual situations, 8) lack of available communication partners for partner-supported communicators, 9) an inadequate support network to assist in message development for generative communicators, and/or 10) lack of communication opportunities because needs are met and anticipated by others. Funding is frequently cited as a barrier, but in fact it is relatively available because of recent changes in Medicare and private insurer funding guidelines (see Chapter 6).

The following interaction with the spouse of a controlled situation communicator reflects some of the attitudinal barriers that family members may initially project when discussing AAC strategy implementation at home:

Clinician: So how has it been going at home?

Spouse: Oh, it's much easier to communicate with Robert now. He really seems to know what's going on.

Clinician: Are you and your sons comfortable with talking more slowly, making sure he understands? Can he clearly tell you "yes" and "no"?

Spouse: Yes, although sometimes he laughs if we go too slowly . . . he'll even make fun of us. But we're doing well there. He really thinks about how he's nodding his head. And he points to what he wants now . . . that really helps.

Clinician: Have you been able to talk about more complicated topics? Like what to get the kids for the holidays, or his opinions on what's happening in the news?

Spouse: No, not really . . . mostly we just talk about what he needs.

Clinician: Have you tried to use the written choice technique we practiced?

Spouse: No, I'm glad I haven't had to resort to that yet . . . .

To promote acceptance of AAC strategies, clinicians may find it helpful to acknowledge their clients' hesitations about communicating using the somewhat unnatural alternatives to speech that constitute AAC. Many of the spouses in the authors' clinics have gradually accepted some level of AAC after several months of simultaneously working on speech recovery and gradually incorporating AAC strategies into conversations. Group therapy, an increasingly funded service, is another positive means of illustrating how AAC and natural communication modalities can blend. Watching other, more "senior" participants converse about old movies or introduce themselves in a simulated social club may be more convincing than academic explanations about the benefits of AAC strategies.

It is also essential that the *content* of an AAC system remain dynamic. As changes occur in the situations and contexts of an individual's life, the AAC system must reflect these changes—otherwise, motivation and interest in using the system will quickly diminish! Continual modification of the content of an AAC system requires that one or more facilitators, usually family members or caregivers, must be trained to monitor and adjust the AAC system. Facilitators must also be able to train new people who enter the aphasic person's life (e.g., a son- or daughter-in-law or a new neighbor), so that they, too, can become effective communication partners. Failure to identify and adequately prepare facilitators is a common reason for AAC intervention failures among people with severe aphasia.

Clearly, the successful integration of AAC interventions depends as well on the flexibility and continuity of service delivery as the individual with aphasia transitions from setting to setting. Professionals, family members, and people with aphasia may wish to team together to create better solutions for management of long-term aphasia. Options could include increasing the emphasis on training partners to use immediate communication strategies early in the individual's recovery, with more intensive involvement of the speech-language pathologist later in the rehabilitation process. It may be useful to schedule clients with aphasia for routine follow-up visits each year when they receive their annual therapy visit allotment from their insurer. Some people with aphasia may benefit from weekly group therapy sessions rather than individual treatment sessions only. Still others may benefit from home visits by a speech-language pathologist as well as other health care professionals, since it is at home that many of the true communication challenges are most visible. With careful planning and extended clinical support, AAC interventions can enrich the communication options for individuals and their communication partners at all stages of their adjustment to a life with aphasia.

CHAPTER 17

ADULTS WITH DEGENERATIVE COGNITIVE/LINGUISTIC DISORDERS

WITH ELIZABETH K. HANSON

The gradual deterioration of communication effectiveness is a commonly reported symptom of various types of degenerative, cognitive/linguistic conditions. The exact pattern of communication deterioration varies in that some people experience cognitive symptoms such as memory loss, impaired judgment, reduced problem solving, or visuospatial orientation before changes in their language are observed. Others demonstrate a gradual deterioration of language as an early symptom. During the past decade, AAC strategies have been implemented to enhance the receptive and expressive communication effectiveness of people with degenerative language and cognitive disorders such as primary progressive aphasia, dementia, and Huntington disease.

PRIMARY PROGRESSIVE APHASIA

Primary progressive aphasia (PPA) is recognized as a distinct clinical condition characterized by a gradual progression of language impairment in the absence of more widespread cognitive and behavioral disturbances for a period of at least 2 years (Mesulam, 2001; Rogers, King, & Alarcon, 2000). Duffy (2000) reported that the mean age of onset is 60.5 years with about a 2 to 1 ratio of men to women. PPA is considered the fifth most common type of dementia. There is no known cause of PPA, although about half of patients with PPA have a family history of dementia and research into a genetic component in PPA is ongoing (Mandell, 2002; Mesulam, 2001). In a recent summary, Duffy (2004) reported that approximately 150 cases of PPA have been described in the literature.

After a history of language symptoms, some individuals with PPA eventually demonstrate other cognitive impairments consistent with a diagnosis of dementia. In 1999, Rogers and Alarcon reviewed 57 articles that described the course of 147 individuals with

PPA. Twenty-five percent of them demonstrated symptoms of fluent aphasia, 60% had symptoms of nonfluent aphasia, and 15% had indeterminate symptoms. Twenty-seven percent of the fluent group, 37% of the nonfluent group, and 77% of the indeterminate group eventually demonstrated symptoms of dementia. Although the initial symptoms of PPA vary among individuals, anomia (i.e., trouble thinking of specific words) is the most commonly reported language symptom. Another common symptom, particularly in the nonfluent group, is slow, hesitant speech with long pauses.

Stages of Intervention

Rogers et al. (2000) recommended the implementation of a proactive intervention plan. In anticipation of future declines in language function, intervention that focuses on early incorporation of AAC strategies into everyday communication is recommended.

Early Stage

During the early stages of PPA, affected individuals continue to use speech to interact with others. However, they may need assistance with word finding (i.e., recall of specific words). Intervention techniques involve many of the strategies identified in Chapter 16 (severe aphasia) under the section for "specific-need communicators." These include booklets or cards with specific information, prepared questions for difficult situations, and gestures (yes, no, left, right, past, and future) to resolve communication breakdowns. The techniques should be introduced gradually and early so that people with PPA and their listeners can become familiar with them and accept this type of communication support.

Middle Stage

People with PPA in the middle stage are considered to be "generative message" or "transitional" communicators (see Chapter 16) in that they need AAC support in most communication contexts. In addition to communication notebooks and cards, these individuals often benefit from photographs of scenes that are familiar to them. Some also benefit from drawing scenes to communicate or clarify messages. For others, spatial representations such as maps, calendars, family trees, and floor plans are helpful to communicate specific content (Cress & King, 1999). Individuals in this stage often need augmented input strategies to enhance their comprehension of spoken information as well. Such strategies may include key words (printed), photos, gestures, drawings, or line drawings.

Late Stage

The severe communication limitations associated with late-stage PPA are often quite similar to the needs of "contextual choice communicators," as described in Chapter 16. These individuals need help both to communicate and to comprehend information about basic needs and routines. Early in this stage, they may continue to use the materials developed in the early and middle stages. However, as they progress further into the late stage, they become "emerging communicators" (Chapter 16), in that they need to be presented with very limited choices in order to communicate about their needs, preferences, and routines.

Development and Use of Communication Notebooks

Communication notebooks are usually small, easy-to-carry binders that contain information that supports the communication efforts of people with complex communication needs. The content of the notebooks is personalized with regard to content and form. For example, these notebooks may contain pictures of individuals who are unable to read or may contain considerable printed information if the individuals can read but have difficulty remembering the names of people, places, and activities. People with PPA usually begin the notebooks early so that they can participate in the selection of content and in the organization of the notebook.

Rogers et al. (2000) presented an excellent discussion of the preparation and maintenance of communication notebooks for people with PPA, including guidelines to enhance the long-term usefulness of such books. These include the following:

1. The communication notebook must reflect the person with PPA; it must be personalized.

2. The person with PPA must take a lead role in determining its content early in the course of the disease.

3. The communication notebook and opportunities to use it must be available consistently throughout the course of PPA.

4. The communication notebook is never finished; it must be dynamic so that it reflects the changing needs and experiences of the person with PPA and his or her social network.

Figure 17.1 provides an example of a communication page described by Cress and King (1999).

It is important to begin AAC intervention as soon as possible for people with PPA because familiarity and context seem to influence the use and retention of AAC strategies. [These individuals] demonstrate . . . their most effective communication using strategies that they . . . generate . . . themselves . . . . If we can provide early guidance and information to facilitate these self-generating strategies, then further intervention can concentrate on maintaining and modifying those strategies or techniques, and providing additional facilitator training as needed . . . (Cress & King, 1999, pp. 254–255)

In summary, PPA is a progressive condition characterized by language impairment at least 2 years prior to the occurrence of other cognitive deficits, which typically lead to dementia. AAC interventions can help individuals with PPA to enhance both expressive and receptive language. AAC strategies should be introduced early in the course of the disease to allow the person with PPA to contribute to the design and content, and to help both the person with PPA and their communication partners to learn how to use the strategies.

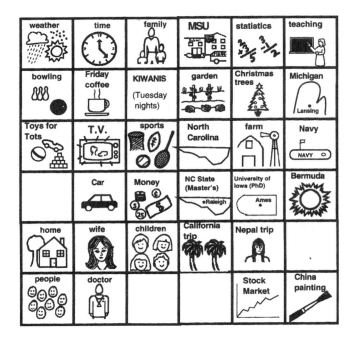

Figure 17.1.   Example of a communication page. (From Cress, C., & King, J. [1999]. AAC strategies for people with primary progressive aphasia without dementia: Two case studies. *Augmentative and Alternative Communication, 15*, 248–259.; reprinted by permission of Taylor & Francis Ltd, http://www.tandf.co.uk/journals.)

DEMENTIA

Dementia is a medical syndrome characterized by an acquired, chronic, cognitive impairment. A diagnosis of dementia requires that the cognitive impairments involve memory and at least one additional cognitive domain, such as language, attention, visuospatial function, praxia (movement), and executive or frontal lobe functions (Fried-Oken, Rau, & Oken, 2000). Dementia is a relatively common syndrome, with a prevalence of 1% of the population for people age 65 and almost 50% for individuals age 90 and older (Jorm & Jolley, 1998). Alzheimer's disease (AD) is the most common form of dementia. The Alzheimer's Association (2001) estimates that AD affects 10% of people age 65 and almost 50% of people age 85 or older.

Memory Strengths and Deficits

Memory deficits in dementia affect various memory domains in different ways. *Episodic memory* about recent events is often impaired quite early in the progression of the syndrome. Thus, memory loss in the early stages includes an inability to recall information such as who has visited, where items were left, what was eaten for breakfast, and so forth. *Semantic memory* involves factual information and general, organized knowledge. There is some debate about whether problems with semantic and other forms of declarative memory have to do with memory loss or with the inability to access and retrieve that type of memory (Bayles & Kim, 2003). Nonetheless, deficits may be evidenced in an inability to remember facts such as the name of the leader of one's country, that bananas are yellow, or that both cats and dogs are animals. *Procedural memory* is often the best preserved of the memory domains. Procedural memory involves retaining the ability to complete common procedures such as shaving, dressing, writing checks, and so forth.

Typically, people with memory deficits due to dementia perform better when using recognition rather than recall memory. Examples of *recognition memory* include people realizing that they know someone when they see him or her, recognizing that a familiar item is out of place, selecting a specific item from among a choice of items, and recognizing a favorite TV channel when they see it. *Recall memory*, on the other hand, relies on one's ability to retrieve "invisible" information that is not concretely represented in some way, such as a person's name, the code for a digital door lock, or the TV channel for a favorite show.

Dementia, which involves the impairment of short-term memory in older people, is a very serious problem for people who develop it and for their family and careers. Short-term memory plays a very important role in human communication. It helps to maintain the thread of a conversation, it ensures that topics are fully discussed, and it allows new topics to be introduced at appropriate times. Impaired short-term memory can therefore have a severe impact on a person's conversations, resulting in topics being repeatedly introduced, and giving the appearance that the person is not listening. This can be very disturbing and frustrating for the conversation partner, and can in turn have a negative effect on the person as he or she becomes aware of a partner's negative emotions but does not understand how they have come about. (CIRCA Web site, 2004)

Communication Strengths and Deficits

Although relative strength and deficit profiles differ widely among people with dementia, there are overall patterns of strengths and deficits that occur with each stage of the condition. Communication strengths and deficits by stage are summarized in Table 17.1.

AAC Interventions

Because AAC intervention for people with dementia is relatively new, there is limited evidence of the effectiveness of these efforts. However, given the prevalence of dementia, the need to develop and evaluate intervention strategies is apparent. In this section, we summarize some clinical guidelines and strategies.

Focus on Strengths

The primary focus of intervention for individuals with dementia is to enhance their strengths at each stage rather than to attempt to remediate their deficits. Thus, materials and training should be provided to frequent communication partners so that they can support people with dementia to use their strengths and allow them to compensate for their particular pattern of deficits. For example, if a person with dementia experiences deficits in recent episodic memory (i.e., remembering what happened yesterday), inter-

Table 17.1.   Communication strengths and deficits of people with dementia by stage

Stage	Strengths		Deficits	
Early stage	1.	Language comprehension	1.	Diminished reading comprehension
	2.	Grammar	2.	Difficulty with written expression
	3.	Syntax	3.	Word finding
	4.	Express needs independently	4.	Reduced verbal output
	5.	Conversations	5.	Pragmatic deficits
	6.	Answer multiple choice and yes/no questions	6.	Distractibility
			7.	Difficulty concentrating
			8.	Confusion
			9.	Disorientation
			10.	Problems managing activities of daily living
Middle stage	1.	Grammar	1.	Pragmatics: topic changes, discourse cohesion and coherence
	2.	Syntax	2.	Poor reading and writing skills
	3.	Reading comprehension for single words	3.	Reduced verbal output
	4.	Express needs with help		
	5.	Follow two-step commands		
	6.	Gestural input helps		
	7.	Recognition memory		
Late stage	1.	Some meaningful words	1.	Dependent
	2.	Maybe read single words	2.	No relevant language
	3.	Social communication (greetings)		
	4.	Attend to pleasant stimuli		

vention might consist of providing him or her with a concrete reminder, such as a memento of a recent event in the form of a remnant or a photograph. Alternatively, training activities designed to strengthen episodic memory are generally not indicated. The following intervention guidelines and strategies focus on the cognitive and communicative strengths of people with dementia:

- **Reduce memory demands.** Because recall memory deficits in particular are so common in dementia, AAC interventions should be designed to reduce demands on recall memory and processing capacity. Bourgeois, Dijkstra, Burgio, and Allen-Burge (2001) described a "memory book" with pages that each contain one sentence or item, such as illustrations to provide graphic information. The memory books typically include autobiographical information, daily schedules, and problem resolution information. Providing information in the form of memory books builds on recognition memory, which takes less effort than recall tasks (Bayles & Kim, 2003). Figure 17.2 shows a sample memory book developed by Bourgeois and colleagues (2001).

- **Reduce distractions.** People with dementia often experience difficulty processing information and interacting in environments that contain distractions. Therefore, their communication partners, including family and caregivers, need to be trained to position themselves in a way that minimizes distractions and optimizes performance.

- **Chunk information.** Organizing information into manageable "chunks" often enhances the communication effectiveness of people with dementia. This can be done

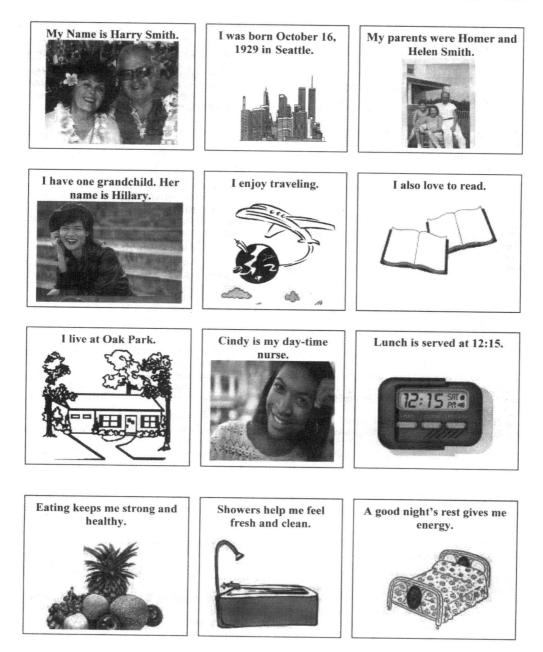

Figure 17.2.   Sample memory book (From Bourgeois, M.S., Dijkstra, K., Burgio, L., & Allen-Burge, R. [2001]. Memory aids as an augmentative and alternative communication strategy for nursing home residents with dementia. *Augmentative and Alternative Communication, 17,* 196–209; reprinted by permission of Taylor & Francis Ltd, http://www.tandf.co.uk/journals.)

using a variety of AAC strategies. For example, if listeners use augmented listening strategies by identifying topics of conversation using pictures, the associated information will often be understood better than if the person with dementia is engaged in a free-flowing conversation that moves from topic to topic without clear demarcation of content.

- **Provide information in alternative forms.** Provision of alternative forms of information allows for redundancy, thereby reducing the information-processing load. Consider the perceptual and cognitive complexity of a family reunion. Photographs will allow a person with dementia to remember more clearly who is related to whom. In addition, a written schedule of activities will allow the person to understand the flow of activities better than verbal descriptions alone.

Bourgeois et al. (2003) examined the effectiveness of two training approaches, *spaced retrieval* and a modified *cueing hierarchy*, to teach individuals with dementia strategies to remember to use external aids such as memory books and memory wallets. Spaced retrieval involves learning to remember information by recalling it over increasingly longer durations of time. Cueing hierarchies are widely used in speech-language therapy to systematically increase or decrease cues or prompts for specific communicative behavior, contingent on performance of the behavior. Twenty-five people with dementia participated in the study. Custom goals were developed to address individual cognitive-communication needs, and each participant was taught one strategy using one training method, and another strategy using the other method. The results demonstrated that both approaches resulted in the participants' ability to learn new strategies that generally lasted for four months after the intervention. However, the spaced retrieval approach yielded better performance than the modified cueing hierarchy approach, overall. This research demonstrates that, contrary to widely held views, new learning that targets procedural and recognition memory is possible for some individuals with dementia.

Represent Language Symbolically

With regard to AAC strategies and options, Fried-Oken and colleagues (2000) suggested that interventionists need to address both language representation and organization. Messages communicated to and by a person with dementia can be represented visually using several levels of symbolization, depending on the person's capabilities. Typically, simple print can be read by many individuals with mild, moderate, and (occasionally) severe dementia. Printed words can be used to label the locations of items, provide memory support, clarify spoken messages, and act as reminders of tasks to be completed. As dementia progresses, printed words can be accompanied by photographs and pictures. For some, objects eventually become the most effective way to represent information. If printed words become ineffective, drawings or photographs may be used to represent language concepts.

Once the language symbolization level of a person with dementia is determined, the range of language content to be represented needs to be identified. Usually, this is a team effort by the person with dementia, caregivers, family members, and others. The content will depend on the person's lifestyle, the settings in which he or she participates, and the supports that are available. The *Social Networks* assessment (Blackstone & Hunt Berg, 2003a, 2003b) may be useful to assist the team to identify communication partners who may contribute to this content.

Lacking specific research in language organization and dementia, Fried-Oken and colleagues (2000) suggested that AAC teams look to related fields, such as aphasia, for insights into the linguistic changes that may result from the neurological changes associated with dementia. Based on the knowledge that people with aphasia sometimes develop different categorization schemes than their typical peers, it may be reasonable to question whether people with dementia experience similar changes in lexical organization. If so, it may be helpful to teach people with dementia to use alternate strategies to access lexical information.

Use a Variety of AAC Strategies

The incorporation of language representation techniques into the lives of people with dementia and the members of their social networks (e.g., caregivers, family, friends, members of the public) can be managed using a number of common AAC strategies. For example, written choice techniques, originally developed for people with aphasia, can be used with print or pictures to provide communication choices that represent the preferences and needs of people with dementia. Communication notebooks or small wallets are also useful in many cases, particularly when they include information represented using digital photography techniques that allow editing, enhancement, sizing, and manipulation of images to support communication. Communication cards and labels are widely employed to strategically locate communication supports for these individuals. For example, photographs placed on doors to identify various rooms of the house, labels placed on cupboards as reminders of the contents, and printed or pictured instructions that act as reminders to flush the toilet or take one's medicine may be helpful.

As noted previously, memory books have probably been the most investigated AAC intervention for people with dementia. Bourgeois and colleagues (Bourgeois, 1990, 1992, 1993, 1996; Bourgeois et al., 2001) reported that the quality of conversational interactions for people with mild and moderate dementia improved significantly when they used personalized memory wallets or books. In addition, Andrews-Salvia, Roy, and Cameron (2003) found that four nursing home residents with severe dementia made more on-topic factual statements when they used memory books than when they did not. An unexpected outcome of this study was that when caregivers allowed additional wait time for responses, some residents who used the memory books made even more on-topic statements than when such wait time was not provided. Bourgeois and colleagues (2001) studied 66 people with dementia (who were residents in one of seven nursing homes) paired with 66 nursing aides. The dyads were randomly assigned to control and treatment groups. All of the dyads participated in 5-minute conversations that were videotaped before the start of an 8-week training program for the nursing aides in the treatment group and then again after the training. Some of the positive outcomes were that after the training, the residents with memory books showed increases in their overall number of utterances as well as the number of positive statements and informative utterances in their conversations. The nursing aides used more facilitative comments when talking to the residents.

Train Communication Partners

As evidenced in the studies by Andrews-Salvia et al. (2003) and Bourgeois et al. (2001), the research emphasizes how important it is that the intervention target both the person with dementia and his or her communication partners (Hopper, 2003). The degenerative nature of this condition requires that the responsibility shared between two communication partners will increasingly fall to the partner without impairment as the capability of the person with dementia decreases. Therefore, the partner must learn strategies that will enhance communication as the disease process progresses. Caregivers, family members, professionals, and friends make up the social networks of most people with dementia, and most of these individuals are used to communicating primarily through speech. Ongoing training must teach them new, more effective ways to communicate with individuals with dementia by shifting their communication patterns to include AAC techniques such as memory aids.

Small, Gutman, Makela, and Hillhouse (2003) studied communication strategies used by 18 married couples that included one spouse with AD, as the dyads communicated about various activities of daily living. The researchers observed the couples and documented the effectiveness or ineffectiveness of 10 strategies that are commonly recommended to increase communicative success for people with dementia. Table 17.2 lists the strategies and illustrates their effectiveness. The researchers also asked the spouses, who did not have impairment, to rate how much they used the strategies and the effectiveness of the resulting interactions. Some of the results were quite surprising. Of the 10 strategies documented, only 3 were found to decrease communication breakdowns: eliminating distractions, speaking in simple sentences, and using yes/no questions. One strategy, using slower speech, appeared to be related to increased communication breakdowns; however, the investigators found that some spouses were not slowing their speaking rate even when they thought they were. In other cases where the rate was slower but still not effective, the researchers postulated that the longer duration of the message increased the burden on the already limited working memory capacities of the spouses with AD, consistent with previous research (Bayles & Kim, 2003; Small, Kemper, & Lyons, 1997; Tomoeda, Bayles, Boone, Kaszniak, & Slauson, 1990).

In response to questionnaires about how much the spouses without impairment used the different strategies and how effective their communication was with their partners who

Table 17.2. Communication strategies commonly recommended for people who care for patients with Alzheimer's disease and their effectiveness

Strategy	Did the strategy decrease communication breakdowns?
Eliminate distractions	Yes
Approach from front slowly/give eye contact	No clear difference
Use short, simple sentences	Yes
Speak slowly	No
One question/instruction at a time	No clear difference
Use yes/no rather than open-ended questions	Yes
Repeat verbatim	No clear difference
Repeat using paraphrase	No clear difference
Avoid interrupting/allow time to respond	No clear difference
Encourage person to describe word, if word finding is a problem	No clear difference

From Small, J.A., Gutman, G., Makela, S., & Hillhouse, B. (2003). Effectiveness of communication strategies used by caregivers of persons with Alzheimer's disease during activities of daily living. *Journal of Speech, Language, and Hearing Research, 46,* 353–367; reprinted by permission.

had impairments, their perceptions did not reflect the actual interactions. In some cases, the spouses reported using strategies frequently (e.g., slow speech and encouraging circumlocution), but in reality the strategies were rarely observed. Conversely, they reported only the occasional use of other strategies (e.g., eliminating distractions and approaching the person slowly), when in fact, these strategies were used quite frequently. Overall, the spouses reported a higher level of communicative effectiveness than was supported by the objective data on communication breakdowns. This study emphasizes the critical need for interventions that target the communication partners of people with dementia.

Bayles and Tomoeda (1998a, 1998b) provide resources for people who support people with dementia in a book entitled *Improving the Ability of Alzheimer's Patients to Communicate* and a videotape entitled *Understanding the Communication Problems of Alzheimer's Patients.* Both are available from Canyonlands Publishing.

A high-tech multimedia system that supports reminiscence or memory book-type interactions for people with dementia is under development by a group of researchers in Scotland (Alm et al., 2003). The premise of the system is that it must be easy to use both for people with dementia and their communication partners, and it must circumvent the typical demands of conversational interactions on short-term memory. The prototype system incorporates a database of general photographs, video or film footage, folk songs, sounds, and text in a presentation system with a touch-screen display. The purpose is to provide an error-free navigational environment that encourages users to talk about topics inspired by the elements of the database. Six participants in a pilot study (including people with dementia and their caregivers) reacted positively, reporting that the system was easy to use and promoted more conversation on a wide range of topics from the participants with dementia. The researchers surmise that the system alleviates the conversational burden that falls on the communication partner by equating the contribution of the person with dementia. Future research will incorporate personalized media into the database for individual users.

In summary, dementia is a syndrome characterized by progressive cognitive impairment affecting memory and at least one other cognitive domain. Distinct communicative strengths and weaknesses are associated with each stage of the syndrome. People with dementia may benefit from AAC strategies that are designed to support and enhance communication strengths rather than remediate communication deficits. Memory books, which enhance communicative interactions, have received much of the research attention as an AAC strategy for dementia. Memory books can serve as alternate forms of communication input, enhance procedural memory for completing daily care activities, and support the communicative intent of a person with dementia who is experiencing expressive language difficulty. A growing body of research confirms the effectiveness of partner training in AAC interventions for dementia. Partner training is critical to the success of AAC interventions, and new investigations are determining which communicative strategies used by partners are actually effective.

HUNTINGTON'S DISEASE

Huntington's disease (HD) is an inherited autosomal dominant degenerative disease, which means that people who have one parent with the disease have a 50–50 chance of inheriting it. The symptoms of HD typically appear in the fourth decade, with death occurring 15–17 years after onset. The National Institute of Neurological Disorders and Stroke (retrieved August 25, 2004) estimates that 30,000 people suffer from HD and another 150,000 have a 50% chance of inheriting the disease. People with HD are often unable to speak functionally by the end stages of the disease (Folstein, 1990). The primary symptoms of HD include chorea (involuntary, irregular spasmodic movements of the limbs or facial muscles), emotional disturbance, and hyperkinetic dysarthria. Early cognitive changes include impaired attention, memory, and cognitive functions with full dementia developing in some patients in later stages (Murray, 2000). The communication impairments associated with HD vary considerably from person to person. Language comprehension deficits associated with HD include high-level processing difficulties with metaphoric or ambiguous sentences or sentences containing implied information or complex grammar. Expressive language deficits include shorter, less complex, and less grammatical utterances (Murray, 2000). For some, abnormal motor movements may be restricted primarily to the lower extremities without obvious speech disorder. For others, speech is so impaired that AAC strategies are required (Klassner & Yorkston, 2000). Klassner and Yorkston (2001) documented a case report in which linguistic and cognitive supplementation strategies were employed to support the communication of a 44-year-old man with HD. Linguistic supplementation through scripting "home to work" conversations involved a notebook in which regular daily activities were described in two or three short sentences. Cognitive supplementation using task lists on tag board sheets were used to support his completion of household activities such as caring for the family pet.

A review of the literature reveals limited successful use of high-tech AAC systems for people with HD. Low-tech AAC strategies that focus primarily on choice making and scheduling should be introduced early in the course of the disease so that people with HD can learn to use them before their cognitive impairments make new learning difficult. Communication partners also require careful training so that they can cue and prompt the individual to use the AAC system in consistent ways.

In summary, individuals with HD may benefit from linguistic and cognitive supplementation strategies that support the procedural memory that underlies activities of daily living. However, the possible improvements realized by AAC strategy use have only begun to be explored in the area of HD.

CHAPTER 18

Individuals with Traumatic Brain Injury

with Susan Fager

Augmentative and alternative communication (AAC) interventions for people who have experienced traumatic brain injury (TBI) have changed dramatically through the years. Until the mid-1990s, AAC interventions occurred primarily with individuals who experienced severe, persistent anarthria or dysarthria following TBI. It was not uncommon for teams to delay AAC interventions until the individual's associated communication disorders "stabilized"; consequently, many people with TBI were unable to communicate functionally for months or even years after their accidents. The justification for this conservative approach had three bases. First, cognitive limitations during early stages of recovery make it difficult for many people with TBI to operate complex AAC technology. Second, because the cognitive and motor performance of a person with TBI changes over time, an appropriate long-term AAC system is difficult to select. Third, clinical observations indicate that some individuals with TBI do recover functional speech and thus do not require long-term AAC systems. With this view, AAC teams often felt that the most conservative approach was the "safest" when recommending an intervention.

Currently, the goal of an AAC team is to provide communication assistance so that people with TBI can participate effectively in a rehabilitation program and are able to communicate their ongoing needs. Thus, the focus of intervention has shifted from providing a single AAC system for long-term use to providing a series of AAC systems designed to meet short-term communication needs while continuing efforts to reestablish natural speech. For example, the changing AAC intervention goals over a 3-year period for Ann, an adolescent with TBI, are illustrated in Table 18.1 (Light, Beesley, & Collier, 1988).

This chapter outlines the general approaches to AAC intervention for individuals with TBI. However, because individuals with brain injuries recover over an extended period of time, it is beyond the scope of this book to detail the extensive AAC intervention concepts, techniques, and strategies developed for these individuals. DeRuyter and Kennedy (1991) and Ladtkow and Culp (1992) have written two in-depth presentations of such information.

Table 18.1.   Principal goals of intervention with Ann over a 3-year period

Phase One: 6–9 months post-trauma
1. To establish consistent and reliable yes/no responses
2. To develop a preliminary communication display as a means to indicate basic needs and wants

Phase Two: 13–16 months post-trauma
1. To provide a means to request attention
2. To encourage more explicit "yes" responses
3. To develop a communication display as a means to share information and express needs and wants

Phase Three: 22–23 months post-trauma
1. To provide access to a microcomputer for written communication
2. To establish more explicit "no" responses for unfamiliar listeners
3. To develop strategies to share information and generate novel vocabulary

Phase Four: 36 months post-trauma
1. To develop breath control, articulation skills, and voicing
2. To develop strategies to interact effectively with unfamiliar partners and in group activities
3. To develop conversation skills around a range of topics
4. To enhance the rate of written expression

Phase Five: 40–44 months post-trauma
1. To continue to develop breath control, articulation skills, and voicing
2. To recognize breakdowns in communication
3. To use clarification strategies to repair communication

From Light, J., Beesley, M., and Collier, B. (1988). Transition through multiple augmentative and alternative communication systems: A three-year case study of a head-injured adolescent. *Augmentative and Alternative Communication, 4,* 3; reprinted by permission of Taylor & Francis Ltd, http://www.tandf.co.uk/journals.

Prevalence and Etiology

Injuries to the head that result in temporary or permanent brain damage are quite common. It is difficult to estimate the number of these injuries that occur each year because many go unreported. Individuals who do not lose consciousness or do so only briefly are rarely admitted to the hospital and may not even go to an emergency room. The incidence of TBI as reported by emergency department records is approximately 200 per 100,000 people (Hux, 2003). Of the 1.5 million individuals who sustain TBI in the United States each year, 230,000 are hospitalized and survive, but 80,000–90,000 survive with impairments that are so severe that they interfere with independent living. One of six individuals are unable to return to school or work when discharged from the hospital or from rehabilitation. People between age 15 and 24 years and those older than age 75 years are at highest risk for TBI (Centers for Disease Control and Prevention, 2001, 2003; Thurman, Alverson, Dunn, Guerrero, & Sniezek, 1999).

> Individuals with TBI do not represent a random sample of the total population. More than twice as many males as females are injured. The risk of TBI is also greater among children from 4 to 5 years of age, males from 15 to 24 years of age, older adults (especially those older than 75 years of age), and individuals who have had previous TBI (Beukelman & Yorkston, 1991).

The causes of TBI are varied. Motor vehicle accidents are the most common cause, firearms are second, and falls of various types are third. Among students, recreational- and sports-related injuries such as those that occur from bicycling, skating, and horseback riding are common. Among adolescents and young adults, assaults are a common cause of TBI (Hux, 2003; Thurman et al., 1999).

As people with TBI recover, they usually progress through a continuum of care that begins in a trauma unit and may include time in a variety of different living situations. Fager (2003) described the experiences of a 36-year-old man who relies on AAC technology to communicate all messages except a few greetings. In the 15 years since his TBI, he has lived in 11 different settings including an acute care hospital, rehabilitation center, assisted living center, his parents' home, independent living with attendant care, and an assisted living center. He has successfully used AAC strategies in each of these settings. However, not all individuals with TBI have adequate support to use AAC technologies consistently. Fager, Hux, Karantounis, and Beukelman (2004) documented long-term AAC use patterns by 25 people with TBI and reported that two of these individuals discontinued use of their AAC systems because they did not receive adequate supports in their living situations. The facilitator support received by people with TBI who successfully use AAC is often extensive. Thus, intervention efforts must focus on facilitator training as these individuals transition through the multiple living situations that they are likely to experience.

Cognitive/Linguistic and Communication Disorders

Several categorical scales have been developed in an effort to describe people with severe TBI. The Levels of Cognitive Functioning scale (Hagen, 1984), which describes cognitive and associated language behaviors that occur during recovery, is presented in Table 18.2. AAC teams use scales such as this to design AAC and other interventions appropriate to each stage.

In general, the communication disorders associated with TBI are the result of impairments in three areas. First, some of the language characteristics of people with TBI are a consequence of cognitive impairments, as summarized in Table 18.2. The level of linguistic performance can vary depending on the individual's cognitive level. Second, language disorders may occur because of damage to specific language processing areas of the brain. Sarno, Buonaguvro, and Levita (1986) evaluated 125 individuals with TBI using the Battery of Language Test and reported that 29% of these individuals exhibited classic symptoms associated with acquired aphasia. An additional 36% exhibited subclinical aphasia, which the researchers defined as "linguistic processing deficits on testing in the absence of clinical manifestations of linguistic impairment" (p. 106).

Third, some communication disorders in TBI are caused by damage to the motor control networks and pathways of the brain that occurred at the time of injury. Dysarthria has often been reported as one of the long-term sequela of TBI. Oliver, Ponford, and Curren (1996) reported that motor speech disorders were present in 34% of their sample 5 years after injury. Yorkston, Honsinger, Mitsuda, and Hammen (1989) surveyed 151 people following TBI and found that prevalence changed as a function of time after

Table 18.2. Levels of cognitive functioning and associated language behaviors

General behaviors	Language behaviors
I. No response Patient appears to be in a deep sleep and is completely unresponsive to any stimuli.	Receptive and expressive: No evidence of processing or verbal or gestural expression.
II. Generalized response Patient reacts inconsistently and nonpurposefully to stimuli in a nonspecific manner. Responses are limited and often the same, regardless of stimulus presented. Responses may be physiologic changes, gross body movements, or vocalization.	Receptive and expressive: No evidence of processing or verbal or gestural expression.
III. Localized response Patient reacts specifically, but inconsistently, to stimuli. Responses are directly related to the type of stimulus presented. May follow simple commands such as "Close your eyes" or "Squeeze my hand" in an inconsistent, delayed manner.	Language begins to emerge. Receptively: Patient progresses from localizing to processing and following simple commands that elicit automatic responses in a delayed and inconsistent manner. Limited reading emerges. Expressively: Automatic verbal and gestural responses emerge in response to direct elicitation. Negative head nods emerge before positive head nods. Utterances are single words serving as "holophrastic" responses.
IV. Confused-agitated Behavior is bizarre and nonpurposeful relative to immediate environment. Does not discriminate among persons or objects; is unable to cooperate directly with treatment efforts; verbalizations are frequently incoherent or inappropriate to the environment; confabulation may be present. Gross attention to environment is very short, and selective attention is often nonexistent. Patient lacks short-term recall.	Severe disruption of frontal–temporal lobes, with the resultant confusion apparent. Receptively: Marked disruption in auditory and visual processing, including inability to order phonemic events, monitor rate, and attend to, retain, categorize, and associate stimuli. Disinhibition interferes with comprehension and ability to inhibit responses to self-generated mental activity. Expressively: Marked disruption of phonologic, semantic, syntactic, and suprasegmental features. Output is bizarre, unrelated to environment, and incoherent. Literal, verbal, and neologistic paraphasias appear with disturbance of logico-sequential features and incompleteness of thought. Monitoring of pitch, rate, intensity, and suprasegmentals is severely impaired.
V. Confused, inappropriate, nonagitated Patient is able to respond to simple commands fairly consistently. However, with increased complexity of commands or lack of any external structure, responses are nonpurposeful, random, or fragmented. Has gross attention to the environment but is highly distractible and lacks ability to focus attention on a specific task; with structure, may be able to converse on a social-automatic level for short periods; verbalization is often inappropriate and confabulatory; memory is severely impaired; often shows inappropriate use of subjects; individual may perform previously learned tasks with structure but is unable to learn new information.	Linguistic fluctuations are in accordance with the degree of external structure and familiarity-predictability of linguistic events. Receptively: Processing has improved, with increased ability to retain temporal order of phonemic events, but semantic and syntactic confusions persist. Only phrases or short sentences are retained. Rate, accuracy, and quality remain significantly reduced. Expressively: Persistence of phonologic, semantic, syntactic and prosodic processes. Disturbances in logicosequential features result in irrelevances, incompleteness, tangents, circumlocutions, and confabulations. Literal paraphasias subside, while neologisms and verbal paraphasias continue. Utterances may be expansive or telegraphic, depending on inhibition–disinhibition factors. Responses are stimulus bound. Word retrieval de-

General behaviors	Language behaviors

ficits are characterized by delays, generalizations, descriptions, semantic associations, or circumlocutions. Disruptions in syntactic features are present beyond concrete levels of expression or with increased length of output. Written output is severely limited. Gestures are incomplete.

VI.   Confused-appropriate

Patient shows goal-directed behavior but depends on external input for direction; follows simple directions consistently and shows carryover for relearned tasks with little or no carryover for new tasks; responses may be incorrect due to memory problems but appropriate to the situation; past memories show more depth and detail than recent memory.

Receptively: Processing remains delayed, with difficulty in retaining, analyzing, and synthesizing. Auditory processing is present for compound sentences, while reading comprehension is present for simple sentences. Self-monitoring capacity emerges.

Expressively: Internal confusion-disorganization is reflected in expression, but appropriateness is maintained. Language is confused relative to impaired new learning and displaced temporal and situational contexts, but confabulation is no longer present. Social–automatic conversation is intact but remains stimulus bound. Tangential and irrelevant responses are present only in open-ended situations requiring referential language. Neologisms are extinguished, with literal paraphasias present only in conjunction with an apraxia. Word retrieval errors occur in conversation but seldom in confrontation naming. Length of utterance reflects inhibitory–initiation mechanisms. Written and gestural expression increases. Prosodic features reflect the "voice of confusion," characterized by monopitch, monostress, and monoloudness.

VII.   Automatic-appropriate

Patient appears appropriate and oriented within hospital and home settings, goes through daily routine automatically, but is frequently robotlike with minimal-to-absent confusion; has shallow recall of activities; shows carryover for new learning but at a decreased rate; with structure, is able to initiate social or recreational activities; judgment remains impaired.

Linguistic behaviors appear "normal" within familiar, predictable, structured settings, but deficits emerge in open-ended communication and less structured settings.

Receptively: Reductions persist in auditory processing and reading comprehension relative to length, complexity, and presence of competing stimuli. Retention has improved to short paragraphs but without the abilities to identify salient features, organize, integrate input, order, and retain detail.

Expressively: Automatic level of language is apparent in referential communication. Reasoning is concrete and self-oriented. Expression becomes tangential and irrelevant when abstract linguistic concepts are attempted. Word retrieval errors are minimal. Length of utterance and gestures approximately normal. Writing is disorganized and simple at a paragraph level. Prosodic features may remain aberrant. Pragmatic features of ritualizing and referencing are present, while other components remain disrupted.

(continued)

Table 18.2.   *(continued)*

General behaviors	Language behaviors
VIII. Purposeful and appropriate Patient is able to recall and integrate past and recent events and is aware of and responsive to the environment, shows carryover for new learning and needs no supervision once activities are learned; may continue to show a decreased ability relative to premorbid abilities in language, abstract reasoning, tolerance for stress, and judgment in emergencies or unusual circumstances.	Language capacities may fall within normal limits. Otherwise, problems persist in competitive situations and in response to fatigue, stress, and emotionality, characterized in reduced effectiveness, efficiency, and quality of performance. Receptively: Rate of processing remains reduced but unremarkable on testing. Retention span remains limited at paragraph level but improved with use of retrieval–organization strategies. Analysis, organization, and integration are reduced in rate and quality. Expressively: Syntactic and semantic features fall within normal limits, while verbal reasoning and abstraction remain reduced. Written expression may fall below premorbid level. Prosodic features are essentially normal. Pragmatic features of referencing, presuppositions, topic maintenance, turn taking, and use of paralinguistic features in context remain impaired.

From Hagen, C. (1984). Language disorders in head trauma. In A. Holland (Ed.). *Language disorders in adults* (pp. 257–258). Austin, TX: PRO-ED; reprinted by permission.

onset. Of those in acute rehabilitation, 45% reported mild to moderate dysarthria and 20% reported severe dysarthria. In outpatient settings, 12% demonstrated mild to moderate dysarthria and 10% demonstrated severe dysarthria. For children, Ylvisaker (1986) reported that 10% of children and 8% of adolescents continued to produce unintelligible speech during follow-up studies. Several different types of dysarthria have been observed following TBI including ataxic, flaccid, spastic, and combinations (Yorkston, Beukelman, Strand, & Bell, 1999).

[Judy] tried to talk several times during the day. Much of it sounded unintelligible, but occasionally we heard a "Where am I?" or other words we could understand. We could not tell if she knew us, or understood anything we said. Then a few days later . . . Judy started trying to answer. . . .We spent the rest of the day hanging over her bed admiring her, as you might hang over the crib of a newborn baby. . . .The next day she responded less. This turned out to be a pattern. Nearly every day on which she showed definite improvement was followed by one of passivity or even apparent regression. It kept us on an emotional roller coaster. (D. Thatch, recounting the first few days in the hospital after her daughter Judy's severe TBI, in Weiss, Thatch, & Thatch, 1987, p. 17)

Recovery from Severe Communication Disorders

Communication disorders of individuals with TBI can change dramatically over the course of their recovery. Limited longitudinal research describes the patterns of these changes; however, some authors have provided insight about the course of recovery.

Ladtkow and Culp (1992) followed 138 people with TBI over an 18-month period. They reported that 29 of these individuals (21%) were judged unable to speak at some point in their recovery. Of these 29, 16 individuals (55%) regained functional speech during the middle stage of recovery (i.e., Levels IV and V in Table 18.2). Thirteen individuals (45%) did not regain functional speech; unfortunately, the description of the cognitive recovery of those who did not regain functional speech is incomplete. The authors merely indicated that only three people (10%) reached the late stage of recovery, corresponding to Levels VI, VII, and VIII.

In a related study, Dongilli, Hakel, and Beukelman (1992) investigated the recovery of 27 people who were unable to speak on admission to inpatient rehabilitation following TBI. Of these, 16 individuals (59%) became functional natural speakers during inpatient rehabilitation, whereas the other 11 (41%) did not. All individuals who became functional speakers did so at Level V or VI. Of the 11 individuals who left inpatient rehabilitation unable to speak, one achieved functional natural speech almost 24 months postinjury, and another was making substantial progress toward becoming a functional speaker 48 months postinjury.

As the Dongilli et al. (1992) study shows, people with TBI may experience severe communication disorders for cognitive- as well as motor-related reasons. Jordan and Murdoch (1990) described a 7-year-old girl who was mute for 10 months subsequent to coma. Following her mutism, the girl demonstrated rapid and unexpected recovery of functional communication skills, although she continued to experience higher-level language impairments.

Adding to this limited information base regarding recovery from communication disorders are two interesting case studies. In one, Workinger and Netsell (1988) described a man who recovered intelligible speech 13 years following injury and used various AAC systems during the intervening years. In addition, Light et al. (1988) described the transitions of an adolescent girl with TBI through approximately 3 years of multiple AAC systems before she became a functional natural speaker (see Table 18.1). Enderby and Crow (1990), who followed four people with severe bulbar dysfunction due to TBI, reported similar outcomes. They reported that although the individuals made few gains within the first 18 months after injury, they made substantial improvements as long as 48 months postinjury.

NATURAL ABILITY INTERVENTIONS RELATED TO SPEECH

As noted in the previous discussion, some individuals with TBI recover natural speech following injury, whereas others do not. As of 2004, the communication disorders field did not have enough information to predict the likelihood of natural speech recovery. Therefore, individuals who experience TBI, their families, and their rehabilitation teams must address natural speech recovery on an individual basis.

Some individuals may be able to produce a number of intelligible words, although they may not develop completely functional speech in all situations. Family members, friends, and team members should encourage the use and improvement of these words if they allow the individuals to manage certain aspects of communication interaction. Others with dysarthria following TBI can say many words, but their words are unintelligible because of impaired motor control. They may call on AAC techniques to augment the intelligibility of their natural speech. In fact, most individuals with TBI use multiple modes of communication at every stage of recovery. Rehabilitation that emphasizes reestablishing natural speech only or AAC only may not meet all the communication needs of a person with TBI.

Topic Supplementation

If a person's speech is marginally intelligible, his or her message can often be understood if the listener is aware of the semantic context or topic. Communication boards containing lists of frequently occurring topics can be used to establish context at the beginning of an interaction and to lessen the likelihood of a communication breakdown. Hanson and colleagues (2004) reviewed the literature on topic supplementation for speakers with various types of dysarthria. They reported that topic supplementation increased word intelligibility by an average of 28% and sentence intelligibility by 10.7%. Use of topic supplementation should be considered after assessment with the technique documents that 1) the individual with TBI can learn to implement it in conversational interactions and 2) the technique has a positive impact on speech intelligibility. In a study involving only individuals with TBI, Beukelman, Fager, Ullman, Hanson, and Logemann (2002) reported intelligibility gains of more than 50% for some speakers and as low as 2.4% for others.

Alphabet Supplementation

Beukelman and Yorkston (1977) reported that a supplemented speech strategy substantially improved the speech intelligibility of speakers with dysarthria. In alphabet supplementation, the speaker identifies the first letter of each word on an alphabet board or other type of AAC display while saying the word. This procedure provides listeners with information that allows them to restrict their word retrieval to words that begin with the letter indicated. In the same study, Beukelman and Yorkston described the impact of alphabet supplementation on the speech of a young man who had sustained a TBI. His habitual sentence intelligibility was 33%, compared with 66% when he used alphabet supplementation. Hanson and colleagues (2004) reported that, across speakers with various types of dysarthria, alphabet supplementation increased sentence intelligibility by 25.5% and single-word intelligibility by 10%. Use of alphabet supplementation should be considered if an assessment confirms that 1) the individual with TBI can learn to implement it in conversational interactions and 2) the technique has a positive impact on speech intelligibility. In a study involving only people with TBI, Beukelman, Fager, and colleagues (2002) reported intelligibility gains of up to 69% for some speakers (see Figure 18.1).

Portable Voice Amplification

Some people with dysarthria following TBI speak so quietly that their speech is difficult to hear, especially in groups of people or noisy environments. These individuals may find it useful to increase the loudness of their speech with a portable speech amplifier (see Chapter 15 for a more extensive discussion of this approach).

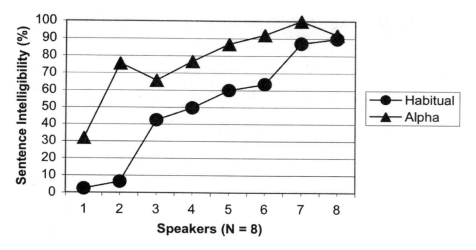

Figure 18.1. Habitual and alphabet-supplemented speech intelligibility for eight speakers with dysarthria due to traumatic brain injury.

AAC ACCEPTANCE AND USE PATTERNS

Outcome studies have described AAC recommendations for individuals with TBI. DeRuyter and Lafontaine (1987) collected data on 63 individuals who were referred to the Non-oral Center at Rancho Los Amigos Medical Center for AAC assessment. AAC recommendations included communication boards ($n = 37$); simple systems other than communication boards, such as yes/no systems, gestures, or writing ($n = 11$); dedicated communication devices ($n = 12$); and no communication system ($n = 3$).

Some studies have described the long-term use of AAC systems. Keenan and Barnhardt (1993) described the long-term AAC use of individuals with TBI after discharge from a rehabilitation facility. Of the 20 individuals that continued to be nonspeaking, one did not use AAC to communicate; seven used yes/no systems alone; nine used simple communication boards; and three used electronic communication devices.

Fager et al. (2004) described the AAC acceptance and use patterns of 25 individuals with TBI. Following AAC assessment, 17 high-tech and 8 low-tech AAC systems were recommended. Fifteen of 17 individuals for whom high-tech AAC was recommended received a device. One individual rejected the recommendation and one did not receive a device due to funding constraints. Thirteen of the 15 individuals who received a high-tech AAC device continued to use their devices for an extended period of time, for an overall acceptance rate of 87%. Two individuals discontinued use of their high-tech AAC systems due to loss of ongoing facilitator support. All individuals for whom low-tech AAC was recommended ($n = 8$) accepted the recommendation. Three of these individuals discontinued use of their systems due to recovery of natural speech. These individuals formulated their messages primarily through letter-by-letter spelling, unless they experienced a preexisting language disorder. Few used encoding strategies. Only one used alpha encoding extensively.

ACCESS ASSESSMENT AND INTERVENTION

AAC teams should base their intervention approaches with people who have TBI on individual levels of cognitive recovery (DeRuyter & Kennedy, 1991; Ladtkow & Culp, 1992). AAC approaches have been described for three general stages of recovery: 1) the early stage, which involves Levels I, II, and III (see Table 18.2); 2) the middle stage, which includes Levels IV and V; and 3) the late stage, which includes Levels VI, VII, and VIII. Assessment and intervention goals and techniques differ considerably in these three stages (see Blackstone, 1989a, for a summary).

Early Stage (Levels I, II, and III)

Assessment

It is almost impossible in the early stage of recovery to assess cognitive, language, or motor control capabilities because the individual may be unable to stay awake or pay attention for any significant amount of time. Thus, at this stage AAC teams attempt very little formal assessment. Instead, team members document systematic observations to identify changes in the individual's response patterns and to identify functional movements that the individual may use in a subsequent AAC program. Family members, friends, and other communication partners can also observe and chart such information if they spend a large amount of time with the individual. Because they know the person well, they are in a good position to document changes and responses.

As individuals with TBI become more alert, they are gradually able to differentiate between two or more people or objects. This is a positive sign, as it is often a precursor to the development of a yes/no response. The response mode for differentiation varies from person to person and may include eye pointing, moving a body part, or activating a beeper. The stimuli to which people recovering from TBI are able to respond must be presented in a careful and controlled manner. Family members and communication partners can usually be trained in this approach. They can also provide information about the interests and preinjury activities of the individual with TBI so that medical and rehabilitation personnel can provide the person with interesting and meaningful stimulation.

AAC Intervention

During the early stages of recovery, people with TBI are unable to speak functionally because of cognitive impairments. Some people may have language or motor control impairments that further contribute to their communication disorder. Ladtkow and Culp suggested that "the primary treatment goal of early stage TBI recovery is for the person to emerge from coma and to begin to respond consistently to simple commands" (1992, p. 154). Given this goal, the purpose of implementing AAC techniques during this stage is to stimulate the individual and to facilitate consistent, purposeful responses.

AAC techniques used at this point vary considerably depending on the individual's overall neurological involvement. For example, consider the individual who is functioning in the range of Levels I–III and who also has considerable motor control impairment. This individual might be unable to respond to stimuli consistently not only because of cognitive problems but also because of his or her motor weakness, spasticity, or lack of coordination. An AAC intervention for such a person might provide an alternative access mode, such as a single switch (Garrett, Schutz-Muehling, & Morrow, 1990). Then, as the individual begins to respond to various stimuli by making purposeful movements, facilitators can encourage contingency awareness (i.e., cause and effect). For example, facilitators might encourage the individual to operate a tape recorder with a single switch to play favorite music or listen to recorded letters from family members or friends. In addition, a single switch with a control unit can be used to activate electrical appliances such as fans, radios, and lamps. As the individual becomes more purposeful, he or she may activate single message tapes containing basic greetings and other social phrases with a single switch and tape recorder (see Chapter 11 for additional suggestions). Then, if motor control permits, facilitators can connect two or more switches to different tape recorders so the individual can choose from among different musical selections or letters. During the early stage of recovery, a limited number of symbols (e.g., one to four) might represent choices. Symbols should be brightly colored or exaggerated (Fried-Oken & Doyle, 1992). AAC teams should take care to understand the visual capabilities of AAC users following TBI, as impairments can range from double vision to cortical blindness.

Keenan and Barnhart (1993) documented the return of yes/no responses in 82 individuals with severe TBI: 49% signaled yes/no with head nods, 26% with motor responses of upper and lower extremities, 15% with eye gaze, and 9% with speech. Individuals with primarily cognitive or hemiplegic impairments developed yes/no responses earlier than those with flexor withdrawal or high or low muscle tone. Twenty-nine percent of the individuals regained yes/no responses within 3 months of onset, 66% within 6 months, and 84% within 9 months.

Middle Stage (Levels IV and V)

Assessment

In the middle stage of recovery, the individual may respond consistently to stimuli while still showing evidence of considerable performance and communication impairments due to attention and memory impairments. Individuals who do not have specific language impairments or severe motor control impairments usually begin to speak functionally during these stages, although they may produce somewhat confused messages (Dongilli et al., 1992; Ladtkow & Culp, 1992). In addition, people with TBI generally begin to indicate their basic needs at this point. These may include comfort messages related to being hot/cold, hurt, or hungry. Individuals may also be able to communicate messages related to their location, time of day, and other personal information. Family members and friends can assist with the selection of topics that are particularly important to people in the middle stages of recovery.

Early in the middle phase of recovery, people with TBI often experience agitation and poor awareness of their communication deficits. Therefore, they may initially have difficulty accepting AAC interventions. This may be reflected in limited willingness to participate in some aspects of AAC assessment.

The aim of assessment in the middle stage is to identify residual capabilities that the individual with TBI can utilize to achieve the specific communication goals mentioned previously. Most of the procedures for this assessment are nonstandardized and informal. The initial assessment often focuses on seating and postural issues, which team members should coordinate with AAC concerns. Proper seating and positioning help to minimize reflex activity, excessive tone, and other movements that may interfere with verbal communication or AAC system usage (DeRuyter & Kennedy, 1991). Specifically, "the overall seating and positioning goals during [this] stage should be to provide for a structurally appropriate and functional position in which minimal or no pain is encountered" (DeRuyter & Kennedy, 1991, p. 342).

Assessment of motor control capability is important to determine the individual's direct selection or scanning options. As discussed in Chapter 7, assessors should consider various access sites in terms of accuracy, efficiency, reliability, and endurance. This assessment may be difficult in some cases because people with TBI may require orthopedic surgical procedures that interfere, either temporarily or permanently, with their ability to use specific motor access sites (DeRuyter & Kennedy, 1991). Thus, it is important for AAC specialists to coordinate communication interventions with medical procedures by working closely with the medical team responsible for the individual's overall care. Assessment should also focus on the memory and attention capabilities of people with TBI. Complex scanning patterns (row-column or group-item) may be too demanding, so AAC teams should limit the individual's early scanning experiences to circular or linear scanning.

People with TBI often experience visual-perceptual and visual acuity disturbances, and these should also be considered in AAC assessment. At lower cognitive levels, assessors can usually determine visual functioning by observing the individual's ocular response to threat, gross focus movements of the eyes, and ability to follow a bright object or familiar face (DeRuyter & Kennedy, 1991). At higher cognitive levels, many visual disturbances can be detected through standard ophthalmologic examinations. A member of the AAC team should accompany the individual to such assessments to encourage the examiner to consider AAC-related issues, such as the optimal size for symbols and the array and the optimal distance between the user and the display.

AAC Intervention

Depending on the nature of the brain injury, AAC teams should choose one or two major communication goals for the middle stages of recovery. The goal may be to help the person compensate for attention and memory impairments. This is particularly relevant for individuals with TBI who begin to speak during this stage because they often need communication techniques to help them remember, for example, the names of important people and their schedule of activities. A second goal of intervention in the middle stage applies specifically to individuals who have sustained damage to language or motor control areas of the brain. These individuals probably will not develop natural speech at this point in their recovery. Thus, AAC interventions should seek to provide these individuals with techniques that support conversational interaction. In Levels IV and V, messages that relate to wants/needs and information sharing are more important to most individuals than are messages that support social closeness and social etiquette (DeRuyter & Kennedy, 1991).

Most AAC interventions during the middle stages of recovery are nonelectronic and include alphabet boards, pictures, word boards, yes/no techniques, and dependent scanning, among others. In an effort to reduce the complexity of communication, AAC teams may elect to use context-specific activity displays at this stage. For example, specific boards might facilitate participation in cognitive rehabilitation activities, recreational events, or daily living routines. Depending on the linguistic capabilities of the individual, photographs, line drawings, or printed words and phrases may symbolize the messages on the activity displays. Interventionists should remember that people in this stage of recovery may experience difficulty visually discriminating similar symbols or symbols with several elements. Individuals might use alphabetic displays, but encoding is almost always too difficult at this stage of recovery (Fried-Oken & Doyle, 1992). To control the complexity of the AAC system, teams may choose small activity displays with specific content, rather than large, complex boards containing multiple areas of content. For those with extensive attention and memory limitations, interventionists might consider written choice strategies (see Chapter 16). During the middle stage, the individual might also use single switches to activate call buzzers or appliances or to run tape recorders. Depending on the physical capabilities of the individual, such switch control activities may serve as training for the operation of a long-term environmental control device.

Communication partners play an important role in structuring communication interactions during the middle stage. For example, partners may need to introduce topics for conversation, suggest the augmentative mode that can be used most productively at a particular time, assist with resolving communication breakdowns, and create motivating communication opportunities. Communication partners should actively help to structure interactions, but they should also be very patient and allow ample time for people with TBI to prepare, clarify, and repair their messages. Perhaps one of the most common partner errors is to rush or offer excessive encouragement during this stage by making multiple suggestions of how to formulate or complete a message. This can be very distracting and frustrating to the individual with TBI who must concentrate very hard in order to think, plan, compose, and finally produce a communicative utterance. At times, partners will also need to learn to provide systematic cuing in order for the person in middle stages to use his or her communication system effectively. In time, individuals with TBI should attempt to phase out partner cuing.

DeRuyter and Donoghue (1989) described in detail the AAC interventions over a 28-week period for a young man who was unable to speak functionally due to TBI. During the first weeks of intervention (8 months postinjury), he established a reliable yes/no response by nodding his head, and he began to learn the visual-perceptual and upper-extremity skills necessary for eventual use of a communication board. In addition, his AAC team initiated interventions designed to encourage the development of natural speech during this time. By the 10th week of intervention, he was able to use a simple alphabet board, 12″ × 18″, with approximately 2-inch letters. Initially, he exhibited "extreme frustration" (p. 52) with the board because of his motor planning deficits. By the 26th week of intervention, however, this young man exhibited "no hesitation in using his alphabet board when he was unable to communicate effectively verbally or gesturally" (1989, p. 53). His team introduced an electronic AAC device with voice output. With very little training on the device, he was able to communicate at a rate of up to eight words per minute. At the time of his discharge from the inpatient rehabilitation facility, he communicated via limited speech, a sophisticated gesturing system, an alphabet board, and an AAC device with an expanded membrane keyboard.

Late Stage (Levels VI, VII, and VIII)

Assessment

By the late stage of recovery, most individuals have regained the cognitive capability to become natural speakers, and those who remain unable to speak usually experience severe specific language or motor control disorders. AAC teams can implement the Participation Model (see Figure 6.1) at this point for effective assessment and intervention planning. Analysis of the participation patterns of individuals with TBI and their families forms a particularly important part of this process. When people with TBI move from acute rehabilitation, to outpatient rehabilitation, to independent living, to employment, their patterns and expectations of participation change dramatically. These expectations greatly affect the nature and extent of their communication needs. It is also important to assess opportunity barriers, in much the same manner as is discussed in Chapter 6. For people with TBI in late-stage recovery, AAC teams often identify communication needs, assess specific capabilities and constraints, and match these to AAC system/device interventions (DeRuyter & Kennedy, 1991; Ladtkow & Culp, 1992).

AAC Interventions

In the late stage of recovery, individuals with TBI are generally oriented and able to demonstrate goal-directed, socially appropriate behavior. However, they may still have difficulties learning new information due to residual cognitive impairments. Some individuals may become natural speakers during Level VI, but by Levels VII and VIII, most individuals who are likely to become natural speakers without extensive intervention have already done so (Dongilli et al., 1992). Thus, by the late stage of recovery, many people with TBI can interact and converse with their families and friends through natural speech. Nevertheless, even those individuals who regain speech may require augmented writing systems for an extended period. In addition, people with residual language and motor control impairments will continue to require long-term communication systems to meet their specific interaction needs. Individuals have many interaction needs at this point, including those related to communicating wants/needs, sharing information, achieving social closeness, and participating in social routines (DeRuyter & Kennedy, 1991).

During the late stage of cognitive recovery, traditional AAC techniques that resemble those used with other individuals who experience physical and cognitive impairments are often appropriate. Although people with TBI who cannot speak usually experience a high incidence of physical problems, one study found that approximately 78% were able to successfully utilize direct selection AAC techniques (DeRuyter & Lafontaine, 1987). Almost 75% of the direct selection users in DeRuyter and Lafontaine's database operated their devices with their fingers or hands, whereas the remainder used eye pointing, headlight pointing, or chin pointing; 16% utilized dependent or independent scanning, and the remainder used other or no AAC techniques.

As social support for health care and rehabilitation decreases in some countries, people with TBI are spending less and less time in intensive rehabilitation programs where AAC services may be available. It is important that people with TBI and their families educate themselves early in the recovery process about available AAC services and how to gain access to such services when they are needed.

It might be assumed that due to the cognitive impairments associated with TBI, individuals will require AAC systems that contain pictorial or other nonorthographic symbols. However, this is often not the case. It is important to remember that even late in the recovery process, cognitive impairments may mask considerable residual skills. One of the most important skills that many people with TBI retain is the ability to read and spell. Thus, many individuals with TBI can utilize AAC systems that employ orthographic symbols, including letters, words, and sentences (Fager et al., 2004; Fried-Oken & Doyle, 1992). In fact in one review, Doyle, Kennedy, Jausalaitis, and Phillips (2000) report that the majority of adults with TBI eventually are candidates for spelling-based systems. AAC teams should take care when introducing encoding strategies, as some people, even in the late stage of recovery, may have difficulty learning and implementing these strategies efficiently. If coding strategies are used they need to be relatively concrete rather than abstract (Doyle et al., 2000). These authors provide a summary of the impact of cognitive limitations on AAC interventions with TBI survivors.

Those who assist people with TBI during the recovery process may be well aware that new learning can be difficult and require considerable time and practice. This is an important consideration for those individuals who require long-term communication systems because some AAC approaches require extensive training for operation. Examples of such methods are those that are technically complex to operate or that require the individual to learn a large number of messages using sequences of alphabetic or iconic codes. The AAC team should exercise caution when introducing such techniques and should be careful not to make frequent changes in a system once the individual has learned it.

CHAPTER 19

AAC in Intensive and Acute Medical Settings

Acute and intensive medical units serve a wide range of individuals who are unable to communicate, either temporarily or permanently. Such communication problems occur as a result of primary medical conditions, such as traumatic brain injury, stroke, myasthenia gravis, oral-laryngeal cancer, and Guillain-Barré syndrome; or as a side effect of interventions such as surgery, intubation, and/or tracheostomy. For most of us, acute medical experiences have been experienced in the form of visiting friends in the hospital or viewing television documentaries. As a result, we think that most individuals (i.e., patients) in these settings are very passive regarding their own care and are "having things done to them" constantly. This perception logically leads to the belief that, because acutely ill patients are so ill and so passive, they do not need to communicate. This is not at all the case, with the exception of people who are unconscious. Most people in acute medical settings need to communicate regularly with hospital staff in order to participate in their own care, and they report an urgent need to communicate with family members at this uncertain and frightening time in their lives. Depending on the length of stay, it may also be necessary for them to communicate about family finances, the operation of a business, the care of dependent children, and other personal matters. When one considers that the term "acute medical" refers to both short- and long-term services for people with complex medical conditions, the need for AAC strategies to support a wide range of communication needs becomes apparent.

For most people in acute medical settings who are unable to use their natural speech to communicate and their families, having a severe communication limitation is a new and unfamiliar condition. Typically, they are unaware of AAC approaches. Other individuals, such as those with progressive disorders like ALS, will have used AAC systems prior to entering the hospital, and both they and their families may be familiar with a wide range of AAC options. In either case, however, hospital staff members are unlikely to be knowledgeable about AAC options and will need to learn about them rather quickly.

It (AAC) allowed him to vent his anger. Every time we would do a procedure he would say "I hate you," and "This sucks," and it would make him feel better. I was glad to hear it every time he pushed the buttons because at least he was clearly expressing how he felt, which makes him feel better. (The mother of a child in an intensive care unit [ICU], in Costello, 2000)

CAUSES OF COMMUNICATION DISORDERS IN ACUTE MEDICAL SETTINGS

Communication disorders in acute medical settings can occur as a result of both primary causes (i.e., those directly related to an individual's illness or condition) and secondary causes (i.e., those related to an individual's need for temporary respiratory support). The primary causes of complex communication needs are discussed throughout this book and will not be reviewed here. However, individuals with a number of different medical conditions may require respiratory support, either temporarily or permanently. These include, for example, people with Guillian-Barré syndrome, botulism, cardiopulmonary insufficiency, and extensive surgical interventions. Such respiratory support often interferes with communication processes and a person's ability to speak. This is particularly true if endotracheal intubation or tracheostomy is required.

Endotracheal Intubation

An endotracheal tube (see Figure 19.1) is designed to transport air from a ventilator to an individual's respiratory system. Endotracheal tubes are usually passed in emergency situations through the person's mouth, pharynx, and larynx into the trachea (i.e., the airway

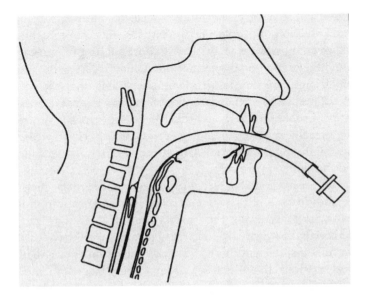

Figure 19.1.   Lateral view of an endotracheal tube.

below the larynx). Oral intubation interferes with communication in several ways. First, because the endotracheal tube passes through the oral cavity, it is impossible to articulate speech accurately. Second, because the endotracheal tube passes between the vocal folds, which are located in the larynx, it is impossible to produce sound (i.e., phonation). Thus, people who are orally intubated are unable to communicate using natural speech.

> When they put the tubes in, you get to the point of being helpless and you feel a need to communicate and talk to someone. You can't move. And you can't talk. And you want to say things. And you think, "Now I'd like to ask some more questions. You explained to me what's going on. But no, I want to know more now. What's going to happen?" And all you can really do is just lay there. That's when you really, really get spooked the most. (Mike S., a 46-year-old man who had Guillian-Barré syndrome, in Fried-Oken et al., 1991, p. 43)

An endotracheal tube may also pass through the nasal cavity into the trachea. Although in this case the tube does not interfere with articulation as occurs when it passes through the mouth, the endotracheal tube does pass between the vocal folds. Therefore, an individual is still unable to produce vocal sounds and efforts to communicate are limited to mouthing messages with the lips.

Tracheostomy

A tracheostomy is another way to transport air from a ventilator to an individual's respiratory system. It is a surgical opening from the front wall of the lower neck into the trachea (i.e., the airway below the larynx). Tracheostomies are usually performed at the level of the second or third tracheal ring. Generally, the opening of the tracheostomy is maintained by inserting a tube or button through the neck wall into the trachea. As illustrated in Figure 19.2, the tracheostomy tube curves to extend down into the trachea to keep it open for the movement of air. The ventilator attaches to the portion of the tube that extends anterior to the neck. An individual with a tracheostomy tube who depends on a ventilator has limited natural speech because air passes from the ventilator through the tube, rather than through the oral cavity and past the vocal folds.

Tracheostomy tubes remain in place when the individual no longer needs ventilator support to maintain an open airway or to permit suction of respiratory secretions. Nonetheless, air passes in and out of the trachea via the tracheostomy tube, bypassing the vocal folds. Thus, no phonation is possible, and messages must be mouthed. However, depending on the respiratory problem, some individuals who do not breathe with ventilator assistance are able to inhale through the tracheostomy tube, then occlude the tube with their fingers or an external valve and exhale through the larynx and the oral cavity. In this way, air moves past the vocal folds on exhalation, and they are able to produce sound and speak naturally. In other cases, individuals who can breathe on their own may be fitted with a tracheal button that maintains the tracheostomy through the neck wall. These in-

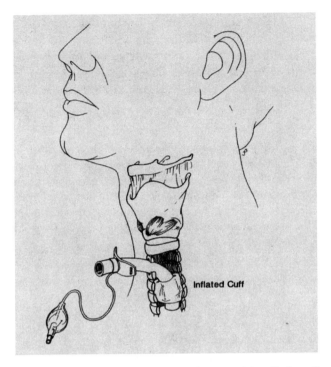

Inflated Cuff

Figure 19.2.   Lateral view of a cuffed tracheostomy tube with the cuff inflated.

dividuals can inhale through the button and then occlude the button with their finger or a valve to direct air past the vocal folds and produce speech.

AAC SERVICE DELIVERY IN ACUTE MEDICAL SETTINGS

> [His] messages were short but effective . . . I remember some of them clearly: Where am I, When, What happened, Move me up/down, Bedpan, More pillow, Get Nurse . . . It was clear that the perceptions of others were influenced by his communication performance . . . The portable typewriter (LightWRITER, ZYGO Industries) with voice output was essential in changing the way people talked to Barry and asked him questions. (Melanie Fried-Oken, 2001, writing about her husband's use of AAC in an ICU following a severe bicycling accident)

Because acute medical settings are so organizationally complex, on-site professionals usually provide the most effective ongoing AAC services. It is much more difficult for a consultant to come intermittently to a hospital to provide AAC services because the individual who requires them may be unavailable, too ill, resting, or receiving other medical treatments that take priority at the time of the consultant's visit. The core AAC team generally includes a speech-language pathologist, a physical therapist, and an occupational therapist who are employed by the hospital. In addition to their roles on the AAC team, these professionals may be responsible for other therapy needs of these individuals. They may consult with personnel from a regional AAC center or with a local AAC specialist in the area.

The delivery of AAC services in acute medical settings is structured differently from typical rehabilitation or educational settings. A successful AAC program in any given setting must accommodate factors specific to these settings in order to be accepted and used by patients and medical personnel.

Patient Issues

Individuals in acute medical settings have serious medical needs that are critical to their survival. The delivery of AAC services simply cannot interfere with the delivery of medical care. Such services must be integrated into the overall care plan for the individual.

The intensity of medical care affects the AAC program in a variety of ways. Medical staff are responsible for establishing and delivering an overall medical plan of which communication intervention may be a small part. Thus, the AAC staff cannot provide services without a request or referral from the medical team. The AAC team must clearly communicate the types of services they can deliver. They must consult with the medical team before and during AAC interventions to ensure that efforts coordinate well with the overall medical plan. If communication specialists do not follow these guidelines, they may fail to meet individuals' AAC needs.

Because individuals in acute medical settings receive such extensive medical support, it is common for as many as 10–25 different professionals as well as visiting family members and friends to have contact with each person during a 24-hour period. Thus, a variety of individuals must be able to understand AAC interventions. Signs on the walls, written messages, or verbal instructions must provide instructions for all these people. AAC interventions must be minimally complex and require minimal training and learning to be successful.

Medical Team Issues

Because nursing personnel are generally responsible for carrying out most day-to-day activities in the medical care plan, they have extensive contact with both individuals with complex communication needs and their family members. Thus, nurses are in an excellent position to assist the AAC team by monitoring an individual's status, coordinating AAC interventions with the medical care plan, documenting the individual's communication needs, and keeping family members informed of changes in the communication plan. The nursing coordinator often assumes the role of patient advocate during communication intervention and actively encourages physicians to request AAC services.

Respiratory therapists deal with a high proportion of the people in acute care units. These therapists are generally responsible for day-to-day management of individuals' respiratory status, including people with endotracheal or tracheostomy tubes. The AAC team must cooperate closely with respiratory therapists for successful intervention. Ongoing physician education is also important, especially in training hospitals where the staff consists of interns and residents as well as senior medical personnel. The AAC team may be invited to present their plan directly to the medical team. Instruction about AAC services, however, usually occurs in the context of ongoing service delivery.

Establishing an AAC Program

It is beyond the scope of this chapter to provide an extensive discussion regarding how to develop an AAC program in an intensive or acute care medical setting (see Costello, 2000, and Mitsuda, Baarslag-Benson, Hazel, & Therriault, 1992, for a detailed descriptions of this process). Mitsuda et al. (1992) noted that AAC teams should pay careful attention to individuals' equipment needs in acute care settings as well as to administrative, organizational, and personnel training issues. They suggested that the following equipment and materials form the basis for many AAC interventions in acute medical settings: 1) a lightweight neck-type electrolarynx (i.e., one that is positioned against the neck and vibrates the air column within the vocal tract); 2) an oral-type electrolarynx (i.e., one that delivers sound into the oral cavity through a tube); 3) materials to construct alphabet boards, word boards, and picture boards; 4) several magic slates (these are generally sold as toys and consist of a sheet of plastic over a piece of coated board that can be written on; when the plastic is lifted, written messages disappear); and 5) a portable mounting system on wheels to hold cardboard message boards or eye-pointing displays. These minimal equipment needs reflect the previously stated philosophy of simplifying AAC interventions in this area and are echoed by Dowden, Beukelman, and Lossing:

> Clinicians with very few communication augmentation systems can nonetheless serve ICU patients quite well . . . The majority of our patients were served with electrolarynges or . . . modified natural speech approaches. With additional access to the least expensive communication systems (plexiglas boards for eye-gaze, . . . paper and pencil, [and a few small typing systems]), we were able to serve all but a few of our patients. This means that even the smallest clinical program should consider serving patients in intensive care units. (1986, p. 43)

More extensive electronic AAC devices may be necessary for people who remain in long-term acute care settings.

AAC INTERVENTION MODEL

Communication specialists have not utilized the Participation Model (see Figure 6.1), which is described in detail in Chapters 6–8, for individuals in the acute medical setting. Instead, a Communication Needs Model has been used more commonly (Dowden, Honsinger, & Beukelman, 1986; Mitsuda et al., 1992). Nevertheless, the Participation Model can be used quite effectively in acute medical setting as the basis for an overall AAC program.

Identify Participation Patterns and Communication Needs

The Participation Model supports the overall delivery of AAC services to people in acute care environments. Interventionists can expect restricted participation patterns because individuals are limited to essentially one communication environment and have limited face-to-face contact with people in their social networks and are not working. However, communication over a telephone remains an option for some as does internet communication for some in long-term acute medical settings. Thus, most individuals in these settings have quite limited communication needs.

> She [a child] came back from the OR [operating room], and she immediately told me [using her AAC system] she needed to be suctioned. We got up all this gunk from her lungs, and otherwise we wouldn't have known she needed it until she was in distress. (An ICU nurse, quoted in Costello, 2000)

Assess Opportunity Barriers and Supports

Individuals in acute medical settings deserve to have access to AAC services to meet their restricted communication needs, and a lack of availability of AAC services can be considered to be an opportunity barrier. Few hospitals appear to have actual policies against AAC services; even so, AAC teams must deal with a number of practice or knowledge barriers. These barriers may include 1) medical teams that do not refer individuals for AAC services, 2) personnel who prefer not to be burdened with additional work in an already busy (and, perhaps, understaffed) workplace, and 3) speech-language pathologists and other professionals who are not familiar with conducting AAC interventions in these settings.

Assess Access Barriers and Capabilities

As with other AAC assessments, those that occur in acute care settings require considerations of specific access barriers and capabilities.

Assess Specific Capabilities: Preliminary Screening

Many individuals in acute medical settings are unable to participate in extensive assessment procedures. The AAC team should conduct a preliminary screening as the first step of an assessment to determine whether the individual is an appropriate candidate for a more complete evaluation (Dowden, Honsinger, et al., 1986). Tasks in the initial screening are shown in Figure 19.3. In order to respond to these tasks, the individual must be able to follow simple directions and have some way of indicating yes and no. This is often the first type of communication that develops between individuals and their staff or family members. Sometimes the first step in assessment is to isolate or identify a yes/no response. Medical teams rarely refer individuals for evaluation unless they can respond in this way.

Dowden, Honsinger, et al. described the use of the screening tasks in Figure 19.3 as follows:

> Patients are eliminated immediately if they are functional speakers or if they do not respond to either touch or their spoken name. Of those who are responsive, some may fail to pass the initial screening procedure, and are eliminated as too confused, agitated, or disoriented to cooperate with the communication augmentation intervention. (1986, p. 25)

Attending behaviors:

Attends to spoken name?   yes   no

Attends to "Look at me"?   yes   no

Orientation questions:

"Is your name (_____)?"   yes   no

"Is the current year (_____)?"   yes   no

"Is (_____) your home town?"   yes   no

"Are you married?"   yes   no

Single-step commands:

"Close your eyes."   yes   no

"Open your mouth."   yes   no

Figure 19.3.   Initial cognitive/linguistic screening tasks for ICU assessment. (From Dowden, P., Honsinger, M., & Beukelman, D. [1986]. Serving non-speaking people in acute care settings. *Augmentative and Alternative Communication, 2,* 31; reprinted by permission of Taylor & Francis Ltd, http://www.tandf.co.uk/journals.)

These authors reported that, of 42 individuals who completed six or more of the screening tasks, 9% were provided with "limited switch approaches" (i.e., electronic scanning devices) that met their communication needs, 53%–68% used oral or direct selection approaches that met their needs, and 70%–82% used several approaches simultaneously to meet their needs. Of eight individuals in their study who completed fewer than six tasks accurately, three did not receive AAC services because they died or were transferred to another hospital. The remaining five underwent further assessment, but the AAC team was completely unsuccessful in providing them with AAC techniques to meet their communication needs. Dowden, Beukelman, et al. drew two conclusions from these findings:

> First, it appears that the percentage of needs met may be related to the patient's cognitive status, as measured grossly by the cognitive screening tasks because on the average, more communication needs were met for Group 2 patients [i.e., those who passed six or more items] than Group 1 patients [i.e., those who passed fewer than six items]. Second, within Group 2, the percentage of needs met appears to change with the type of intervention. For example, it appears that serving patients with multiple systems meets, on the average, more communication needs than serving the patient with a single system. (1986, p. 43)

Extended Capability Assessment and AAC Intervention

Individuals who successfully complete preliminary screening tasks undergo a more extensive assessment of their capabilities. Mitsuda et al. (1992) provided a flowchart to guide

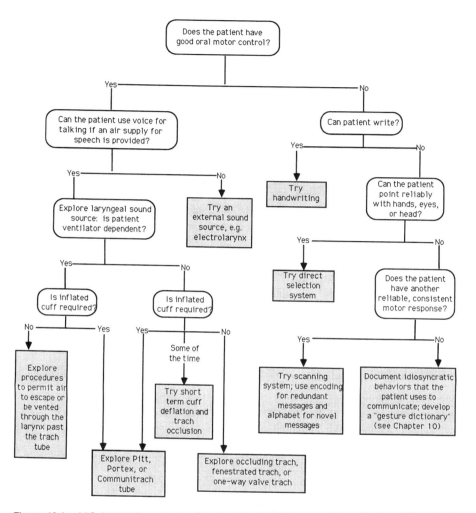

Figure 19.4. AAC intervention planning flowchart for intensive care unit applications. (Mitsuda, P., Baarslag-Benson, R., Hazel, K., & Therriault, T. [1992]. Augmentative communication in intensive and acute care settings. In K. Yorkston (Ed.), *Augmentative communication in the medical setting* (pp. 5–58). Tucson, AZ: Communication Skill Builders; adapted by permission.)

the decision-making process, which we have modified and present in Figure 19.4. Discussion of an extended capability assessment and related interventions follows.

People with Sufficient Oral-Motor Control for Speech   Many individuals in acute medical settings have sufficient motor control for speech, provided that they have an adequate sound source for voicing. Thus, the first step in evaluation should be assessment of oral-motor capabilities. If these are adequate to support speech, assessors should explore oral communication options. If oral-motor control is inadequate, assessors must explore other communication options.

Voicing Capabilities   Many individuals who have adequate oral-motor control for speech are unable to produce sound (i.e., voice) for one of several reasons. Some lack airflow past their vocal folds because of a tracheostomy but are able to produce vocal sounds if this airflow can be reestablished temporarily. Other individuals may experience severe respiratory problems or require ventilator supports that preclude any airflow past the vocal folds. We discuss interventions related to these two options later in this chapter.

Still other people may not have the motor control necessary to produce voicing. For these individuals, one of two types of electrolarynges often serves as an effective intervention device. A "neck-type" electrolarynx (see Figure 19.5) is positioned against the exterior neck wall and vibrates the air column within the vocal tract. "Mouthing words" then produces audible speech. The second, an oral-type electrolarynx (see Figure 19.6), delivers sound into the oral cavity through a tube or a catheter. The oral-type electrolarynx is useful for individuals who cannot use a neck-type electrolarynx due to extensive tissue damage, swelling, or surgical tenderness in the neck area or because they must wear cervical collars that obscure their necks.

Reestablishing the Airflow for Voicing   The first step in initiating an intervention to reestablish the flow of air past the vocal folds is to determine if the individual requires a cuffed tracheostomy tube and whether the cuff must be inflated. (A cuffed tracheostomy tube is shown in Figure 19.2.) The air supply for respiration passes through the cuffed tube into the lungs. The cuff around the tube inflates against the wall of the trachea to prevent air from escaping from the ventilator and lungs through the mouth and to prevent food or liquid from moving through the mouth and pharynx into the respiratory system. Many individuals require the cuff to be inflated at all times. Some devices, however, allow the airflow to be directed through the vocal folds on exhalation although the cuffed tracheostomy tube is in place. An external valve that directs the air stream usually operates these "talking tracheostomy" products. Individuals who can tolerate the deflation of their tracheostomy cuffs for brief periods may achieve phonation by allowing air to escape from the respiratory system past the deflated cuff and vocal folds. They are able to produce natural speech in this way.

Another option is to use a tracheostomy tube that does not involve a cuff. This option may be appropriate for someone who requires a tracheostomy to maintain an open

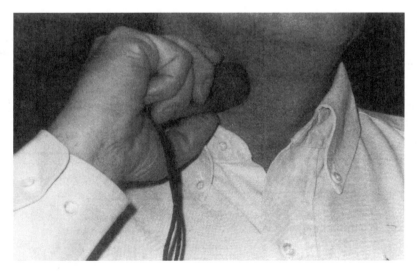

Figure 19.5.   A neck-type (Romet) electrolarynx.

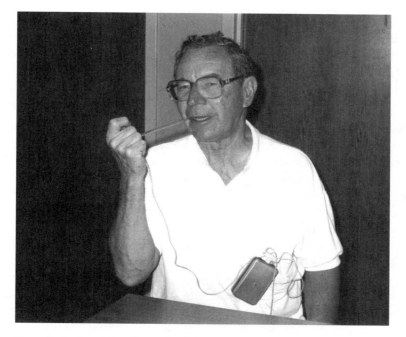

Figure 19.6.   An oral-type (CooperRand) electrolarynx.

airway because of swelling or trauma to the neck area but who does not depend on a ventilator. In this case, the individual can direct air past the vocal folds by 1) learning to occlude the tube with a finger during exhalation, 2) utilizing a fenestrated tracheostomy tube that has an opening on the top in the trachea, or 3) using a one-way valve that permits inhalation through the tube and exhalation through the vocal tract.

Individuals with Insufficient Oral-Motor Control for Speech   The flowchart assessment (see Figure 19.4) may reveal insufficient oral-motor control for speech. If this is the case, individuals may require communication systems that use writing, direct selection, and/or scanning, as discussed in the following sections.

Writing Options   Handwriting can serve as an effective communication mode because many people are comfortable and familiar with this mode of communication. Some individuals prefer to use a pencil and tablet so that as they write and save messages, they can begin to construct their own communication book. Then, rather than writing the same message again and again, they can simply refer to a question or a comment they have communicated previously. Others prefer to use a magic slate so that they can erase messages when they are finished and thus maintain privacy.

I think that board [a magic slate] was my preference over everything. You could communicate quickly and say what you wanted to say. You can write your letters and separate your words, like in normal writing. And it was much quicker and easier to understand by other people. I think they probably like it the best, too. So the Magic board was the best one, once I could start using my hands again.

> When I was unable to use my hands, of course the alphabet board [for dependent scanning] was the best, assuming that the other person understood how to use it, which many didn't. (Alec K., a 35-year-old man who had GBS, in Fried-Oken et al., 1991, p. 47)

Options for People Who Cannot Write   Some individuals are unable to write by hand, but they can point accurately with their hands, eyes, or head. AAC teams generally encourage these individuals to use a direct selection communication system. This direct selection system can be as simple as an alphabet board with some words or phrases on it. Other individuals may prefer a small typing system. Usually, individuals in acute medical settings do not have the time or motivation to use an encoding strategy. Therefore, some prefer to type their messages.

If available, voice output may be preferred by some individuals. Costello (2000) described the use of "voice banking" for children scheduled in advance for major surgical procedures such as facial reconstruction. Prior to their surgeries, the children recorded messages that were later transferred to simple speech-generating devices (SGDs) that they used in ICU. Thus, the children were able to use "their own voices" to "talk" during this difficult and stressful time. Small, portable, digitized SGDs that contain 30–60 easily accessible messages are convenient for this purpose. If the individual has insufficient hand or arm control to use these options, he or she may use a headlight pointer to indicate words or letters on a wall or ceiling chart or on a communication board placed on a mounting stand.

> George was unable to communicate, except to move his head slightly side-to-side to signal no and to point with his eyes. With a diagnosis of severe myasthenia gravis, he faced an extended hospital stay. An observant nurse informed us that he could move his right foot a bit, so we mounted a safe-laser device on his big toe and a communication device at the foot of his bed. With his head propped up slightly so he could see the device, George spelled his messages by moving his foot. Six weeks later, he recovered sufficiently to return home, speaking once again.

Some individuals may be limited to eye pointing in one of two forms. The first form is conventional eye pointing, in which the individual selects and gazes at a message on a display that is mounted on a transparent plastic board. The communication partner then interprets the direction of the individual's eye gaze and reads the related message. The second form, a technique known as *eye linking*, may be used. In eye linking, the individual looks at the desired message, and the partner (who is positioned opposite the individual on the other side of the transparent communication board) moves the board until his or her eyes are "linked" directly across from the individual's. At that point, the message that the individual wants to convey lies between the two people. Many individuals find this to be easier than eye pointing.

Options for People Who Cannot Use Direct Selection   Some individuals do not have the motor capability to engage in direct selection communication. If they have other reliable, consistent motor responses, individuals may be able to successfully use a scanning communication option. Many families can learn to use dependent scanning, in which an array of letters or messages is displayed on a communication board. The communication partner points to various message options, and the individual sends a yes signal when a desired message is reached by making a gesture or eye blink or by activating a beeper with a switch. Independent (i.e., electronic) scanning is more difficult to implement in these settings, and, as noted previously, this difficulty may cause a low rate of success with this option (Dowden, Beukelman, et al., 1986). Most individuals generally are unfamiliar with this type of communication, and the learning requirements for scanning may be too great for effective application of this option in acute medical environments.

Assess Constraints

The two most common constraints that affect AAC interventions are related to funding and listener instruction. We discuss these briefly in the following sections.

Funding

Individuals encounter different constraints in acute medical settings than those experienced by individuals in other environments. Fortunately, the same resources that are responsible for hospitalization fees usually fund all medical-related services, including AAC services.

Instruction of Listeners

The short-term acute medical environment imposes quite extensive learning constraints. First, individuals are very ill and under a considerable amount of stress. Many individuals in these settings demonstrate little ability or tolerance for learning. Second, many professionals and others interact with these individuals over the course of their stay. Thus, the most effective AAC interventions are those that require minimal listener training. As noted previously, individuals and their medical teams tend not to use complicated AAC systems in short-term acute medical environments.

References

AAC Feature Match [Computer software]. (1996). Arlington, TX: Doug Dodgen & Associates.

AAT Assessment Tool [Computer software]. (1998). Arlington, TX: Doug Dodgen & Associates.

Abdala, C. (1999). Pediatric audiology: Evaluating infants. In D. Chen (Ed.), *Essential elements in early intervention* (pp. 246–284). New York: AFB Press.

Adams, L. (1998). Oral-motor and motor-speech characteristics of children with autism. *Focus on Autism and Other Developmental Disabilities, 13,* 108–112.

Adams, M.J. (1990). *Beginning to read: Thinking and learning about print.* Cambridge, MA: MIT Press.

Adamson, L., & Dunbar, B. (1991). Communication development of young children with tracheostomies. *Augmentative and Alternative Communication, 7,* 275–283.

Alant, E. (1993). *Towards community-based communication intervention for severely handicapped children.* Pretoria, South Africa: Human Sciences Research Council.

Alant, E. (1996). Augmentative and alternative communication in developing countries: Challenge of the future. *Augmentative and Alternative Communication, 12,* 1–12.

Alant, E. (1999). Students with little or no functional speech in schools for students with mental retardation in South Africa. *Augmentative and Alternative Communication, 15,* 83–94.

Alant, E., & Emmett, T. (1995). *Breaking the silence: Communication and education for children with severe handicaps.* Pretoria, South Africa: Human Sciences Research Council.

Alant, E., & Lloyd, L.L. (2005). *Augmentative and alternative communication: Beyond poverty.* London: Whurr Publishers.

Alm, N., Gowans, G., Astell, A., Dye, R., Campbell, J., & Ellis, M. (2003). *Helping people with dementia to have a satisfying conversation with a multi-media communication system.* Proceedings of Communication Matters CM2003 National Symposium (p. 910), September 14–16, 2003, Lancaster University.

Alm, N., & Parnes, P. (1995). Augmentative and alternative communication: Past, present, and future. *Folia Phoniatrica et Logopaedica, 47,* 165–192.

Alper, S. (2003). The relationship between inclusion and other trends in education. In D. Ryndak & S. Alper (Eds.), *Curriculum and instruction for students with significant disabilities in inclusive settings* (2nd ed., pp. 13–30). Boston: Allyn & Bacon.

Alzheimer's Association, Inc. (2001). *An overview of Alzheimer's disease and related dementias.* Retrieved from http://www.alz.org

American Psychiatric Association. (1994). *Diagnostic and statistical manual of mental disorders* (4th ed.). Washington, DC: Author.

American Speech-Language-Hearing Association. (2004). Roles and responsibilities of speech-language pathologists with respect to augmentative and alternative communication: Technical report. *ASHA Supplement, 24,* 1–17.

American Speech-Language-Hearing Association. (2005). *Roles and responsibilities of speech-language pathologists with respect to alternative communication: Position statement.* Retrieved from http://www.asha.org/NR/rdonlyres/BA19B90C-1C17-4230-86A8-83B4E12E4365/0/v3PSaac.pdf

Americans with Disabilities Act of 1990, PL 101-336, 42 U.S.C. §§ 12101 *et seq.*

Anderson, R.C., Hiebert, E.H., Scott, J.A., & Wilkinson, I.A.G. (1985). *Becoming a nation of readers: The report of the commission on reading.* Washington, DC: The National Institute of Education.

Andrews-Salvia, M., Roy, N., & Cameron, R.M. (2003). Evaluating the effects of memory books for individuals with severe dementia. *Journal of Medical Speech-Language Pathology, 11*(1), 51–59.

Angelo, D. (1998). Impact of augmentative and alternative communication devices on families. *Augmentative and Alternative Communication, 16,* 37–47.

Angelo, D., Jones, S., & Kokoska, S. (1995). Family perspective on augmentative and alternative communication: Families of young children. *Augmentative and Alternative Communication, 11,* 193–201.

Angelo, D., Kokoska, S., & Jones, S. (1996). Family perspective on augmentative and alternative communication: Families of adolescents and young adults. *Augmentative and Alternative Communication, 12,* 13–22.

Angelo, J. (1987). *A comparison of three coding methods for abbreviation expansion in acceleration vocabularies.* Unpublished doctoral dissertation, University of Wisconsin–Madison.

Aram, D., & Nation, J. (1982). *Child language.* St. Louis: Mosby.

Arnott, J., & Javed, M. (1992). Probabilistic character disambiguation for reduced keyboards using small text samples. *Augmentative and Alternative Communication, 8,* 215–223.

Assistive Technology Act Amendments of 2004, PL 105-394, 29 U.S.C. §§ 3001 *et seq.*

Assistive Technology Assessment Questionnaire. (2002). Retrieved February 24, 2004, from http://www.techconnections.org/training/march2002/AssessProtocol.pdf

Assistive Technology Inc. (1999). EvaluWare™ [Computer software]. Newton, MA: Author.

Atwell, N. (1987). *In the middle: Writing, reading, and learning with adolescents.* Portsmouth, NH: Boynton/Cook.

Ault, M., Guy, B., Guess, D., Bashinski, S., & Roberts, S. (1995). Analyzing behavior state and learning environments: Application in instructional settings. *Mental Retardation, 33,* 304–326.

Autism Society of America. (2004). *Common characteristics of autism.* Retrieved May 20, 2004, from http://www.autism-society.org/

Bailey, B., & Downing, J. (1994). Using visual accents to enhance attending to communication symbols for students with severe multiple disabilities. *RE:view, 26*(3), 101–118.

Bak, T.H., & Hodges, J.R. (2001). Motor neuron disease, dementia and aphasia: Coincidence, co-occurrence or continuum? *Journal of Neurology, 248,* 260–270.

Baker, B. (1982, September). Minspeak: A semantic compaction system that makes self-expression easier for communicatively disabled individuals. *Byte, 7,* 186–202.

Baker, B. (1986). Using images to generate speech. *Byte, 11,* 160–168.

Baker, K., & Chaparro, C. (2003). *Schedule it! Sequence it!* Solana Beach. CA: Mayer-Johnson, Inc.

Balandin, S., & Iacono, T. (1998a). A few well-chosen words. *Augmentative and Alternative Communication, 14,* 147–161.

Balandin, S., & Iacono, T. (1998b). Topics of meal-break conversations. *Augmentative and Alternative Communication, 14,* 131–146.

Balandin, S., & Morgan, J. (2001). Preparing for the future: Aging and augmentative and alternative communication. *Augmentative and Alternative Communication, 17,* 99–108.

Ball, L. (2003). AAC transition for adults: Maximizing communication and participation. *ASHA Leader, 8,* 141.

Ball, L., Beukelman, D.R., & Pattee, G. (2001). A protocol for identification of early bulbar signs in ALS. *Journal of Neurological Sciences, 191,* 43–53.

Ball, L., Beukelman, D.R., & Pattee, G. (2002). Timing of speech deterioration in people with amyotrophic lateral sclerosis. *Journal of Medical Speech-Language Pathology, 10,* 231–235.

Ball, L., Beukelman, D.R., & Pattee, G. (2003, November). *AAC transitions for adults I: Maximizing communication and participation (AAC transitions for persons with ALS).* Presentation at the annual convention of the American Speech-Language-Hearing Association, Chicago, IL.

Ball, L., Beukelman, D.R., & Pattee, G. (2004). Acceptance of augmentative and alternative communication technology by persons with amyotrophic lateral sclerosis. *Augmentative and Alternative Communication, 20*, 113–122.

Ball, L., Marvin, C., Beukelman, D.R., Lasker, J., & Rupp, D. (1997). *"Generic small talk" use by preschool children.* Manuscript submitted for publication, University of Nebraska–Lincoln.

Bambara, L., Spiegel-McGill, P., Shores, R., & Fox, J. (1984). A comparison of reactive and nonreactive toys on severely handicapped children's manipulative play. *Journal of The Association for Persons with Severe Handicaps, 9*, 142–149.

Banajee, M., Dicarlo, C., & Stricklin, S. (2003). Core vocabulary determination for toddlers. *Augmentative and Alternative Communication, 19*, 67–73.

Bankson, N., & Bernthal, J. (1990). *Bankson–Bernthal Test of Phonology.* Austin, TX: PRO-ED.

Barraga, N. (2001). *Visual handicaps and learning* (4th ed.). Austin, TX: Exceptional Resources.

Barrera, R., Lobato-Barrera, D., & Sulzer-Azaroff, B. (1980). A simultaneous treatment comparison of three expressive language training programs with a mute autistic child. *Journal of Autism and Developmental Disorders, 10*, 21–38.

Barritt, L., & Kroll, B. (1978). Some implications of cognitive developmental psychology for research in composing. In C. Cooper & L. Odell (Eds.), *Research on composing: Points of departure* (pp. 49–57). Urbana, IL: National Council of Teachers of English.

Bashir, A., Grahamjones, F., & Bostwick, R. (1984). A touch-cue method of therapy for developmental verbal apraxia. *Seminars in Speech and Language, 5*(2), 127–128.

Basil, C. (1992). Social interaction and learned helplessness in severely disabled children. *Augmentative and Alternative Communication, 8*, 188–199.

Basil, C., & Soro-Camats, E. (1996). Supporting graphic language acquisition by a girl with multiple impairments. In S. von Tetzchner & M.H. Jensen (Eds.), *Augmentative and alternative communication: European perspectives* (pp. 270–291). London: Whurr Publishers.

Bates, E. (1979). *The emergence of symbols: Cognition and communication in infancy.* San Diego: Academic Press.

Batshaw, M.L., & Shapiro, B. (2002). Mental retardation. In M.L. Batshaw (Ed.), *Children with disabilities* (5th ed., pp. 287–305). Baltimore: Paul H. Brookes Publishing Co.

Bauby, J.-D. (1997). *The diving bell and the butterfly* (Jeremy Leggatt, Trans). New York: Alfred A. Knopf.

Bauer, A.M., & Matuszek, K. (2001). Designing and evaluating accommodations and adaptations. In A.M. Bauer & G.M. Brown (Eds.), *Adolescents and inclusion: Transforming secondary schools* (pp. 139–166). Baltimore: Paul H. Brookes Publishing Co.

Baumann, J.F., Hoffman, J.V., Duffy-Hester, A.M., & Moon Ro, J. (2000). The first R yesterday and today: U.S. elementary reading instruction practices reported by teachers and administrators. *Reading Research Quarterly, 35*(3), 338–377.

Baumann, J.F., Hoffman, J.V., Moon Ro, J., & Duffy-Hester, A.M. (1998). Where are the teachers' voices in the phonics/whole language debate? Results from a survey of U.S. elementary classroom teachers. *The Reading Teacher, 51*(8), 636–650.

Baumgart, D., Johnson, J., & Helmstetter, E. (1990). *Augmentative and alternative communication systems for persons with moderate and severe disabilities.* Baltimore: Paul H. Brookes Publishing Co.

Bayles, K.A., & Kim, E.S. (2003). Improving the functioning of individuals with Alzheimer's disease: Emergence of behavioral interventions. *Journal of Communication Disorders, 36*, 327–343.

Bayles, K.A., & Tomoeda, C.K. (1998a). *Improving the ability of Alzheimer's patients to communicate.* Phoenix, AZ: Canyonlands Publishing.

Bayles, K.A., & Tomoeda, C.K. (1998b). *Understanding the communication problems of Alzheimer's patients* [Videotape]. Phoenix, AZ: Canyonlands Publishing.

Bayles, K., Tomoeda, C., Wood, J., Montgomery, E., Cruz, R., Azuma, T., & McGeagh, A. (1996). Changes in cognitive function in idiopathic Parkinson's disease. *Archives of Neurology, 53*, 1140–1146.

Beck, A., Bock, S., Thompson, J., & Kosuwan, K. (2002). Influence of communicative competence and augmentative and alternative communication technique on children's attitudes toward a peer who uses AAC. *Augmentative and Alternative Communication, 18*, 217–227.

Beck, A., & Dennis, M. (1996). Attitudes of children toward a similar-aged child who uses augmentative communication. *Augmentative and Alternative Communication, 12,* 78–87.

Beck, A., & Fritz, H. (1998). Can people with aphasia learn iconic codes? *Augmentative and Alternative Communication, 14,* 184–195.

Beck, A., Fritz, H., Keller, A., & Dennis, M. (2000). Attitudes of school-aged children toward their peers who use AAC. *Augmentative and Alternative Communication, 16,* 13–26.

Beck, A., & Fritz-Verticchio, H. (2003). The influence of information and role-playing experiences on children's attitudes toward peers who use AAC. *American Journal of Speech-Language Pathology, 12,* 51–60.

Beck, A., Kingsbury, K., Neff, A., & Dennis, M. (2000). Influence of length of augmented message on children's attitudes towards peers who use augmentative and alternative communication. *Augmentative and Alternative Communication, 16,* 239–249.

Beck, A., Thompson, J., & Clay, S. (2000). The effect of icon prediction on college students' recall of icon codes. *Journal of Special Education Technology, 15,* 17–23.

Beckman, P., & Kohl, F. (1984). The effects of social and isolated toys on the interactions and play of integrated and nonintegrated groups of preschoolers. *Education and Training of the Mentally Retarded, 19,* 169–174.

Bedrosian, J. (1997). Language acquisition in young AAC system users: Issues and directions for future research. *Augmentative and Alternative Communication, 13,* 179–185.

Bedrosian, J. (1999). AAC efficacy research: Challenges for the new century. *Augmentative and Alternative Communication, 15,* 2–3.

Bedrosian, J., Hoag, L., Calculator, S., & Molineux, B. (1992). Variables influencing perceptions of the communicative competence of an adult augmentative and alternative communication system user. *Journal of Speech and Hearing Research, 35,* 1105–1113.

Bedrosian, J., Hoag, L., Johnson, D., & Calculator, S. (1998). Communicative competence as perceived by adults with severe speech impairments associated with cerebral palsy. *Journal of Speech, Language, and Hearing Research, 41,* 667–675.

Bedrosian, J., Hoag, L., & McCoy, K. (2003). Relevance and speed of message delivery trade-offs in augmentative and alternative communication. *Journal of Speech, Language, and Hearing Research, 46,* 800–817.

Bellugi, U., & Fischer, S. (1972). A comparison of sign language and spoken language. *Cognition, 1,* 173–200.

Bereiter, C. (1980). Development in writing. In L.W. Gregg & E.R. Steinberg (Eds.), *Cognitive processes in writing* (pp. 73–93). Hillsdale, NJ: Lawrence Erlbaum Associates.

Berlowitz, C. (1991, January 13). Ana begins to speak. *This World,* 16.

Berninger, V.W. (2000). Development of language by hand and its connections with language by ear, mouth, and eye. *Topics in Language Disorders, 20*(4), 65–84.

Berninger, V., & Gans, B. (1986). Language profiles in nonspeaking individuals of normal intelligence with severe cerebral palsy. *Augmentative and Alternative Communication, 2,* 45–50.

Bernthal, J., & Bankson, N. (1988). *Articulation and phonological disorders* (2nd ed.). Upper Saddle River, NJ: Prentice Hall.

Beukelman, D.R. (1987). When you have a hammer, everything looks like a nail. *Augmentative and Alternative Communication, 3,* 94–95.

Beukelman, D.R. (1991). Magic and cost of communicative competence. *Augmentative and Alternative Communication, 7,* 2–10.

Beukelman, D.R. (with Garrett, K.L.). (1998). Adults with severe aphasia. In D.R. Beukelman & P. Mirenda, *Augmentative and alternative communication: Management of severe communication disorders in children and adults* (pp. 465–499). Baltimore: Paul H. Brookes Publishing Co.

Beukelman, D.R., Ball, L., & Pattee, G. (2004). Intervention decision making for persons with amyotrophic lateral sclerosis. *ASHA Leader, 9,* 4–5.

Beukelman, D.R., Burke, R., Ball, L., & Horn, C. (2002). Augmentative and alternative communication technology learning, Part 2: Preprofessional students. *Augmentative & Alternative Communication, 18,* 250–254.

Beukelman, D.R., Fager, S., Ball, L., Prentice, C., Jakobs, T., & Caves, K. (2003). New AAC interfaces: Field test results. *ASHA Leader, 8*, 144.

Beukelman, D.R., Fager, S., Ullman, C., Hanson, E., & Logemann, J. (2002). The impact of speech
supplementation and clear speech on the intelligibility and speaking rate of people with traumatic brain injury. *Journal of Medical Speech-Language Pathology, 10*, 237–242.

Beukelman, D.R., & Garrett, K. (1988). Augmentative and alternative communication for adults
with acquired severe communication disorders. *Augmentative and Alternative Communication, 4*,
104–121.

Beukelman, D.R., Hanson, E., Hiatt, E., Fager, S., & Bilyeu, D. (in press). AAC technology learning: Part 3—Regular AAC team members. *Augmentative and Alternative Communication.*

Beukelman, D.R., Jones, R., & Rowan, M. (1989). Frequency of word usage by nondisabled peers
in integrated preschool classrooms. *Augmentative and Alternative Communication, 5*, 243–248.

Beukelman, D.R., Kraft, G., & Freal, J. (1985). Expressive communication disorders in persons
with multiple sclerosis: A survey. *Archives of Physical Medicine and Rehabilitation, 66*, 675–677.

Beukelman, D.R., & Mirenda, P. (1988). Communication options for persons who cannot speak:
Assessment and evaluation. In C.A. Coston (Ed.), *Proceedings of the National Planners Conference
on Assistive Device Service Delivery* (pp. 151–165). Washington, DC: Association for the Advancement of Rehabilitation Technology.

Beukelman, D.R., & Yorkston, K. (1977). A communication system for the severely dysarthric
speaker with an intact language system. *Journal of Speech and Hearing Disorders, 42*, 265–270.

Beukelman, D.R., & Yorkston, K. (1978). A series of communication options for individuals with
brain stem lesions. *Archives of Physical Medicine and Rehabilitation, 59*, 337–342.

Beukelman, D.R., & Yorkston, K. (1984). Computer enhancement of message formulation and presentation for communication augmentation system users. *Seminars in Speech and Language, 5*, 1–10.

Beukelman, D.R., & Yorkston, K. (Eds.). (1991). Traumatic brain injury changes the way we live.
In *Communication disorders following traumatic brain injury: Management of cognitive, language, and
motor impairments* (pp. 1–14). Austin, TX: PRO-ED.

Beukelman, D.R., Yorkston, K., & Dowden, P. (1985). *Communication augmentation: A casebook of clinical management.* Austin, TX: PRO-ED.

Beukelman, D.R., Yorkston, K., Poblete, M., & Naranjo, C. (1984). Frequency of word occurrence
in communication samples produced by adult communication aid users. *Journal of Speech and
Hearing Disorders, 49*, 360–367.

Bevan-Brown, J. (2001). Evaluating special education services for learners from ethnically diverse
groups: Getting it right. *Journal of The Association for Persons with Severe Handicaps, 26*, 138–147.

Biklen, D. (1990). Communication unbound: Autism and praxis. *Harvard Educational Review, 60*,
291–314.

Biklen, D. (1992). *Schooling without labels.* Philadelphia: Temple University Press.

Biklen, D. (1993). *Communication unbound.* New York: Teachers College Press.

Biklen, D. (1996). No time for silence. *TASH Newsletter, 22*(12), 20–23.

Biklen, D., & Cardinal, D. (1997). *Contested words, contested science: Unraveling the facilitated communication controversy.* New York: Teachers College Press.

Binger, C., & Light, J. (2003, November). *Grammar assessment and intervention with individuals who
use AAC.* Paper presented at the annual convention of the American Speech-Language-Hearing
Association, Chicago, IL.

Bird, F., Dores, P., Moniz, D., & Robinson, J. (1989). Reducing severe aggressive and self-injurious
behaviors with functional communication training. *American Journal on Mental Retardation, 94*,
37–48.

Bishop, D.V.M., Byers Brown, B., & Robson, J. (1990). The relationship between phoneme discrimination, speech production, and language comprehension in cerebral-palsied individuals.
Journal of Speech and Hearing Research, 33, 210–219.

Bishop, D.V.M., & Robson, J. (1989a). Accurate non-word spelling despite congenital inability to
speak: Phoneme-grapheme conversion does not require subvocal articulation. *British Journal of
Psychology, 80*, 1–13.

Bishop, D.V.M., & Robson, J. (1989b). Unimpaired short-term memory and rhyme judgment in congenitally speechless individuals: Implications for the notion of "articulatory coding." *Quarterly Journal of Experimental Psychology, 40A*, 123–140.

Bishop, D. (2003). *Test for Reception of Grammar–Version 2 (TROG-2)*. San Antonio, TX: Harcourt Assessment.

Bishop, K., Rankin, J., & Mirenda, P. (1994). Impact of graphic symbol use on reading acquisition. *Augmentative and Alternative Communication, 10*, 113–125.

Blackburn, D., Bonvillian, J., & Ashby, R. (1984). Manual communication as an alternative mode of language instruction for children with severe reading disabilities. *Language, Speech, and Hearing Services in Schools, 15*, 22–31.

Blackman, L. (1999). *Lucy's story: Autism & other adventures*. Brisbane, Australia: Book in Hand.

Blackstien-Adler, S. (2003). *Training school teams to use the Participation Model: Evaluation of a train-the-trainer model*. Unpublished master's thesis, Ontario Institute for the Study of Education, University of Toronto.

Blackstone, S. (1989a). For consumers: Societal rehabilitation. *Augmentative Communication News, 2*(3), 1–3.

Blackstone, S. (1989b). M & Ms: Meaningful, manageable measurement. *Augmentative Communication News, 2*(3), 3–5.

Blackstone, S. (1989c). The 3 R's: Reading, writing, and reasoning. *Augmentative Communication News, 2*(1), 1–6, 8.

Blackstone, S. (1990). Populations and practices in AAC. *Augmentative Communication News, 3*(4), 1–3.

Blackstone, S. (1991). Telecommunication technologies. *Augmentative Communication News, 4*(4), 3–8.

Blackstone, S. (1993). Cultural sensitivity and AAC services. *Augmentative Communication News, 6*(2), 3–5.

Blackstone, S. (1994a). Auditory scanning. *Augmentative Communication News, 7*(2), 6–7.

Blackstone, S. (1994b). Equipment loan programs: A rationale. *Augmentative Communication News, 7*(1), 4.

Blackstone, S. (1997). Time study and caseload allocation: Three examples. *Augmentative Communication News, 9*(5), 1–8.

Blackstone, S. (2001). Assessment protocol for SGDs. *Augmentative Communication News, 13*(6) and *14*(1), 1–16.

Blackstone, S. (2002). On the web: EBP websites. *Augmentative Communication News, 14*(4 and 5), 4–5.

Blackstone, S. (2004). Clinical news: Visual scene displays. *Augmentative Communication News, 16*(2), 1–8.

Blackstone, S.W., Cassatt-James, E.L., & Bruskin, D. (Eds.). (1988). *Augmentative communication: Implementation strategies*. Rockville, MD: American Speech-Language-Hearing Association.

Blackstone, S., & Hunt Berg, M. (2003a). *Social networks: A communication inventory for individuals with complex communication needs and their communication partners—Inventory Booklet*. Monterey, CA: Augmentative Communication, Inc.

Blackstone, S., & Hunt Berg, M. (2003b). *Social networks: A communication inventory for individuals with complex communication needs and their communication partners—Manual*. Monterey, CA: Augmentative Communication, Inc.

Blackstone, S., & Pressman, H. (1995). *Outcomes in AAC conference report: Alliance '95*. Monterey, CA: Augmentative Communication.

Blackstone, S., Williams, M., & Joyce, M. (2002). Future AAC technology needs: Consumer perspectives. *Assistive Technology, 14*, 3–16.

Blischak, D. (1994). Phonologic awareness: Implications for individuals with little or no functional speech. *Augmentative and Alternative Communication, 10*, 245–254.

Blischak, D.M. (1995). Thomas the writer: Case study of a child with severe speech and physical impairments. *Language Speech and Hearing Services in Schools, 25*, 11–20.

Blischak, D., Lombardino, L., & Dyson, A. (2003). Use of speech generating devices: In support of natural speech. *Augmentative and Alternative Communication, 19*, 29–36.

Bliss, C. (1965). *Semantography*. Sydney, Australia: Semantography Publications.

Blissymbolics Communication International. (1984). *Picture your Blissymbols*. Toronto: Author.

Blockberger, S. (1995). AAC intervention and early conceptual and lexical development. *Journal of Speech-Language Pathology and Audiology, 19*, 221–232.

Blockberger, S., Armstrong, R., & O'Connor, A. (1993). Children's attitudes toward a nonspeaking child using various augmentative and alternative communication techniques. *Augmentative and Alternative Communication, 9*, 243–250.

Blockberger, S., & Johnston, J. (2003). Grammatical morphology acquisition by children with complex communication needs. *Augmentative and Alternative Communication, 19*, 207–221.

Blockberger, S., & Kamp, L. (1990). The use of voice output communication aids (VOCAs) by ambulatory children. *Augmentative and Alternative Communication, 6*, 127–128.

Blockberger, S., & Sutton, A. (2003). Toward linguistic competence: Language experiences and knowledge of children with extremely limited speech. In J.C. Light, D.R. Beukelman, & J. Reichle (Eds.), *Communicative competence for individuals who use AAC: From research to effective practice* (pp. 63–106). Baltimore: Paul H. Brookes Publishing Co.

Bloomberg, K. (1990). Computer pictographs for communication. *Communication Outlook, 12*(1), 17–18.

Bloomberg, K. (1996). *PrAACtically speaking* [Videotape]. Melbourne, Australia: Yooralla Society.

Bloomberg, K., & Johnson, H. (1990). A statewide demographic survey of people with severe communication impairments. *Augmentative and Alternative Communication, 6*, 50–60.

Bloomberg, K., Karlan, G., & Lloyd, L. (1990). The comparative translucency of initial lexical items represented by five graphic symbol systems and sets. *Journal of Speech and Hearing Research, 33*, 717–725.

Bloomberg, K., & West, D. (1999). *The Triple C: Manual and video*. Box Hill, Victoria, BC: Scope Communication Resource Centre.

Bloomberg, K., West, D., Johnson, H., & Caithness, T. (2001). *InterAACtion strategies for intentional communicators* [Videotape]. St. Kilda, Victoria, Australia: Severe Communication Impairment Outreach Program.

Boden, D., & Bielby, D. (1983). The way it was: Topical organization in elderly conversation. *Language and Communication, 6*(1/2), 73–79.

Bogdan, R., & Taylor, S. (1994). *The social meaning of mental retardation: Two life stories*. New York: Teachers College Press.

Bölte, S., & Poustka, F. (2002). The relation between general cognitive level and adaptive behavior domains in individuals with autism with and without co-morbid mental retardation. *Child Psychiatry & Human Development, 33*, 165–172.

Bolton, S., & Dashiell, S. (1991). *Interaction Checklist for Augmentative Communication—Revised Edition*. Austin, TX: PRO-ED.

Bondy, A., & Frost, L. (1994). The Picture Exchange Communication System. *Focus on Autistic Behavior, 9*, 1–19.

Bondy, A., & Frost, L. (1998). The Picture Exchange Communication System. *Topics in Language Disorders, 19*, 373–390.

Bondy, A., & Frost, L. (2001). *A picture's worth: PECS and other visual communication strategies in autism*. Bethesda, MD: Woodbine.

Bonvillian, J., & Friedman, R. (1978). Language development in another mode: The acquisition of signs by a brain-damaged adult. *Sign Language Studies, 19*, 111–120.

Bonvillian, J., & Nelson, K. (1978). Development of sign language in autistic children and other language-handicapped individuals. In P. Siple (Ed.), *Understanding language through sign language research* (pp. 187–209). New York: Academic Press.

Bonvillian, J., & Siedlecki, T., Jr. (1996). Young children's acquisition of the location aspect of American Sign Language: Parental report findings. *Journal of Communication Disorders, 29*, 13–35.

Bonvillian, J., & Siedlecki, T., Jr. (1998). Young children's acquisition of the movement aspect of American Sign Language: Parental report findings. *Journal of Speech, Language, and Hearing Research, 41*, 588–602.

Bopp, K., Brown, K., & Mirenda, P. (2004). Speech-language pathologists' roles in the delivery of positive behavior support for individuals with developmental disabilities. *American Journal of Speech-Language Pathology, 13,* 5–19.

Bornman, J., & Alant, E. (1999). Training teachers to facilitate interaction with autistic children using digital voice output devices. *South African Journal of Education, 19,* 364–373.

Bornman, J., Alant, E., & Meiring, E. (2001). The use of a digital voice output device to facilitate language development in a child with developmental apraxia of speech: A case study. *Disability and Rehabilitation, 23,* 623–634.

Bornstein, H. (1990). Signed English. In H. Bornstein (Ed.), *Manual communication: Implications for education* (pp. 128–138). Washington, DC: Gallaudet University Press.

Bornstein, H., Saulnier, L., & Hamilton, L. (1983). *The comprehensive Signed English dictionary.* Washington, DC: Gallaudet University Press.

Bourgeois, M. (1990). Caregiver training, generalization, and maintenance of communicative behaviors in patients with Alzheimer's disease. Treatment efficacy research in communication disorders. *Asha, 32,* 65.

Bourgeois, M.S. (1992). Evaluating memory wallets in conversation with persons with dementia. *Journal of Speech and Hearing Research, 35*(6), 1344–1357.

Bourgeois, M.S. (1993). Effects of memory aids on the dyadic conversation of individuals with dementia. *Journal of Applied Behavior Analysis, 26,* 77–87.

Bourgeois, M.S. (1996). Memory wallet intervention in an adult day-care setting. *Behavioral Interventions, 11*(1), 3–18.

Bourgeois, M.S., Camp, C., Rose, M., White, B., Malone, M., Carr, J., & Rovine, M. (2003). A comparison of training strategies to enhance use of external aids by persons with dementia. *Journal of Communication Disorders, 36,* 361–378.

Bourgeois, M.S., Dijkstra, K., Burgio, L., & Allen-Burge, R. (2001). Memory aids as an augmentative and alternative communication strategy for nursing home residents with dementia. *Augmentative and Alternative Communication, 17,* 196–209.

Bracken, B.A., & McCallum, R.S. (1998). *Universal Nonverbal Intelligence Test (UNIT).* Itasca, IL: Riverside.

Bracken, B.B. (1998). *Bracken Basic Concept Scale–Revised.* San Antonio, TX: Harcourt Assessment.

Brady, D., & Smouse, A. (1978). A simultaneous comparison of three methods for language training with an autistic child: An experimental single case analysis. *Journal of Autism and Childhood Schizophrenia, 8,* 271–279.

Brady, N. (2000). Improved comprehension of object names following voice output communication aid use: Two case studies. *Augmentative and Alternative Communication, 16,* 197–204.

Brady, N.C., & Halle, J.W. (2002). Breakdowns and repairs in conversations between beginning AAC users and their partners. In J. Reichle, D.R. Beukelman, & J.C. Light (Eds.), *Exemplary practices for beginning communicators: Implications for AAC* (pp. 323–351). Baltimore: Paul H. Brookes Publishing Co.

Brady, N., & McLean, L. (2000). Emergent symbolic relations in speakers and nonspeakers. *Research in Developmental Disabilities, 21,* 197–214.

Brahne, C., & Hall, V. (1995). One life to live. *Communication Outlook, 17*(1), 9–10.

Brandenberg, S., & Vanderheiden, G. (1988). Communication board design and vocabulary selection. In L. Bernstein (Ed.), *The vocally impaired: Clinical practice and research* (3rd ed., pp. 84–135). Needham Heights, MA: Allyn & Bacon.

Braun, U., & Stuckenschneider-Braun, M. (1990). Adapting "Words Strategy" to the German culture and language. *Augmentative and Alternative Communication, 6,* 115.

Bridges, S. (2000, May). Delivery of AAC services to a rural American Indian community. *ASHA Special Interest Division 12 Newsletter, 9*(2), 6–9.

Brigance, A. (1999). *Brigance Comprehensive Inventory of Basic Skills–Revised (CIBS-R).* North Billerica, MA: Curriculum Associates.

Bristow, D., & Fristoe, M. (1984, November). *Systematic evaluation of the nonspeaking child.* Miniseminar presented at the annual convention of the American Speech-Language-Hearing Association, San Francisco, CA.

Bristow, D., & Fristoe, M. (1987, November). *Effects of test adaptations on test performance.* Paper presented at the annual convention of the American Speech-Language-Hearing Association, New Orleans, LA.

Broderick, A., & Kasa-Hendrickson, C. (2001). "SAY JUST ONE WORD AT FIRST": The emergence of reliable speech in a student labeled with autism. *Journal of The Association for Persons with Severe Handicaps, 26,* 13–24.

Brodin, J. (1991). *To interpret children's signals: Play and communication in profoundly mentally retarded and multiply handicapped children.* Unpublished doctoral dissertation, University of Stockholm, Sweden.

Brookshire, R.H. (2003). *An introduction to neurogenic communication disorders* (6th ed.). St. Louis: Mosby-Year Book.

Brown, C. (1954). *My left foot.* London: Secker & Warburg.

Brown, F. (1991). Creative daily scheduling: A nonintrusive approach to challenging behaviors in community residences. *Journal of The Association for Persons with Severe Handicaps, 16,* 75–84.

Brown, K.A., Wacker, D.P., Derby, K.M., Peck, S.M., Richman, D.M., Sasso, G.M., Knutson, C.L., & Harding, J.W. (2000). Evaluating the effects of functional communication training in the presence and absence of establishing operations. *Journal of Applied Behavior Analysis, 33,* 53–71.

Brown, L., Sherbenou, R.J., & Johnsen, S.K. (1997). *TONI-3: Test of Nonverbal Intelligence* (3rd ed.). Circle Pines, MN: American Guidance Service.

Brown, R. (1977, May–June). *Why are signed languages easier to learn than spoken languages?* Keynote address at the National Association of the Deaf Symposium on Sign Language Research and Teaching, Chicago.

Brown, V., Hammill, D., & Wiederholt, J.L. (1995). *Test of Reading Comprehension* (3rd ed.). Austin, TX: PRO-ED.

Bruno, J. (1989). Customizing a Minspeak system for a preliterate child: A case example. *Augmentative and Alternative Communication, 5,* 89–100.

Bruno, J., & Dribbon, M. (1998). Outcomes in AAC: Evaluating the effectiveness of a parent training program. *Augmentative and Alternative Communication, 14,* 59–70.

Bruno, J., & Trembath, D. (2004). *Use of aided language stimulation to improve syntactic performance during a weeklong intervention program.* Manuscript submitted for publication.

Bryen, D., Carey, A., & Frantz, B. (2003). Ending the silence: Adults who use augmentative communication and their experiences as victims of crimes. *Augmentative and Alternative Communication, 19,* 125–134.

Bryen, D., & Joyce, D. (1985). Language intervention with the severely handicapped: A decade of research. *Journal of Special Education, 19,* 7–39.

Burke, R., Beukelman, D.R., Ball, L., & Horn, C. (2002). AAC technology learning: Part I—AAC intervention specialists. *Augmentative and Alternative Communication, 18,* 242–249.

Burkhart, L. (1993). *Total augmentative communication in the early childhood classroom.* Solana Beach, CA: Mayer-Johnson Co.

Burkhart, L. (1994, October). *Organizing vocabulary on dynamic display devices: Practical ideas and strategies.* Paper presented at the sixth biennial conference of the International Society for Augmentative and Alternative Communication, Maastricht, the Netherlands.

Buzolich, M., King, J., & Baroody, S. (1991). Acquisition of the commenting function among system users. *Augmentative and Alternative Communication, 7,* 88–99.

Buzolich, M., & Lunger, J. (1995). Empowering system users in peer training. *Augmentative and Alternative Communication, 11,* 37–48.

Cafiero, J. (1998). Communication power for individuals with autism. *Focus on Autism and Other Developmental Disabilities, 13,* 113–121.

Cafiero, J. (2001). The effect of an augmentative communication intervention on the communication, behavior, and academic program of an adolescent with autism. *Focus on Autism and Other Developmental Disabilities, 16,* 179–189.

Calculator, S. (1991). Evaluating the efficacy of AAC intervention for children with severe disabilities. In J. Brodin & E. Björck-Åkesson (Eds.), *Methodological issues in research in augmentative and alternative communication: Proceedings from the First ISAAC Research Symposium* (pp. 22–31). Stockholm: The Swedish Handicap Institute.

Calculator, S. (1999a). AAC outcomes for children and youths with severe disabilities: When seeing is believing. *Augmentative and Alternative Communication, 15,* 4–12.

Calculator, S. (1999b). Look who's pointing now: Cautions related to the use of facilitated communication. *Language, Speech, and Hearing Services in Schools, 30,* 408–414.

Calculator, S. (2002). Use of enhanced natural gestures to foster interactions between children with Angelman syndrome and their parents. *American Journal of Speech-Language Pathology, 11,* 340–355.

Calculator, S., & Bedrosian, J. (1988). *Communication assessment and intervention for adults with mental retardation.* San Diego: College-Hill Press.

Calculator, S., & Dollaghan, C. (1982). The use of communication boards in a residential setting. *Journal of Speech and Hearing Disorders, 14,* 281–287.

Caldwell, B. (1997). Educating children who are deaf or hard of hearing: Cued speech. *ERIC Digest* #E555, Report Number: EDO-EC-97-2. Reston, VA: ERIC Clearinghouse on Disabilities and Gifted Education.

Cali, K., & Sturm, J. (March, 2003). *The development of narrative and non-narrative writing genres in beginning writers.* Paper presented at the annual meeting of the North Carolina Association for Research in Education, Apex, NC.

Calkins, L.M. (1994). *The art of teaching writing* (New edition). Portsmouth, NH: Heinemann Educational Books.

Callaghan, T. (1999). Early understanding and production of graphic symbols. *Child Development, 70,* 1314–1324.

Cambridge, P., & Forrester-Jones, R. (2003). Using individualized communication for interviewing people with intellectual disability: A case study of user-centred research. *Journal of Intellectual and Developmental Disability, 28,* 5–23.

Campbell, C.R., & Jackson, S.T. (1995). Transparency of one-handed Amer-Ind hand signals to nonfamiliar viewers. *Journal of Speech and Hearing Research, 38,* 1284–1289.

Canfield, H., & Locke, P. (1997). *A book of possibilities: Activities using simple technology.* Minneapolis, MN: AbleNet, Inc.

Capone, N., & McGregor, K. (2004). Gesture development: A review for clinical and research practices. *Journal of Speech, Language, and Hearing Research, 42,* 173–186.

Cardinal, D., Hanson, D., & Wakeham, J. (1996). An investigation of authorship in facilitated communication. *Mental Retardation, 34,* 231–242.

Cardona, G.W. (2000). Spaghetti talk. In M. Fried-Oken & H.A. Bersani, Jr. (Eds.), *Speaking up and spelling it out: Personal essays on augmentative and alternative communication* (pp. 237–244). Baltimore: Paul H. Brookes Publishing Co.

Carey, S. (1978). The child as word learner. In M. Halle, J. Bresnan, & G. Miller (Eds.), *Linguistic theory and psychological reality* (pp. 264–293). Cambridge, MA: MIT Press.

Carey, S., & Bartlett, E. (1978). Acquiring a single new word. *Papers and Reports on Child Language Development, 15,* 17–29.

Carlson, F. (1981). A format for selecting vocabulary for the nonspeaking child. *Language, Speech, and Hearing Services in Schools, 12,* 140–145.

Carlson, F. (1985). *Picsyms categorical dictionary.* Lawrence, KS: Baggeboda Press.

Carr, E. (1982). Sign language. In R. Koegel, A. Rincover, & A. Egel (Eds.), *Educating and understanding autistic children* (pp. 142–157). San Diego: College-Hill Press.

Carr, E., Binkoff, J., Kologinsky, E., & Eddy, M. (1978). Acquisition of sign language by autistic children: I. Expressive labeling. *Journal of Applied Behavior Analysis, 11,* 459–501.

Carr, E., & Dores, P. (1981). Patterns of language acquisition following simultaneous communication with autistic children. *Analysis and Intervention in Developmental Disabilities, 1,* 1–15.

Carr, E., & Kologinsky, E. (1983). Acquisition of sign language by autistic children: II. Spontaneity and generalization. *Journal of Applied Behavior Analysis, 16,* 297–314.

Carr, E., Pridal, C., & Dores, P. (1984). Speech versus sign comprehension in autistic children: Analysis and prediction. *Journal of Experimental Child Psychology, 37,* 587–597.

Carr, E., Robinson, S., & Palumbo, L. (1990). The wrong issue: Aversive versus nonaversive treatment. The right issue: Functional versus nonfunctional treatment. In A. Repp & N. Singh (Eds.),

Perspectives on the use of nonaversive and aversive interventions for persons with developmental disabilities (pp. 361–380). Sycamore, IL: Sycamore Publishing.

Carr, E.G., Levin, L., McConnachie, G., Carlson, J.I., Kemp, D.C., & Smith, C.E. (1994). *Communication-based intervention for problem behavior: A user's guide for producing positive change.* Baltimore: Paul H. Brookes Publishing Co.

Carrow-Woolfolk, E. (1999). *Test for Auditory Comprehension of Language–Third Edition (TACL-3).* Austin, TX: PRO-ED.

Carter, M. (2003a). Communicative spontaneity of children with high support needs who use augmentative and alternative communication systems I: Classroom spontaneity, mode, and function. *Augmentative and Alternative Communication, 19,* 141–154.

Carter, M. (2003b). Communicative spontaneity of children with high support needs who use augmentative and alternative communication systems II: Antecedents and effectiveness of communication. *Augmentative and Alternative Communication, 19,* 155–169.

Carter, M., & Grunsell, J. (2001). The behavior chain interruption strategy: A review of research and discussion of future directions. *Journal of the Association for Persons with Severe Handicaps, 26,* 37–49.

Carter, M., Hotchkis, G., & Cassar, M. (1996). Spontaneity of augmentative and alternative communication in persons with intellectual disabilities: A critical review. *Augmentative and Alternative Communication, 12,* 97–109.

Carter, M., & Iacono, T. (2002). Professional judgments of the intentionality of communicative acts. *Augmentative and Alternative Communication, 18,* 177–191.

Caselli, R.J., Windebank, A.J., Petersen, R.C., Komori, T., Parisi, J.E., Okazaki, H., et al. (1993). Rapidly progressive aphasic dementia and motor neuron disease. *Annals of Neurology, 33*(2), 200–207.

Casey, L. (1978). Development of communicative behavior in autistic children: A parent program using manual signs. *Journal of Autism and Childhood Schizophrenia, 8,* 45–59.

Centers for Disease Control and Prevention (CDC). (2001–2002). *Injury fact book 2001–2002.* Atlanta, GA: Centers for Disease Control and Prevention.

Centers for Disease Control and Prevention (CDC). (2003). Public health and aging: Nonfatal fall-related traumatic brain injury among older adults—California, 1996–1999. *MMWR, 52,* 276–278.

Chadsey-Rusch, J., Drasgow, E., Reinoehl, B., Halle, J., & Collet-Klingenberg, L. (1993). Using general-case instruction to teach spontaneous and generalized requests for assistance to learners with severe disabilities. *Journal of The Association for Persons with Severe Handicaps, 18,* 177–187.

Chadsey-Rusch, J., & Halle, J. (1992). The application of general-case instruction to the requesting repertoires of learners with severe disabilities. *Journal of The Association for Persons with Severe Handicaps, 17,* 121–132.

Chakrabarti, S., & Fombonne, E. (2001). Pervasive developmental disorders in preschool children. *Journal of the American Medical Association, 285,* 3093–3097.

Chaney, C. (1990). Evaluating the whole language approach to language arts: The pros and cons. *Language, Speech, and Hearing Services in Schools, 21,* 244–249.

Chapey, R., & Hallowell, B. (2001). Introduction to language intervention strategies in adult aphaisa. In R. Chapey (Ed.), *Language intervention strategies in aphasia and related neurogenic disorders* (4th ed., pp. 3–17). Baltimore: Lippincott Williams & Wilkins.

Chapman, R., Kay-Raining Bird, E., & Schwartz, S. (1990). Fast mapping in event contexts by children with Down syndrome. *Journal of Speech and Hearing Disorders, 55,* 761–770.

Chapple, D. (2000). Empowerment. In M. Fried-Oken & H.A. Bersani, Jr. (Eds.), *Speaking up and spelling it out: Personal essays on augmentative and alternative communication* (pp. 153–159). Baltimore: Paul H. Brookes Publishing Co.

Charlop-Christy, M., Carpenter, M., Le, L., LeBlanc, L., & Kellet, K. (2002). Using the Picture Exchange Communication System (PECS) with children with autism: Assessment of PECS acquisition, speech, social-communicative behavior, and problem behavior. *Journal of Applied Behavior Analysis, 35,* 213–231.

Chen, D. (1999). Beginning communication with infants. In D. Chen (Ed.), *Essential elements in early intervention: Visual impairment and multiple disabilities* (pp. 337–377). New York: AFB Press.

Cipiani, E. (1988). The missing item format. *Teaching Exceptional Children, 21,* 25–27.

CIRCA: Computer interactive reminiscence and conversation aid. (2004). Retrieved August 25, 2004, from http://www.computing.dundee.ac.uk/projects/circa/

Clay, M. (1991). *Becoming literate: The construction of inner control.* Portsmouth, NH: Heinemann.

Clay, M.M. (1993). *An observational survey of literacy achievement.* Portsmouth, NH: Heinemann.

Clay, M.M. (2002). *An observational survey of literacy achievement* (2nd ed.). Portsmouth, NH: Heinemann.

Clendon, S., Sturm, J., & Cali, K. (2003, November). *The vocabularies of beginning writers: Implications for students who use AAC.* Research presented at the annual convention of the American Speech-Language-Hearing Association, Chicago, IL.

Cline, D., Hofstetter, H., & Griffin, J. (1980). *Dictionary of visual science* (3rd ed.). Radnor, PA: Chilton Book Co.

Coelho, C., & Duffy, R.J. (1987). The relationship of the acquisition of manual signs to severity of aphasia: A training study. *Brain and Language, 31,* 328–345.

Cohen, C., & Light, J. (2000). Use of electronic communication to develop mentor-protégé relationships between adolescent and adult users: Pilot study. *Augmentative and Alternative Communication, 16,* 227–238.

Cohen, C., & Palin, M. (1986). Speech syntheses and speech recognition devices. In M. Grossfeld & C. Grossfeld (Eds.), *Microcomputer applications in rehabilitation of communication disorders* (pp. 183–211). Rockville, MD: Aspen Publishers.

Cohen, E., Allgood, M., Heller, K.W., & Castelle, M. (2001). Use of picture dictionaries to promote written communication by students with hearing and cognitive impairments. *Augmentative and Alternative Communication, 17,* 245–254.

Cole, S., Horvath, B., Chapman, C., Deschenes, C., Ebeling, D., & Sprague, J. (2000). *Adapting curriculum and instruction in inclusive classrooms* (2nd ed.). Port Chester, NY: National Professional Resources.

Coleman, P.P. (1991). *Literacy lost: A qualitative analysis of the early literacy experiences of preschool children with severe speech and physical impairments.* Unpublished doctoral dissertation, University of North Carolina at Chapel Hill.

Collier, B.M. (2000). *See what we say: Situational vocabulary for adults who use augmentative and alternative communication.* Baltimore: Paul H. Brookes Publishing Co.

Collins, M. (1986). *Diagnosis and treatment of global aphasia.* San Diego: College-Hill Press.

Collins, S. (1996). Referring expressions in conversations between aided and natural speakers. In S. von Tetzchner & M.H. Jensen (Eds.), *Augmentative and alternative communication: European perspectives* (pp. 89–100). London: Whurr Publishers.

Cook, A.M., & Hussey, S.M. (2002). *Assistive technologies: Principles and practice* (2nd ed.). St. Louis: Mosby.

Cossette, L., & Duclos, E. (2003). *A profile of disability in Canada, 2001.* Ottawa: Statistics Canada.

Costello, J. (2000). Intervention in the intensive care unit: The Children's Hospital Boston model. *Augmentative and Alternative Communication, 16,* 137–153.

Costello, J., & Shane, H. (1994, November). *Augmentative communication assessment and the feature matching process.* Miniseminar presented at the annual convention of the American Speech-Language-Hearing Association, New Orleans, LA.

Crais, E. (1992). Fast mapping: A new look at word learning. In R. Chapman (Ed.), *Processes in language acquisition and disorders* (pp. 159–185). St. Louis: Mosby.

Crary, M. (1987). *A neurolinguistic model of articulatory/phonological disorders.* Paper presented at the Boy's Town Institute Communication Series, Omaha, NE.

Creech, R., Kissick, L., Koski, M., & Musselwhite, C. (1988). Paravocal communicators speak out: Strategies for encouraging communication aid use. *Augmentative and Alternative Communication, 4,* 168.

Creedon, M. (1973). *Language development in nonverbal autistic children using a simultaneous communication system.* Paper presented at the meeting of the Society for Research in Child Development, Philadelphia.

Cregan, A. (1993). Sigsymbol system in a multimodal approach to speech elicitation: Classroom project involving an adolescent with severe mental retardation. *Augmentative and Alternative Communication, 9*, 146–160.

Cress, C., & King, J. (1999). AAC strategies for people with primary progressive aphasia without dementia: Two case studies. *Augmentative and Alternative Communication, 15*, 248–259.

Cress, C., & Marvin, C. (2003). Common questions about AAC services in early intervention. *Augmentative and Alternative Communication, 19*, 254–272.

Cress, C., Sterup, G., & Hould, T. (2003, November). *Adapted phonological assessment for young children with severe impairments.* Paper presented at the American Speech-Language-Hearing Association Convention, Chicago. (available at http://www.unl.edu/barkley/present/cress/847.pdf)

Cress, P., Spellman, C., DeBriere, T., Sizemore, A., Northam, J., & Johnson, J. (1981). Vision screening for persons with severe handicaps. *Journal of The Association for Persons with Severe Handicaps, 6*(3), 41–50.

Crossley, R. (1988). *Unexpected communication attainment by persons diagnosed as autistic and intellectually impaired.* Paper presented at the third biennial conference of the International Society for Augmentative and Alternative Communication, Anaheim, CA.

Crossley, R. (1990, September). *Communication training involving facilitated communication.* Paper presented to the Australian Association of Special Education, Canberra, Australia.

Crossley, R. (1991). Communication training involving facilitated communication. *Communicating Together, 9*(2), 19–22.

Crossley, R., & McDonald, A. (1984). *Annie's coming out.* New York: Viking Penguin.

Crystal, D. (1987). Teaching vocabulary: The case for a semantic curriculum. *Child Language Teaching and Therapy, 3*, 40–56.

Culp, D. (1987). Outcome measurement: The impact of communication augmentation. *Seminars in Speech and Language, 8*, 169–181.

Culp, D. (1989). Developmental apraxia and augmentative or alternative communication: A case example. *Augmentative and Alternative Communication, 5*, 27–34.

Culp, D., & Carlisle, M. (1988). *PACT: Partners in augmentative communication training.* Tucson, AZ: Communication Skill Builders.

Culp, D., & Effinger, J. (1996). *ChalkTalk: Augmentative communication in the classroom.* Anchorage: The Assistive Technology Library of Alaska.

Culp, D., & Ladtkow, M. (1992). Locked-in syndrome and augmentative communication. In K. Yorkston (Ed.), *Augmentative communication in the medical setting* (pp. 59–138). San Antonio, TX: Harcourt Assessment.

Cumley, G. (1997). *Introduction of augmentative and alternative modality: Effects on the quality and quantity of communication interactions of children with severe phonological disorders.* Unpublished doctoral dissertation, University of Nebraska–Lincoln.

Cumley, G., & Swanson, S. (1997). *Case studies: Augmentative and alternative communication options for children with developmental apraxia of speech.* Manuscript submitted for publication.

Cumley, G., & Swanson, S. (1999). Augmentative and alternative communication options for children with developmental apraxia of speech: Three case studies. *Augmentative and Alternative Communication, 15*, 110–125.

Cunningham, J.W. (1993). Whole-to-part reading diagnosis. *Reading and Writing Quarterly, 9*, 31–49.

Cunningham, P.M. (1999). What should we do about phonics? In L.B. Gambrell, L.M. Morrow, S.B. Neuman, & M. Pressley (Eds.), *Best practices in literacy instruction* (pp. 68–89). New York: The Guilford Press.

Cunningham, P., Hall, D., & Sigmon, C. (1999). *The teacher's guide to the four blocks: A multimethod, multilevel framework for grades 1–3.* Greensboro, NC: Carson-Dellosa Publishing.

Curcio, F. (1978). Sensorimotor functioning and communication in mute autistic children. *Journal of Autism and Childhood Schizophrenia, 8*, 181–189.

Dahlgren Sandberg, A. (2001). Reading and spelling, phonological awareness, and working memory in children with severe speech impairments: A longitudinal study. *Augmentative and Alternative Communication, 17*, 11–25.

Dahlgren Sandberg, A., & Hjelmquist, E. (1996a). A comparative, descriptive study of reading and writing skills among non-speaking children: A preliminary study. *European Journal of Disorders of Communication, 31,* 289–308.

Dahlgren Sandberg, A., & Hjelmquist, E. (1996b). Phonologic awareness and literacy abilities in nonspeaking preschool children with cerebral palsy. *Augmentative and Alternative Communication, 12,* 138–154.

Dahlgren Sandberg, A., & Hjelmquist, E. (1997). Language and literacy in nonvocal children with cerebral palsy. *Reading and Writing: An Interdisciplinary Journal, 8,* 453–485.

Daniloff, J., Lloyd, L., & Fristoe, M. (1983). Amer-Ind transparency. *Journal of Speech and Hearing Disorders, 48,* 103–110.

Daniloff, J., Noll, J., Fristoe, M., & Lloyd, L. (1982). Gesture recognition in patients with aphasia. *Journal of Speech and Hearing Disorders, 47,* 43–56.

Daniloff, J., & Shafer, A. (1981). A gestural communication program for severely-profoundly handicapped children. *Language, Speech, and Hearing Services in Schools, 12,* 258–268.

Daniloff, J., & Vergara, D. (1984). Comparison between the motoric constraints for Amer-Ind and ASL sign formation. *Journal of Speech and Hearing Research, 27,* 76–88.

Darley, F., Aronson, A., & Brown, J. (1975). *Motor speech disorders.* Philadelphia: W.B. Saunders.

Darley, F., Brown, J., & Goldstein, N. (1972). Dysarthria in multiple sclerosis. *Journal of Speech and Hearing Research, 15,* 229–245.

Dattilo, J., & Camarata, S. (1991). Facilitating conversation through self-initiated augmentative communication treatment. *Journal of Applied Behavior Analysis, 24,* 369–378.

Day, H.M., Horner, R., & O'Neill, R. (1994). Multiple functions of problem behaviors: Assessment and intervention. *Journal of Applied Behavior Analysis, 27,* 279–290.

Day, H., & Jutai, J. (1996). Measuring the psychosocial impact of assistive devices: The PIADS. *Canadian Journal of Rehabilitation, 9,* 159–168.

DeCoste, D.C. (1997a). Augmentative and alternative communication assessment strategies: Motor access and visual considerations. In S.L. Glennen & D.C. DeCoste (Eds.), *The handbook of augmentative and alternative communication* (pp. 243–282). San Diego: Singular Publishing Group.

DeCoste, D.C. (1997b). The role of literacy in augmentative and alternative communication. In S.L. Glennen & D.C. DeCoste (Eds.), *The handbook of augmentative and alternative communication* (pp. 283–333). San Diego: Singular Publishing Group.

Delange, F. (2000). The role of iodine in brain development. *Proceedings of the Nutrition Society, 59*(1), 75–79.

DeLoache, J., Miller, K., & Rosengren, K. (1997). The credible shrinking room: Very young children's performance with symbolic and nonsymbolic relations. *Psychological Science, 8,* 308–313.

DeLoache, J., Pierroutsakos, S., & Troseth, G. (1997). The three 'R's' of pictorial competence. In R. Vasta (Ed.), *Annals of child development: A research annual* (Vol. 12, pp. 1–48). Philadelphia: Jessica Kingsley Publishers.

DeLoache, J., Pierroutsakos, S., & Uttal, D. (2003). The origins of pictorial competence. *Current Directions in Psychological Science, 12,* 114–118.

Delsandro, E. (1997). AAC for adults with developmental disabilities. In S.L. Glennen & D. DeCoste (Eds.), *Handbook of augmentative and alternative communication* (pp. 637–673). San Diego: Singular Publishing Group.

Demers, L., Weiss-Lambrou, R., & Ska, B. (1996). Development of the Quebec User Evaluation of Satisfaction with Assistive Technology (QUEST). *Assistive Technology, 8,* 1–13.

Dennis, R., Reichle, J., Williams, W., & Vogelsberg, R.T. (1982). Motoric factors influencing the selection of vocabulary for sign production programs. *Journal of The Association for Persons with Severe Handicaps, 7*(1), 20–32.

DePaepe, P., Reichle, J., & O'Neill, R. (1993). Applying general-case instructional strategies when teaching communicative alternatives to challenging behavior. In J. Reichle & D.P. Wacker (Eds.), *Communicative alternatives to challenging behavior: Integrating functional assessment and intervention strategies* (pp. 237–262). Baltimore: Paul H. Brookes Publishing Co.

DeRuyter, F. (1995). Only the lead dog sees the scenery? In S. Blackstone & H. Pressman (Eds.), *Outcomes in AAC conference report: Alliance '95* (pp. 13–14). Monterey, CA: Augmentative Communication.

DeRuyter, F., & Donoghue, K. (1989). Communication and traumatic brain injury: A case study. *Augmentative and Alternative Communication, 5,* 49–54.

DeRuyter, F., & Kennedy, M. (1991). Augmentative communication following traumatic brain injury. In D.R. Beukelman & K. Yorkston (Eds.), *Communication disorders following traumatic brain injury: Management of cognitive, language, and motor impairments* (pp. 317–365). Austin, TX: PRO-ED.

DeRuyter, F., & Lafontaine, L. (1987). The nonspeaking brain injured: A clinical and demographic database report. *Augmentative and Alternative Communication, 3,* 18–25.

Deshler, K., & Schumaker, J. (1988). An instructional model for teaching students how to learn. In J. Graden, J. Zins, & M. Curtis (Eds.), *Alternative educational delivery systems: Enhancing instructional options for all students* (pp. 391–411). Washington, DC: National Association of School Psychologists.

DeThorne, K., & Schaefer, B. (2004). A guide to child nonverbal IQ measures. *American Journal of Speech-Language Pathology, 13,* 275–290.

Diamanti, T. (2000). Get to know me. In M. Williams & C. Krezman (Eds.), *Beneath the surface: Creative expressions of augmented communicators* (pp. 98–99). Toronto: ISAAC Press.

DiCarlo, C., Stricklin, S., Banajee, M., & Reid, D. (2001). Effects of manual signing on communicative verbalizations by toddlers with and without disabilities in inclusive classrooms. *Journal of The Association for Persons with Severe Handicaps, 26,* 120–126.

Dixon, L.S. (1981). A functional analysis of photo-object matching skills of severely retarded adolescents. *Journal of Applied Behavior Analysis, 14,* 465–478.

Doherty, J. (1985). The effects of sign characteristics on sign acquisition and retention: An integrative review of the literature. *Augmentative and Alternative Communication, 1,* 108–121.

Doherty, J., Daniloff, J., & Lloyd, L. (1985). The effect of categorical presentation on Amer-Ind transparency. *Augmentative and Alternative Communication, 1,* 10–16.

Dollaghan, C. (1987). Fast mapping in normal and language impaired children. *Journal of Speech and Hearing Disorders, 52,* 218–222.

Dongilli, P., Hakel, M., & Beukelman, D.R. (1992). Recovery of functional speech following traumatic brain injury. *Journal of Head Trauma Rehabilitation, 7,* 91–101.

Donnellan, A. (1984). The criterion of the least dangerous assumption. *Behavior Disorders, 9,* 141–150.

Donnellan, A., Mirenda, P., Mesaros, R., & Fassbender, L. (1984). Analyzing the communicative functions of aberrant behavior. *Journal of The Association for Persons with Severe Handicaps, 9,* 201–212.

Douglas, M., & Shane, H. (2002, November). *Application of "intelligent agents" in children evidencing autism.* Paper presented at the annual conference of the American Speech-Language-Hearing Association, Atlanta, GA.

Dowden, P. (1997). Augmentative and alternative communication decision making for children with severely unintelligible speech. *Augmentative and Alternative Communication, 13,* 48–58.

Dowden, P., Beukelman, D.R., & Lossing, C. (1986). Serving non-speaking patients in acute care settings: Intervention outcomes. *Augmentative and Alternative Communication, 2,* 38–44.

Dowden, P., & Cook, A.M. (2002). Choosing effective selection techniques for beginning communicators. In J. Reichle, D.R. Beukelman, & J.C. Light (Eds.), *Exemplary practices for beginning communicators: Implications for AAC* (pp. 395–429). Baltimore: Paul H. Brookes Publishing Co.

Dowden, P., Honsinger, M., & Beukelman, D.R. (1986). Serving non-speaking patients in acute care settings: An intervention approach. *Augmentative and Alternative Communication, 2,* 25–32.

Downing, J. (2002). *Including students with severe and multiple disabilities in typical classrooms: Practical strategies for teachers* (2nd ed.). Baltimore: Paul H. Brookes Publishing Co.

Doyle, M., Kennedy, M.R.T., Jausalaitis, G., & Phillips, B. (2000). AAC and traumatic brain injury. In D.R. Beukelman, K.M. Yorkston, & J. Reichle (Eds.), *Augmentative and alternative communication for adults with acquired neurologic disorders* (pp. 271–304). Baltimore: Paul H. Brookes Publishing Co.

Drager, K., Hustad, K., & Gable, K. (2004). Telephone communication: Synthetic and dysarthric speech intelligibility and listener preferences. *Augmentative and Alternative Communication, 20,* 103–112.

Drager, K., Light, J., Carlson, R., D'Silva, K., Larsson, B., Pitkin, L., & Stopper, G. (2004). Learning of dynamic display AAC technologies by typically developing 3-year-olds: Effect of different layouts and menu approaches. *Journal of Speech, Language, and Hearing Research, 47,* 1133–1148.

Drager, K., Light, J., Speltz, J., Fallon, K., & Jeffries, L. (2003). The performance of typically developing 2 1/2-year-olds on dynamic display AAC technologies with different system layouts and language organizations. *Journal of Speech, Language, and Hearing Research, 46,* 298–312.

Drasgow, E., Halle, J.W., & Ostrosky, M.M. (1998). Effects of differential reinforcement on the generalization of a replacement mand in three children with severe language delays. *Journal of Applied Behavior Analysis, 31,* 357–374.

Drasgow, E., Halle, J.W., Ostroksy, M., & Harbers, H. (1996). Using behavioral indication and functional communication training to establish an initial sign repertoire with a young child with severe disabilities. *Topics in Early Childhood Special Education, 16,* 500–521.

Duchan, J. (1987). Perspectives for understanding children with communicative disorders. In P. Knoblock (Ed.), *Understanding exceptional children and youth* (pp. 163–199). Boston: Little, Brown.

Duchan, J. (1995). *Supporting language learning in everyday life.* San Diego: Singular Publishing Group.

Duchan, J. (1999). Views of facilitated communication: What's the point? *Language, Speech, and Hearing Services in Schools, 30,* 401–407.

Duffy, J. (2000). Primary progressive aphasia. *ASHA Leader, 5,* 94.

Duffy, J. (2004). Primary progressive aphasia and primary progressive apraxia of speech: An update. *ASHA Leader, 9,* 120.

Dugan, E., Kamps, D., Leonard, B., Watkins, N., Rheinberger, A., & Stackhaus, J. (1995). Effects of cooperative learning groups during social studies for students with autism and fourth-grade peers. *Journal of Applied Behavior Analysis, 28,* 175–188.

Duker, P., & Jutten, W. (1997). Establishing gestural yes-no responding with individuals with profound mental retardation. *Education and Training in Mental Retardation and Developmental Disabilities, 32,* 59–67.

Duker, P.C., Kraaykamp, M., & Visser, E. (1994). A stimulus control procedure to increase requesting with individuals who are severely/profoundly intellectually disabled. *Journal of Intellectual Disability Research, 38,* 177–186.

Dunham, J. (1989). The transparency of manual signs in a linguistic and an environmental nonlinguistic context. *Augmentative and Alternative Communication, 5,* 214–225.

Dunn, L.M., & Dunn, L.M. (1981). *Peabody Picture Vocabulary Test–Revised.* Circle Pines, MN: American Guidance Service.

Dunn, L.M., & Dunn, L.M. (1997). *Peabody Picture Vocabulary Test–III (PPVT-III).* Circle Pines, MN: American Guidance Service.

Dunn, M. (1982). *Pre-sign language motor skills.* Tucson, AZ: Communication Skill Builders.

Durand, V.M. (1990). *Severe behavior problems.* New York: Guilford Press.

Durand, V.M. (1993). Functional communication training using assistive devices: Effects on challenging behavior. *Augmentative and Alternative Communication, 9,* 168–176.

Durand, V.M. (1999). Functional communication training using assistive devices: Recruiting natural communities of reinforcement. *Journal of Applied Behavior Analysis, 32,* 247–267.

Durand, V.M., & Carr, E. (1991). Functional communication training to reduce challenging behavior: Maintenance and application in new settings. *Journal of Applied Behavior Analysis, 24,* 251–264.

Durand, V.M., & Carr, E.G. (1987). Social influences on self-stimulatory behavior: Analysis and treatment application. *Journal of Applied Behavior Analysis, 20,* 119–132.

Durand, V.M., & Kishi, G. (1987). Reducing severe behavior problems among persons with dual sensory impairments: An evaluation of a technical assistance model. *Journal of The Association for Persons with Severe Handicaps, 12,* 2–10.

Dworkin, J., Aronson, A., & Mulder, D. (1980). Tongue force in normals and in dysarthric patients with amyotrophic lateral sclerosis. *Journal of Speech and Hearing Research, 23,* 828–837.

Dyches, T. (1998). Effects of switch training on the communication of children with autism and severe disabilities. *Focus on Autism and Other Developmental Disabilities, 13*, 151–162.

Dye, R., Alm, N., Arnott, J.L., Harper, G., & Morrison, A. (1998). A script-based AAC system for transactional interaction. *Natural Language Engineering, 4*, 57–71.

Dykens, E.M., Hodapp, R.M., & Finucane, B.M. (2000). *Genetics and mental retardation syndromes: A new look at behavior and interventions.* Baltimore: Paul H. Brookes Publishing Co.

Dyson, A.H. (1986). Transitions and tensions: Interrelationships between the drawing, talking, and dictating of young children. *Research in the Teaching of English, 20*, 379–409.

Easton, J. (1989). Oh, the frustration! *Communication Outlook, 10*(3), 16–17.

Edman, P. (1991). Relief Bliss: A low tech technique. *Communicating Together, 9*(1), 21–22.

Edmonds, R. (1979). Some schools work and more can. *Social Policy, 9*(5), 25–29.

Egof, D. (1988). *Coding communication devices: The effects of symbol set selection and code origin on the recall of utterances.* Paper presented at the third annual Council for Exceptional Children conference, Baltimore, MD.

Ehri, L.C. (1992). Reconceptualizing the development of sight word reading and its relationship to recoding. In P.B. Gough, L.C. Ehri, & R. Treiman (Eds.), *Reading acquisition* (pp. 107–143). Hillsdale, NJ: Lawrence Erlbaum Associates.

Ekman, P. (1976). Movements with precise meanings. *Journal of Communication, 26*, 14–26.

Ekman, P., & Friesen, W. (1969). The repertoire of nonverbal behavior: Categories, origin, usage, and coding. *Semiotica, 1*, 49–98.

Elder, P., & Goossens', C. (1994). *Engineering training environments for interactive augmentative communication: Strategies for adolescents and adults who are moderately/severely developmentally delayed.* Birmingham, AL: Southeast Augmentative Communication Conference Publications.

Elder, P., & Goossens', C. (1996). *Communication overlays for engineering training environments: Overlays for adolescents and adults who are moderately/severely developmentally delayed.* Solana Beach, CA: Mayer-Johnson, Inc.

Elder, P., Goossens', C., & Bray, N. (1989). *Semantic compaction proficiency profile (Experimental edition).* Birmingham, AL: Southeast Augmentative Communication Conference Publications.

Emery, A., & Holloway, S. (1982). Familial motor neuron diseases. In L. Rowland (Ed.), *Human motor neuron diseases.* New York: Raven Press.

Enderby, P., & Crow, E. (1990). Long-term recovery patterns of severe dysarthria following head injury. *British Journal of Disorders of Communication, 25*, 341–354.

Enderby, P., & Philipp, R. (1986). Speech and language handicap: Towards knowing the size of the problem. *British Journal of Disorders of Communication, 21*, 151–165.

English braille–American edition. (1994). Retrieved January 26, 2005, from http://www.brl.org/ebae/

Erickson, K.A. (2000). All children are ready to learn: An emergent versus readiness perspective in early literacy assessment. *Seminars in Speech and Language, 21*(3), 193–203.

Erickson, K. (2003, June 24). Reading comprehension in AAC. *The ASHA Leader, 8*(12), 6–9.

Erickson, K., & Baker, B. (1996, August). *Language, literacy, and semantic compaction.* Paper presented at the seventh biennial conference of the International Society for Augmentative and Alternative Communication, Vancouver, British Columbia.

Erickson, K.A., & Koppenhaver, D.A. (1995). Developing a literacy program for children with severe disabilities. *The Reading Teacher, 48*(8), 676–684.

Erickson, K.A., & Koppenhaver, D.A. (2000). *Emergent literacy intervention for preschoolers with autism.* Seminar presented at the Biennial Conference for the International Society for Augmentative and Alternative Communication, Crystal City, VA.

Erickson, K.A., Koppenhaver, D.A., & Yoder, D.E. (2002). *Waves of words: Augmented communicators read and write.* Toronto: International Society for Augmentative and Alternative Communication.

Erickson, K.A., Koppenhaver, D.A., Yoder, D.E., & Nance, J. (1997). Integrated communication and literacy instruction for a child with multiple disabilities. *Focus on Autism and Other Developmental Disabilities, 12*(3), 142–150.

Erickson, K., Koppenhaver, D., Yoder, D., & Nance, J. (2001). Integrated communication and literacy instruction for a child with multiple disabilities. *Focus on Autism and Other Developmental Disabilities, 12,* 142–150.

Estrella, G. (2000). Confessions of a blabber finger. In M. Fried-Oken & H.A. Bersani, Jr. (Eds.), *Speaking up and spelling it out: Personal essays on augmentative and alternative communication* (pp. 31–45). Baltimore: Paul H. Brookes Publishing Co.

Evans, R., & Bilsky, L. (1979). Clustering and categorical list retention in the mentally retarded. In N. Ellis (Ed.), *Handbook of mental deficiency: Psychological research and theory.* Hillsdale, NJ: Lawrence Erlbaum Associates.

Fager, S. (2003, November). *AAC use across multiple settings.* Unpublished presentation at the annual convention of the American Speech-Language-Hearing Association, Philadelphia, PA.

Fager, S., Beukelman, D.R., & Jakobs, T. (2002). AAC intervention for locked in syndrome using the safe laser system. *Perspectives on Augmentative and Alternative Communication, 11*(1), 4–7.

Fager, S., Hux, K., Karantounis, R., & Beukelman, D.R. (2004). AAC use and acceptance by adults with traumatic brain injury, *Augmentative and Alternative Communication.* Submitted for publication.

Fallon, K., Light, J., & Achenbach, A. (2003). The semantic organization patterns of young children: Implications for augmentative and alternative communication. *Augmentative and Alternative Communication, 19,* 74–85.

Fallon, K., Light, J., & Paige, T. (2001). Enhancing vocabulary selection for preschoolers who require augmentative and alternative communication (AAC). *American Journal of Speech-Language Pathology, 10,* 81–94.

Falvey, M.A. (1986). *Community-based curriculum: Instructional strategies for students with severe handicaps.* Baltimore: Paul H. Brookes Publishing Co.

Falvey, M., Forest, M., Pearpoint, J., & Rosenberg, R. (1994). *All my life's a circle: Using the tools of circles, MAPS, and PATHS.* Toronto: Inclusion Press.

Farrier, L., Yorkston, K., Marriner, N., & Beukelman, D.R. (1985). Conversational control in non-impaired speakers using an augmentative communication system. *Augmentative and Alternative Communication, 1,* 65–73.

Fay, W., & Schuler, A. (1980). *Emerging language in autistic children.* Baltimore: University Park Press.

Fenson, L., Dale, P., Reznick, S., Thal, D., Bates, E., Hartung, J., Pethick, S., & Reilly, J. (1993). *MacArthur-Bates Communicative Development Inventory: Words and Sentences.* Baltimore: Paul H. Brookes Publishing Co.

Ferketic, M., Fratalli, C., Holland, A., Thompson, C., & Wohl, C. (2004). *Functional Assessment of Communication Skills for Adults (ASHA FACS).* Rockville, MD: American Speech-Language-Hearing Association.

Ferm, U., Amberntson, B., & Thunberg, G. (2001). Development and evaluation of a Minspeak application using Blissymbols: Experiences from two case studies. *Augmentative and Alternative Communication, 17,* 233–244.

Ferroli, L., & Shanahan, T. (1987). Kindergarten spelling: Explaining its relationship to first grade reading. In J.E. Readence & R.S. Baldwin (Eds.), *Research in literacy: Merging perspectives* (36th Yearbook of the National Reading Conference). Rochester, NY: National Reading Conference.

Feys, P., Romberg, A., Ruutiainen, J., Davies-Smith, A., Jones, R., Avizzano, C., Bergamasco, M., & Ketelaer, P. (2001). Assistive technology to improve PC interaction for people with intention tremor. *Journal of Rehabilitation Research and Development, 38,* 235–243.

File, P., & Todman, J. (2002). Evaluation of the coherence of computer-aided conversations. *Augmentative and Alternative Communication, 18,* 228–241.

Fisher, D., & Ryndak, D. (2001). *Inclusive education: A compendium of articles on effective strategies to achieve inclusive education.* Baltimore: TASH.

Fisher, R., Ury, W., & Patton, B. (1991). *Getting to yes: Negotiating agreement without giving in.* New York: Penguin Books.

Flannery, B., & Horner, R. (1994). The relationship between predictability and problem behavior for students with severe disabilities. *Journal of Behavioral Education, 4,* 157–176.

Flouriot, M., & DeSerres, L. (2000). Commun.i.mage: A multilingual picture symbol system developed by professionals. In *Proceedings of the 9th biennial conference of the International Society for Augmentative and Alternative Communication* (pp. 324–325). Washington, DC: ISAAC Press.

Flower, L.S., & Hayes, J.R. (1981). A cognitive process theory of writing. *College Composition, 32,* 365–387.

Foley, B., & Pollatsek, A. (1999). Phonological processing and reading abilities in adolescents and adults with severe congenital speech impairments. *Augmentative and Alternative Communication, 15,* 156–173.

Foley, B.E. (1993). The development of literacy in individuals with severe congenital speech and motor impairments. *Topics in Language Disorders, 13*(2), 16–32.

Folstein, S.E. (1990). *Huntington disease: A disorder of families.* Baltimore: Johns Hopkins University Press.

Fombonne, E. (1999). Epidemiological surveys of autism: A review. *Psychological Medicine, 29,* 769–786.

Foorman, B., & Torgesen, J. (2001). Critical elements of classroom and small-group instruction promote reading success in all children. *Learning Disabilities Research and Practice, 16*(4), 203–212.

Ford, A., & Mirenda, P. (1984). Community instruction: A natural cues and corrections decision model. *Journal of The Association for Persons with Severe Handicaps, 9,* 79–87.

Foreman, P., & Crews, G. (1998). Using augmentative communication with infants and young children with Down syndrome. *Down Syndrome Research and Practice, 5,* 16–25.

Fossett, B., Smith, V., & Mirenda, P. (2003). Facilitating oral language and literacy development during general education activities. In D. Ryndak & S. Alper (Eds.), *Curriculum and instruction for students with significant disabilities in inclusive settings* (2nd ed., pp. 173–205). Boston: Allyn & Bacon.

Foster, C. (1989). *Shakespeare for children: Romeo and Juliet.* Chandler, AZ: Five Star Publishers.

Foster, C., Shakespeare, W., & Howey, P. (2000). *Sixty-minute Shakespeare: Romeo and Juliet* (2nd ed). Chandler, AZ: Five Star Publishers.

Foulds, R. (1980). Communication rates of nonspeech expression as a function in manual tasks and linguistic constraints. In *Proceedings of the International Conference on Rehabilitation Engineering* (pp. 83–87). Toronto: RESNA Press.

Foulds, R. (1985). Observations on interfacing in nonvocal communication. In C. Barry & M. Byrne (Eds.), *Proceedings of the Fourth International Conference on Communication Through Technology for the Physically Disabled* (pp. 46–51). London: The International Cerebral Palsy Association.

Foulds, R. (1987). Guest editorial. *Augmentative and Alternative Communication, 3,* 169.

Fox, L., & Fried-Oken, M. (1996). AAC aphasiology: Partnership for future research. *Augmentative and Alternative Communication, 12,* 257–271.

Fox, L., Sohlberg, M.M., & Fried-Oken, M. (2001). Effects of conversational topic choice on outcomes of an augmentative communication intervention for adults with aphasia. *Aphasiology, 15,* 171–200.

Fox, M.J. (2002). *Lucky man: A memoir.* New York: Random House.

Francis, W., Nail, B., & Lloyd, L. (1990, November). *Mentally retarded adults' perception of emotions represented by pictographic symbols.* Paper presented at the annual convention of the American Speech-Language-Hearing Association, Seattle, WA.

Franklin, N.K., Mirenda, P., & Phillips, G. (1994). Comparisons of five symbol assessment protocols with nondisabled preschoolers and learners with severe intellectual disabilities. *Augmentative and Alternative Communication, 12,* 73–77.

Fraser, B.A., Hensinger, R.N., & Phelps, J.A. (1990). *Physical management of multiple handicaps: A professional's guide* (2nd ed.). Baltimore: Paul H. Brookes Publishing Co.

Frea, W.D., Arnold, C.L., & Vittemberga, G.L. (2001). A demonstration of the effects of augmentative communication on extreme aggressive behavior of a child with autism within an integrated preschool setting. *Journal of Positive Behavioral Interventions, 3*(4), 194–198.

French, J.L. (2001). *The Pictorial Test of Intelligence* (2nd ed.). Austin, TX: PRO-ED.

Fried-Oken, M. (1989, June). *Sentence recognition for auditory and visual scanning techniques in electronic augmentative communication devices.* Paper presented at the Rehabilitation Engineering and

Assistive Technology Association (RESNA)/United States Society for Augmentative and Alternative Communication annual conference, New Orleans, LA.

Fried-Oken, M. (1995). Story telling as an augmentative communication approach for a man with severe apraxia of speech and expressive aphasia. *Augmentative and Alternative Communication (American Speech-Language-Hearing Association Special Interest Division #12 Newsletter), 4*, 3–4.

Fried-Oken, M. (2001). Been there, done that: A very personal introduction to the special issues on *Augmentative and Alternative Communication, 17*, 138–140.

Fried-Oken, M., Ball, L., Golinker, L., Lasker, J., Mathy, P., & Ourand, P. (2002, November). *AAC challenges in adults with acquired neurological impairment.* Session presented at the American Speech-Language-Hearing Association Convention, Atlanta, GA.

Fried-Oken, M., & Bersani, H.A., Jr. (Eds.). (2000). *Speaking up and spelling it out: Personal essays on augmentative and alternative communication.* Baltimore: Paul H. Brookes Publishing Co.

Fried-Oken, M., & Doyle, M. (1992). Language representation for the augmentative and alternative communication of adults with traumatic brain injury. *Journal of Head Trauma Rehabilitation, 7*(3), 59–69.

Fried-Oken, M., Howard, J., & Prillwitz, D. (1988). Establishing initial communicative control with a loop-tape system. In S.W. Blackstone, E.L. Cassatt-James, & D. Bruskin (Eds.), *Augmentative communication: Implementation strategies* (pp. 5.1–45–5.1–51). Rockville, MD: American Speech-Language-Hearing Association.

Fried-Oken, M., Howard, J., & Stewart, S. (1991). Feedback on AAC intervention from adults who are temporarily unable to speak. *Augmentative and Alternative Communication, 7*, 43–50.

Fried-Oken, M., & More, L. (1992). An initial vocabulary for nonspeaking preschool children based on developmental and environmental language sources. *Augmentative and Alternative Communication, 8*, 41–56.

Fried-Oken, M., Rau, M., Fox, L., Tulman, J., & Hindal, M. (2004). ALS, AAC technology and caregivers: Attitudes, skills, and role strain. *ASHA Leader, 9*, 98.

Fried-Oken, M., Rau, M.T., & Oken, B.S. (2000). AAC and dementia. In D.R. Beukelman, K.M. Yorkston, & J. Reichle (Eds.), *Augmentative and alternative communication for adults with acquired neurologic disorders* (pp. 375–406). Baltimore: Paul H. Brookes Publishing Co.

Frith, U. (2003). *Autism: Explaining the enigma* (2nd ed.). Oxford, UK: Blackwell.

Frost, L., & Bondy, A. (2002). *Picture exchange communication system training manual* (2nd ed.). Newark, DE: Pyramid Education Products.

Fuller, D., & Lloyd, L. (1991). Toward a common usage of iconicity terminology. *Augmentative and Alternative Communication, 7*, 215–220.

Fuller, D., Lloyd, L., & Schlosser, R. (1992). Further development of an augmentative and alternative communication symbol taxonomy. *Augmentative and Alternative Communication, 8*, 67–74.

Fuller, D., Lloyd, L., & Stratton, M. (1997). Aided AAC symbols. In L. Lloyd, D. Fuller, & H. Arvidson (Eds.), *Augmentative and alternative communication: Principles and practice* (pp. 48–79). Needham Heights, MA: Allyn & Bacon.

Galvin, J., & Donnell, C. (2002). Educating the consumer and caretaker on assistive technology. In M. Scherer (Ed.), *Assistive technology: Matching device and consumer for successful rehabilitation* (pp. 153–167). Washington, DC: American Psychological Association.

Galvin, J., & Scherer, M. (1996). *Evaluating, selecting, and using appropriate assistive technology.* Gaithersberg, MD: Aspen Publications.

Garrett, K. (1993). *Changes in the interaction patterns of individuals with severe aphasia given three types of partner support.* Doctoral dissertation, University of Nebraska–Lincoln.

Garrett, K. (2001, November). *Referential skills and expressive communication in severe aphasia: Treatment implications.* Seminar presented at the annual convention of the American Speech-Language Hearing Association, New Orleans, LA.

Garrett, K., & Beukelman, D.R. (1992). Augmentative communication approaches for persons with severe aphasia. In K. Yorkston (Ed.), *Augmentative communication in the medical setting* (pp. 245–338). Tucson, AZ: Communication Skill Builders.

Garrett, K., & Beukelman, D.R. (1995). Changes in the interaction patterns of an individual with severe aphasia given three types of partner support. In M. Lemme (Ed.), *Clinical aphasiology* (Vol. 23). Austin, TX: PRO-ED.

Garrett, K., Beukelman, D.R., & Low-Morrow, D. (1989). A comprehensive augmentative communication system for an adult with Broca's aphasia. *Augmentative and Alternative Communication, 5,* 55–61.

Garrett, K., & Huth, C. (2002). The impact of graphic contextual information and instruction on the conversational behaviors of an individual with severe aphasia. *Aphasiology, 16,* 523–536.

Garrett, K.L., & Kimelman, M.D.Z. (2000). AAC and aphasia: Cognitive-linguistic considerations. In D.R. Beukelman, K.M. Yorkston, & J. Reichle (Eds.), *Augmentative and alternative communication for adults with acquired neurologic disorders* (pp. 339–374). Baltimore: Paul H. Brookes Publishing Co.

Garrett, K., & Lasker, J. (2004). Website materials: http://aac.unl.edu/

Garrett, K., Schutz-Muehling, L., & Morrow, D. (1990). Low level head injury: A novel AAC approach. *Augmentative and Alternative Communication, 6,* 124.

Garrett, K., Staab, L., & Agocs, L. (1996, November). *Perceptions of scaffolded letters generated by a person with aphasia.* Paper presented at the annual convention of the American Speech-Language-Hearing Association, Seattle, WA.

Garrett, S. (1986). A case study in tactile Blissymbols. *Communicating Together, 4*(2), 16.

Garrison-Harrell, L., Kamps, D., & Kravits, T. (1997). The effects of peer networks on social-communicative behaviors for students with autism. *Focus on Autism and Other Developmental Disabilities, 12,* 241–254.

Gates, C. (1985). Survey of multiply handicapped visually impaired children in the Rocky Mountain/Great Plains region. *Journal of Visual Impairment and Blindness, 79,* 385–391.

Gee, J.B. (1999). Language and communication: The key is effectiveness. *Disability Solutions, 3*(5–6), 18–22.

Gee, K., Graham, N., Goetz, L., Oshima, G., & Yoshioka, K. (1991). Teaching students to request the continuation of routine activities by using time delay and decreasing physical assistance in the context of chain interruption. *Journal of The Association for Persons with Severe Handicaps, 16,* 154–167.

Gerra, L., Dorfman, S., Plaue, E., Schlackman, S., & Workman, D. (1995). Functional communication as a means of decreasing self-injurious behavior: A case study. *Journal of Visual Impairment and Blindness, 89,* 343–347.

Giangreco, M. (2000). Related services research for students with low-incidence disabilities: Implications for speech-language pathologists in inclusive classrooms. *Language, Speech, and Hearing Services in Schools, 31,* 230–239.

Giangreco, M.F. (1996a). Choosing options and accommodations for children (COACH): Curriculum planning for students with disabilities in general education. In S. Stainback & W. Stainback (Eds.), *Inclusion: A guide for educators* (pp. 237–254). Baltimore: Paul H. Brookes Publishing Co.

Giangreco, M.F. (1996b). *VISTA: Vermont interdependent services team approach. A guide to coordinating support services.* Baltimore: Paul H. Brookes Publishing Co.

Giangreco, M.F., Cloninger, C.J., & Iverson, V.S. (1998). *Choosing outcomes and accommodations for children (COACH): A guide to educational planning for students with disabilities* (2nd ed.). Baltimore: Paul H. Brookes Publishing Co.

Gillette, Y. (2003). *Achieving communication independence: A comprehensive guide to assessment and intervention.* Eau Claire, WI: Thinking Publications.

Gillon, G., Clendon, S., Cupples, L., Flynn, M., Iacono, T., Schmidkie, T., Yoder, D., & Young, A. (2004). Phonological awareness development in children with physical, sensory, or intellectual impairment. In G. Gillon (Ed.), *Phonological awareness: From research to practice* (pp. 183–224). New York: Guilford Press.

Glennen, S. (1997). Augmentative and alternative communication assessment strategies. In S.L. Glennen & D. DeCoste (Eds.), *The handbook of augmentative and alternative communication* (pp. 149–192). San Diego: Singular Publishing Group.

Glennen, S.L., & DeCoste, D. (1997). *The handbook of augmentative and alternative communication.* San Diego: Singular Publishing Group.

Gleser, G., Gottschalk, L., & John, W. (1959). The relationship of sex and intelligence to choice words: A normative study of verbal behavior. *Journal of Clinical Psychology, 15,* 182–191.

Gloeckler, T., & Simpson, C. (1988). *Exceptional students in regular classrooms: Challenges, services, and methods.* Mountain View, CA: Mayfield Publishing.

Goetz, L., Gee, K., & Sailor, W. (1983). Crossmodal transfer of stimulus control: Preparing students with severe multiple disabilities for audiological assessment. *Journal of The Association for Persons with Severe Handicaps, 8,* 3–13.

Goldman, H. (2002). *Augmentative Communication Assessment Profile.* London: Speechmark Publishing.

Goldman-Eisler, F. (1986). *Cycle linguistics: Experiments in spontaneous speech.* New York: Academic Press.

Goldman, R., & Fristoe, M. (2000). *Goldman-Fristoe Test of Articulation–Second Edition.* Circle Pines, MN: AGS Publishing.

Goldstein, H. (2002). Communication intervention for children with autism: A review of treatment efficacy. *Journal of Autism and Developmental Disorders, 32,* 373–396.

Goodenough-Trepagnier, C., Tarry, E., & Prather, P. (1982). Derivation of an efficient nonvocal communication system. *Human Factors, 24,* 163–172.

Goodglass, H. (1980). Naming disorders and aging. In L. Obler & M. Alberts (Eds.), *Language and communication* (pp. 35–47). Lexington, MA: Lexington Books.

Goodglass, H. (1993). *Understanding aphasia.* San Diego: Academic Press.

Goodglass, H., & Kaplan, E. (1983). *Boston Diagnostic Aphasia Examination, Second Edition.* Philadelphia: Lea & Febiger.

Goodman, J., & Remington, B. (1993). Acquisition of expressive signing: Comparison of reinforcement strategies. *Augmentative and Alternative Communication, 9,* 26–35.

Goossens', C. (1989). Aided communication intervention before assessment: A case study of a child with cerebral palsy. *Augmentative and Alternative Communication, 5,* 14–26.

Goossens', C., & Crain, S. (1986a). *Augmentative communication assessment resource.* Wauconda, IL: Don Johnston.

Goossens', C., & Crain, S. (1986b). *Augmentative communication intervention resource.* Wauconda, IL: Don Johnston.

Goossens', C., & Crain, S. (1987). Overview of nonelectronic eye-gaze communication devices. *Augmentative and Alternative Communication, 3,* 77–89.

Goossens', C., & Crain, S. (1992). *Utilizing switch interfaces with children who are severely physically challenged.* Austin, TX: PRO-ED.

Goossens', C., Crain, S., & Elder, P. (1992). *Engineering the preschool environment for interactive, symbolic communication.* Birmingham, AL: Southeast Augmentative Communication Conference Publications.

Goossens', C., Crain, S., & Elder, P. (1994). *Communication displays for engineered preschool environments: Books 1 and 2.* Solana Beach, CA: Mayer-Johnson Inc.

Gorenflo, C., & Gorenflo, D. (1991). The effects of information and augmentative communication technique on attitudes toward nonspeaking individuals. *Journal of Speech and Hearing Research, 34,* 19–26.

Goswami, U., & Mead, F. (1992). Onset and rime awareness and analogies in reading. *Reading Research Quarterly, 27,* 150–162.

Graham, S., & Harris, K.R. (1989). A component analysis of cognitive strategy instruction: Effects of LD students' compositions and self-efficacy. *Journal of Educational Psychology, 81*(3), 353–361.

Graham, S., & Harris, K.R. (1993). Self-regulated strategy development: Helping students with learning problems develop as writers. *The Elementary School Journal, 94*(2), 169–181.

Graham, S., & Harris, K.R. (1997). Whole language and process writing: Does one approach fit all? In J. Lloyd, E. Kameenui, & D. Chard (Eds.), *Issues in educating students with disabilities* (pp. 239–258). Mahwah, NJ: Lawrence Erlbaum Associates.

Graham, S., & Harris, K.R. (2005). *Writing better: Effective strategies for teaching students with learning difficulties.* Baltimore: Paul H. Brookes Publishing Co.

Graham, S., MacArthur, C., Schwartz, S., & Page-Voth, V. (1992). Improving the compositions of students with learning disabilities using a strategy involving product and process goal setting. *Exceptional Children, 58*(4), 322–334.

Grandin, T. (1995). *Thinking in pictures and other reports from my life with autism.* New York: Vintage Books.

Grandin, T., & Scariano, M. (1986). *Emergence: Labeled autistic.* Novato, CA: Arena Press.

Granlund, M., & Blackstone, S. (1999). Outcomes measurement in AAC. In F.T. Loncke, J. Clibbens, H. Arvidson, & L.L. Lloyd (Eds.), *Augmentative and alternative communication: New directions in research and practice* (pp. 207–227). London: Whurr Publishers.

Granlund, M., & Olsson, C. (1987). *Talspråksalternativ kommunikation och begåvningshandikapp* [Alternative communication and mental retardation]. Stockholm: Stiftelsen ALA.

Granlund, M., Ström, E., & Olsson, C. (1989). Iconicity and productive recall of a selected sample of signs from Signed Swedish. *Augmentative and Alternative Communication, 5,* 173–182.

Graves, D.H. (1994). *A fresh look at writing.* Portsmouth, NH: Heinemann.

Green, G., & Shane, H. (1994). Science, reason, and facilitated communication. *Journal of The Association for Persons with Severe Handicaps, 19,* 151–172.

Greenspan, S., & Weider, S. (1999). A functional developmental approach to autism spectrum disorders. *Journal of The Association for Persons with Severe Handicaps, 24,* 147–161.

Gregory, C., & McNaughton, S. (1993, September). Language! Welcoming a parent's perspective. *Communicating Together, 11*(3), 21–23.

Grove, N., & Walker, M. (1990). The Makaton Vocabulary: Using manual signs and graphic symbols to develop interpersonal communication. *Augmentative and Alternative Communication, 6,* 15–28.

Guralnick, M.J. (2001). Social competence with peers and early childhood inclusion: Need for alternative approaches. In M.J. Guralnick (Ed.), *Early childhood inclusion: Focus on change* (pp. 481–502). Baltimore: Paul H. Brookes Publishing Co.

Gustason, G. (1990). Signing Exact English. In H. Bornstein (Ed.), *Manual communication: Implications for education* (pp. 108–127). Washington, DC: Gallaudet University Press.

Gustason, G., Pfetzing, D., & Zawolkow, E. (1980). *Signing Exact English* (3rd ed.). Los Alamitos, CA: Modern Signs Press.

Gutmann, M. (1999, November). *The communication continuum in ALS: Client preferences and communication competence.* Paper presented at the annual convention of the American Speech-Language-Hearing Association, San Francisco, CA.

Gutmann, M., & Gryfe, P. (1996, August). *The communication continuum in ALS: Critical paths and client preferences.* Proceedings of the seventh biennial conference of the International Society of Augmentative and Alternative Communication (ISAAC), Vancouver.

Guyette, T., & Diedrich, W. (1981). A critical review of developmental apraxia of speech. In N. Lass (Ed.), *Speech and language advances in basic research and practice* (Vol. 5). New York: Academic Press.

Haaf, R. (1994). Technology in transition: Colin. *Communicating Together, 12*(3), 11–13.

Haaf, R., Millin, N., & Verberg, G. (1994). Sheila. *Communicating Together, 12*(2), 4–6.

Hagen, C. (1984). Language disorders in head trauma. In A. Holland (Ed.), *Language disorders in adults* (pp. 245–281). Austin, TX: PRO-ED.

Hall, P. (2001a). A letter to the parent(s) of a child with developmental apraxia of speech, Part 1: Speech characteristics of the disorder. *Language, Speech, and Hearing Services in Schools, 31,* 169–172.

Hall, P. (2001b). A letter to the parent(s) of a child with developmental apraxia of speech, Part 2: The nature and causes of DAS. *Language, Speech, and Hearing Services in Schools, 31,* 173–175.

Hall, P. (2001c). A letter to the parent(s) of a child with developmental apraxia of speech, Part 3: Other problems often associated with DAS. *Language, Speech, and Hearing Services in Schools, 31,* 176–178.

Hall, P. (2001d). A letter to the parent(s) of a child with developmental apraxia of speech, Part 4: Treatment of DAS. *Language, Speech, and Hearing Services in Schools, 31,* 179–181.

Hall, P., Jordan, L., & Robin, D. (1992). *Developmental apraxia of speech: Theory and clinical practice.* Austin, TX: PRO-ED.

Halle, J.W. (1987). Teaching language in the natural environment: An analysis of spontaneity. *Journal of The Association for Persons with Severe Handicaps, 12,* 28–37.

Halle, J., Baer, D., & Spradlin, J. (1981). Teacher's generalized use of delay as a stimulus control procedure to increase language use in handicapped children. *Journal of Applied Behavior Analysis, 14,* 389–409.

Halle, J., Brady, N., & Drasgow, E. (2004). Enhancing socially adaptive communicative repairs of beginning communicators with disabilities. *American Journal of Speech-Language Pathology, 13,* 43–54.

Halle, J., & Drasgow, E. (1995). Teaching social communication to young children with severe disabilities. *Topics in Early Childhood Special Education, 15,* 164–186.

Hamilton, B., & Snell, M. (1993). Using the milieu approach to increase spontaneous communication book use across environments by an adolescent with autism. *Augmentative and Alternative Communication, 9,* 259–272.

Hamm, B., & Mirenda, P. (2004). *Post-school quality of life of individuals with complex communication needs.* Manuscript in preparation, University of British Columbia.

Hammill, D., & Newcomer, P.L. (1996). *Test of Language Development-Primary–Third Edition (TOLD-P:3).* Circle Pines, MN: AGS Publishing.

Hammill, D.D., Pearson, N.S., & Wiederholt, J.L. (2001). *CTONI: Comprehensive Test of Nonverbal Intelligence.* Circle Pines, MN: American Guidance Service.

Hanley, G., Iwata, B., & Thompson, R. (2001). Reinforcement schedule thinning following treatment with functional communication training. *Journal of Applied Behavior Analysis, 34,* 17–38.

Hanson, E., Yorkston, K., & Beukelman, D.R. (2004). Speech supplementation techniques for dysarthria: A systematic review. *Journal of Medical Speech Language Pathology. 12,* ix–xxix.

Hardy, J. (1983). *Cerebral palsy.* Upper Saddle River, NJ: Prentice Hall.

Harrington, D. (1976). *The visual fields: A textbook and atlas of clinical perimetry* (4th ed.). St. Louis: Mosby.

Harris, J., Hartshorn, N., Jess, T., Mar, H., Rowland, C., Sall, N., et al. (n.d.). *Home talk: A family assessment of children who are deafblind.* Monmouth, OR: National Information Clearinghouse on Children Who Are Deafblind.

Harris, K.R., & Graham, S. (1996). *Making the writing process work: Strategies for composition and self-regulation.* Cambridge, MA: Brookline Books.

Harris, L., Doyle, E.S., & Haaf, R. (1996). Language treatment approach for users of AC: Experimental single-subject investigation. *Augmentative and Alternative Communication, 12,* 230–243.

Harris, M., & Reichle, J. (2004). The impact of aided language stimulation on symbol comprehension and production in children with moderate cognitive disabilities. *American Journal of Speech-Language Pathology, 13,* 155–167.

Harris, T.L., & Hodges, R.E. (1995). *The literacy dictionary: The vocabulary of reading and writing.* Newark, DE: International Reading Association.

Harrison-Harris, O. (2002). AAC, literacy, and bilingualism. *ASHA Leader Online, 20* (November 5, 2002). Retrieved March 18, 2004, from http://www.asha.org/about/publications/leader-online/archives/2002/q4/f021105.htm

Hart, B., & Risley, T.R. (1995). *Meaningful differences in the everyday experience of young American children.* Baltimore: Paul H. Brookes Publishing Co.

Hart, B., & Risley, T.R. (1999). *The social world of children learning to talk.* Baltimore: Paul H. Brookes Publishing Co.

Hart, V. (1977). The use of many disciplines with the severely and profoundly handicapped. In E. Sontag, J. Smith, & N. Certo (Eds.), *Educational programming for the severely and profoundly handicapped* (pp. 391–396). Reston, VA: Council for Exceptional Children.

Hartelius, L., & Svensson, P. (1994). Speech and swallowing symptoms associated with Parkinson's disease and multiple sclerosis: A survey. *Folia Phoniatrica et Logopaedica, 46,* 9–17.

Hawking, S. (1995). Professor Stephen Hawking [On-line]. Available from http://www.hawking.org.uk/home/hindex.html

Hawking, S. (2003). Intel Worldwide Employee Communications, 2003.

Hayden, D., & Square, P. (1994). Motor speech treatment hierarchy: A systems approach. *Clinics in Communication Disorders, 4,* 162–174.

Haynes, S. (1985). Developmental apraxia of speech: Symptoms and treatment. In D.F. Johns (Ed.), *Clinical management of neurogenic communicative disorders* (pp. 259–266). Boston: Little, Brown.

Heaton, E., Beliveau, C., & Blois, T. (1995). Outcomes in assistive technology. *Journal of Speech-Language Pathology and Audiology, 19,* 233–240.

Hedrick, D., Prather, E., & Tobin, A. (1984). *Sequenced Inventory of Communication Development—Revised.* East Aurora, NY: Slosson Educational Publications.

Hedrick, W.B., Katims, D.S., & Carr, N.J. (1999). Implementing a multimethod, multilevel literacy program for students with mental retardation. *Focus on Autism and Other Developmental Disabilities, 14*(4), 231–239.

Heimann, M., Nelson, K.E., Tjus, T., & Gillberg, C. (1995). Increasing reading and communication skills in children with autism through an interactive multimedia computer program. *Journal of Autism and Developmental Disorders, 25,* 459–480.

Heine, K., Wilkerson, R., & Kennedy, T. (1996, May). *Unity now and later: Equipping a two-year-old now, while preparing in the future.* Paper presented at the 1996 Minspeak conference, Wooster, OH.

Helfrich-Miller, K. (1994). A clinical perspective: Melodic intonation therapy for developmental apraxia. *Clinics in Communication Disorders, 4,* 175–182.

Heller, K., Allgood, M., Ware, S., Arnold, S., & Castelle, M. (1996). Initiating requests during community-based vocational training by students with mental retardation and sensory impairments. *Research in Developmental Disabilities, 17,* 173–184.

Heller, K., Ware, S., Allgood, M., & Castelle, M. (1994). Use of dual communication boards with students who are deaf-blind. *Journal of Visual Impairment and Blindness, 88,* 368–376.

Helm-Estabrooks, N. (1984). Severe aphasia. In A. Holland (Ed.), *Language disorders in adults* (pp. 159–176). San Diego: College-Hill Press.

Helm-Estabrooks, N. (2001). *Cognitive Linguistic Quick Test.* San Antonio, TX: Harcourt Assessment.

Helm-Estabrooks, N., Ramsberger, G., Morgan, A., & Nicholas, M. (1989). *Boston Assessment of Severe Aphasia.* Austin, TX: PRO-ED.

Hetzroni, O. (2002). Augmentative and alternative communication in Israel: Results from a family survey. *Augmentative and Alternative Communication, 18,* 255–266.

Hetzroni, O., Rubin, C., & Konkol, O. (2002). The use of assistive technology for symbol identification by children with Rett syndrome. *Journal of Intellectual and Developmental Disability, 27,* 57–71.

Hetzroni, O., & Tannous, J. (2004). Effects of a computer-based intervention program on the communicative functions of children with autism. *Journal of Autism and Developmental Disorders, 34,* 95–113.

Hetzroni, R., & Harris, O. (1996). Cultural aspects in the development of AAC users. *Augmentative and Alternative Communication, 12,* 52–58.

Higginbotham, D. (1989). The interplay of communication device output mode and interaction style between nonspeaking persons and their speaking partners. *Journal of Speech and Hearing Disorders, 54,* 320–333.

Higginbotham, D.J. (2001, December). Introduction: Research on utterance-based communication. *ASHA Special Interest Division 12 Newsletter, 10*(4), 2–5.

Higginbotham, D.J., Moulton, B., Lesher, G., Wilkins, D., & Cornish, J. (2000). Frametalker: Development of a frame-based communication system. In *Proceedings of the 2000 CSUN Annual Conference.* Northridge, CA: California State University at Northridge.

Higginbotham, D.J., Wilkins, D., Lesher, G., & Moulton, B. (1999). Frametalker: A communication frame and utterance-based augmentative communication device. In *Proceedings of the RESNA Annual Conference* (pp. 52–54). Arlington, VA: RESNA Press.

Hill, K. (2004). *AAC Performance Report Tool (PeRT) to support evidence-based practice.* Paper presented at the Technology and Persons with Disabilities Conference, California State University at Northridge.

Hill, K., & Romich, B. (2002). A rate index for augmentative and alternative communication. *International Journal of Speech Technology, 5,* 57–64.

Hirdes, J., Ellis-Hale, K., & Pearson Hirdes, B. (1993). Prevalence and policy implications of communication disabilities among adults. *Augmentative and Alternative Communication, 9,* 273–280.

Ho, K., Weiss, S., Garrett, K., & Lloyd, L. (in press). The effect of remnant and pictographic books on the communicative interaction of individuals with global aphasia. *Augmentative and Alternative Communication.*

Hoag, L., & Bedrosian, J. (1992). The effects of speech output type, message length, and reauditorization on perceptions of communicative competence of an adult AAC user. *Journal of Speech and Hearing Research, 35,* 1363–1366.

Hoag, L., Bedrosian, J., Johnson, D., & Molineux, B. (1994). Variables affecting perceptions of social aspects of the communicative competence of an adult AAC user. *Augmentative and Alternative Communication, 10,* 129–137.

Hoag, L., Bedrosian, J., McCoy, K., & Johnson, D. (2004). Trade-offs between informativeness and speed of message delivery in augmentative and alternative communication. *Journal of Speech, Language, and Hearing Research, 47,* 1270–1285.

Hochstein, D., McDaniel, M., & Nettleton, S. (2004). Recognition of vocabulary in children and adolescents with cerebral palsy: A comparison of two speech coding schemes. *Augmentative and Alternative Communication, 20,* 45–62.

Hochstein, D., McDaniel, M., Nettleton, S., & Neufeld, K. (2003). The fruitfulness of a nomothetic approach to investigating AAC: Comparing two speech encoding schemes across cerebral palsied and nondisabled children. *American Journal of Speech-Language Pathology, 12,* 110–122.

Hodgdon, L. (1996). *Visual strategies for improving communication.* Troy, MI: QuirkRoberts Publishing.

Hodges, P., & Schwethelm, B. (1984). A comparison of the effectiveness of graphic symbol and manual sign training with profoundly retarded children. *Applied Psycholinguistics, 5,* 223–253.

Hodson, B. (1986). *The Assessment of Phonological Processes–Revised Edition.* Austin. TX: PRO-ED.

Hoffmeister, R. (1990). ASL and its implications for education. In H. Bornstein (Ed.), *Manual communication: Implications for education* (pp. 81–107). Washington, DC: Gallaudet University Press.

Holland, A. (1998). Why can't clinicians talk to aphasic adults? Comments on supported conversation for adults with aphasia: Methods and resources for training conversational partners. *Aphasiology, 12,* 844–847.

Holland, A., Fromm, D., DeRuyter, F., & Stein, M. (1996). Treatment efficacy: Aphasia. *Journal of Speech and Hearing Research, 39,* S27–S36.

Honsinger, M. (1989). Midcourse intervention in multiple sclerosis: An inpatient model. *Augmentative and Alternative Communication, 5,* 71–73.

Hooper, J., Connell, T., & Flett, P. (1987). Blissymbols and manual signs: A multimodal approach to intervention in a case of multiple disability. *Augmentative and Alternative Communication, 3,* 68–76.

Hopper, T.L. (2003). "They're just going to get worse anyway": Perspectives on rehabilitation for nursing home residents with dementia. *Journal of Communication Disorders, 36,* 345–359.

Horn, E., & Jones, H. (1996). Comparison of two selection techniques used in augmentative and alternative communication. *Augmentative and Alternative Communication, 12,* 23–31.

Horner, R.H., McDonnell, J.J., & Bellamy, G.T. (1986). Teaching generalized skills: Instruction in simulation and community settings. In R.H. Horner, L.H. Meyer, & H.D.B. Fredericks (Eds.), *Education of learners with severe handicaps: Exemplary service strategies* (pp. 289–314). Baltimore: Paul H. Brookes Publishing Co.

Hoskins, B. (1990). Collaborative consultation: Designing the role of the speech-language pathologist in a new educational context. In W. Secord (Ed.), *Best practices in school speech-language pathology* (pp. 29–38). San Antonio, TX: Harcourt Assessment.

Houghton, J., Bronicki, B., & Guess, D. (1987). Opportunities to express preferences and make choices among students with severe disabilities in classroom settings. *Journal of The Association for Persons with Severe Handicaps, 11,* 255–265.

Hsieh, M-C., & Luo, C-H. (1999). Morse code typing of an adolescent with cerebral palsy using microcomputer technology: Case study. *Augmentative and Alternative Communication, 15,* 216–221.

Hudson, A.J. (1981). Amyotrophic lateral sclerosis and its association with dementia, parkinsonism and other neurologic disorders: A review. *Brain, 104*(2), 217–247.

Huebner, K. (1986). Curricula adaptations. In G.T. Scholl (Ed.), *Foundations of education for blind and visually handicapped children and youth: Theory and practice* (pp. 363–404). New York: American Foundation for the Blind.

Huer, M.B. (1997). Culturally inclusive assessments for children using augmentative and alternative communication (AAC). *Journal of Children's Communication Development, 19*, 23–34.

Huer, M.B. (2000). Examining perceptions of graphic symbols across cultures: Preliminary study of the impact of culture/ethnicity. *Augmentative and Alternative Communication, 16*, 180–185.

Huer, M.B. (2003). Individuals from diverse cultural and ethnic backgrounds may perceive graphic symbols differently: Response to Nigam. *Augmentative and Alternative Communication, 19*, 137–140.

Huer, M.B., Parette, H.P., & Saenz, T. (2001). Conversations with Mexican Americans regarding children with disabilities and augmentative and alternative communication. *Communication Disorders Quarterly, 22*, 197–206.

Huer, M.B., Saenz, T., & Doan, J.H.D. (2001). Understanding the Vietnamese American community: Implications for training educational personnel providing services to children with disabilities. *Communication Disorders Quarterly, 23*, 27–39.

Huer, M.B., & Wyatt, T. (1999). Cultural factors in the delivery of AAC services to the African-American community. *Multicultural Electronic Journal of Communication Disorders, 2.* Retrieved August 30, 2004, from http://www.asha.ucf.edu/huer.wyatt.html

Hunt, P., Alwell, M., Farron-Davis, F., & Goetz, L. (1996). Creating socially supportive environments for fully included students who experience multiple disabilities. *Journal of The Association for Persons with Severe Handicaps, 21*, 53–71.

Hunt, P., Alwell, M., & Goetz, L. (1988). Acquisition of conversation skills and the reduction of inappropriate social interaction behaviors. *Journal of The Association for Persons with Severe Handicaps, 13*, 20–27.

Hunt, P., Alwell, M., & Goetz, L. (1990). *Teaching conversation skills to individuals with severe disabilities with a communication book adaptation.* Unpublished manuscript. (Available from P. Hunt, San Francisco State University, 14 Tapia Street, San Francisco, CA 94132)

Hunt, P., Alwell, M., & Goetz, L. (1991a). Establishing conversational exchanges with family and friends: Moving from training to meaningful communication. *Journal of Special Education, 25*, 305–319.

Hunt, P., Alwell, M., & Goetz, L. (1991b). Interacting with peers through conversation turn taking with a communication book adaptation. *Augmentative and Alternative Communication, 7*, 117–126.

Hunt, P., Soto, G., Maier, J., Müller, E., & Goetz, L. (2002). Collaborative teaming to support students with augmentative and alternative communication needs in general education classrooms. *Augmentative and Alternative Communication, 18*, 20–35.

Hunt, P., Staub, D., Alwell, M., & Goetz, L. (1994). Achievement by all students within the context of cooperative learning groups. *Journal of The Association for Persons with Severe Handicaps, 19*, 290–301.

Hunt Berg, M. (in press). The Bridge School: Educational inclusion outcomes over fifteen years. *Augmentative and Alternative Communication.*

Huntley Bahr, R., Velleman, S., & Ziegler, M.A. (1999). Meeting the challenge of suspected developmental apraxia of speech through inclusion. *Topics in Language Disorders, 19*, 19–35.

Hurlbut, B., Iwata, B., & Green, J. (1982). Nonvocal language acquisition in adolescents with severe physical disabilities: Blissymbol versus iconic stimulus formats. *Journal of Applied Behavior Analysis, 15*, 241–258.

Hustad, K.C., & Shapley, K.L. (2003). AAC and natural speech in individuals with developmental disabilities. In J.C. Light, D.R. Beukelman, & J. Reichle (Eds.), *Communicative competence for individuals who use AAC: From research to effective practice* (pp. 41–62). Baltimore: Paul H. Brookes Publishing Co.

Hux, K. (Ed.). (2003). Epidemiology of traumatic brain injury. In *Assisting survivors of traumatic brain injury: The role of speech-language pathologists.* Austin, TX: PRO-ED.

Hwa-Froelich, D., & Westby, C. (2003). Frameworks of education: Perspectives of Southeast Asian parents and Head Start staff. *Language, Speech, and Hearing Services in Schools, 34,* 299–319.

Hymes, D. (1972). On communicative competence. In J.B. Pride & J. Holmes (Eds.), *Sociolinguistics* (pp. 269–293). London: Penguin Books.

Iacono, T.A. (2003). Pragmatic development in individuals with developmental disabilities who use AAC. In J.C. Light, D.R. Beukelman, & J. Reichle (Eds.), *Communicative competence for individuals who use AAC: From research to effective practice* (pp. 323–360). Baltimore: Paul H. Brookes Publishing Co.

Iacono, T., & Cupples, L. (2004). Assessment of phonemic awareness and word reading skills of people with complex communication needs. *Journal of Speech, Language, and Hearing Research, 47,* 437–449.

Iacono, T., Carter, M., & Hook, J. (1998). Identification of intentional communication in students with severe and multiple disabilities. *Augmentative and Alternative Communication, 14,* 102–114.

Iacono, T., & Duncum, J. (1995). Comparisons of sign alone and in combination with an electronic communication device in early language intervention: A case study. *Augmentative and Alternative Communication, 11,* 249–259.

Iacono, T., Mirenda, P., & Beukelman, D.R. (1993). Comparison of unimodal and multimodal AAC techniques for children with intellectual disabilities. *Augmentative and Alternative Communication, 9,* 83–94.

Iacono, T., & Parsons, C. (1986). A survey of the use of signing with the intellectually disabled. *Australian Communication Quarterly, 2,* 21–25.

Iacono, T., & Waring, R. (1996, August). *A case study of a parent-implemented AAC language intervention comparing signs versus sign+aid.* Paper presented at the seventh biennial conference of the International Society for Augmentative and Alternative Communication, Vancouver, British Columbia.

Ivers, R., & Goldstein, N. (1963). Multiple sclerosis: A current appraisal of symptoms and signs. *Proceedings of the Staff Meetings of the Mayo Clinic, 38,* 457–466.

Jennische, M. (1993, June). There are still reasons for concern. *Communicating Together, 11*(2), 21–22.

Jensema, C. (1982). Communication methods and devices for deaf-blind persons. *Directions, 3,* 60–69.

Jinks, A., & Sinteff, B. (1994). Consumer response to AAC devices: Acquisition, training, use, and satisfaction. *Augmentative and Alternative Communication, 10,* 184–190.

Johns, J. (2001). *Basic reading inventory* (8th ed.). Boston: Allyn & Bacon.

Johnson, D., & Johnson, R. (1987a). *Joining together: Group theory and skills* (2nd ed.). Upper Saddle River, NJ: Prentice Hall.

Johnson, D., & Johnson, R. (1987b). *Learning together and alone: Cooperation, competition, and individualization* (2nd ed.). Upper Saddle River, NJ: Prentice Hall.

Johnson, D., Johnson, R., & Holubec, E. (1993). *Circles of learning: Cooperation in the classroom* (4th ed.). Edina, MN: Interaction Book Co.

Johnson, D., Johnson, R., Holubec, E., & Roy, P. (1994). *The new circles of learning: Cooperation in the classroom and school.* Alexandra, VA: Association for Supervision and Curriculum Development.

Johnson, J. (1986). *Self-talk: Communication boards for children and adults.* Tucson, AZ: Communication Skill Builders.

Johnson, R. (1994). *The Picture Communication Symbols combination book.* Solana Beach, CA: Mayer-Johnson Co.

Johnston, J., & Wong, M.-Y. (2002). Cultural differences in beliefs and practices concerning talk to children. *Journal of Speech, Language, and Hearing Research, 42,* 916–926.

Johnston, S., Nelson, C., Evans, J., & Palazolo, K. (2003). The use of visual supports in teaching young children with autism spectrum disorder to initiate interactions. *Augmentative and Alternative Communication, 19,* 86–103.

Jolleff, N., & Ryan, M. (1993). Communication development in Angelman syndrome. *Archives of Disease in Childhood, 69,* 148–150.

Jolly, A., Test, D., & Spooner, F. (1993). Using badges to increase initiations of children with severe disabilities in a play setting. *Journal of The Association for Persons with Severe Handicaps, 18,* 46–51.

Jordan, F., & Murdoch, B. (1990). Unexpected recovery of functional communication following a prolonged period of mutism post-head injury. *Brain Injury, 4,* 101–108.

Jorgensen, C.M. (1998). *Restructuring high schools for all students: Taking inclusion to the next level.* Baltimore: Paul H. Brookes Publishing Co.

Jorm, A., & Jolly, D. (1998). The incidence of dementia: A meta-analysis. *Neurology, 51,* 728–733.

Jose, R.T. (Ed.). (1983). *Understanding low vision.* New York: American Foundation for the Blind.

Judd-Wall, J. (1995). *Assistive Technology Screener©.* Retrieved February 24, 2004, from http://www.taicenter.com/test_pretty/screeners/screener%20text.html

Judge, S.L., & Parette, H.P. (Eds.). (1998). *Assistive technology for young children with disabilities.* Cambridge, MA: Brookline Books.

Jutai, J., & Day, H. (2002). Psychological impact of Assistive Devices Scale (PIADS). *Technology and Disability, 14,* 107–111.

Kagan, A. (1995). Revealing the competence of aphasic adults through conversation: A challenge to health professionals. *Topics in Stroke Rehabilitation, 2,* 15–28.

Kagan, A. (1998). Supported conversation for adults with aphasia: Methods and resources for training conversation partners. *Aphasiology, 12,* 816–830.

Kagan, A., Black, S., Duchan, J., Simmons-Mackie, N., & Square, P. (2001). Training volunteers as conversation partners using "Supported Conversation for Adults with Aphasia" (SCA): A controlled trial. *Journal of Speech, Language, and Hearing Research, 44,* 624–638.

Kaiser, A.P., Yoder, P.J., & Keetz, A. (1992). Evaluating milieu teaching. In S.F. Warren & J. Reichle (Eds.), *Communication and language intervention series: Vol. 1. Causes and effects in communication and language intervention* (pp. 9–47). Baltimore: Paul H. Brookes Publishing Co.

Kalman, S., & Pajor, A. (1996). Some psychological and psychosocial aspects of introducing augmentative and alternative communication in Hungary: Tales, facts, and numbers. In S. von Tetzchner & M.H. Jensen (Eds.), *Augmentative and alternative communication: European perspectives* (pp. 355–372). London: Whurr Publishers.

Kame'enui, E., & Simmons, J. (1999). *Toward successful inclusion of students with disabilities: The architecture of instruction.* Reston, VA: Council for Exceptional Children.

Kangas, K., & Lloyd, L. (1988). Early cognitive skills as prerequisites to augmentative and alternative communication use: What are we waiting for? *Augmentative and Alternative Communication, 4,* 211–221.

Karlan, G. (1990). Manual communication with those who can hear. In H. Bornstein (Ed.), *Manual communication: Implications for education* (pp. 151–185). Washington, DC: Gallaudet University Press.

Karuth, D. (1985). If I were a car, I'd be a lemon. In A. Brightman (Ed.), *Ordinary moments: The disabled experience* (pp. 9–31). Syracuse, NY: Human Policy Press.

Kates, B., & McNaughton, S. (1975). *The first application of Blissymbolics as a communication medium for nonspeaking children: History and development, 1971–1974.* Don Mills, Ontario, Canada: Easter Seals Communication Institute.

Katims, D.S. (1991). Emergent literacy in childhood special education: Curriculum and education. *Topics in Early Childhood Special Education, 11*(1), 69–84.

Katz, J., & Mirenda, P. (2002). Including students with developmental disabilities in general education classrooms: Social benefits. *International Journal of Special Education, 17,* 25–35.

Katz, J., Mirenda, P., & Auerbach, S. (2002). Instructional strategies and educational outcomes for students with developmental disabilities in inclusive "multiple intelligences" and typical inclusive classrooms. *Research and Practice for Persons with Severe Disabilities, 27,* 227–238.

Katz, R., Haig, A., Clark, B., & DiPaola, R. (1992). Long-term survival, prognosis and life-care planning for 29 patients with chronic locked-in syndrome. *Archives of Physical Medical Rehabilitation, 73,* 403–408.

Kearns, T. (1990). Training families as effective sign communication partners and teachers. *Augmentative and Alternative Communication, 6,* 103.

Keen, D., Sigafoos, J., & Woodyatt, G. (2001). Replacing prelinguistic behaviors with functional communication. *Journal of Autism and Developmental Disorders, 31,* 385–398.

Keenan, J., & Barnhart, K. (1993). Development of yes/no systems in individuals with severe traumatic brain injuries. *Augmentative and Alternative Communication, 9,* 184–190.

Kelford Smith, A., Thurston, S., Light, J., Parnes, P., & O'Keefe, B. (1989). The form and use of written communication produced by physically disabled individuals using microcomputers. *Augmentative and Alternative Communication, 5,* 115–124.

Kemper, S. (1988). Geriatric psycholinguistics: Syntactic limitations of oral and written language. In L. Light & D. Burke (Eds.), *Language, memory, and aging* (pp. 58–76). Cambridge, UK: Cambridge University Press.

Kennedy, C.H., Meyer, K.A., Knowles, T., & Shulka, S. (2000). Analyzing the multiple functions of stereotypical behavior for students with autism: Implications for assessment and treatment. *Journal of Applied Behavior Analysis, 33,* 559–571.

Kent, R., Miolo, G., & Bloedel, S. (1994). The intelligibility of children's speech: A review of evaluation procedures. *American Journal of Speech-Language Pathology, 3,* 81–95.

Kent-Walsh, J., & Light, J. (2003). General education teachers' experiences with inclusion of students who use augmentative and alternative communication. *Augmentative and Alternative Communication, 19,* 104–124.

Keogh, W., & Reichle, J. (1985). Communication intervention for the "difficult-to-teach" severely handicapped. In S.F. Warren & A.K. Rogers-Warren (Eds.), *Teaching functional language* (pp. 157–194). Austin, TX: PRO-ED.

Kertesz, A. (1982). *Western Aphasia Battery.* Orlando, FL: Grune & Stratton.

Kiernan, C. (1983). The use of nonvocal communication techniques with autistic individuals. *Journal of Child Psychology and Psychiatry, 24,* 339–375.

Kiernan, C., Reid, B., & Jones, M. (1982). *Signs and symbols: Use of non-vocal communication systems.* Portsmouth, NH: Heinemann.

Kiernan, J.A., & Hudson, A.J. (1994). Frontal lobe atrophy in motor neuron diseases. *Brain, 117,* 747–757.

King, J., & Hux, K. (1995). Intervention using talking word processing software: An aphasia case study. *Augmentative and Alternative Communication, 11,* 187–192.

King, J., Spoeneman, T., Stuart, S., & Beukelman, D.R. (1995). Small talk in adult conversations. *Augmentative and Alternative Communication, 11,* 244–248.

Kipila, E., & Williams-Scott, B. (1990). Cued speech. In H. Bornstein (Ed.), *Manual communication: Implications for education* (pp. 139–150). Washington, DC: Gallaudet University Press.

Kirstein, I. (1981). *Oakland Schools Picture Dictionary.* Wauconda, IL: Don Johnston.

Klassner, E.R., & Yorkston, K.M. (2000). AAC for Huntington disease and Parkinson's disease: Planning for change. In D.R. Beukelman, K.M. Yorkston, & J. Reichle (Eds.), *Augmentative and alternative communication for adults with acquired neurologic disorders* (pp. 233–270). Baltimore: Paul H. Brookes Publishing Co.

Klassner, E.R., & Yorkston, K.M. (2001). Linguistic and cognitive supplementation strategies as augmentative and alternative communication techniques in Huntington's disease: Case report. *Augmentative and Alternative Communication, 17,* 154–160.

Klick, S. (1985). Adapted cuing technique for use in treatment of dyspraxia. *Language, Speech, and Hearing Services in Schools, 16,* 256–259.

Klick, S. (1994). Adapted cuing technique: Facilitating sequential phoneme production. *Clinics in Communication Disorders, 4,* 183–189.

Kliewer, C., & Biklen, D. (1996). Labeling: Who wants to be called retarded? In W. Stainback & S. Stainback (Eds.), *Controversial issues in special education* (pp. 83–95). Needham Heights, MA: Allyn & Bacon.

Kliewer, C., & Biklen, D. (2001). "School's not really a place for reading": A research synthesis of the literacy lives of students with severe disabilities. *Journal of The Association for Persons with Severe Handicaps, 26,* 1–12.

Kluth, P. (2003). *"You're going to love this kid!": Teaching students with autism in the inclusive classroom.* Baltimore: Paul H. Brookes Publishing Co.

Knapp, M. (1980). *Essentials of nonverbal communication.* New York: Holt, Rinehart & Winston.

Kochmeister, S. (1997). Excerpts from *Shattering walls. Facilitated Communication Digest, 5*(3), 10–12.

Koehler, L., Lloyd, L., & Swanson, L. (1994). Visual similarity between manual and printed alphabet letters. *Augmentative and Alternative Communication, 10,* 87–95.

Koenig, A., & Holbrook, M.C. (1995). *Learning media assessment of students with visual impairments: A resource guide for teachers.* Austin, TX: Texas School for the Blind and Visually Impaired.

Koester, H., & Levine, S. (1996). Effect of a word prediction feature on user performance. *Augmentative and Alternative Communication, 12,* 155–168.

Koester, H., & Levine, S. (1998). Model simulations of user performance with word prediction. *Augmentative and Alternative Communication, 14,* 25–35.

Koke, S., & Neilson, J. (1987). *The effect of auditory feedback on the spelling of nonspeaking physically disabled individuals.* Unpublished master's thesis. University of Toronto.

Konstantareas, M. (1984). Sign language as a communication prosthesis with language-impaired children. *Journal of Autism and Developmental Disorders, 14,* 9–23.

Konstantareas, M., Oxman, J., & Webster, C. (1978). Iconicity: Effects of the acquisition of sign language by autistic and other severely dysfunctional children. In P. Siple (Ed.), *Understanding language through sign language research* (pp. 213–237). New York: Academic Press.

Koppenhaver, D.A. (2000). Literacy in AAC: What should be written on the envelope we push? *Augmentative and Alternative Communication, 16,* 267–277.

Koppenhaver, D.A., Coleman, P.P., Kalman, S.L., & Yoder, D.E. (1991). The implications of emergent literacy research for children with developmental disabilities. *American Journal of Speech-Language Pathology, 1*(1), 38–44.

Koppenhaver, D.A., & Erickson, K.E. (2003). Natural emergent literacy supports for preschoolers with autism and severe communication impairments. *Topics in Language Disorders, 23*(4), 283–292.

Koppenhaver, D.A., Erickson, K.A., Harris, B., McLellan, J., Skotko, B.G., & Newton, R.A. (2001). Storybook-based communication intervention for girls with Rett syndrome and their mothers. *Disability and Rehabilitation, 23*(3/4), 149–159.

Koppenhaver, D., Erickson, K., & Skotko, B. (2001). Supporting communication of girls with Rett syndrome and their mothers in storybook reading. *International Journal of Disability, Development, and Education, 48,* 395–410.

Koppenhaver, D., Evans, D., & Yoder, D. (1991). Childhood reading and writing experiences of literate adults with severe speech and motor impairments. *Augmentative and Alternative Communication, 7,* 20–33.

Koppenhaver, D.A., & Yoder, D.E. (1988). Study of a spelling strategy for physically disabled augmentative communication users. *Communication Outlook, 10*(3), 10–12.

Koppenhaver, D., & Yoder, D. (1990, July–August). *A descriptive analysis of classroom reading and writing instruction for adolescents with severe speech and physical impairments.* Paper presented at the International Special Education Conference, Cardiff, Wales.

Koppenhaver, D., & Yoder, D. (1992a). Literacy issues in persons with severe physical and speech impairments. In R. Gaylord-Ross (Ed.), *Issues and research in special education* (Vol. 2, pp. 156–201). New York: Teachers College Press.

Koppenhaver, D., & Yoder, D. (1992b). Literacy learning of children with severe speech and physical impairments in school settings. *Seminars in Speech and Language, 13*(2), 143–153.

Koppenhaver, D., & Yoder, D. (1993). Classroom literacy instruction for children with severe speech and physical impairments (SSPI): What is and what might be. *Topics in Language Disorders, 13*(2), 1–15.

Koul, R. (2003). Synthetic speech perception in individuals with and without disabilities. *Augmentative and Alternative Communication, 19,* 29–36.

Koul, R., & Corwin, M. (2003). Efficacy of AAC intervention in individuals with chronic severe aphasia. In R. Schlosser, H. Arvidson, & L. Lloyd (Eds.), *The efficacy of augmentative and alternative communication: Toward evidence-based practice* (pp. 449–470). New York: Elsevier.

Koul, R., & Harding, R. (1998). Identification and production of graphic symbols by individuals with aphasia: Efficacy of a software application. *Augmentative and Alternative Communication, 14,* 11–23.

Kovach, T.M., & Kenyon, P.B. (2003). Visual issues and access to AAC. In J.C. Light, D.R. Beukelman, & J. Reichle (Eds.), *Communicative competence for individuals who use AAC: From research to effective practice* (pp. 277–319). Baltimore: Paul H. Brookes Publishing Co.

Kovarsky, D., Culatta, B., Franklin, A., & Theadore, G. (2001). "Communicative participation" as a way of facilitating and ascertaining communicative outcomes. *Topics in Language Disorders, 21*(4), 1–20.

Kozleski, E. (1991a). Expectant delay procedure for teaching requests. *Augmentative and Alternative Communication, 7*, 11–19.

Kozleski, E. (1991b). Visual symbol acquisition by students with autism. *Exceptionality, 2*, 175–194.

Kraat, A. (1985). *Communication interaction between aided and natural speakers: A state of the art report.* Toronto: Canadian Rehabilitation Council for the Disabled.

Kraat, A. (1990). Augmentative and alternative communication: Does it have a future in aphasia rehabilitation? *Aphasiology, 4*, 321–338.

Kraft, G. (1981). Multiple sclerosis. In W. Stolov & M. Clowers (Eds.), *Handbook of severe disability* (pp. 111–118). Washington, DC: U.S. Department of Education.

Kravits, T.R., Kamps, D.M., Kemmerer, K., & Potucek, J. (2002). Brief report: Increasing communication skills for an elementary-aged student with autism using the Picture Exchange Communication System. *Journal of Autism and Developmental Disorders, 32*, 225–230.

Kravitz, E., & Littman, S. (1990). A communication system for a nonspeaking person with hearing and cognitive impairments. *Augmentative and Alternative Communication, 6*, 100.

Kumin, L. (2002). You said it just yesterday, why not now? Developmental apraxia of speech in children and adults with Down syndrome. *Disability Solutions, 5*(2), 1–13.

Kunc, N., & Van der Klift, E. (1995). Beyond benevolence: Friendship and the politics of help. In J.S. Thousand, R.A. Villa, & A.I. Nevin (Eds.), *Creativity and collaborative learning* (pp. 391–401). Baltimore: Paul H. Brookes Publishing Co.

Kynette, D., & Kemper, S. (1986). Aging and loss of grammatical forms: A cross-sectional study of language performance. *Language and Communication, 6*(1/2), 65–72.

Ladtkow, M., & Culp, D. (1992). Augmentative communication with the traumatically brain injured population. In K. Yorkston (Ed.), *Augmentative communication in the medical setting* (pp. 139–243). Tucson, AZ: Communication Skill Builders.

Lafontaine, L., & DeRuyter, F. (1987). The nonspeaking cerebral palsied: A clinical and demographic database report. *Augmentative and Alternative Communication, 3*, 153–162.

Lahey, M., & Bloom, L. (1977). Planning a first lexicon: Which words to teach first. *Journal of Speech and Hearing Disorders, 42*, 340–349.

Lalli, J., Browder, D., Mace, C., & Brown, D. (1993). Teacher use of descriptive analysis data to implement interventions to decrease students' problem behaviors. *Journal of Applied Behavior Analysis, 25*, 227–238.

Lalli, J., Casey, S., & Kates, K. (1995). Reducing escape behavior and increasing task completion with functional communication training, extinction, and response chaining. *Journal of Applied Behavior Analysis, 28*, 261–268.

Lancioni, G., O'Reilly, M., & Basili, G. (2001). Use of microswitches and speech output systems with people with severe/profound intellectual or multiple disabilities: A literature review. *Research in Developmental Disabilities, 22*, 21–40.

Lancioni, G., Singh, N., O'Reilly, M., & Oliva, D. (2003a). Extending microswitch-based programs for people with multiple disabilities: Use of words and choice opportunities. *Research in Developmental Disabilities, 24*, 139–148.

Lancioni, G., Singh, N., O'Reilly, M., & Oliva, D. (2003b). Some recent research efforts on microswitches for persons with multiple disabilities. *Journal of Child and Family Studies, 12*, 251–256.

Lancioni, G., Singh, N., O'Reilly, M., Oliva, D., Dardanelli, E., & Pirani, P. (2003). Adapting the use of microswitches to foster response awareness and word association: Two case evaluations. *Journal of Positive Behavior Interventions, 5*, 153–157.

Landman, C., & Schaeffler, C. (1986). Object communication boards. *Communication Outlook, 8*(1), 7–8.

Lasker, J., Ball, L., Bringewatt, J., Stuart, S., & Marvin, M. (1996, November). *Small talk across the lifespan: AAC vocabulary selection.* Paper presented at the annual convention of the American Speech-Language-Hearing Association, Seattle, WA.

Lasker, J.P., & Bedrosian, J.L. (2001). Promoting acceptance of augmentative and alternative communication by adults with acquired communication disorders. *Augmentative and Alternative Communication, 17*(3), 141–153.

Lasker, J., & Beukelman, D.R. (1999). Peers' perceptions of storytelling by an adult with aphasia. *Aphasiology, 13*, 857–869.

Lasker, J., & Garrett, K. (2004). Website materials available from http://aac.unl.edu/

Lasker, J., Hux, K., Garrett, K., Moncrief, E., & Eischeid, T. (1997). Variations on the written choice communication strategy for individuals with severe aphasia. *Augmentative and Alternative Communication, 13*, 108–116.

Lawson, W. (1998). *Life behind glass: A personal account of autism spectrum disorder.* London: Jessica Kingsley.

Leaf, R., & McEachin, J. (1999). *A work in progress: Behavior management strategies and a curriculum for intensive behavioral treatment of autism.* New York: DRL Books.

Lee, J.H., Larson, S., Lakin, C., Anderson, L., Lee, N.K., & Anderson, D. (2001). Prevalence of mental retardation and developmental disabilities: Estimates from the 1994/1995 National Health Interview Survey Disability Supplements. *American Journal on Mental Retardation, 106*, 231–252.

Lee, K., & Thomas, D. (1990). *Control of computer-based technology for people with physical disabilities: An assessment manual.* Toronto: University of Toronto Press.

Leese, B., Wright, K., Hennessy, S., Tolley, K., Chamberlain, M.A., Stowe, J., & Rowley, C. (1993). How do communication aid centres provide services to their clients? *European Journal of Disorders of Communication, 28*, 263–272.

Leonhart, W., & Maharaj, S. (1979). *A comparison of initial recognition and rate of acquisition of Pictogram Ideogram Communication (PIC) and Blissymbols with institutionalized severely retarded adults.* Unpublished manuscript, Pictogram Centre, Saskatoon, Saskatchewan, Canada.

Lerner, J. (1988). *Learning disabilities: Theories, diagnosis, and teaching strategies.* Boston: Houghton Mifflin.

Lesher, G., Moulton, B., & Higginbotham, D.J. (1998a). Optimal character arrangements for ambiguous keyboards. *IEEE Transactions on Rehabilitation Engineering, 6*, 415–423.

Lesher, G., Moulton, B., & Higginbotham, D.J. (1998b). Techniques for augmenting scanning communication. *Augmentative and Alternative Communication, 14*, 81–101.

Lesher, G., Moulton, B., Higginbotham, D.J., & Alsofrom, B. (2002). Acquisition of scanning skills: The use of an adaptive scanning delay algorithm across four scanning displays. In *Proceedings of the 25th Annual Conference on Rehabilitation Engineering.* Washington, DC: RESNA Press.

Lesher, G., Moulton, B., Rinkus, G., & Higginbotham, D.J. (2000). *A universal logging format for augmentative communication.* Paper presented at the Technology and Persons With Disabilities Conference, California State University at Northridge. Retrieved February 23, 2004, from http://www.csun.edu/cod/conf/2000/proceedings/0088Lesher.htm

Lesher, G., & Rinkus, G. (2002). Leveraging word prediction to improve character prediction in a scanning configuration. In *Proceedings of the 25th Annual Conference on Rehabilitation Engineering.* Washington, DC: RESNA Press.

Levine, S., Goodenough-Trepagnier, C., Getschow, C., & Minneman, S. (1987). Multi-character key text entry using computer disambiguation. In *Proceedings of the 10th Annual Conference on Rehabilitation Engineering* (pp. 177–179). Washington, DC: RESNA Press.

Lewis, B., Freebairn, L., Hansen, A., Iyengar, S., & Taylor, H.G. (2004). School-age follow-up of children with childhood apraxia of speech. *Language, Speech, and Hearing Services in Schools, 35*, 122–140.

Light, J. (1988). Interaction involving individuals using augmentative and alternative communication systems: State of the art and future directions. *Augmentative and Alternative Communication, 4*, 66–82.

Light, J. (1989a). *Encoding techniques for augmentative communication systems: An investigation of the recall performance of nonspeaking physically disabled adults.* Unpublished doctoral dissertation, University of Toronto.

Light, J. (1989b). Toward a definition of communicative competence for individuals using augmentative and alternative communication systems. *Augmentative and Alternative Communication, 5*, 137–144.

Light, J. (1993). Teaching automatic linear scanning for computer access: A case study of a preschooler with severe physical and communication disabilities. *Journal of Special Education Technology, 2*, 125–134.

Light, J. (1996). *Exemplary practices to develop the communicative competence of students who use augmentative and alternative communication: Final grant report.* University Park, PA: The Pennsylvania State University.

Light, J. (1997). Communication is the essence of human life: Reflections on communication competence. *Augmentative and Alternative Communication, 13,* 61–70.

Light, J., Adkins, D., Ahmon, C., Jordan, J., Moulton, J., & Seich, A. (1998). *The effect of nonverbal feedback on the communicative competence of individuals who use AAC.* Manuscript in preparation.

Light, J.C., Arnold, K.B., & Clark, E.A. (2003). Finding a place in the "social circle of life." In J.C. Light, D.R. Beukelman, & J. Reichle (Eds.), *Communicative competence for individuals who use AAC: From research to effective practice* (pp. 361–397). Baltimore: Paul H. Brookes Publishing Co.

Light, J., Beer, D., Buchert, L., Casey, E., DiMarco, R., & Dolan, K. (1995, December). *The effect of grammatical completeness on the communicative competence of AAC users.* Poster presented at the national convention of the American Speech-Language-Hearing Association, Orlando, FL.

Light, J., Beesley, M., & Collier, B. (1988). Transition through multiple augmentative and alternative communication systems: A three-year case study of a head-injured adolescent. *Augmentative and Alternative Communication, 4,* 2–14.

Light, J.C., Beukelman, D.R., & Reichle, J. (Eds.). (2003). *Communicative competence for individuals who use AAC: From research to effective practice.* Baltimore: Paul H. Brookes Publishing Co.

Light, J.C., & Binger, C. (1998). *Building communicative competence with individuals who use augmentative and alternative communication.* Baltimore: Paul H. Brookes Publishing Co.

Light, J., Binger, C., Agate, T., & Ramsay, K. (1999). Teaching partner-focused questions to enhance the communicative competence of individuals who use AAC. *Journal of Speech, Language, and Hearing Research, 42,* 241–255.

Light, J., Binger, C., Bailey, M., & Millar, D. (1997). *Teaching the use of nonobligatory turns to enhance the communicative competence of individuals who use AAC.* Unpublished manuscript, The Pennsylvania State University.

Light, J., Binger, C., Dilg, H., & Livelsberger, B. (1996, August). *Use of an introduction strategy to enhance communication competence.* Paper presented at the seventh biennial conference of the International Society for Augmentative and Alternative Communication, Vancouver.

Light, J., Binger, C., & Kelford Smith, A. (1994). Story reading interactions between preschoolers who use AAC and their mothers. *Augmentative and Alternative Communication, 10,* 255–268.

Light, J., Collier, B., & Parnes, P. (1985a). Communication interaction between young nonspeaking physically disabled children and their primary caregivers: Part I. Discourse patterns. *Augmentative and Alternative Communication, 1,* 74–83.

Light, J., Collier, B., & Parnes, P. (1985b). Communication interaction between young nonspeaking physically disabled children and their primary caregivers: Part II. Communicative functions. *Augmentative and Alternative Communication, 1,* 98–107.

Light, J., Collier, B., & Parnes, P. (1985c). Communication interaction between young nonspeaking physically disabled children and their primary caregivers: Part III. Modes of communication. *Augmentative and Alternative Communication, 1,* 125–133.

Light, J., Corbett, M.B., Gullapalli, G., and Lepowski, S. (1995, December). *Other orientation and the communicative competence of AAC users.* Poster presented at the annual convention of the American Speech-Language-Hearing Association, Orlando, FL.

Light, J., Dattilo, J., English, J., Gutierrez, L., & Hartz, J. (1992). Instructing facilitators to support the communication of people who use augmentative communication systems. *Journal of Speech and Hearing Research, 35,* 865–875.

Light, J., & Drager, K. (2002). Improving the design of augmentative and alternative communication technologies for young children. *Assistive Technology, 14,* 17–32.

Light, J., & Drager, K. (2004). Re-thinking access to AAC technologies for young children: Simplifying the learning demands. *Perspectives on Augmentative and Alternative Communication, 13,* 5–12.

Light, J., Drager, K., D'Silva, K., Burki, B., Hanner, C., Kristiansen, L., & Worah, S. (2004). *Developmental and cultural influences on children's graphic representations of early emerging language concepts: Implications for AAC.* Manuscript in preparation, The Pennsylvania State University.

Light, J., Drager, K., Haley, A., & Hartnett, R. (2004). *Drawing of early emerging language concepts by children with disabilities.* Manuscript in preparation, The Pennsylvania State University.

Light, J., Drager, K., McCarthy, J., Mellott, S., Millar, D., Parrish, C., et al. (2004). Performance of typically developing four- and five-year-old children with AAC systems using different language organization techniques. *Augmentative and Alternative Communication, 20,* 63–88.

Light, J., & Kelford Smith, A. (1993). The home literacy experiences of preschoolers who use augmentative communication systems and their nondisabled peers. *Augmentative and Alternative Communication, 9,* 10–25.

Light, J., & Lindsay, P. (1991). Cognitive science and augmentative and alternative communication. *Augmentative and Alternative Communication, 7,* 186–203.

Light, J., & Lindsay, P. (1992). Message-encoding techniques for augmentative communication systems: The recall performances of adults with severe speech impairments. *Journal of Speech and Hearing Research, 35,* 853–864.

Light, J., Lindsay, P., Siegel, L., & Parnes, P. (1990). The effects of message and coding techniques on recall by literate adults using AAC systems. *Augmentative and Alternative Communication, 6,* 184–201.

Light, J., & McNaughton, D. (1993). Literacy and augmentative and alternative communication (AAC): The expectations and priorities of parents and teachers. *Topics in Language Disorders, 13*(2), 33–46.

Light, J., McNaughton, D., Krezman, C., Williams, M., & Gulens, M. (2000). The mentor project. *Proceedings of the International Society of Augmentative and Alternative Communication, 9,* 73–75.

Light, J., McNaughton, D., & Parnes, P. (1986). *A protocol for the assessment of the communicative interaction skills of nonspeaking severely handicapped adults and their facilitators.* Toronto: Augmentative Communication Service, Hugh MacMillan Medical Centre.

Light, J.C., Parsons, A.R., & Drager, K. (2002). "There's more to life than cookies": Developing interactions for social closeness with beginning communicators who use AAC. In J. Reichle, D.R. Beukelman, & J.C. Light (Eds.), *Exemplary practices for beginning communicators: Implications for AAC* (pp. 187–218). Baltimore: Paul H. Brookes Publishing Co.

Light, J., Roberts, B., Dimarco, R., & Greiner, N. (1998). Augmentative and alternative communication to support receptive and expressive communication for people with autism. *Journal of Communication Disorders, 31,* 153–180.

Lilienfeld, M., & Alant, E. (2002). Attitudes of children toward an unfamiliar peer using an AAC device with and without voice output. *Augmentative and Alternative Communication, 18,* 91–101.

Lloyd, C.M., Richardson, M.P., Brooks, D.J., Al-Chalabi, A., & Leigh, P.N. (2000). Extramotor involvement in ALS: PET studies with the GABAa ligand (11C)flumazenil. *Brain, 123*(11), 2289–2296.

Lloyd, L., & Blischak, D. (1992). AAC terminology policy and issues update. *Augmentative and Alternative Communication, 8,* 104–109.

Lloyd, L., & Fuller, D. (1986). Toward an augmentative and alternative communication symbol taxonomy: A proposed superordinate classification. *Augmentative and Alternative Communication, 2,* 165–171.

Lloyd, L., & Karlan, G. (1984). Nonspeech communication symbols and systems: Where have we been and where are we going? *Journal of Mental Deficiency Research, 38,* 3–20.

Locke, P., & Mirenda, P. (1988). A computer-supported communication approach for nonspeaking child with severe visual and cognitive impairments: A case study. *Augmentative and Alternative Communication, 4,* 15–22.

Locke, P., & Mirenda, P. (1992). Roles and responsibilities of special education teachers serving on teams delivering AAC services. *Augmentative and Alternative Communication, 8,* 200–214.

Locke, P., & Piché, L. (1994). Inclusion + technology = friendships. *Communication Outlook, 16*(4), 5–8.

Loeding, B., Zangari, C., & Lloyd, L. (1990). A "working party" approach to planning inservice training in manual signs for an entire public school staff. *Augmentative and Alternative Communication, 6,* 38–49.

Logemann, J.A., Fisher, H.B., Boshes, B., & Blonsky, E. (1978). Frequency and cooccurrence of vocal tract dysfunction in the speech of a large sample of Parkinson patients. *Journal of Speech and Hearing Disorders, 43,* 47–57.

Lohman, D.F., & Hagen, E.P. (2001). *Cognitive Abilities Test (CogAT), Form 6.* Itasca, IL: Riverside.

Lomen-Hoerth, C. (2004). Characterization of amyotrophic lateral sclerosis and frontotemporal dementia. *Dementia and Geriatric Cognitive Disorders, 17*(4), 337–341.

Lomen-Hoerth, C., Murphy, J., Langmore, S., Kramer, J.H., Olney, R.K., & Miller, B. (2003). Are amyotrophic lateral sclerosis patients cognitively normal? *Neurology, 60*(7), 1094–1097.

Lovaas, O.I. (2003). *Teaching individuals with developmental delays.* Austin, TX: PRO-ED.

Luckasson, R., Borthwick-Duffy, S., Buntinx, W.H.E., Coulter, D.L., Craig, E.M., Reeve, A., et al. (2002). *Mental retardation: Definition, classification, and systems of supports* (10th ed.). Washington, DC: AAMR.

Lueck, A. (2004). *Functional vision: A practitioner's guide to evaluation and intervention.* New York: AFB Press.

Luftig, R. (1984). An analysis of initial sign lexicons as a function of eight learnability variables. *Journal of The Association for Persons with Severe Handicaps, 9,* 193–200.

Lund, S.K. (2001). Fifteen years later: Long-term outcomes for individuals who use augmentative and alternative communication. *Dissertations Abstracts International* (UMI No. 3036075).

Lund, S., & Light, J. (2003). The effectiveness of grammar instruction for individuals who use augmentative and alternative communication systems: A preliminary study. *Journal of Speech, Language, and Hearing Research, 46,* 1110–1123.

Lund, S., Millar, D., Herman, M., Hinds, A., & Light, J. (November, 1998). *Children's pictorial representations of early emerging concepts: Implications for AAC.* Paper presented at the annual convention of the American Speech-Language-Hearing Association, San Antonio, TX.

Lunn, J., Coles, E., File, P., & Todman, J. (2003, September). *Making contact in the workplace.* Paper presented at the Communication Matters National Symposium, Lancaster, UK.

Lyon, J. (1992). Communication use and participation in life for adults with aphasia in natural settings: The scope of the problem. *American Journal of Speech-Language Pathology, 1,* 7–14.

Lyon, J. (1995). Drawing: Its value as a communication aid for adults with aphasia. *Aphasiology, 9,* 33–94.

MacArthur, C., Harris, K., & Graham, S. (1994). Improving students' planning process through cognitive strategy instruction. *Advances in Cognition and Educational Practice, 2,* 173–198.

MacDonald, J. (2004). *Communicating partners: Developmental guidelines for professionals and parents.* London: Jessica Kingsley Publishers.

MacDonald, J., & Gillette, Y. (1986). *Ecological communication system (ECO).* Columbus: Ohio State University, Nisonger Center.

MacGinitie, W., MacGinitie, R., Maria, K., & Dreyer, L. (2000). *Gates-MacGinitie Reading Tests®* (4th ed.). Itasca, IL: Riverside Publishing.

Magito-McLaughlin, D., Mullen-James, K., Anderson-Ryan, K., & Carr, E.G. (2002). Best practices: Finding a new direction for Christos. *Journal of Positive Behavior Interventions, 4,* 156–164.

Maharaj, S. (1980). *Pictogram ideogram communication.* Regina, Saskatchewan, Canada: The George Reed Foundation for the Handicapped.

Mandell, A. (2002, Fall). Diagnosing primary progressive aphasia. *National Aphasia Association Newsletter, 14*(2). Retrieved from http://www.aphasia.org/newsletter/Fall2002/DiagnosingPPA .html

Markwardt, F., Jr. (1998). *Peabody Individual Achievement Test–Revised-Normative Update (PIAT-R/NU).* Circle Pines, MN: American Guidance Service.

Marriner, N., Beukelman, D.R., Wilson, W., & Ross, A. (1989). *Implementing Morse Code in an augmentative communication system for ten nonspeaking individuals.* Unpublished manuscript, University of Washington, Seattle.

Martin, B., Jr. (1967). *Brown bear, brown bear, what do you see?* New York: Henry Holt & Co.

Marvin, C., & Privratsky, A. (1999). After-school talk: The effects of materials sent home from preschool. *American Journal of Speech-Language Pathology, 8,* 231–240.

Marvin, C.A., Beukelman, D.R., & Bilyeu, D. (1994). Vocabulary-use patterns in preschool children: Effects of context and time sampling. *Augmentative and Alternative Communication, 10,* 224–236.

Matas, J., Mathy-Laikko, P., Beukelman, D.R., & Legresley, K. (1985). Identifying the nonspeaking population: A demographic study. *Augmentative and Alternative Communication, 1,* 17–31.

Mathy, P., Yorkston, K.M., & Gutmann, M.L. (2000). AAC for individuals with amyotrophic lateral sclerosis. In D.R. Beukelman, K.M. Yorkston, & J. Reichle (Eds.), *Augmentative and alternative communication for adults with acquired neurologic disorders* (pp. 183–232). Baltimore: Paul H. Brookes Publishing Co.

Mathy-Laikko, P., Iacono, T., Ratcliff, A., Villarruel, F., Yoder, D., & Vanderheiden, G. (1989). Teaching a child with multiple disabilities to use a tactile augmentative communication device. *Augmentative and Alternative Communication, 5,* 249–256.

Mathy-Laikko, P., Ratcliff, A.E., Villarruel, F., & Yoder, D.E. (1987). Augmentative communication systems. In M. Bullis (Ed.), *Communication development in young children with deaf-blindness: III. Literature review* (pp. 205–241). Monmouth: Communication Skills Center for Young Children with Deaf-Blindness, Teaching Research Division, Oregon State System of Higher Education.

McCarthy, C.F., McLean, L.K., Miller, J., Paul-Brown, D., Romski, M.A., Rourk, J.D., & Yoder, D.E. (1998). *Communication supports checklist for programs serving individuals with severe disabilities.* Baltimore: Paul H. Brookes Publishing Co.

McClannahan, L.E., & Krantz, P.J. (1999). *Activity schedules for children with autism: Teaching independent behavior.* Bethesda, MD: Woodbine House.

McCloskey, S., & Zabala, J. (2003). Using quality indicators to improve service delivery for assistive technology services in educational settings. *Perspectives on Augmentative and Alternative Communication, 11*(3), 3–6.

McCord, M.S., & Soto, G. (2004). Perceptions of AAC: An ethnographic investigation of Mexican-American families. *Augmentative and Alternative Communication, 20,* 209–227.

McDonald, A. (1994). Readers write. *Communicating Together, 12*(4), 15.

McDonald, E., & Schultz, A. (1973). Communication boards for cerebral palsied children. *Journal of Speech and Hearing Disorders, 38,* 73–88.

McEwen, I., & Lloyd, L.L. (1990). Positioning students with cerebral palsy to use augmentative and alternative communication. *Language, Speech, and Hearing Services in Schools, 21,* 15–21.

McGee, G., Morrier, M., & Daly, T. (1999). An incidental teaching approach to early intervention for toddlers with autism. *Journal of The Association for Persons with Severe Handicaps, 24,* 133–146.

McGinnis, J. (1991). *Development of two source lists for vocabulary selection in augmentative communication: Documentation of the spoken and written vocabulary of third grade students.* Unpublished doctoral dissertation, University of Nebraska–Lincoln.

McGregor, G., & Vogelsberg, R.T. (1998). *Inclusive schooling practices: Pedagogical and research foundations—A synthesis of the literature that informs best practices about inclusive schooling.* Baltimore: Paul H. Brookes Publishing Co.

McLean, J., McLean, L., Brady, N., & Etter, R. (1991). Communication profiles of two types of gestures using nonverbal persons with severe to profound mental retardation. *Journal of Speech and Hearing Research, 34,* 294–308.

McNaughton, D., & Light, J. (1989). Teaching facilitators to support the communication skills of an adult with severe cognitive disabilities: A case study. *Augmentative and Alternative Communication, 5,* 35–41.

McNaugthon, D., Light, J., & Arnold, K. (2002). "Getting your wheel in the door": Successful full-time employment experiences of individuals with cerebral palsy who use augmentative and alternative communication. *Augmentative and Alternative Communication, 18,* 59–76.

McNaughton, D., Light, J., & Groszyk, L. (2001). "Don't give up": Employment experiences of individuals with amyotrophic lateral sclerosis who use augmentative and alternative communication. *Augmentative and Alternative Communication, 17,* 179–195.

McNaughton, S. (1990a). Introducing AccessBliss. *Communicating Together, 8*(2), 12–13.

McNaughton, S. (1990b). StoryBliss. *Communicating Together, 8*(1), 12–13.

McNaughton, S. (1993). Graphic representational systems and literacy learning. *Topics in Language Disorders, 13*(2), 58–75.

McNaughton, S., & Lindsay, P. (1995). Approaching literacy with AAC graphics. *Augmentative and Alternative Communication, 11,* 212–228.

McNeil, M. (1983). Aphasia: Neurological considerations. *Topics in Language Disorders, 3,* 1–19.

Medicare Funding of AAC Technology, Assessment/Application Protocol. (2001). Retrieved February 24, 2004, from the AAC-RERC Web site, http://www.aac-rerc.com/archive_aac-rerc/pages/MCsite/MCAppProtocol.html, supported in part by the National Institute on Disability and Rehabilitation Research (NIDRR).

Mergler, N., & Goldstein, M. (1983). Why are there old people? *Human Development, 26,* 130–143.

Mesibov, G., Browder, D., & Kirkland, C. (2002). Using individualized schedules as a component of positive behavioral support for students with developmental disabilities. *Journal of Positive Behavior Interventions, 4,* 73–79.

Mesulam, M. (2001). Primary progressive aphasia. *Annals of Neurology, 49*(4), 425–432.

Meyer, L.H., Peck, C.A., & Brown, L. (Eds.). (1991). *Critical issues in the lives of people with severe disabilities.* Baltimore: Paul H. Brookes Publishing Co.

Michael, P. (1981). *Multiple sclerosis: A dragon with a hundred heads.* Port Washington, NY: Ashley Books.

Mike, D.G. (1995). Literacy and cerebral palsy: Factors influencing literacy learning in a self-contained setting. *Journal of Literacy Research, 27,* 627–642.

Millar, D., Light, J., & Schlosser, R. (1999, November). *The impact of augmentative and alternative communication (AAC) on natural speech development: A meta-analysis.* Poster session presented at the American Speech-Language-Hearing Association annual conference, San Francisco.

Miller, J., & Paul, R. (1995). *Clinical assessment of language comprehension.* Baltimore: Paul H. Brookes Publishing Co.

Millin, N. (1995). Developing our own voices. *Communicating Together, 12*(1), 2–4.

Mineo Mollica, B. (2003). Representational competence. In J.C. Light, D.R. Beukelman, & J. Reichle (Eds.), *Communicative competence for individuals who use AAC: From research to effective practice* (pp. 107–145). Baltimore: Paul H. Brookes Publishing Co.

Mirenda, P. (1985). Designing pictorial communication systems for physically able-bodied students with severe handicaps. *Augmentative and Alternative Communication, 1,* 58–64.

Mirenda, P. (1993). AAC: Bonding the uncertain mosaic. *Augmentative and Alternative Communication, 9,* 3–9.

Mirenda, P. (1997). Supporting individuals with challenging behaviour through functional communication training and AAC: A research review. *Augmentative and Alternative Communication, 13,* 207–225.

Mirenda, P. (1999). Augmentative and alternative communication in inclusive classrooms. *Disability Solutions, 3*(4), 1–9.

Mirenda, P. (2001). Autism, augmentative communication, and assistive technology: What do we really know? *Focus on Autism and Other Developmental Disabilities, 16,* 141–151.

Mirenda, P. (2003a). "He's not really a reader . . . . ": Perspectives on supporting literacy development in individuals with autism. *Topics in Language Disorders, 23,* 270–281.

Mirenda, P. (2003b). Toward functional augmentative and alternative communication for students with autism: Manual signs, graphic symbols, and voice output communication aids. *Language, Speech, and Hearing Services in Schools, 34,* 202–215.

Mirenda, P. (2003c). Using AAC to replace problem behavior. *Augmentative Communication News, 15*(4), 10–11.

Mirenda, P., & Bopp, K.D. (2003). "Playing the game": Strategic competence in AAC. In J.C. Light, D.R. Beukelman, & J. Reichle (Eds.), *Communicative competence for individuals who use AAC: From research to effective practice* (pp. 401–437). Baltimore: Paul H. Brookes Publishing Co.

Mirenda, P., & Calculator, S. (1993). Enhancing curricula design. *Clinics in Communication Disorders, 3*(2), 43–58.

Mirenda, P., & Dattilo, J. (1987). Instructional techniques in alternative communication for learners with severe intellectual disabilities. *Augmentative and Alternative Communication, 3,* 143–152.

Mirenda, P., & Erickson, K. (2000). Augmentative communication and literacy. In A.M. Wetherby & B.M. Prizant (Eds.), *Autism spectrum disorders: A transactional developmental perspective* (pp. 333–367). Baltimore: Paul H. Brookes Publishing Co.

Mirenda, P., & Locke, P. (1989). A comparison of symbol transparency in nonspeaking persons with intellectual disabilities. *Journal of Speech and Hearing Disorders, 54*, 131–140.

Mirenda, P., MacGregor, T., & Kelly-Keough, S. (2002). Teaching communication skills for behavioral support in the context of family life. In J.M. Lucyshyn, G. Dunlap, & R.W. Albin (Eds.), *Families and positive behavior support: Addressing the challenge of problem behaviors in family contexts* (pp. 185–208). Baltimore: Paul H. Brookes Publishing Co.

Mirenda, P., Malette, P., & MacGregor, T. (1994, October). *Multicomponent, integrated communication systems for persons with severe intellectual disabilities.* Paper presented at the sixth biennial conference of the International Society for Augmentative and Alternative Communication, Maastricht, the Netherlands.

Mirenda, P., & Mathy-Laikko, P. (1989). Augmentative and alternative communication applications for persons with severe congenital communication disorders: An introduction. *Augmentative and Alternative Communication, 5*, 3–13.

Mirenda, P., & Santogrossi, J. (1985). A prompt-free strategy to teach pictorial communication system use. *Augmentative and Alternative Communication, 1*, 143–150.

Mirenda, P., & Schuler, A. (1988). Teaching individuals with autism and related disorders to use visual-spatial symbols to communicate. In S. Blackstone, E. Cassatt-James, & D. Bruskin (Eds.), *Augmentative communication: Intervention strategies* (pp. 5.1–17–5.1–25). Rockville, MD: American Speech-Language-Hearing Association.

Mirenda, P., & Schuler, A. (1989). Augmenting communication for persons with autism: Issues and strategies. *Topics in Language Disorders, 9*, 24–43.

Mirenda, P., Wilk, D., & Carson, P. (2000). A retrospective analysis of technology use patterns in students with autism over a five-year period. *Journal of Special Education Technology, 15*, 5–16.

Mitsuyama, Y., Kogoh, H., & Ata, K. (1985). Progressive dementia with motor neuron disease. An additional case report and neuropathological review of 20 cases in Japan. *European Archives of Psychiatry and Neurological Sciences, 235*(1), 1–8.

Mitsuda, P., Baarslag-Benson, R., Hazel, K., & Therriault, T. (1992). Augmentative communication in intensive and acute care settings. In K. Yorkston (Ed.), *Augmentative communication in the medical setting* (pp. 5–58). Tucson, AZ: Communication Skill Builders.

Mizuko, M. (1987). Transparency and ease of learning of symbols represented by Blissymbols, PCS, and Picsyms. *Augmentative and Alternative Communication, 3*, 129–136.

Mizuko, M., & Esser, J. (1991). The effect of direct selection and circular scanning on visual sequential recall. *Journal of Speech and Hearing Research, 34*, 43–48.

Mizuko, M., & Reichle, J. (1989). Transparency and recall of symbols among intellectually handicapped adults. *Journal of Speech and Hearing Disorders, 54*, 627–633.

Mizuko, M., Reichle, J., Ratcliff, A., & Esser, J. (1994). Effects of selection techniques and array sizes on short-term visual memory. *Augmentative and Alternative Communication, 10*, 237–244.

Montgomery, G.K., & Erickson, L.M. (1987). Neuropsychological perspectives in amyotrophic lateral sclerosis. *Neurologic Clinics, 5*(1), 61–81.

Morrow, D., Beukelman, D.R., Mirenda, P., & Yorkston, K. (1993). Vocabulary selection for augmentative communication systems: A comparison of three techniques. *American Journal of Speech-Language Pathology, 2*, 19–30.

Moster, D., Lie, R., Irgens, L., Bjerkedal, T., & Markestad, T. (2001). The association of Apgar score with subsequent death and cerebral palsy: A population-based study in infants. *Journal of Pediatrics, 138*, 791–792.

Mount, B., & Zwernik, K. (1988). *It's never too early, it's never too late* (Pub. No. 421–88–109). St. Paul, MN: Metropolitan Council.

Moustafa, M. (1995). Children's productive phonological recoding. *Reading Research Quarterly, 30*, 464–476.

Müller, E., & Soto, G. (2002). Conversation patterns of three adults using aided speech: Variations across partners. *Augmentative and Alternative Communication, 18*, 77–90.

Murdoch, B.E., & Lethlean, J.B. (2000). High-level language, naming and discourse abilities in multiple sclerosis. In B. Murdoch & D.G. Theodoros (Eds.), *Speech and language disorders in multiple sclerosis* (pp. 131–155). London: Whurr Publishers.

Murphy, J., Marková, I., Collins, S., & Moodie, E. (1996). AAC systems: Obstacles to effective use. *European Journal of Disorders of Communication, 31*, 31–44.

Murphy, J., Marková, I., Moodie, E., Scott, J., & Boa, S. (1995). Augmentative and alternative communication systems used by people with cerebral palsy in Scotland: Demographic survey. *Augmentative and Alternative Communication, 11*, 26–36.

Murray, L.L. (2000). Spoken language production in Huntington's and Parkinson's diseases. *Journal of Speech, Language, and Hearing Research, 43*, 1350–1366.

Murray-Branch, J., Udvari-Solner, A., & Bailey, B. (1991). Textured communication systems for individuals with severe intellectual and dual sensory impairments. *Language, Speech, and Hearing Services in Schools, 22*, 260–268.

Musselwhite, C. (1985). *Songbook: Signs and symbols for children.* Wauconda, IL: Don Johnston.

Musselwhite, C. (1986). *Adaptive play for special needs children: Strategies to enhance communication and learning.* San Diego: Singular Publishing Group.

Musselwhite, C. (1990, August). *Topic setting: Generic and specific strategies.* Paper presented at the fourth biennial conference of the International Society for Augmentative and Alternative Communication, Stockholm.

Musselwhite, C., & King-DeBaun, P. (1997). *Emerging literacy success: Merging whole language and technology for students with disabilities.* Park City, UT: Creative Communicating.

Musselwhite, C., & Ruscello, D. (1984). Transparency of three symbol communication systems. *Journal of Speech and Hearing Research, 27*, 436–443.

Musselwhite, C., & St. Louis, K. (1988). *Communication programming for persons with severe handicaps* (2nd ed.). Austin, TX: PRO-ED.

Nagi, S. (1991). Disability concepts revisited: Implications for prevention. In A. Pope & A. Tarlov (Eds.), *Disability in America: Toward a national agenda for prevention* (pp. 309–327). Washington, DC: National Academy Press.

Naglieri, J.A. (2000). *Naglieri Nonverbal Ability Test–Individual.* San Antonio, TX: Harcourt Assessment.

Nakamura, K., Newell, A., Alm, N., & Waller, A. (1998). How do members of different language communities compose sentences with a picture-based communication system? A cross-cultural study of picture-based sentences constructed by English and Japanese speakers. *Augmentative and Alternative Communication, 14*, 71–80.

National Aphasia Association. (1988). *Impact of aphasia on patients and family: Results of a needs survey.* Retrieved from National Aphasia Association Web site: http://www.aphasia.org

National Institute of Neurological Disorders and Stroke. (n.d.) *Guillain-Barré syndrome fact sheet.* Retrieved June 17, 1997, from http://www.ninds.nih.gov/

National Institute of Neurological Disorders and Stroke. (n.d.). *Huntington's disease—Hope through research.* Retrieved August 25, 2004, from http://www.ninds.nih.gov/health_and_medical/pubs/huntington_disease-htr.htm

National Joint Committee for the Communication Needs of Persons with Severe Disabilities. (2003a). Position statement on access to communication services and supports: Concerns regarding the application of restrictive "eligibility" policies. *ASHA Supplement, 23*, 19–20.

National Joint Committee for the Communication Needs of Persons with Severe Disabilities. (2003b). Supporting documentation for the position statement on access to communication services and supports: Concerns regarding the application of restrictive "eligibility" policies. *ASHA Supplement, 23*, 73–81.

National Research Council. (2001). *Educating children with autism.* Committee on Educational Interventions for Children with Autism, Division of Behavioral and Social Sciences and Education. Washington, DC: National Academy Press.

Needs First [Computer software]. (1996). Poughkeepsie, NY: Computer Options for the Exceptional.

Nelson, C., & van Dijk, J. (2001). Child-guided strategies for assessing children who are deafblind or have multiple disabilities [Computer software]. St. Michielsgestel, The Netherlands: Aap-NootMuis.

Nelson, N. (1992). Performance is the prize: Language competence and performance among AAC users. *Augmentative and Alternative Communication, 8,* 3–18.

Nelson, N.W., Bahr, C., & Van Meter, A. (2004). *The writing lab approach to language instruction and intervention.* Baltimore: Paul H. Brookes Publishing Co.

Newkirk, T. (1989). *More than stories: The range of children's writing.* Portsmouth, NH: Heinemann.

Nicholas, M., Sinotte, M., & Helm-Estabrooks, N. (2003) *Alternative communication computer treatment for aphasia: Who succeeds and why?* A seminar presented at the annual meeting of the American Speech-Language-Hearing Association, Chicago, IL.

Nickels, C. (1996). A gift from Alex: The art of belonging. In L.K. Koegel, R. Koegel, & G. Dunlap (Eds.), *Positive behavioral support* (pp. 123–144). Baltimore: Paul H. Brookes Publishing Co.

Nigam, R. (2003). Do individuals from diverse cultural and ethnic backgrounds perceive graphic symbols differently? *Augmentative and Alternative Communication, 19,* 135–136.

Nijland, L., Maassen, B., & van der Meilen, S. (2003). Evidence of motor programming deficits in children diagnosed with DAS. *Journal of Speech, Language, and Hearing Research, 46,* 437–450.

Northup, J., Wacker, D., Berg, W., Kelly, L., Sasso, G., & DeRaad, A. (1994). The treatment of severe behavior problems in school settings using a technical assistance model. *Journal of Applied Behavior Analysis, 27,* 33–48.

O'Brien, J., & Lyle O'Brien, C. (2002). *Implementing person-centered planning: Voices of experience.* Toronto: Inclusion Press.

O'Brien, J., & Pearpoint, J. (n.d.). *Person-centered planning with MAPS and PATH: A workbook for facilitators.* Toronto: Inclusion Press.

O'Keefe, B., Brown, L., & Schuller, R. (1998). Identification and rankings of communication aid features by five groups. *Augmentative and Alternative Communication, 14,* 37–50.

O'Keefe, B., & Dattilo, J. (1992). Teaching the response-recode form to adults with mental retardation using AAC systems. *Augmentative and Alternative Communication, 8,* 224–233.

Olaszi, P., Koutny, I., & Kálmán, S. (2002). From Blissymbols to grammatically correct voice out-out: A communication tool for people with disabilities. *International Journal of Speech Technology, 5,* 49–56.

Oliver, J., Ponford, J., & Curren, C. (1996). Outcomes following traumatic brain injury. A comparison between 2 and 5 years after injury. *Brain Injury, 10,* 841–848.

Olmos-Lau, N., Ginsberg, M., & Geller, J. (1977). Aphasia in multiple sclerosis. *Neurology, 27,* 623–626.

Olshan, M. (2000, February). Voice lessons: Speaking with ALS. *Asha Leader,* 4–5.

Olsson, C., & Granlund, M. (2003). Communication intervention for pre-symbolic communication. In R. Schlosser (Ed.), *Efficacy research in augmentative and alternative communication.* New York: Elsevier.

O'Neill, R., Horner, R., Albin, R., Sprague, J., Storey, K., & Newton, S. (1997). *Functional assessment and program development for problem behavior: A practical handbook* (2nd ed.). Pacific Grove, CA: Brooks/Cole.

Orel-Bixler, D. (1999). Clinical vision assessment for infants. In D. Chen (Ed.), *Essential elements in early intervention* (pp. 107–156). New York: AFB Press.

Orelove, F.P., & Sobsey, D. (1996). *Educating children with multiple disabilities: A transdisciplinary approach* (3rd ed.). Baltimore: Paul H. Brookes Publishing Co.

Osborn, A. (1963). *Applied imagination: Principles and procedures of creative problem-solving.* New York: Charles Scribner's Sons.

Osterling, J., Dawson, G., & Munson, J. (2002). Early recognition of 1-year-old infants with autism spectrum disorder versus mental retardation. *Development & Psychopathology, 14,* 239–251.

Owens, R.E. (2004). *Language disorders: A functional approach to assessment and intervention* (4th ed.). New York: Merrill/Macmillan.

Oxley, J., & Norris, J. (2000). Children's use of memory strategies: Relevance to voice output communication aid use. *Augmentative and Alternative Communication, 16,* 79–94.

Oxley, J., & von Tetzchner, S. (1999). Reflections on the development of alternative language forms. In F.T. Loncke, J. Clibbens, H. Arvidson, & L.L. Lloyd (Eds.), *Augmentative and alternative communication: New directions in research and practice* (pp. 62–74). London: Whurr Publishers.

Parette, P., Chuang, S.J., & Huer, M.B. (2004). First generation Chinese family attitudes regarding disabilities and educational interventions. *Focus on Autism and Other Developmental Disabilities, 19,* 114–123.

Parette, P., & Huer, M.B. (2002). Working with Asian American families whose children have augmentative and alternative communication needs. *Journal of Special Education Technology, 17*(4), 5–13.

Parette, P., Huer, M.B., & Wyatt, T. (2002). Young African American children with disabilities and augmentative and alternative communication issues. *Early Childhood Journal, 29,* 210–227.

Parette, P., VanBiervliet, A., & Hourcade, J. (2000). Family-centered decision making in assistive technology. *Journal of Special Education Technology, 15,* 45–55.

Park, C.C. (1982). *The siege.* Boston: Little, Brown.

Parnes, P. (1995). "Oh, Wow Days are gone forever," Canadian administrator reports. In S. Blackstone & H. Pressman (Eds.), *Outcomes in AAC conference report: Alliance '95* (pp. 21–22). Monterey, CA: Augmentative Communication.

Parnes, S. (1985). *A facilitating style of leadership.* Buffalo, NY: The Creative Education Foundation.

Parnes, S. (1988). *Visioning: State-of-the-art process for encouraging innovative excellence.* East Aurora, NY: DOK Publishers.

Parsons, C., & LaSorte, D. (1993). The effect of computers with synthesized speech and no speech on the spontaneous communication of children with autism. *Australian Journal of Human Communication Disorders, 21,* 12–31.

Paul, D., Frattali, C., Holland, A., Thompson, C., Caperton, C., & Slater, S. (2004). *Quality of Communication Life Scale (ASHA QCL).* Rockville, MD: American Speech-Language-Hearing Association.

Paul, R. (1997). Facilitating transitions in language development for children using AAC. *Augmentative and Alternative Communication, 13,* 141–148.

Pearpoint, J., Forest, M., & O'Brien, J. (1996). MAPs, Circles of Friends, and PATH: Powerful tools to help build caring communities. In S. Stainback & W. Stainback (Eds.), *Inclusion: A guide for educators* (pp. 67–86). Baltimore: Paul H. Brookes Publishing Co.

Pearpoint, J., O'Brien, J., & Forest, M. (2001). *PATH: A workbook for planning positive possible futures.* Toronto: Inclusion Press.

Peck, S., Wacker, D., Berg, W., Cooper, L., Brown, K., Richman, D., McComas, J., Frischmeyer, P., & Millard, T. (1996). Choice-making treatment of young children's severe behavior problems. *Journal of Applied Behavior Analysis, 29,* 263–290.

Peck Peterson, S.M., Derby, K.M., Harding, J.W., Weddle, T., & Barretto, A. (2002). Behavioral support for school-age children with developmental disabilities and problem behavior. In J.M. Lucyshyn, G. Dunlap, & R.W. Albin (Eds.), *Families and positive behavior support: Addressing problem behaviors in family contexts* (pp. 287–304). Baltimore: Paul H. Brookes Publishing Co.

Pellegrino, L. (2002). Cerebral palsy. In M.L. Batshaw (Ed.), *Children with disabilities* (5th ed., pp. 443–466). Baltimore: Paul H. Brookes Publishing Co.

Pepper, J., & Weitzman, E. (2004). *It takes two to talk: A practical guide for parents of children with language delays.* Toronto: The Hanen Centre.

Pierce, P., Steelman, J., Koppenhaver, D., & Yoder, D. (1993, March). Linking symbols with language. *Communicating Together, 11*(1), 18–19.

Pierce, P.L., & McWilliam, P.J. (1993). Emerging literacy and children with severe speech and physical impairments (SSPI): Issues and possible intervention strategies. *Topics in Language Disorders, 13*(2), 47–57.

Poeck, K., Huber, W., & Willmes, K. (1989). Outcome of intensive language treatment in aphasia. *Journal of Speech and Hearing Disorders, 54,* 471–479.

Poole, M. (1979). Social class, sex, and linguistic coding. *Language and Speech, 22,* 49–67.

Porter, P. (1989). Intervention in end stage of multiple sclerosis. *Augmentative and Alternative Communication, 5,* 125–127.

Poser, C.M. (Ed.). (1984). *The diagnosis of multiple sclerosis.* New York: Thieme-Stratton.

Pressley, M., & McCormick, C. (1995). *Advanced educational psychology: For educators, researchers, and policy makers.* New York: HarperCollins.

Pressley, M., Wharton-McDonald, R., Mistretta-Hampston, J., & Echevarria, M. (1998). Literacy instruction in 10 fourth- and fifth-grade classrooms in upstate New York. *Scientific Studies of Reading, 2*(2), 159–194.

Pressley, M., Wharton-McDonald, R., Rankin, J., Mistretta, J., Yokoi, L., & Ettenberger, S. (1996). The nature of outstanding primary grades literacy instruction. In E. McIntyre & M. Pressley (Eds.), *Balanced instruction: Strategies and skills in whole language* (pp. 251–276). Norwood, MA: Christopher-Gordon.

Pressley, M., & Woloshyn, V. (1995). *Cognitive strategy instruction that really improves academic performance* (2nd ed.). Cambridge, MA: Brookline Books.

Price, S.P. (2000). My early life and education. In M. Fried-Oken & H.A. Bersani, Jr. (Eds.), *Speaking up and spelling it out: Personal essays on augmentative and alternative communication* (pp. 105–114). Baltimore: Paul H. Brookes Publishing Co.

Prizant, B. (1983). Language and communicative behavior in autism: Toward an understanding of the "whole" of it. *Journal of Speech and Hearing Disorders, 46,* 241–249.

Prizant, B.M., Wetherby, A., Rubin, E., & Laurent, A. (2003). The SCERTS Model: A transactional, family-centered approach to enhancing communication and socioemotional abilities of children with autism spectrum disorder. *Infants and Young Children, 16,* 296–316.

Prizant, B.M., Wetherby, A.M., Rubin, E., Laurent, A.C., & Rydell, P.J. (2005a). *The SCERTS™ Model: A comprehensive educational approach for children with autism spectrum disorders. Vol. I: Assessment.* Baltimore: Paul H. Brookes Publishing Co.

Prizant, B.M., Wetherby, A.M., Rubin, E., Laurent, A.C., & Rydell, P.J. (2005b). *The SCERTS™ Model: A comprehensive educational approach for children with autism spectrum disorders. Vol. II: Program planning and intervention.* Baltimore: Paul H. Brookes Publishing Co.

Pugliese, M. (2001). *Stages: Software solutions for special needs.* Newton, MA: Assistive Technologies.

Pulli, T., & Jaroma, M. (1990). Exploring novel solutions for motivating simplified signing, pictorializing, and vocalizing. *Augmentative and Alternative Communication, 6,* 103.

Putnam, J.W. (1998). *Cooperative learning and strategies for inclusion: Celebrating diversity in the classroom* (2nd ed.). Baltimore: Paul H. Brookes Publishing Co.

QIAT Consortium. (2003). *Quality indicators for assistive technology services in schools.* Retrieved August 28, 2004, from http://www.qiat.org

Rackowska, M. (2000). The different one in society. In M. Williams & C. Krezman (Eds.), *Beneath the surface: Creative expressions of augmented communicators* (p. 88). Toronto: ISAAC Press.

Radell, U. (1997). Augmentative and alternative communication assessment strategies: Seating and positioning. In S.L. Glennen & D. DeCoste (Eds.), *The handbook of augmentative and alternative communication* (pp. 193–242). San Diego: Singular Publishing Group.

Raghavendra, P., & Fristoe, M. (1990). "A spinach with a V on it": What 3-year-olds see in standard and enhanced Blissymbolics. *Journal of Speech and Hearing Disorders, 55,* 149–159.

Raghavendra, P., & Fristoe, M. (1995). "No shoes; they walked away?": Effects of using enhancements on learning and using Blissymbols by normal 3-year-old children. *Journal of Speech and Hearing Research, 38,* 174–188.

Rainforth, B., & York-Barr, J. (1997). *Collaborative teams for students with severe disabilities* (2nd ed.). Baltimore: Paul H. Brookes Publishing Co.

Rakowicz, W.P., & Hodges, J.R. (1998). Dementia and aphasia in motor neuron disease: An underrecognized association? *Journal of Neurology, Neurosurgery, and Psychiatry, 65,* 881–889.

Ramig, L.O., Pawlas, A.A., & Countryman, S. (1995). *The Lee Silverman Voice Treatment.* Iowa City, IA: National Center for Voice and Speech.

Ramig, L.O., Sapir, S., Countryman, S., Pawlas, A., O'Brien, C., Hoehn, M., & Thompson, L. (2001). Intensive voice treatment (LSVT) for individuals with Parkinson disease: A two-year follow-up. *Journal of Neurology, Neuropsychiatry, and Psychiatry, 71,* 493–498.

Ramig, L.O., Sapir, S., Fox, C., & Countryman, S. (2001). Changes in vocal intensity following intensive voice treatment (LSVT) in individuals with Parkinson disease: A comparison with untreated patients and normal age-matched controls. *Movement Disorders, 16*(1), 79–83.

Raney, C., & Silverman, F. (1992). Attitudes toward nonspeaking individuals who use communication boards. *Journal of Speech and Hearing Research, 35*, 1269–1271.

Rankin, J.L., Harwood, K., & Mirenda, P. (1994). Influence of graphic symbol use on reading comprehension. *Augmentative and Alternative Communication, 10*, 269–281.

Rao, P. (1994). Introducing a communication board for child-to-child conversations. *Communication Outlook, 16*(2), 10–12.

Rao, S.M. (1995). Neuropsychology of multiple sclerosis. *Current Opinion in Neurology, 8*, 216–220.

Rasmussen, P., Börjesson, O., Wentz, E., & Gillberg, C. (2001). Autistic disorders in Down syndrome: Background factors and clinical correlates. *Developmental Medicine and Child Neurology, 43*, 750–754.

Ratcliff, A. (1994). Comparison of relative demands implicated in direct selection and scanning: Considerations from normal children. *Augmentative and Alternative Communication, 10*, 67–74.

Redmond, S., & Johnston, S. (2001). Evaluating the morphological competence of children with severe speech and physical impairments. *Journal of Speech, Language, and Hearing Research, 44*, 1362–1375.

Reed, C., Delhorne, L., Durlach, N., & Fischer, S. (1990). A study of the tactual and visual reception of fingerspelling. *Journal of Speech and Hearing Research, 33*, 786–797.

Reed, C., Delhorne, L., Durlach, N., & Fischer, S. (1995). A study of the tactual reception of sign language. *Journal of Speech and Hearing Research, 38*, 477–489.

Reed, P. (1998). Assistive technology: Putting the puzzle together. *Disability Solutions, 3*(2), 1–6.

Rees, N. (1982). Language intervention with children. In J. Miller, D. Yoder, & R. Schiefelbusch (Eds.), *Contemporary issues in language intervention* (American Speech-Language-Hearing Association Report No. 12, pp. 309–316). Rockville, MD: American Speech-Language-Hearing Association.

Rehfeldt, R., Kinney, E., Root, S., & Stromer, R. (2004). Creating activity schedules using Microsoft® Powerpoint®. *Journal of Applied Behavior Analysis, 37*, 115–128.

Reichle, J., & Brown, L. (1986). Teaching the use of a multipage direct selection communication board to an adult with autism. *Journal of The Association for Persons with Severe Handicaps, 11*, 68–73.

Reichle, J., Dettling, E., Drager, K., & Leiter, A. (2000). Comparison of correct responses and response latency for fixed and dynamic displays: Performance of a learner with severe developmental disabilities. *Augmentative and Alternative Communication, 16*, 154–163.

Reichle, J., & Johnston, S. (1999). Teaching the conditional use of communicative requests to two school-age children with severe developmental disabilities. *Language, Speech, and Hearing Services in Schools, 30*, 324–334.

Reichle, J., & Karlan, G. (1985). The selection of an augmentative system of communication intervention: A critique of decision rules. *Journal of The Association for Persons with Severe Handicaps, 10*, 146–156.

Reichle, J., Rogers, N., & Barrett, C. (1984). Establishing pragmatic discrimination among the communicative functions of requesting, rejecting, and commenting in an adolescent. *Journal of The Association for Persons with Severe Handicaps, 9*, 31–36.

Reichle, J., Sigafoos, J., & Piché, L. (1989). Teaching an adolescent with blindness and severe disabilities: A correspondence between requesting and selecting preferred objects. *Journal of The Association for Persons with Severe Handicaps, 14*, 75–80.

Reichle, J., & Wacker, D.P. (Eds.). (1993). *Communication and language intervention series: Vol. 3. Communicative alternatives to challenging behavior: Integrating functional assessment and intervention strategies.* Baltimore: Paul H. Brookes Publishing Co.

Reichle, J., & Ward, M. (1985). Teaching the discriminative use of an encoding electronic communication device and Signing Exact English to a moderately handicapped child. *Language, Speech, and Hearing Services in Schools, 16*, 58–63.

Reichle, J., & Yoder, D. (1985). Communication board use in severely handicapped learners. *Language, Speech, and Hearing Services in Schools, 16*, 146–157.

Reichle, J., York, J., & Sigafoos, J. (1991). *Implementing augmentative and alternative communication: Strategies for learners with severe disabilities.* Baltimore: Paul H. Brookes Publishing Co.

Reif, L. (1992). *Seeking diversity: Language arts with adolescents.* Portsmouth, NH: Heinemann.

Remington, B. (1994). Augmentative and alternative communication and behavior analysis: A productive partnership? *Augmentative and Alternative Communication, 10,* 3–13.

Remington, B., & Clarke, S. (1993a). Simultaneous communication and speech comprehension: Part I. Comparison of two methods of teaching expressive signing and speech comprehension skills. *Augmentative and Alternative Communication, 9,* 36–48.

Remington, B., & Clarke, S. (1993b). Simultaneous communication and speech comprehension: Part II. Comparison of two methods overcoming selective attention during expressive sign training. *Augmentative and Alternative Communication, 9,* 49–60.

Remington, B., Watson, J., & Light, J. (1990). Beyond the single sign: A matrix-based approach to teaching productive sign combinations. *Mental Handicap Research, 3,* 33–50.

Renwick, R., Rudman, D., Raphael, D., & Brown, I. (1998). *Quality of life profile: People with physical and sensory disabilities.* Toronto: University of Toronto, Centre for Health Promotion.

Rescorla, L., Alley, A., & Christine, J. (2001). Word frequencies of toddlers' lexicons. *Journal of Speech, Language, and Hearing Research, 44,* 598–609.

Richter, M., Ball, L., Beukelman, D.R., Lasker, J., & Ullman, C. (2003). Attitudes toward communication odes and message formulation techniques used for storytelling by people with amyotrophic lateral sclerosis. *Augmentative and Alternative Communication, 19,* 170–186.

Riemer-Reiss, M., & Wacker, R. (2000). Factors associated with assistive technology discontinuance among individuals with disabilities. *Journal of Rehabilitation, 66,* 44–50.

Robbins, A.M., & Osberger, M.J. (1992). *Meaningful use of speech scale.* Indianapolis, IN: Indiana University School of Medicine.

Roberts, W., & Brian, J. (2004, March). *Challenges in ASD intervention: Research to practice to research.* Paper presented at the Research to Policy and Care Conference, Richmond, British Columbia.

Robin, D. (1992). Developmental apraxia of speech: Just another motor problem. *American Journal of Speech-Language Pathology, 1,* 19–22.

Robinson, J., & Griffith, P. (1979). On the scientific status of iconicity. *Sign Language Studies, 25,* 297–315.

Rogers, M.A., & Alarcon, N.B. (1999). Characteristics and management of primary progressive aphasia. *Neurophysiology and Neurogenic Speech and Language Disorders Newsletter, 9,* 12–26.

Rogers, M.A., King, J.M., & Alarcon, N.B. (2000). Proactive management of primary progressive aphasia. In D.R. Beukelman, K.M. Yorkston, & J. Reichle (Eds.), *Augmentative and alternative communication for adults with acquired neurologic disorders* (pp. 305–337). Baltimore: Paul H. Brookes Publishing Co.

Roid, G.H., & Miller, L.J. (1997). *Leiter International Performance Scale–Revised.* Wood Dale, IL: Stoelting.

Roid, G.H., & Miller, L.J. (1999). *Stoelting Brief Nonverbal Intelligence Test (S-BIT).* Wood Dale, IL: Soelting.

Romich, B., Hill, K., Miller, D., Adamson, J., Anthony, A., & Sunday, J. (2004). U-LAM: Universal Language Activity Monitor. In *Proceedings of the 2004 RESNA Conference.* Arlington, VA: RESNA Press. Retrieved February 23, 2004, from http://www.aacinstitute.org/Resources/ProductsandServices/U-LAM/papers/Romich,et.al.(2004).html

Romski, M.A., & Ruder, K. (1984). Effects of speech and speech and sign instruction on oral language learning and generalization of object + action combinations by Down's syndrome children. *Journal of Speech and Hearing Disorders, 49,* 293–302.

Romski, M., & Sevcik, R. (1988a). Augmentative and alternative communication systems: Considerations for individuals with severe intellectual disabilities. *Augmentative and Alternative Communication, 4,* 83–93.

Romski, M., & Sevcik, R. (1988b, November). *Speech output communication systems: Acquisition/use by youngsters with retardation.* Miniseminar presented at the annual convention of the American Speech-Language-Hearing Association, Boston, MA.

Romski, M.A., & Sevcik, R.A. (1992). Developing augmented language in children with severe mental retardation. In S.F. Warren & J. Reichle (Eds.), *Communication and language intervention series: Vol. 1. Causes and effects in communication and language intervention* (pp. 113–130). Baltimore: Paul H. Brookes Publishing Co.

Romski, M.A., & Sevcik, R.A. (1993). Language learning through augmented means: The process and its products. In A.P. Kaiser & D.B. Gray (Eds.), *Communication and language intervention series: Vol. 2. Enhancing children's communication: Research foundations for intervention* (pp. 85–104). Baltimore: Paul H. Brookes Publishing Co.

Romski, M.A., & Sevcik, R.A. (1996). *Breaking the speech barrier: Language development through augmented means.* Baltimore: Paul H. Brookes Publishing Co.

Romski, M.A., & Sevcik, R. (1999, May). Speech comprehension and early augmented language intervention: Concepts, measurement, and clinical considerations. *ASHA Special Interest Division 12 Newsletter, 8*(2), 7–10.

Romski, M.A., & Sevcik, R.A. (2003). Augmented input: Enhancing communication development. In J.C. Light, D.R. Beukelman, & J. Reichle (Eds.), *Communicative competence for individuals who use AAC: From research to effective practice* (pp. 147–162). Baltimore: Paul H. Brookes Publishing Co.

Romski, M.A., Sevcik, R.A., & Adamson, L.B. (1999a). Communication patterns of youth with mental retardation with and without their speech-output communication devices. *American Journal on Mental Retardation, 104,* 249–259.

Romski, M.A., Sevcik, R.A., & Adamson, L.B. (1999b, March). *Toddlers with developmental disabilities who are not speaking: Vocabulary growth and augmented language intervention.* Paper presented at the Gatlinburg Conference on Research and Theory in Mental Retardation and Developmental Disabilities, Charleston, SC.

Romski, M.A., Sevcik, R.A., Adamson, L.B., & Bakeman, R.A. (2005). Communication patterns of augmented communicators, nonspeakers and speakers: Interactions with unfamiliar partners. *American Journal on Mental Retardation, 110,* 226–239.

Romski, M.A., Sevcik, R.A., Adamson, L.B., & Cheslock, M. (2002, August). *Exploring communication development in toddlers who are not speaking.* Paper presented at the biennial meeting of the International Society for Augmentative and Alternative Communication, Odense, Denmark.

Romski, M.A., Sevcik, R.A., & Forrest, S.C. (2001). Assistive technology and augmentative and alternative communication in inclusive early childhood programs. In M.J. Guralnick (Ed.), *Early childhood inclusion: Focus on change* (pp. 465–479). Baltimore: Paul H. Brookes Publishing Co.

Romski, M., Sevcik, R., & Pate, J. (1988). Establishment of symbolic communication in persons with severe retardation. *Journal of Speech and Hearing Disorders, 53,* 94–107.

Romski, M.A., Sevcik, R., Robinson, B., Mervis, C., & Bertrand, J. (1995). Mapping the meanings of novel visual symbols by youth with moderate or severe mental retardation. *American Journal on Mental Retardation, 100,* 391–402.

Romski, M., White, R., Millen, C., & Rumbaugh, D. (1984). Effects of computer keyboard teaching on symbolic communication of severely retarded persons: Five case studies. *The Psychological Record, 34,* 39–54.

Rose, D., & Meyer, A. (2002). *Teaching every student in the digital age: Universal design for learning.* Washington, DC: Association for Supervision and Curriculum Development (ASCD).

Roseberry-McKinnon, C. (2000). "Mirror, mirror on the wall": Reflections of a "third culture" American. *Communication Disorders Quarterly, 22,* 56–60.

Rosen, M., & Goodenough-Trepagnier, C. (1981). Factors affecting communication rate in nonvocal communication systems. In *Proceedings of the Fourth Annual Conference on Rehabilitation Engineering* (pp. 194–195). Washington, DC: RESNA Press.

Rosenbek, J., LaPointe, L., & Wertz, R. (1989). *Aphasia: A clinical approach.* Austin, TX: PRO-ED.

Rosenberg, S., & Beukelman, D.R. (1987). The participation model. In C.A. Coston (Ed.), *Proceedings of the national planners conference on assistive device service delivery* (pp. 159–161). Washington, DC: The Association for the Advancement of Rehabilitation Technology.

Rosenthal, R., & Rosenthal, K. (1989). *A model for mainstreaming handicapped kids: Handicapped kids are regular kids, too!* Lincoln, NE: Meadowlane Elementary School.

Roth, F., & Cassatt-James, E. (1989). The language assessment process: Clinical implications for individuals with severe speech impairments. *Augmentative and Alternative Communication, 5,* 165–172.

Rotholz, D., Berkowitz, S., & Burberry, J. (1989). Functionality of two modes of communication in the community by students with developmental disabilities: A comparison of signing and communication books. *Journal of The Association for Persons with Severe Handicaps, 14,* 227–233.

Rowland, C. (1990). Communication in the classroom for children with dual sensory impairments: Studies of teacher and child behavior. *Augmentative and Alternative Communication, 6,* 262–274.

Rowland, C. (1996, 2004). *Communication matrix.* Portland, OR: Oregon Health and Science University.

Rowland, C., & Schweigert, P. (1989). Tangible symbols: Symbolic communication for individuals with multisensory impairments. *Augmentative and Alternative Communication, 5,* 226–234.

Rowland, C., & Schweigert, P. (1990). *Tangible symbol systems: Symbolic communication for individuals with multisensory impairments.* Tucson, AZ: Communication Skill Builders.

Rowland, C., & Schweigert, P. (1991). *The early communication process using microswitch technology.* Tucson, AZ: Communication Skill Builders.

Rowland, C., & Schweigert, P. (1996). *Tangible symbol systems* (Rev. ed.) [Videotape]. San Antonio, TX: Harcourt Assessment.

Rowland, C., & Schweigert, P. (2000a). Tangible symbols, tangible outcomes. *Augmentative and Alternative Communication, 16,* 61–78, 205.

Rowland, C., & Schweigert, P. (2000b). *Tangible symbol systems* (2nd ed.). Portland, OR: Oregon Health & Science University.

Rowland, C., & Schweigert, P. (2002). *Problem solving skills.* Portland, OR: Design to Learn.

Rowland, C., & Schweigert, P.D. (2003). Cognitive skills and AAC. In J.C. Light, D.R. Beukelman, & J. Reichle (Eds.), *Communicative competence for individuals who use AAC: From research to effective practice* (pp. 241–275). Baltimore: Paul H. Brookes Publishing Co.

Rowland, C., & Schweigert, P. (2004). *First things first: Early communication for the pre-symbolic child with severe disabilities.* Portland, OR: Design to Learn.

Rubin, S. (1998). Castigating assumptions about mental retardation and low functioning autism. *Facilitated Communication Digest, 7*(1), 2–5.

Ruiter, I. (2000). *Allow me: A guide to promoting communication skills in adults with developmental delays.* Toronto: The Hanen Centre.

Rumbaugh, D. (1977). *Language learning by a chimpanzee: The LANA project.* New York: Academic Press.

Ryndak, D., & Alper, S. (Eds.). (2003). *Curriculum and instruction for students with significant disabilities in inclusive settings* (2nd ed.). Boston: Allyn & Bacon.

Ryndak, D., Morrison, A., & Sommerstein, L. (1999). Literacy before and after inclusion in general education settings: A case study. *Journal of The Association for Persons with Severe Handicaps, 24,* 5–22.

Sadowsky, A. (1985). Visual impairment among developmentally disabled clients in California regional centers. *Journal of Visual Impairment and Blindness, 79,* 199–202.

Sainato, D.M., & Morrison, R.S. (2001). Transition to inclusive environments for young children with disabilities: Toward a seamless system of service delivery. In M.J. Guralnick (Ed.), *Early childhood inclusion: Focus on change* (pp. 293–306). Baltimore: Paul H. Brookes Publishing Co.

Sarno, M., Buonaguvro, A., & Levita, E. (1986). Characteristics of verbal impairment in closed head injured patients. *Archives of Physical Medicine and Rehabilitation, 67,* 400–405.

Saunders, C., Walsh, T., & Smith, M. (1981). Hospice care in the motor neuron diseases. In C. Saunders & J. Teller (Eds.), *Hospice: The living idea.* London: Edward Arnold.

Sax, C. (2001). Using technology to support belonging and achievement. In C.H. Kennedy & D. Fisher (Eds.), *Inclusive middle schools* (pp. 89–103). Baltimore: Paul H. Brookes Publishing Co.

Schaeffer, B. (1980). Spontaneous language through signed speech. In R. Schiefelbusch (Ed.), *Nonspeech language and communication* (pp. 421–446). Baltimore: University Park Press.

Schank, R. (1990). *Tell me a story: A new look at real and artificial memory.* New York: Charles Scribner's Sons.

Schepis, M., & Reid, D. (2003). Issues affecting staff enhancement of speech-generating device use among people with severe cognitive disabilities. *Augmentative and Alternative Communication, 19,* 59–65.

Schepis, M., Reid, D., Behrmann, M., & Sutton, K. (1998). Increasing communicative interactions of young children with autism using a voice output communication aid and naturalistic teaching. *Journal of Applied Behavior Analysis, 31,* 561–578.

Scherer, M. (1994). *Matching person and technology.* Webster, NY: The Institute for Matching Person & Technology, Inc.

Scherer, M. (1997). *Matching assistive technology and child.* Webster, NY: The Institute for Matching Person & Technology, Inc.

Schlosser, R. (1999a). Nomenclature of category levels in graphic symbols, Part I: Is a flower a flower a flower? *Augmentative and Alternative Communication, 13,* 4–13.

Schlosser, R. (1999b). Nomenclature of category levels in graphic symbols, Part I: The role of similarity in categorization. *Augmentative and Alternative Communication, 13,* 14–29.

Schlosser, R. (Ed.). (2003a). Effects of AAC on natural speech development. In *The efficacy of augmentative and alternative communication* (pp. 403–425). New York: Elsevier.

Schlosser, R. (Ed.). (2003b). Efficacy and outcomes measurement in augmentative and alternative communication. In *The efficacy of augmentative and alternative communication: Toward evidence-based practice* (pp. 13–25). New York: Elsevier.

Schlosser, R. (Ed.). (2003c). *The efficacy of augmentative and alternative communication.* New York: Elsevier.

Schlosser, R.W. (Ed.). (2003d). Outcomes measurement in AAC. In J.C. Light, D.R. Beukelman, & J. Reichle (Eds.), *Communicative competence for individuals who use AAC: From research to effective practice* (pp. 479–513). Baltimore: Paul H. Brookes Publishing Co.

Schlosser, R. (2003e). Roles of speech output in augmentative and alternative communication: Narrative review. *Augmentative and Alternative Communication, 19,* 5–27.

Schlosser, R. (Ed.). (2003f). Selecting graphic symbols for an initial request lexicon. *The efficacy of augmentative and alternative communication: Toward evidence-based practice* (pp. 347–402). New York: Elsevier.

Schlosser, R., Belfiore, P., Nigam, R., Blischak, D., & Hetzroni, O. (1995). The effects of speech output technology on the learning of graphic symbols. *Journal of Applied Behavior Analysis, 28,* 537–549.

Schlosser, R., & Blischak, D. (2001). Is there a role for speech output in interventions for persons with autism? A review. *Focus on Autism and Other Developmental Disabilities, 16,* 170–178.

Schlosser, R., Blischak, D., Belfiore, P., Bartley, C., & Barnett, N. (1998). The effectiveness of synthetic speech output and orthographic feedback in a student with autism: A preliminary study. *Journal of Autism and Developmental Disorders, 28,* 309–319.

Schlosser, R., Blischak, D., & Koul, R. (2003). Roles of speech output in AAC. In R. Schlosser (Ed.), *The efficacy of augmentative and alternative communication: Toward evidence-based practice* (pp. 472–532). New York: Elsevier.

Schlosser, R., & Lee, D. (2000). Promoting generalization and maintenance in augmentative and alternative communication: A meta-analysis of 20 years of effectiveness research. *Augmentative and Alternative Communication, 16,* 208–226.

Schlosser, R., McGhie-Richmond, D., Blackstien-Adler, S., Mirenda, P., Antonius, K., & Janzen, P. (2000). Training a school team to integrate technology meaningfully into the curriculum: Effects on student participation. *Journal of Special Education Technology, 15,* 31–44.

Schlosser, R., & Raghavendra, P. (2003). Toward evidence-based practice in AAC. In R. Schlosser (Ed.), *The efficacy of augmentative and alternative communication: Toward evidence-based practice* (pp. 260–297). New York: Elsevier.

Schlosser, R., & Sigafoos, J. (2002). Selecting graphic symbols for an initial request lexicon: Integrative review. *Augmentative and Alternative Communication, 18,* 102–123.

Schnorr, R. (1990). "Peter? . . . He comes and goes . . . ": First graders' perspectives on a part-time mainstream student. *Journal of The Association for Persons with Severe Handicaps, 15,* 231–240.

Schnorr, R. (1997). From enrollment to membership: "Belonging" in middle and high school classes. *Journal of The Association for Persons with Severe Handicaps, 22,* 1–15.

Scholl, G. (1986). What does it mean to be blind? Definitions, terminology, and prevalence. In G. Scholl (Ed.), *Foundations of education for blind and visually handicapped children and youth: Theory and practice* (pp. 23–35). New York: American Foundation for the Blind.

Schuler, A., Peck, C., Willard, C., & Theimer, K. (1989). Assessment of communicative means and functions through interview: Assessing the communicative capabilities of individuals with limited language. *Seminars in Speech and Language, 19,* 54.

Schumm, J., Vaughn, S., & Leavell, A. (1994). Planning pyramid: A framework for planning for diverse students' needs during content area instruction. *The Reading Teacher, 47,* 608–615.

Schwartz, I., Garfinkle, A., & Bauer, J. (1998). The Picture Exchange Communication System: Communicative outcomes for young children with disabilities. *Topics in Early Childhood Special Education, 18,* 144–159.

Seidenberg, P.L. (1988). Cognitive and academic instructional intervention for learning-disabled adolescents. *Topics in Language Disorders, 8*(3), 56–71.

Seligman, M. (1975). *Helplessness: On depression, development, and death.* San Francisco: W.H. Freeman.

Semel, E., Wiig, E., & Secord, W. (2003). *Clinical Evaluation of Language Fundamentals–Fourth Edition (CELF-4).* San Antonio, TX: Harcourt Assessment.

Sergiovanni, T. (1990). *Value-added leadership: How to get extraordinary performance in schools.* San Diego: Harcourt Brace Jovanovich.

Sevcik, R., & Romski, M. (1986). Representational matching skills of persons with severe retardation. *Augmentative and Alternative Communication, 2,* 160–164.

Sevcik, R.A., & Romski, M.A. (in press). *A school district's guide to augmentative communication service delivery.* Baltimore: Paul H. Brookes Publishing Co.

Sevcik, R.A., Romski, M.A., & Adamson, L.B. (2005). Augmentative communication and preschool children: Case example and research directions. *Disability and Rehabilitation, 26,* 1323–1329.

Sevcik, R., Romski, M.A., & Wilkinson, K. (1991). Roles of graphic symbols in the language acquisition process for persons with severe cognitive disabilities. *Augmentative and Alternative Communication, 7,* 161–170.

Shakespeare, W.T., & Muir, C.K. (Ed.). (1982). *Troilus and Cressida.* New York: Oxford University Press.

Shane, H., & Cohen, C. (1981). A discussion of communicative strategies and patterns by nonspeaking persons. *Language, Speech, and Hearing Services in Schools, 12,* 205–210.

Sheehan, C., & Matuozzi, R. (1996). Validation of facilitated communication. *Mental Retardation, 34,* 94–107.

Shelton, I., & Garves, M. (1985). Use of visual techniques in therapy for developmental apraxia of speech. *Language, Speech, and Hearing Services in Schools, 16,* 129–131.

Shevin, M., & Schubert, A. (2000). Message-passing: Part of the journey to empowered communication. *Facilitated Communication Digest, 8*(3), 3–12.

Shriberg, L. (1994). Five subtypes of developmental phonological disorders. *Clinics in Communication Disorders, 4,* 38–53.

Shriberg, L., Aram, D., & Kwiatowksi, J. (1997a). Developmental apraxia of speech: I. Descriptive and theoretical perspectives. *Journal of Speech, Language, and Hearing Research, 40,* 273–285.

Shriberg, L., Aram, D., & Kwiatowksi, J. (1997b). Developmental apraxia of speech: II. Toward a diagnostic marker. *Journal of Speech, Language, and Hearing Research, 40,* 286–312.

Shriberg, L., Aram, D., & Kwiatowksi, J. (1997c). Developmental apraxia of speech: III. A subtype marked by inappropriate stress. *Journal of Speech, Language, and Hearing Research, 40,* 313–337.

Shroyer, E.H. (1982). *Signs of the times.* Washington, DC: Gallaudet College Press.

Siedlecki, T., Jr., & Bonvillian, J. (1997). Young children's acquisition of the handshape aspect of American Sign Language: Parental report findings. *Applied Psycholinguistics, 18,* 17–39.

Siegel, E., & Bashinski, S. (1997). Enhancing initial communication and responsiveness of learners with multiple disabilities: A tri-focus framework for partners. *Focus on Autism and Other Developmental Disabilities, 12,* 105–120.

Siegel, E.B., & Cress, C.J. (2002). Overview of the emergence of early AAC behaviors: Progression from communicative to symbolic skills. In J. Reichle, D.R. Beukelman, & J.C. Light (Eds.), *Exemplary practices for beginning communicators: Implications for AAC* (pp. 25–57). Baltimore: Paul H. Brookes Publishing Co.

Siegel, E., & Wetherby, A. (2000). Nonsymbolic communication. In M. Snell (Ed.), *Instruction of students with severe disabilities* (5th ed., pp. 409–451). Columbus, OH: Merrill.

Siegel, L., & Linder, B. (1984). Short term memory processes in children with reading and arithmetic disabilities. *Developmental Psychology, 20,* 200–207.

Siegel-Causey, E., & Guess, D. (1989). *Enhancing nonsymbolic communication interactions among students with severe disabilities.* Baltimore: Paul H. Brookes Publishing Co.

Sienkiewicz-Mercer, R., & Kaplan, S. (1989). *I raise my eyes to say yes.* Boston: Houghton Mifflin.

Sigafoos, J. (1998). Assessing conditional use of graphic mode requesting in a young boy with autism. *Journal of Developmental and Physical Disabilities, 10,* 133–151.

Sigafoos, J. (1999). Creating opportunities for augmentative and alternative communication: Strategies for involving people with developmental disabilities. *Augmentative and Alternative Communication, 15,* 183–190.

Sigafoos, J., Arthur, M., & O'Reilly, M. (2003). *Challenging behavior and developmental disability.* Baltimore: Paul H. Brookes Publishing Co.

Sigafoos, J., & Couzens, D. (1995). Teaching functional use of an eye gaze communication board to a child with multiple disabilities. *British Journal of Developmental Disabilities, 16,* 114–125.

Sigafoos, J., Couzens, D., Roberts, D., Phillips, C., & Goodison, K. (1996). Teaching requests for food and drink to children with multiple disabilities in a graphic communication mode. *Journal of Developmental and Physical Disabilities, 8,* 247–262.

Sigafoos, J., Didden, R., & O'Reilly, M. (2003). Effects of speech output on maintenance of requesting and frequency of vocalizations in three children with developmental disabilities. *Augmentative and Alternative Communication, 19,* 37–47.

Sigafoos, J., & Drasgow, E. (2001). Conditional use of aided and unaided AAC: A review and clinical case demonstration. *Focus on Autism and Other Developmental Disabilities, 16,* 152–161.

Sigafoos, J., Drasgow, E., Reichle, J., O'Reilly, M., & Tait, K. (2004). Tutorial: Teaching communicative rejecting to children with severe disabilities. *American Journal of Speech-Language Pathology, 13,* 31–42.

Sigafoos, J., Drasgow, E., & Schlosser, R. (2003). Strategies for beginning communicators. In R. Schlosser (Ed.), *The efficacy of augmentative and alternative communication* (pp. 323–346). New York: Elsevier.

Sigafoos, J., Kerr, M., Roberts, D., & Couzens, D. (1994). Increasing opportunities for requesting in classrooms serving children with developmental disabilities. *Journal of Autism and Developmental Disabilities, 24,* 631–645.

Sigafoos, J., Laurie, S., & Pennell, D. (1995). Preliminary assessment of choice making among children with Rett syndrome. *Journal of The Association for Persons with Severe Handicaps, 20,* 175–184.

Sigafoos, J., Laurie, S., & Pennell, D. (1996). Teaching children with Rett syndrome to request preferred objects using aided communication: Two preliminary studies. *Augmentative and Alternative Communication, 12,* 88–96.

Sigafoos, J., & Meikle, B. (1996). Functional communication training for the treatment of multiply determined challenging behavior in two boys with autism. *Behavior Modification, 20,* 60–84.

Sigafoos, J., & Mirenda, P. (2002). Strengthening communicative behaviors for gaining access to desired items and activities. In J. Reichle, D.R. Beukelman, & J.C. Light (Eds.), *Exemplary practices for beginning communicators: Implications for AAC* (pp. 123–156). Baltimore: Paul H. Brookes Publishing Co.

Sigafoos, J., O'Reilly, M.F., Drasgow, E., & Reichle, J. (2002). Strategies to achieve socially acceptable escape and avoidance. In J. Reichle, D.R. Beukelman, & J.C. Light (Eds.), *Exemplary prac-*

tices for beginning communicators: Implications for AAC (pp. 157–186). Baltimore: Paul H. Brookes Publishing Co.

Sigafoos, J., & Reichle, J. (1992). Comparing explicit to generalized requesting in an augmentative communication mode. *Journal of Developmental and Physical Disabilities, 4,* 167–188.

Sigafoos, J., Roberts, D., Couzens, D., & Kerr, M. (1993). Providing opportunities for choice-making and turn-taking to adults with multiple disabilities. *Journal of Developmental and Physical Disabilities, 5,* 297–310.

Sigafoos, J., Roberts, D., Kerr, M., Couzens, D., & Baglioni, A. (1994). Opportunities for communication in classrooms serving children with developmental disabilities. *Journal of Autism and Developmental Disabilities, 24,* 259–279.

Sigafoos, J., & Roberts-Pennell, D. (1999). Wrong-item format: A promising intervention for teaching socially appropriate forms of rejecting to children with developmental disabilities. *Augmentative and Alternative Communication, 15,* 135–140.

Sigafoos, J., Woodyatt, G., Tucker, M., Roberts-Pennell, D., Keen, D., Tait, K., & Pittendreigh, N. (1998). *Inventory of Potential Communicative Arts.* Queensland, Australia: University of Queensland.

Silverman, F. (1995). *Communication for the speechless* (3rd ed.). Needham Heights, MA: Allyn & Bacon.

Silverstein, S. (1974). *Where the sidewalk ends.* New York: Harper & Row.

Simmons, N., & Johnston, J. (2004, February). *Cultural differences in beliefs and practices concerning talk to children: East-Indian and Western mothers.* Poster presented at the 4th Early Years Conference, Vancouver, British Columbia.

Simpson, K. (1996). *Interaction patterns of four students with severe expressive communication impairments in regular classroom settings.* Unpublished doctoral dissertation, University of Nebraska–Lincoln.

Simpson, K., Beukelman, D.R., & Sharpe, T. (2000). An elementary student with severe expressive communication impairment in a general education classroom: Sequential analysis of interactions. *Augmentative and Alternative Communication, 16,* 107–121.

Singh, N., Lancioni, G., O'Reilly, M., Molina, E., Adkins, A., & Oliva, D. (2003). Self-determination during mealtimes through microswitch choice-making by an individual with complex multiple disabilities and profound mental retardation. *Journal of Positive Behavior Interventions, 5,* 209–215.

Skelly, M. (1979). *Amer-Ind gestural code based on universal American Indian hand talk.* Amsterdam: Elsevier/North Holland.

Skelly, M., Schinsky, L., Smith, R., Donaldson, R., & Griffin, P. (1975). American Indian sign: A gestural communication for the speechless. *Archives of Physical and Rehabilitation Medicine, 56,* 156–160.

Skelly, M., Schinsky, L., Smith, R., & Fust, R. (1974). American Indian sign (Amer-Ind) as a facilitator of verbalization in the oral apraxic. *Journal of Speech and Hearing Disorders, 39,* 445–456.

Skotko, B., Koppenhaver, D., & Erickson, K. (2004). Parent reading behaviors and communication outcomes in girls with Rett syndrome. *Exceptional Children, 70*(2), 145–166.

Slesaransky-Poe, G.L. (1997). Does the use of voice output communication make a difference in the communicative effectiveness and the quality of life of people with significant speech disabilities? *Dissertations Abstracts International* (UMI No. 9724281).

Small, J., Kemper, S., & Lyons, K. (1997). Sentence comprehension in Alzheimer's disease: Effects of grammatical complexity, speech rate and repetition. *Psychology and Aging, 12*(1), 3–11.

Small, J.A., Gutman, G., Makela, S., & Hillhouse, B. (2003). Effectiveness of communication strategies used by caregivers of persons with Alzheimer's disease during activities of daily living. *Journal of Speech, Language, and Hearing Research, 46,* 353–367.

Smebye, H. (1990, August). *A theoretical basis for early communication intervention.* Paper presented at the fifth biennial conference of the International Society for Augmentative and Alternative Communication, Stockholm.

Smith, A., Thurston, S., Light, J., Parnes, P., & O'Keefe, B. (1989). The form and use of written communication produced by physically disabled individuals using microcomputers. *Augmentative and Alternative Communication, 5,* 115–124.

Smith, M. (1992). Reading abilities of nonspeaking students: Two case studies. *Augmentative and Alternative Communication, 8,* 57–66.

Smith, M. (1996). The medium or the message: A study of speaking children using communication boards. In S. von Tetzchner & M.H. Jensen (Eds.), *Augmentative and alternative communication: European perspectives* (pp. 119–136). London: Whurr Publishers.

Smith, M., & Grove, N. (1999). The bimodal situation of children learning language using manual and graphic signs. In F.T. Loncke, J. Clibbens, H. Arvidson, & L.L. Lloyd (Eds.), *Augmentative and alternative communication: New directions in research and practice* (pp. 8–30). London: Whurr Publishers.

Smith, M.M., & Grove, N.C. (2003). Asymmetry in input and output for individuals who use AAC. In J.C. Light, D.R. Beukelman, & J. Reichle (Eds.), *Communicative competence for individuals who use AAC: From research to effective practice* (pp. 163–195). Baltimore: Paul H. Brookes Publishing Co.

Smith-Lewis, M., & Ford, A. (1987). A user's perspective on augmentative communication. *Augmentative and Alternative Communication, 3,* 12–17.

Smith, T. (2001). Discrete trial training in the treatment of autism. *Focus on Autism and Other Developmental Disabilities, 16,* 86–92.

Snell, M. (2002). Using dynamic assessment with learners who communicate nonsymbolically. *Augmentative and Alternative Communication, 18,* 163–176.

Snell, M., Caves, K., McLean, L., Mineo Mollica, B., Mirenda, P., Paul-Brown, D., et al. (2003). Concerns regarding the application of restrictive "eligibility" policies to individuals who need communication services and supports: A response by the National Joint Committee for the Communication Needs of Persons with Severe Disabilities. *Research and Practice for Persons with Severe Disabilities, 28,* 70–78.

Snyder-McLean, L., Solomonson, B., McLean, J., & Sack, S. (1984). Structuring joint action routines: A strategy for facilitating language and communication development in the classroom. *Seminars in Speech and Language, 5,* 213–228.

Sobsey, D., & Wolf-Schein, E. (1996). Children with sensory impairments. In F.P. Orelove & D. Sobsey (Eds.), *Educating children with multiple disabilities: A transdisciplinary approach* (3rd ed., pp. 411–450). Baltimore: Paul H. Brookes Publishing Co.

Soderholm, S., Meinander, M., & Alaranta, H. (2001). Augmentative and alternative communication methods in locked-in syndrome. *Journal of Rehabilitation Medicine, 33*(5), 235–239.

Sonnenmeier, R., & McSheehan, M. (in press). Beyond access: A model for supporting augmentative and alternative communication and learning of the general education curriculum by persons with the most significant disabilities. *Augmentative and Alternative Communication.*

Soto, G. (1996, August). *Multi-unit utterances and syntax in graphic symbol communication.* Paper presented at the fourth biennial research symposium of the International Society for Augmentative and Alternative Communication, Vancouver, British Columbia.

Soto, G. (1997). Special education teacher attitudes toward AAC: Preliminary survey. *Augmentative and Alternative Communication, 13,* 186–197.

Soto, G. (1999). Understanding the impact of graphic sign use on the message structure. In F.T. Loncke, J. Clibbens, H. Arvidson, & L.L. Lloyd (Eds.), *Augmentative and alternative communication: New directions in research and practice* (pp. 40–48). London: Whurr Publishers.

Soto, G., Müller, E., Hunt, P., & Goetz, L. (2001a). Critical issues in the inclusion of students who use augmentative and alternative communication: An educational team perspective. *Augmentative and Alternative Communication, 17,* 62–72.

Soto, G., Müller, E., Hunt, P., & Goetz, L. (2001b). Professional skills for serving students who use AAC in general education classrooms: A team perspective. *Language, Speech, and Hearing Services in Schools, 32,* 51–56.

Soto, G., & Toro-Zambrana, W. (1995). Investigation of Blissymbol use from a language research paradigm. *Augmentative and Alternative Communication, 11,* 118–130.

Spiegel, B., Benjamin, B., & Spiegel, S. (1993). One method to increase spontaneous use of an assistive communication device: A case study. *Augmentative and Alternative Communication, 9,* 111–118.

Spragale, D., & Micucci, S. (1990). Signs of the week: A functional approach to manual sign training. *Augmentative and Alternative Communication, 6,* 29–37.

Staehely, J. (2000). Prologue: The communication dance. In M. Fried-Oken & H.A. Bersani, Jr. (Eds.), *Speaking up and spelling it out: Personal essays on augmentative and alternative communication* (pp. 1–12). Baltimore: Paul H. Brookes Publishing Co.

Stainback, W., & Stainback, S. (1990). *Support networks for inclusive schooling: Interdependent integrated education.* Baltimore: Paul H. Brookes Publishing Co.

State of New Hampshire, Department of Health and Human Services. (1999). *Guidelines for the use of facilitated communication.* Concord, NH: Author.

Stedt, J., & Moores, D. (1990). Manual codes on English and American Sign Language: Historical perspectives and current realities. In H. Bornstein (Ed.), *Manual communication: Implications for education* (pp. 1–20). Washington, DC: Gallaudet University Press.

Steege, M., Wacker, D., Cigrand, K., Berg, W., Novak, C., Reimers, T., Sasso, G., & DeRaad, A. (1990). Use of negative reinforcement in the treatment of self-injurious behavior. *Journal of Applied Behavior Analysis, 23,* 459–468.

Stephenson, J., & Linfoot, K. (1996). Pictures as communication symbols for students with severe intellectual disability. *Augmentative and Alternative Communication, 12,* 244–256.

Sternberg, L. (1982). Communication instruction. In L. Sternberg & G. Adams (Eds.), *Educating severely and profoundly handicapped students* (pp. 209–241). Rockville, MD: Aspen Publishers.

Stillman, R., & Battle, C. (1984). Developing prelanguage communication in the severely handicapped: An interpretation of the Van Dijk method. *Seminars in Speech and Language, 5,* 159–170.

Storey, K., & Provost, O. (1996). The effect of communication skills instruction on the integration of workers with severe disabilities in supported employment settings. *Education and Training in Mental Retardation and Developmental Disabilities, 31,* 123–141.

Strauss, D., & Shavelle, R. (1998). Life expectancy of adults with cerebral palsy. *Developmental Medicine and Child Neurology, 40,* 369–375.

Strickland, D., & Cullinan, B. (1990). Afterword. In M. Adams (Ed.), *Beginning to read: Thinking and learning about print* (pp. 425–433). Cambridge, MA: MIT Press.

Stromswold, K. (1994, January). *Language comprehension without production: Implications for theories of language acquisition.* Paper presented at the Boston University Conference on Language Development, Boston.

Stuart, S. (1988). Expanding sequencing, turn-taking and timing skills through play acting. In S. Blackstone, E. Cassatt-James, & D. Bruskin (Eds.), *Augmentative communication: Implementation strategies* (pp. 5.8–21–5.8–26). Rockville, MD: American Speech-Language-Hearing Association.

Stuart, S. (1991). *Topic and vocabulary use patterns of elderly men and women in two age cohorts.* Unpublished doctoral dissertation, University of Nebraska–Lincoln.

Stuart, S., Lasker, J.P., & Beukelman, D.R. (2000). AAC message management. In D.R. Beukelman, K.M. Yorkston, & J. Reichle (Eds.), *Augmentative and alternative communication for adults with acquired neurologic disorders* (pp. 25–54). Baltimore: Paul H. Brookes Publishing Co.

Stuart, S., Vanderhoof, D., & Beukelman, D.R. (1993). Topic and vocabulary use patterns of elderly women. *Augmentative and Alternative Communication, 9,* 95–110.

Sturm, J.M. (2003, September 9). Writing in AAC. *ASHA Leader, 8*(16), 8–9, 26–27.

Sturm, J.M., & Clendon, S.A. (2004). AAC, language, and literacy: Fostering the relationship. *Topics in Language Disorders, 24*(1), 76–91.

Sturm, J.M., Erickson, K.A., & Yoder, D.E. (2003). State of the science: Enhancing literacy participation through AAC technologies. *Journal of Assistive Technology, 14,* 45–54.

Sturm, J., & Nelson, N. (1997). Formal classroom lessons: New perspectives on a familiar discourse event. *Language, Speech, and Hearing Services in Schools, 28,* 255–273.

Sturm, J.M., Rankin, J.L., Beukelman, D.R., & Schutz-Meuhling, L. (1997). How to select appropriate software for computer assisted writing. *Intervention in School and Clinic, 32,* 148–161.

Sturm, J., Spadorcia, S., Cunningham, J., Cali, K., Staples, A., Erickson, K., Yoder, D., & Koppenhaver, D. (in press). What happens to reading between first and third grade? Implications for students who use AAC. *Augmentative and Alternative Communication.*

Sulzby, E., & Teale, W. (1996). Emergent literacy. In R. Barr, M.L. Kamil, P. Mosenthal, & P.D. Pearson (Eds.), *Handbook of reading research* (Vol. II, pp. 727–757). Mahwah, NJ: Lawrence Erlbaum Associates.

Sundberg, M. (1993). Selecting a response form for nonverbal persons: Facilitated communication, pointing systems, or sign language. *Analysis of Verbal Behavior, 11,* 99–116.

Sundberg, M.L., & Partington, J.W. (1998). *Teaching language to children with autism or other developmental disabilities (version 7.1)*. Pleasant Hill, CA: Behavior Analysts.

Sussman, F. (1999). *More than words: Helping parents to promote communication and social skills in children with autism spectrum disorder*. Toronto: The Hanen Centre.

Sutton, A. (1999). Linking language learning experiences and grammatical acquisition. In F.T. Loncke, J. Clibbens, H. Arvidson, & L.L. Lloyd (Eds.), *Augmentative and alternative communication: New directions in research and practice* (pp. 49–61). London: Whurr Publishers.

Sutton, A., & Gallagher, T. (1993). Verb class distinctions and AAC language-encoding limitations. *Journal of Speech and Hearing Research, 36*, 1216–1226.

Sutton, A., & Gallagher, T. (1995). Comprehension assessment of a child using an AAC system. *American Journal of Speech-Language Pathology, 4*, 60–69.

Sutton, A., Gallagher, T., Morford, J., & Shahnaz, N. (2000). Constituent order patterns and syntactic distinctions in relative clause sentences produced using AAC systems. *Applied Psycholinguistics, 21*, 473–486.

Sutton, A., & Morford, J. (1998). Constituent order in picture pointing sequences produced by speaking children using AAC. *Applied Psycholinguistics, 19*, 526–536.

Sutton, A., Soto, G., & Blockberger, S. (2002). Grammatical issues in graphic symbol communication. *Augmentative and Alternative Communication, 18*, 192–204.

Swengel, K., & Marquette, J. (1997). Service delivery in AAC. In S.L. Glennen & D. DeCoste (Eds.), *The handbook of augmentative and alternative communication* (pp. 21–58). San Diego: Singular Publishing Group.

Szeto, A., Allen, E., & Littrell, M. (1993). Comparison of speed and accuracy for selected electronic communication devices and input methods. *Augmentative and Alternative Communication, 9*, 229–242.

Teale, W.H. (1995). Emergent literacy. In T.L. Harris & R.E. Hodges (Eds.), *The literacy dictionary: The vocabulary of reading and writing* (pp. 71–72). Newark, DE: International Reading Association.

Thousand, J.S., & Villa, R.A. (2000). Collaborative teams: A powerful tool in school restructuring. In R.A. Villa & J.S. Thousand (Eds.), *Restructuring for caring and effective education: Piecing the puzzle together* (pp. 254–292). Baltimore: Paul H. Brookes Publishing Co.

Thurman, D., Alverson, C., Dunn, K., Guerrero, J., & Sniezek, J. (1999). Traumatic brain injury in the United States: A public health perspective. *Journal of Head Trauma and Rehabilitation, 14*, 602–615.

Tirosh, E., & Canby, J. (1993). Autism with hyperlexia: A distinct syndrome? *American Journal on Mental Retardation, 98*, 84–92.

Tjus, T., Heimann, M., & Nelson, K. (1998). Gains in literacy through the use of a specially developed multimedia computer strategy. *Autism, 2*(2), 139–156.

Todman, J. (2000). Rate and quality of conversations using a text-storage AAC system: Single-case training study. *Augmentative and Alternative Communication, 16*, 164–179.

Todman, J., & Alm, N. (1997). TALKboards for social conversation. *Communication Matters, 11*, 13–15.

Todman, J., & Alm, N. (2003). Modelling conversational pragmatics in communication aids. *Journal of Pragmatics, 35*, 523–538.

Todman, J., & Lewins, E. (1996). Conversational rate of a non-vocal person with motor neurone disease using the 'TALK' system. *International Journal of Rehabilitation Research, 19*, 285–287.

Todman, J., Rankin, D., & File, P. (1999). The use of stored text in computer-aided conversation: A single-case experiment. *Journal of Language and Social Psychology, 18*, 287–309.

Todman, J., & Rzepecka, H. (2003). Effect of pre-utterance pause length on perceptions of communicative competence in AAC-aided social conversations. *Augmentative and Alternative Communication, 19*, 222–234.

Tomoeda, C.K., Bayles, K.A., Boone, D.R., Kaszniak, A.W., & Slauson, T.J. (1990). Speech rate and syntactic complexity effects on the auditory comprehension of Alzheimer patients. *Journal of Communication Disorders, 23*, 151–161.

Tonsing, K., & Alant, E. (2004). Topics of social conversation in the work place: A South African perspective. *Augmentative and Alternative Communication, 20*, 89–102.

Topor, I. (1999). Functional vision assessments and early interventions. In D. Chen (Ed.), *Essential elements in early intervention* (pp. 157–206). New York: AFB Press.

Torgesen, J.K., & Bryant, B.R. (1994). *Test of Phonological Awareness.* Austin, TX: PRO-ED.

"Traci." (2003, January). Success comes in all sizes. *Apraxia-Kids Monthly, 4*(1), 7.

Treiman, R. (1985). Onsets and rimes as units of spoken syllables: Evidence from children. *Journal of Experimental Child Psychology, 39*, 161–181.

Treviranus, J., & Roberts, V. (2003). Supporting competent motor control of AAC systems. In J.C. Light, D.R. Beukelman, & J. Reichle (Eds.), *Communicative competence for individuals who use AAC: From research to effective practice* (pp. 199–240). Baltimore: Paul H. Brookes Publishing Co.

"Trina." (2004, March). Success comes in all sizes. *Apraxia-Kids Monthly, 5*(3), 5–6.

Tscuchiya, K., Ozawa, E., Fukushima, J., Yasui, H., Kondo, H., Nakano, I., & Ikeda, K. (2000). Rapidly progressive aphasia and motor neuron disease: A clinical, radiological, and pathological study of an autopsy case with circumscribed lobar atrophy. *Acta Neuropathologica (Berlin), 99*, 81–87.

Tunmer, W.E., & Nesdale, A.R. (1985). Phonemic segmentation skill and beginning reading. *Journal of Educational Psychology, 77*, 417–427.

Turner, E., Barrett, C., Cutshall, A., Lacy, B.K., Keiningham, J., & Webster, M.K. (1995). The user's perspective of assistive technology. In K.F. Flippo, K.J. Inge, & J.M. Barcus (Eds.), *Assistive technology: A resource for school, work, and community* (pp. 283–290). Baltimore: Paul H. Brookes Publishing Co.

Udwin, O., & Yule, W. (1990). Augmentative communication systems taught to cerebral palsied children: A longitudinal study: I. The acquisition of signs and symbols, and syntactic aspects of their use over time. *British Journal of Disorders of Communication, 25*, 295–309.

Udwin, O., & Yule, W. (1991). Augmentative communication systems taught to cerebral palsied children: A longitudinal study: II. Pragmatic features of sign and symbol use. *British Journal of Disorders of Communication, 26*, 137–148.

Ulatowska, H., Cannito, M., Hayashi, M., & Fleming, S. (1985). *The aging brain: Communication in the elderly.* San Diego: College-Hill Press.

U.S. Census Bureau. (1996). *Disability status of persons (SIPP).* Washington, DC: U.S. Government Printing Office.

U.S. Department of Education. (2000). *Twenty-second annual report to Congress on the implementation of the Individuals with Disabilities Education Act.* Washington, DC: U.S. Government Printing Office.

University of Kentucky. (2002). *University of Kentucky Assistive Technology (U-KAT) Toolkit.* Retrieved February 24, 2004, from http://serc.gws.uky.edu/www/ukatii/toolkit/index.html

Utley, B.L. (2002). Visual assessment considerations for the design of AAC systems. In J. Reichle, D.R. Beukelman, & J.C. Light (Eds.), *Exemplary practices for beginning communicators: Implications for AAC* (pp. 353–394). Baltimore: Paul H. Brookes Publishing Co.

Utley, B., & Rapport, M.J.K. (2002). Essential elements of effective teamwork: Shared understanding and differences between special educators and related service providers. *Physical Disabilities: Education and Related Services, 20*, 9–47.

Valentic, V. (1991). Successful integration from a student's perspective. *Communicating Together, 9*(2), 9.

Van Acker, R., & Grant, S. (1995). An effective computer-based requesting system for persons with Rett syndrome. *Journal of Childhood Communication Disorders, 16*, 31–38.

van Balkom, H., & Welle Donker-Gimbrère, M. (1996). A psycholinguistic approach to graphic language use. In S. von Tetzchner & M.H. Jensen (Eds.), *Augmentative and alternative communication: European perspectives* (pp. 153–170). London: Whurr Publishers.

VanBiervliet, A., & Parette, P. (1999). Families, Cultures, and AAC [Computer software]. Little Rock, AR: Southeast Missouri State University and University of Arkansas for Medical Services.

Vandercook, T., York, J., & Forest, M. (1989). The McGill action planning system (MAPS): A strategy for building the vision. *Journal of The Association for Persons with Severe Handicaps, 14*, 205–215.

Vanderheiden, G., & Kelso, D. (1987). Comparative analysis of fixed-vocabulary communication acceleration techniques. *Augmentative and Alternative Communication, 3*, 196–206.

Vanderheiden, G.C., & Lloyd, L. (1986). Communication systems and their components. In S. Blackstone (Ed.), *Augmentative communication: An introduction* (pp. 49–162). Rockville, MD: American Speech-Language-Hearing Association.

Vanderheiden, G., & Yoder, D. (1986). Overview. In S. Blackstone (Ed.), *Augmentative communication: An introduction* (pp. 1–28). Rockville, MD: American Speech-Language-Hearing Association.

Vandervelden, M., & Siegel, L. (1999). Phonological processing and literacy in AAC users and students with motor speech impairments. *Augmentative and Alternative Communication, 15,* 191–211.

Vandervelden, M., & Siegel, L. (2001). Phonological processing in written word learning: Assessment for children who use augmentative and alternative communication. *Augmentative and Alternative Communication, 17,* 37–51.

Van Dijk, J. (1966). The first steps of the deaf-blind child towards language. *International Journal for the Education of the Blind, 15*(4), 112–114.

Van Oosterum, J., & Devereux, K. (1985). *Learning with rebuses.* Black Hill, Ely, Cambridgeshire, UK: EARO, The Resource Centre.

Van Tatenhove, G. (1996). *Field of dreams: Sowing language and reaping communication.* Paper presented at the 1996 Minspeak conference, Wooster, OH.

Vaughn, B., & Horner, R. (1995). Effects of concrete versus verbal choice systems on problem behavior. *Augmentative and Alternative Communication, 11,* 89–92.

Velleman, S., & Strand, K. (1994). Developmental verbal dyspraxia. In J.E. Bernthal & N.W. Bankson (Eds.), *Child phonology: Characteristics, assessment, and intervention with special populations* (pp. 110–139). New York: Thieme Medical Publishers.

Venkatagiri, H. (1993). Efficiency of lexical prediction as a communication acceleration technique. *Augmentative and Alternative Communication, 12,* 161–167.

Venkatagiri, H. (1999). Efficient keyboard layouts for sequential access in augmentative and alternative communication. *Augmentative and Alternative Communication, 15,* 126–134.

Venkatagiri, H., & Ramabadran, T. (1995). Digital speech synthesis: A tutorial. *Augmentative and Alternative Communication, 11,* 14–25.

Vicker, B. (1996). *Using tangible symbols for communication purposes: An optional step in building the two-way communication process.* Bloomington, IN: Indiana University, Indiana Resource Center for Autism.

Villa, R.A., & Thousand, J.S. (2000). *Restructuring for caring and effective education: Piecing the puzzle together* (2nd ed.). Baltimore: Paul H. Brookes Publishing Co.

Villa, R.A., Thousand, J.S., Stainback, W., & Stainback, S. (Eds.). (1992). *Restructuring for caring and effective education: An administrative guide to creating heterogeneous schools.* Baltimore: Paul H. Brookes Publishing Co.

von Tetzchner, S., & Jensen, M.H. (1996). *Augmentative and alternative communication: European perspectives.* London: Whurr Publishers.

von Tetzchner, S., & Martinsen, H. (1992). *Introduction to symbolic and augmentative communication.* London: Whurr Publishers.

Wacker, D.P., Berg, W.K., & Harding, J.W. (2002). Replacing socially unacceptable behavior with acceptable communication responses. In J. Reichle, D.R. Beukelman, & J.C. Light (Eds.), *Exemplary practices for beginning communicators: Implications for AAC* (pp. 97–122). Baltimore: Paul H. Brookes Publishing Co.

Wacker, D., Steege, M., Northup, J., Sasso, G., Berg, W., Reimers, T., et al. (1990). A component analysis of functional communication training across three topographies of severe behavior problems. *Journal of Applied Behavior Analysis, 23,* 417–429.

Wagner, R., & Torgeson, J. (1987). The nature of phonological processing skills in early literacy: A developmental approach. *Psychological Bulletin, 101,* 192–212.

Walker, M. (1987, March). *The Makaton Vocabulary: Uses and effectiveness.* Paper presented at the first international AFASIC Symposium, University of Reading, UK.

Waller, A., Dennis, F., Brodie, J., & Cairns, A. (1998). Evaluating the use of TalksBac, a predictive communication device for non-fluent adults with aphasia. *International Journal of Language and Communication Disorders, 33,* 45–70.

Waller, A., O'Mara, D.A., Tait, L., Booth, L., Brophy-Arnott, B., & Hood, H.E. (2001). Using written stories to support the use of narrative in conversational interactions: Case study. *Augmentative and Alternative Communication, 17,* 221–232.

Weiss, L., Thatch, D., & Thatch, J. (1987). *I wasn't finished with life.* Dallas, TX: E-Heart Press.

Weiss, M., Wagner, S., & Bauman, M. (1996). A case of validated facilitated communication. *Mental Retardation, 34,* 220–230.

Weiss-Lambrou, R. (2002). Satisfaction and comfort. In M. Scherer (Ed.), *Assistive technology: Matching device and consumer for successful rehabilitation* (pp. 77–94). Washington, DC: American Psychological Association.

Welland, R. (1999). Effects of Amer-Ind gestural code on spoken language comprehension in dementia of the Alzheimer type (DAT). *Dissertation Abstracts International, 60,* 2096.

Wertz, R., Weiss, D., Aten, J., Brookshire, R., Garcia-Bunuel, L., Holland, A., et al. (1986). Comparison of clinic, home, and deferred language treatment for aphasia: A Veterans Administration cooperative study. *Archives of Neurology, 43,* 653–658.

West, C.M., Bilyeu, D.D., & Brune, P.J. (1996, November). *AAC strategies for the preschool classroom: Developing communication and literacy.* Short course presented at the annual convention of the American Speech-Language-Hearing Association, Seattle, WA.

Westby, C. (1985). Learning to talk—Talking to learn: Oral-literate language differences. In C. Simon (Ed.), *Communication skills and classroom success: Therapy methodologies for language-learning disabled students* (pp. 181–213). San Diego: College-Hill Press.

Wetherby, A. (1989). Language intervention for autistic children: A look at where we have come in the past 25 years. *Journal of Speech-Language Pathology and Audiology, 13*(4), 15–28.

Wetherby, A., & Prizant, B. (1993). *Communication and Symbolic Behavior Scales (CSBS).* Baltimore: Paul H. Brookes Publishing Co.

Wetherby, A.M., & Prizant, B.M. (Eds.) (2000). *Autism spectrum disorders: A transactional developmental perspective.* Baltimore: Paul H. Brookes Publishing Co.

Wetherby, A.M., & Prizant, B.M. (2002). *Communication and Symbolic Behavior Scales Developmental Profile™ (CSBS DP™).* Baltimore: Paul H. Brookes Publishing Co.

Wetherby, A., & Prutting, C. (1984). Profiles of communicative and cognitive-social abilities in autistic children. *Journal of Speech and Hearing Research, 27,* 364–377.

Wetherby, A.M., Warren, S.F., & Reichle, J. (Eds.). (1998). Introduction. *Transitions in prelinguistic communication* (pp. 1–11). Baltimore: Paul H. Brookes Publishing Co.

Wiig, E.H., Secord, W., & Semel, E. (1992). *Clinical Evaluation of Language Fundamentals–Preschool (CELF-Preschool).* San Antonio, TX: Harcourt Assessment.

Wikstrom, J., Poser, S., & Ritter, G. (1980). Optic neuritis as an initial symptom in multiple sclerosis. *Acta Neurologica Scandinavica, 61,* 178–185.

Wilbur, R., & Peterson, L. (1998). Modality interactions of speech and signing in simultaneous communication. *Journal of Speech, Language, and Hearing Research, 41,* 200–212.

Wilcox, K., & Sherrill, M. (1999). *Children's Speech Intelligibility Measure.* Austin, TX: PRO-ED.

Wilcox, M.J., Bacon, C., & Shannon, M.S. (1995, December). *Prelinguistic intervention: Procedures for young children with disabilities.* Paper presented at the ASHA Annual Convention, Orlando, FL.

Wilkinson, G. (1993). *Wide Range Achievement Test–Third Revision (WRAT-3).* Wilmington, DE: Jastak Associates.

Wilkinson, K. (2005). Disambiguation and mapping of new word meanings by individuals with intellectual/developmental disabilities. *American Journal on Mental Retardation, 110,* 71–86.

Wilkinson, K., & Albert, A. (2001). Adaptations of fast mapping for vocabulary intervention with augmented language users. *Augmentative and Alternative Communication, 17,* 120–132.

Wilkinson, K., & Green, G. (1998). Implications of fast mapping for vocabulary expansion in individuals with mental retardation. *Augmentative and Alternative Communication, 14,* 162–170.

Wilkinson, K., & Jagaroo, V. (2004). Contributions of cognitive science to AAC display design. *Augmentative and Alternative Communication, 20,* 123–136.

Wilkinson, K., Romski, M.A., & Sevcik, R. (1994). Emergence of visual-graphic symbol combinations by youth with moderate or severe mental retardation. *Journal of Speech and Hearing Research, 37,* 883–985.

Williams, B. (2000). More than an exception to the rule. In M. Fried-Oken & H.A. Bersani, Jr. (Eds.), *Speaking up and spelling it out: Personal essays on augmentative and alternative communication* (pp. 245–254). Baltimore: Paul H. Brookes Publishing Co.

Williams, K.T. (2001). *Group Reading Assessment and Diagnostic Evaluation*. Circle Pines, MN: American Guidance Service.

Williams, M. (1995, March). Whose outcome is it anyway? *Alternatively Speaking, 2*(1), 1–2, 6.

Williams, M., & Krezman, C. (Eds.). (2000). *Beneath the surface: Creative expressions of augmented communicators*. Toronto: ISAAC Press.

Williams, W.B., Stemach, G., Wolfe, S., & Stanger, C. (1998). Lifespace Access Profile [Computer software]. Volo, IL: Don Johnston, Inc.

Wilson, R., Teague, G., & Teague, M. (1984). The use of signing and fingerspelling to improve spelling performance with hearing children. *Reading Psychology, 5*, 267–273.

Windsor, J., & Fristoe, M. (1989). Key word signing: Listeners' classification of signed and spoken narratives. *Journal of Speech and Hearing Disorders, 54*, 374–382.

Windsor, J., & Fristoe, M. (1991). Key word signing: Perceived and acoustic differences between signed and spoken narratives. *Journal of Speech and Hearing Research, 34*, 260–268.

Wing, L. (1996). *The autistic spectrum: A guide for parents and professionals*. London: Constable.

Winter, S., Autry, A., Boyle, C., & Yeargin-Allsopp, M. (2002). Trends in the prevalence of cerebral palsy in a population-based study. *Pediatrics, 110*, 1220–1225.

Wisconsin Assistive Technology Initiative. (2004). *W.A.T.I. Assistive Technology Assessment*. Retrieved February 24, 2004, from http://www.wati.org/pdf/Assessmentforms2004.pdf

Wood, L.A., Lasker, J., Siegel-Causey, E., Beukelman, D.R., & Ball, L. (1998). Input framework for augmentative and alternative communication. *Augmentative and Alternative Communication, 14*, 261–267.

Woodcock, R., Clark, C., & Davies, C. (1968). *Peabody Rebus Reading Program*. Circle Pines, MN: AGS Publishing.

Woodcock, R., McGrew, K., & Mather, N. (2001). *Woodcock–Johnson® III (WJ III)*. Itasca, IL: Riverside Publishing.

Woodward, J. (1990). Sign English in the education of deaf students. In H. Bornstein (Ed.), *Manual communication: Implications for education* (pp. 67–80). Washington, DC: Gallaudet University Press.

Workinger, M., & Netsell, R. (1988). *Restoration of intelligible speech 13 years post-head injury*. Unpublished manuscript, Boys Town National Communication Institute, Omaha, NE.

World Health Organization. (1992). *International statistical classification of diseases and related health problems* (10th ed.). Geneva: Author.

World Health Organization. (2001). *The World Health report 2001—Mental illness: New understanding, new hope*. Geneva: Author. Retrieved April 10, 2004, from http://www.who.int/whr2001/2001/

Writer, J. (1987). A movement-based approach to the education of students who are sensory impaired/multihandicapped. In L. Goetz, D. Guess, & K. Stremel-Campbell (Eds.), *Innovative program design for individuals with dual sensory impairments* (pp. 191–223). Baltimore: Paul H. Brookes Publishing Co.

Wylie, R.E., & Durrell, D.D. (1970). Teaching vowels through phonograms. *Elementary English, 47*, 787–791.

Yaden, D.B., Rowe, D.W., & MacGillivray, L. (2000). Emergent literacy: A matter of (polyphony) of perspectives. In M.L. Kamil, P.B. Mosenthal, P.D. Pearson, & R. Barr (Eds.), *Handbook of reading research* (Vol. III, pp. 425–454). Mahwah, NJ: Lawrence Erlbaum Associates.

Yamamoto, J., & Mochizuki, A. (1988). Acquisition and functional analysis of manding with autistic children. *Journal of Applied Behavior Analysis, 21*, 57–64.

Ylvisaker, M. (1986). Language and communication disorders following pediatric head injury, *Journal of Head Trauma Rehabilitation, 1*, 48–56.

Yoder, D., & Kraat, A. (1983). Intervention issues in nonspeech communication. In J. Miller, D. Yoder, & R.L. Schiefelbusch (Eds.), *Contemporary issues in language intervention* (pp. 27–51). ASHA Reports, 12. Rockville, MD: American Speech-Language-Hearing Association.

Yoder, P., & Warren, S. (1998). Maternal responsivity predicts the prelinguistic communication intervention that facilitates generalized intentional communication. *Journal of Speech, Language, and Hearing Research, 41*, 1207–1219.

Yoder, P., & Warren, S. (1999). Maternal responsivity mediates the relationship between prelinguistic intentional communication and later language. *Journal of Early Intervention, 22,* 126–136.

Yoder, P., & Warren, S. (2001). Relative treatment effects of two prelinguistic communication interventions on language development in toddlers with developmental delays vary by maternal characteristics. *Journal of Speech, Language, and Hearing Research, 44,* 224–237.

Yoder, P., & Warren, S. (2002). Effects of prelinguistic milieu teaching and parent responsivity education on dyads involving children with intellectual disabilities. *Journal of Speech, Language, and Hearing Research, 45,* 1158–1174.

York, J., & Weimann, G. (1991). Accommodating severe physical disabilities. In J. Reichle, J. York, & J. Sigafoos (Eds.), *Implementing augmentative and alternative communication: Strategies for learners with severe disabilities* (pp. 239–256). Baltimore: Paul H. Brookes Publishing Co.

Yorkston, K. (1989). Early intervention in amyotrophic lateral sclerosis: A case presentation. *Augmentative and Alternative Communication, 5,* 67–70.

Yorkston, K. (Ed.). (1992). *Augmentative communication in the medical setting.* Austin, TX: PRO-ED.

Yorkston, K., Beukelman, D.R., Strand, E., & Bell, K. (1999). *Management of motor speech disorders in children and adults.* Austin, TX: PRO-ED.

Yorkston, K., Beukelman, D.R., & Tice, R. (1996). Sentence Intelligibility Test (Version 1.0) [Computer software]. Lincoln, NE: Communication Disorders Software.

Yorkston, K., Beukelman, D.R., & Tice, R. (1997). *Pacer/Tally.* Lincoln, NE: Tice Technology Services.

Yorkston, K., Fried-Oken, M., & Beukelman, D.R. (1988). Single word vocabulary needs: Studies from various nonspeaking populations. *Augmentative and Alternative Communication, 4,* 149.

Yorkston, K., Honsinger, M., Mitsuda, P., & Hammen, V. (1989). The relationship between speech and swallowing disorders in head-injured patients. *Journal of Head Trauma Rehabilitation, 4,* 1–16.

Yorkston, K., & Karlan, G. (1986). Assessment procedures. In S. Blackstone (Ed.), *Augmentative communication: An introduction* (pp. 163–196). Rockville, MD: American Speech-Language-Hearing Association.

Yorkston, K.M., Klasner, E.R., & Swanson, K.M. (2001). Communication in context: A qualitative study of the experiences of individuals with multiple sclerosis. *American Journal of Speech-Language Pathology, 10*(2), 126–137.

Yorkston, K.M., Miller, R., & Strand, E.A. (2004). *Management of speech and swallowing in degenerative diseases* (2nd ed.). Austin, TX: PRO-ED.

Yorkston, K., Smith, K., & Beukelman, D.R. (1990). Extended communication samples of augmented communicators: I. A comparison of individualized versus standard vocabularies. *Journal of Speech and Hearing Disorders, 55,* 217–224.

Yorkston, K., Strand, E., & Kennedy, M. (1996). Comprehensibility of dysarthric speech: Implications for assessment and treatment planning. *American Journal of Speech-Language Pathology, 5,* 55–66.

Yoss, K., & Darley, F. (1974). Therapy in developmental apraxia of speech. *Language, Speech, and Hearing Services in Schools, 5,* 23–31.

Zabala, J., Blunt, M., Carl, D., Davis, S., Deterding, C., Foss, T., et al. (2000). Quality indicators for assistive technology services in school settings. *Journal of Special Education Technology, 15,* 5–26.

Zagare, F. (1984). *Game theory: Concepts and applications.* Thousand Oaks, CA: Sage Publications.

Zangari, C., Lloyd, L., & Vicker, B. (1994). Augmentative and alternative communication: An historic perspective. *Augmentative and Alternative Communication, 10,* 27–59.

Resources and Web Links

AAC-RERC: http://aac-rerc.com/
AAC Intervention: http://aacintervention.com
AapNootMuis: http://www.aapnootmuis.com/
AbleNet, Inc.: http://www.ablenetinc.com
Adaptivation, Inc.: http://www.adaptivation.com
AGS Publishing: http://www.agsnet.com/
American Printing House for the Blind, Inc.: http://www.aph.org/
The Amyotrophic Lateral Sclerosis Association: http://www.alsa.org/
Aphasia Institute: http://www.aphasia.ca/training/index.html
Apraxia-Kids: http://www.apraxia-kids.org/index.html
Assistive Technology, Inc.: http://www.assistivetech.com
Assistive Technology Library of Alaska:
    http://www.callier.utdallas.edu/ACT/ChalkTalk.html.
Association for Supervision and Curriculum Development (ASCD):
    http://www.ascd.org/
Attainment Company: http://www.attainmentcompany.com/
Augmentative Communication, Inc.: www.augcominc.com.
Autism Spectrum Disorders-Canadian American Research Consortium (ASD-
    CARC): http://www.autismresearch.ca/
Barkley Augmentative and Alternative Communication Centers: http://aac.unl.edu/
Blissymbolics Communication International: http://home.istar.ca/~bci/
Center for Applied Special Technology (CAST): http://www.cast.org/
Center for Effective Collaboration and Practice: http://cecp.air.org/
Center for Evidence Based Practice for Young Children with Challenging Behavior:
    http://challengingbehavior.fmhi.usf.edu/
Center for Literacy and Disability Studies at the University of North Carolina–
    Chapel Hill: http://www.med.unc.edu/ahs/clds/
Center on Positive Behavioral Interventions and Supports: http://www.pbis.org
Centre Québécois de Communication Non Orale: http://www.cqcno.com
CIRCA (Computer Interactive Reminiscence and Conversation Aid):
    http://www.computing.dundee.ac.uk/projects/circa/

Closing the Gap: http://www.closingthegap.com/

Communication Aid Users Society (Australia):
http://www.users.bigpond.com/causinc/

Communication and Assistive Device Laboratory, State University of New York at
Buffalo: http://www.cadl.buffalo.edu/

Communication Matrix: http://www.communicationmatrix.org

Communication Resource Center (COMPICs): http://www.compic.com/

Computer Options for the Exceptional: http://www.c-o-e.com/Products.html

Creative Communicating: http://www.creativecommunicating.com/

Crestwood Communication Aids, Inc.:
http://www.communicationaids.com/products.htm

Cure Autism Now!: http://www.canfoundation.org/

Design to Learn: http://www.designtolearn.com/

Disability Solutions: http://www.disabilitysolutions.org/

Division of Applied Computing, University of Dundee:
http://www.computing.dundee.ac.uk/external.asp

Don Johnston, Inc.: http://www.donjohnston.com/

Do2Learn: http://www.dotolearn.com/

Doug Dodgen & Associates: http://www.dougdodgen.com/index.html

Down Syndrome Research and Practice: http://www.downsed.org/publishing/
periodicals/dsrp

DynaVox Systems LLC: http://www.dynavoxsys.com/cgi-bin/lava/cgi/index.cgi/
4c158b2c307c5a91d288c534e2932b8e?rm=content&contentid=1

Early Learning Images: http://www.elliecards.com/

Elearning Design Lab: http://www.elearndesign.org/resources.html

Enabling Devices: http://www.enablingdevices.com

Facilitated Communication Institute: http://soeweb.syr.edu/thefci

Gallaudet University Press: http://gupress.gallaudet.edu

Giving Greetings: http://www.givinggreetings.com/index.html

Gus Communications, Inc.: http://www.gusinc.com/index.html

Handicom: http://www.handicom.nl

The Hanen Centre: http://www.hanen.org

Harcourt Assessment (The Psychological Corporation, Canada):
http://www.psych.utoronto.ca/~dgoldst/
The%20Psychological%20Corporation,%20Canada.htm

Huntington's Disease Society of America: http://www.hdsa.org/

Indiana Resource Center for Autism: http://www.iidc.indiana.edu/irca/fmain1.html

Institute on Disabilities, Temple University: http://disabilities.temple.edu/

Institute on Disability, University of New Hampshire:
http://www.iod.unh.edu/projects/early_childhood.html#BeyondAccess

Institute for Matching Person & Technology, Inc.:
http://members.aol.com/IMPT97/MPT.html

IntelliTools: http://www.intellitools.com

International Council on English Braille: http://iceb.org

International Society for Augmentative and Alternative Communication (ISAAC): http://www.isaac-online.org/select_language.html

Lámh Development Office, City Enterprise Centre, Waterford Business Park, Cork Road, Waterford, Ireland. Tel. No.: (051) 845454; Fax No.: (051) 845454.

Let's Play!: http://letsplay.buffalo.edu

Madonna Rehabilitation Hospital: http://www.madonna.org/res_software.htm.

Makaton Vocabulary Development Project: http://www.makaton.org/index.htm

Marsha Forest Centre/Inclusion Press: http://www.inclusion.com.

Mayer-Johnson, Inc.: http://www.mayer-johnson.com/main/index.html

Medicare Funding of AAC Technology Assessment/Application Protocol: http://www.aac-rerc.com/archive_aac-rerc/pages/MCsite/MCAppProtocol.html

Microsystems Software, Ltd.: http://www.microsys.com

Modern Signs Press: http://www.modsigns.com/

Multiple Sclerosis: http://www-medlib.med.utah.edu/kw/ms/

National Alliance of Autism Research (NAAR): http://www.naar.org/

National Aphasia Association Newsletter: http://www.aphasia.org/newsletter/Fall2002/DiagnosingPPA.html

National Center for Treatment Effectiveness in Communication Disorders: http://www.asha.org/members/research/NOMS/

National Center to Improve the Tools of Educators (NCITE): http://idea.uoregon.edu/~ncite/

National Cued Speech Association: http://www.cuedspeech.org/

National Information Clearinghouse on Children Who Are Deaf-Blind: http://www.tr.wou.edu/dblink/

National Joint Committee (NJC) for the Communication Needs of Persons with Severe Disabilities: http://www.asha.org/NJC/default.htm.

National Parkinson's Disease Foundation: http://www.parkinson.org/

Oakland Schools: http://www.oakland.k12.mi.us/index.html

Online Academy for Positive Behavioral Support: http://onlineacademy.org/

Paul H. Brookes Publishing Co.: http://www.brookespublishing.com/

Poppin and Company: http://www.poppinandcompany.com

Prentke Romich Co.: http://www.prentrom.com

PRO-ED: http://www.proedinc.com/store/

Program Development Associates: http://www.pdassoc.com.

PROMPT© Institute: http://www.promptinstitute.com/

Quality Indicators for Assistive Technology (QIAT) Consortium: http://www.qiat.org

Quality of Life Research Unit at the Canadian Center for Health Promotion: http://www.utoronto.ca/qol/

Rehabilitation Engineering Research Center on Communication Enhancement-AAC: http://www.aac-rerc.com/

Rehabilitation Research and Training Center on Positive Behavior Support: http://rrtcpbs.fmhi.usf.edu

Riverside Publishing: http://www.riverpub.com/

Saltillo Corporation: http://www.saltillo.com

Scope Communication Resource Centre:
   http://www.scopevic.org.au/therapy_crc.html
S.E.E. Center for the Advancement of Deaf Children: http://www.seecenter.org/
Sign-It! (board game for learning American Sign Language):
   http://www.signit-original.com/
Silver Lining Multimedia, Inc.: http://www.silverliningmm.com/
Simplified Technology: http://www.lburkhart.com/main.htm
Speaking Differently: http://pages.istar.ca/~marshall/Speaking_Differently/
Speak Up: http://www.aacsafeguarding.ca
Special Communications Books: http://aacintervention.com/caroline.htm
Speechmark Publishing Ltd.: http://www.speechmark.net/index.htm
Stoelting Company: http://www.stoeltingco.com/
Studies to Advance Autism Research and Treatment (STAART):
   http://www.nimh.nih.gov/autismiacc/staart.cfm
Support Helps Others Use Technology (SHOUT): http://www.minspeak.com/shout
Tech Connections: http://www.techconnections.org/training/dec2002/SHOUTinfo.pdf
Technology and Inclusion Center, Assistive Technology Screener Information:
   http://www.taicenter.com/test_pretty/screeners/screener%20text.html
University of Kentucky Assistive Technology (UKAT) Project:
   http://serc.gws.uky.edu/www/ukatii/index.html
WesTest Engineering Corporation: http://www.westest.com/darci/usbindex.html
Whurr Publishers: http://www.whurr.co.uk/
Widgit Software, Ltd.: http://www.widgit.com/index.htm
Wisconsin Assistive Technology Initiative (WATI):
   http://www.wati.org/Materials/assessments.html
Words+, Inc.: http://www.words-plus.com
ZYGO Industries: http://www.zygo-usa.com/

Index

Page numbers followed by *f* indicate figures; those followed by *t* indicate tables.

AAC, *see* Augmentative and alternative communication
AAC Categorical Assessment for Communicators
    with aphasia, 497–498
AAC Feature Match, 163*t*
AAC Intervention, 262
AAC-RERC, *see* Rehabilitation Engineering
    Research Center-Augmentative and Alter-
    native Communication
AAMR, *see* American Association on Mental Retar-
    dation
AAT Assessment Tool, 164*t*
Abbreviation expansion, 72
ABC-Link, 207
Abstract symbol systems, 62–63
Academic workload adaptations, 417–418
Acceptance signals
    aphasia and, 473, 473*t*
    of nonsymbolic communicators, 274*t*, 275, 277
    scripted routines for practicing, 279, 280*t*,
        281–283, 282*t*
    see also Rejection signals; Yes/no questions
Access barriers
    current communication, assessing, 145–146, 146*t*,
        147*f*
    defined, 141–142
    environmental adaptations, 150
    potential for natural speech, 146, 148–150
    potential to use AAC, 150–157
AccessBliss, 107
Accessible Word Reading Intervention (AWRI), 207
Accountability, of intervention team members,
    130–131
ACES, *see* Augmentative Communication Empower-
    ment Supports
Achieving Communication Independence (ACI), 146*t*
ACI, *see* Achieving Communication Independence
ACQUA, *see* Augmentative Communication Quanti-
    tative Analysis software
Acting, play activities, 263–264, 292
Activation strategies
    activation feedback, 101
    assessment, 181–182, 184–185
    direct selection, 96–97
Active educational participation, 399–400
Activity boards/displays
    with Fitzgerald key, 336
    grid displays, 336–338, 337*f*, 339*f*
    organizing, 26
    see also Communication boards/displays; Display
        devices
Activity schedules, *see* Visual schedules
Acute medical settings

assessment in, 538–545, 540*f*, 541*f*
    AAC devices in, 533, 538, 541–545
    barriers, 539, 545
    communication needs in, 533, 534–536
    intervention planning flowchart, 541*f*
    "limited-use" policies, 142
ADA, *see* Americans with Disabilities Act of 1990
    (PL 101-336)
Adaptations
    academic workload, 417–418
    assessment, 189, 191
    choice making, 300–301
    classroom interactions, 428–429
    communication boards/displays
        alphabet boards, 459, 460*f*, 524, 529, 544
        conversation displays, 318–319
        with conversational coaching, 313–314
        dual boards, 319
        speech production and, 148
        topic boards, 459, 460*f*, 524
        for writing support, 386, 387*f*, 388
    emergent literacy, assessment, 363, 363*t*
    environmental adaptations, 150, 225, 412, 417
    in inclusive classrooms, 414, 416–419, 416*t*
    language comprehension, 422*t*–423*t*, 427
    P-switches, 443, 443*f*
    reading instruction, 376, 384
    response modes, 388*t*, 422*t*–423*t*, 423*t*, 427
    telephone, 446, 458, 492
    time constraints, managing, 418–419
    toys and play materials, 261–264, 263*f*, 264*t*
    types of, 416*t*
    vocabulary, 422*t*–423*t*, 427
    writing instruction, 382–383, 383*f*, 383*t*, 386,
        387*f*, 388
    see also Pointing methods; Positioning; Switches
Adapted cueing technique, 250
Adapted Strategic Instruction Model (A-SIM),
    311–312
Adaptive play, 261–264, 263*f*, 264*t*
Adaptor nonverbal behaviors, 40–41
Adolescents, attitudes about AAC, 155–156
Adults
    as beginning communicators, 268–269,
        270*f*–271*f*, 271
    consensus building, 437–438
    scripted routines for, 282*t*
    vocabulary and language usage, 23–24
    see also specific disorders
Affect displays, 40
Affective learning, 412
Affirmation signals, *see* Acceptance signals

Age
    appropriateness of choice-making options, 296
    influence on message selection, 16, 18, 19–20, 470
    and prevalence of communication disorders, 5
    storytelling in later years, 470–471
    symbol learning and, 37–38
    vocabulary and, 23–24
Agencies
    documentation of effectiveness, 439
    policies and practices as barriers, 142–143, 160,
        220, 539
Aggression, 277
    see also Problem behavior
Agraphia, 491–495
Agreement signals, see Acceptance signals
Aided language stimulation, 109–110, 344–348,
        345t, 346f, 347f
Aided symbols
    abstract symbols, 62–63
    in choice making, 298
    defined, 36
    input and output displays, 108, 109–110
    orthographic symbols, 63–64
    representational symbols, 53–62
    tangible symbols, 51–53
All My Words software, 372
Alliance '95, 228, 230
Alliteration, assessment, 209t
ALL-Link, 207
Allow Me!, 273, 344
Alpha (letter) codes
    message coding, 71–72
    word coding, 69
Alphabet boards, 459, 460f, 524, 529, 544
    see also Communication boards/displays
Alphanumeric codes
    message coding, 72
    word coding, 69, 70–71
ALS, see Amyotrophic lateral sclerosis
Alter adaptor nonverbal behavior, 41
Alternative access, see Adaptations; Augmentative
        and alternative communication
Alzheimer's Association, 508
Alzheimer's disease, see Dementia
American Association on Mental Retardation
        (AAMR), 240
American Sign Language (ASL)
    guessability levels, 43, 108
    overview, 47
American Speech-Language-Hearing Association
        (ASHA)
    communication bill of rights, 220, 220t
    definition of augmentative and alternative com-
        munication, 3–4
    endorsement of Participation Model of assess-
        ment, 136
    Functional Assessment of Communication Skills
        for Adults (ASHA FACS), 191
    Quality of Communication Life Scale, 230, 231
Americans with Disabilities Act (ADA) of 1990 (PL
        101-336), 144, 219
Amer-Ind (Hand Talk), 42–43, 108
Amplification, voice, 458, 524
Amyotrophic lateral sclerosis (ALS)

assessment, 441–445
    clinical illustrations, 184t, 186, 435, 437
    described, 439–440
    intervention staging, 445–447
    planning for, 226–227, 438
Anarthria, 453, 460
Angelman syndrome (AS), 39, 242
Anglo-European culture, attitudes about AAC,
        151–152
Ankles, positioning, 173t
Anomic aphasia, 468
Anticipatory repair strategy, 323
AOS, see Apraxia of speech
APAR, see Assessment of Phonological Awareness
        and Reading
Aphasia
    with amyotrophic lateral sclerosis (ALS), 442
    assessment, 191, 495–501
    auditory processing problems, 104, 468, 478–479
    challenges, 468, 501–504
    communication profiles
        contextual choice communicators, 475–481,
            477f, 478f, 479f
        emerging communicators, 472–475, 473f, 475f
        generative message communicators, 487–492,
            488t, 489f, 491f
        specific-need communicators, 492–495, 493f,
            494f, 495t
        stored message communicators, 484–487, 485f,
            486f, 486t
        transitional communicators, 482–484, 483t, 484f
    described, 467–469
    facilitators, assessing, 157
    with multiple sclerosis (MS), 450
    Photographic Communication Resources
        (PCRs), 62
    primary progressive aphasia (PPA), 505–507
    research reviews, 223t
    situation training, 485–486, 486f, 486t,
        493–494, 495t
    with traumatic brain injury (TBI), 519
    visual input, 109–110
    writing skills, 491–492, 493–495, 494f
Apraxia of speech (AOS)
    aphasia and, 468
    see also Developmental apraxia of speech (DAS)
Apraxia-Kids, 250
Arms, positioning, 172f, 173t
Arrays, choice-making, 297
Arthrogryposis, 353
Articulation errors, see Developmental apraxia of
        speech (DAS)
AS, see Angelman syndrome
ASCD, see Association for Supervision and Curricu-
        lum Development
ASD, see Autism
ASD–CARC, see Autism Spectrum
        Disorders–Canadian American Research
        Consortium
ASHA, see American Speech-Language-Hearing
        Association
A-SIM, see Adapted Strategic Instruction Model
ASL, see American Sign Language
Asperger syndrome, characteristics, 243, 246

Assessment
  in acute medical settings, 538–545, 539–545,
    540*f*, 541*f*
  adaptations, 189, 191
  adults with acquired disabilities, 436–439
  amyotrophic lateral sclerosis (ALS), 441–445
  aphasia, 495–501
  models of, 133–136, 137*f*
  multiple sclerosis (MS), 449–451
  Participation Model
    access barriers, 145–157, 153*f*, 154*t*
    current communication, 145–146, 146*t*, 147*f*
    environmental adaptations, 150
    opportunity barriers, 140*f*, 141–144
    Participation Inventory, 139, 140*f*, 141
    participation patterns, identifying, 139, 140*f*,
      141, 257–258, 260*t*, 436, 469, 496
    potential for natural speech, 146, 148–150
    potential to use AAC, 150–157, 497–498,
      501–502
  phases of, 138–139
  traumatic brain injury (TBI), 191, 526,
    527–528, 530
  types of, 159–161
  see also Capability assessment; Outcomes
Assessment of Phonological Awareness and Reading
  (APAR), 207
Assessment of Phonological Processes–Revised, 149
Assistance, *see* Support
Assistive Technology Act Amendments of 2004 (PL
  105-394), 161, 219
Assistive Technology Assessment Questionnaire, 162*t*
Assistive technology (AT), *see* Augmentative and
  alternative communication
Assistive technology (AT) centers, 161
Assistive Technology Predisposition Assessment, 162*t*
Assistive Technology Screener, 162*t*
Assistivetech.net, 161
Association for Supervision and Curriculum Devel-
  opment (ASCD), 414
Association of symbols, 201–203
Asymmetrical tonic neck reflex (ATNR), 165–166, 167*f*
Ataxic cerebral palsy, 236
Athetoid cerebral palsy, 184*t*, 185, 236
ATNR, *see* Asymmetrical tonic neck reflex
Attention-getting signals
  nonsymbolic communicators, 274, 274*t*, 275–276
  in requesting routine, 302, 303*t*
  scripted routines for practicing, 279, 280*t*,
    281–283, 282*t*
Attitudes
  about AAC, 155–156, 438–439, 444, 457, 503
  about disabilities, 151–152
  about importance of literacy, 357
  about low-tech devices, 156, 438
  about technology, 154–155, 444
  as barriers, 144, 221, 503
  belief that intervention will discourage natural abili-
    ties, 146, 148, 155, 224–225, 250, 253–254
  of children and adolescents, 155–156
  physician resistance to intervention, 444
Audiovisual media for enhancing language comprehension and vocabulary, 422*t*–423*t*, 426–427
Auditory brain-stem response, 217

Auditory displays, 83, 90
Auditory feedback
  activation feedback, 101
  emergent literacy instruction, 368
  hearing assessment, need for, 217
  message feedback, 102
Auditory processing problems, 104, 468, 478–479
  see also Hearing impairments
Auditory scanning
  compared with visual scanning, 103
  group–item scanning, 99
  linear scanning, 98
  size and complexity of displays, 90
  visual impairment and, 41–42
Augmentative and alternative communication (AAC)
  attitudes about, 155–156, 438–439, 444, 457, 503
  changing nature of communication needs, 138,
    223, 224*f*, 227, 231, 503–504
  components of communication competence,
    10–14, 136
  prevalence of use, 4–5
  research, integrative reviews, 222, 223*t*
  terminology, 3–4
  word-based versus phrase-based approaches, 18
Augmentative and alternative communication (AAC)
  devices and systems
  acceptance of, 444
  in acute medical settings, 533, 538, 541–545
  components, 4
  desired characteristics of, 226
  feedback methods, 101–102
  influence on language development, 334–341
  low-tech methods compared with electronic
    devices, 156, 438–439
  perceived interference with speech development,
    146, 148, 155, 224–225, 250, 253–254
  performance measurement and analysis technol-
    ogy, 30
  portability, 251, 252, 290
  preferences about, 151–155
  preprogrammed messages, 83–84, 485
  relevance versus rate of communication, 315
  as secondary strategy, 250–251
  see also Display devices; Selection sets; Symbols
Augmentative and alternative communication (AAC)
  users
  consumer satisfaction, 229–230
  first-person accounts, 5–8, 6*t*, 119, 144, 238, 325,
    328, 447
  individual education programs (IEPs) for, 189
  as informants, 30, 31
  preferences of, 151–155
  training for, 227–228, 285, 545
*Augmentative and Alternative Communication: Beyond
  Poverty*, 154
Augmentative and Alternative Communication (journal)
  efficacy research, 228
  headquarters, 111
  language assessment, 205
  speech output, 106
Augmentative Communication Assessment Profile,
  162*t*
Augmentative Communication Empowerment Supports (ACES), 285

Augmentative Communication in the Medical Setting, 188*t*
Augmentative Communication Online User's Group, 236
Augmentative Communication Quantitative Analysis (ACQUA) software, 205
Augmented communication input, *see* System for Augmenting Language (SAL)
Augmented comprehension (input) techniques, 476*t*, 478–481, 480*f*, 483*f*
Augmented writing approach, 443, 493–495, 494*f*
Australia
    AAC use, 238
    manual sign systems, 43
    prevalence of communication disorders, 5
Author's Chair, 380, 386
Autism
    AAC issues, 246–249
    described, 243–246
    facilitated communication (FC) with, 323–324
    literacy learning issues, 355
    manual sign systems, use of, 43, 44, 50–51
    pictogram symbols with, 58
    Picture Exchange Communication System (PECS), 305
    research reviews, 223*t*
    tangible symbols for, 53
    visuospatial information, 109
Autism Spectrum Disorders–Canadian American Research Consortium (ASD-CARC), 244
Automatic scanning
    described, 100
    skill requirements, 182, 184, 184*t*
Automatic word recognition, 373–374
Averaged activation, 97
Awareness, role in cognitive/communication development, 186–187
AWRI, *see* Accessible Word Reading Intervention

Balanced Literacy software, 372
Bankson-Bernthal Test of Phonology, 149
Barriers to AAC
    access barriers, 141–142, 145–146, 146*t*, 147*f*, 148–157
    in acute medical settings, 533, 539, 545
    attitude barriers, 144, 503
    funding, 157, 439, 545
    interventions for, 219–221
    knowledge barriers, 143, 221, 539
    opportunity barriers, 141, 142–144, 160, 219–221, 241, 353, 539
    policy barriers, 142, 160, 219
    practice barriers, 143, 160, 220, 539
Basic choice communicators, *see* Emerging communicators
Battery of Language Test, 519
Bauby, Jean-Dominique, 465–466
Beginning communicators
    adults, 268–269, 270*f*–271*f*, 271
    choice making, teaching about, 295–301
    conversation skills, 310–323, 313*f*, 317*t*
    defined, 255
    facilitated communication (FC), 323–326

    importance of inclusive communication opportunities, 271–272
    nonsymbolic communication, 273–278
    preschool children, 258–265
    rejecting, teaching about, 307–309
    requesting, teaching about, 293, 301–307, 303*t*, 304*t*
    research reviews, 223*t*
    school-age children, 265–268
    sensitizing facilitators to, 272–278, 274*t*
    "talking switch" techniques, 289–292
    visual schedules, 287–289, 288*t*, 289*f*, 290*f*
    "yes" and "no," teaching about, 309–310
Behavior chain interruption strategy
    attention-getting instruction, 276
    requesting instruction, 304*t*
    research reviews, 223*t*
Behavior problems, *see* Problem behavior
Beliefs, *see* Attitudes
Beyond Access Model, 402–403
BIGmack switches, 289–290, 369
Bilingualism, 153–154
Blind spots, 214
Blindness, *see* Visual impairments
Bliss for Windows, 60
BlissInternet, 60
Blissvox, 60
BlissWrite software, 60
Blissymbolics
    compared with other systems, 55, 57, 58
    hard copy output, 107
    language development and, 330, 334
    need for instruction, 360
    overview, 59–60, 60*f*
    with visual impairments, 53
Boardmaker software program, 54–55, 107
Books
    adaptations, 262
    communication notebooks, 485, 485*f*, 507, 508*f*, 513
    remnant books, 316, 317*t*
Boston Assessment of Severe Aphasia, 497
Boston Diagnostic Aphasia Exam, 497
Botulism, 454
Bracken Basic Concept Scale, 188*t*, 203
Braille, 63–64, 63*f*, 216, 384
Brain injury, *see* Traumatic brain injury (TBI)
Brain-stem strokes, 460–465
BRIGANCE® Comprehensive Inventory of Basic Skills, 210
Broca's aphasia, 468
Buddy system, 429
Butterfly harness, 171*f*

Calendar systems, *see* Visual schedules
CAN, *see* Cure Autism Now
Canada, manual sign systems, 47
Candidacy models of assessment, 133–134
Capability assessment
    in acute medical settings, 539–545, 540*f*, 541*f*
    adults with acquired disabilities, 438
    amyotrophic lateral sclerosis (ALS), 441–443
    aphasia, 497–502

brain-stem strokes, 462
clinical illustrations, 184*t*, 185–186
cognitive/linguistic skills, *see under* Cognitive/
    linguistic capabilities
hearing, 217
language, 203–206
literacy skills, 206–207, 208*t*, 209*t*, 210–211
motor skills, *see* Motor skills
multiple sclerosis (MS), 450–451
overview, 159–161
Parkinson's disease (PD), 456–567
positioning and seating, *see* Positioning
tools for, 162*t*–164*t*
vision, 211–217, 212*f*, 213*f*
Caregivers, *see* Facilitators; Families
CASE, *see* Conceptually Accurate Signed English
Case examples, intervention teams, 117–118
CAST, *see* Center for Applied Special Technology
Categorization
    assessment of, 498
    in dementia, 513
    of symbols, 201–203
    taxonomic grids, 336
CCP, *see* Circles of communication partners
Cellular technology, adults with acquired disabili-
    ties, 437
Center for Applied Special Technology (CAST), 414
Center for Effective Collaboration and Practice,
    256, 404
Center for Evidence-Based Practice: Young Chil-
    dren with Challenging Behavior, 404
Center for Literacy and Disability Studies (Univer-
    sity of North Carolina), 364
Cerebral palsy
    AAC issues, 237–239
    described, 235–237, 356
    literacy learning issues, 353
    use of cued speech, 50–51
Chairs
    positioning in, 170*f*, 171*f*, 172*f*, 173*t*
    supports, 175*f*, 176*f*, 177*f*
Chalk Talk, 146*t*, 426
Chalkboards, 388*t*
Challenging behavior, *see* Problem behavior
Chart-based coding strategies, 68, 68*f*, 70–71
Chatbox, 85
ChatBox Deluxe, 301
Cheap Talk 8, 85
Cheap Talk 4 Inline with Jacks, 301
Cheap Talk 4 Square with Jacks, 301
Checklist of Communication Competencies, see
    The Triple C
Checklists, for vocabulary selection, 32
Childhood apraxia, *see* Developmental apraxia of
    speech (DAS)
Children
    attitudes about AAC, 155–156
    vision assessment, 216
    see also Preschool children; School-age children
Children's Speech Intelligibility Measure, 149
China, manual sign systems, 47
Choice making
    aphasia and, 473, 473*t*
    brain-stem strokes and, 464

continuum of formats, 292–293, 294*t*
    teaching about, 295–301
    see also Direct selection methods; Scanning tech-
        niques; Yes/no questions
Choosing Outcomes and Accommodations for
    Children (COACH), 267–268
Circles of communication partners (CCP), 404, 405*f*
Circles of Friends, 266–267, 271
Circular scanning, 97–98, 98*f*
Clarification strategies, 253
Classrooms
    adaptations, 150, 382–384, 383*f*, 383*t*, 428–429
    expected student interaction patterns, 422*t*–423*t*,
        425–426
    instructional arrangements, 420–421, 422*t*–423*t*,
        424–427
    microswitch technology, 264*t*
    routines, importance of, 261
    special education classrooms, 396
    time spent in, 396
    universal design for learning, 412–414, 428–429
    see also Inclusion
Clicker 4 software, 372
Clinical Assessment of Language Comprehension, 203
Clinical Evaluation of Language Fundamentals, 204
Closing the Gap, 414
COACH, *see* Choosing Outcomes and Accomm-
    odations for Children
Coaching, conversational, 312–314, 313*f*
Cognitive Abilities Test™, 190*t*
Cognitive impairment, *see* Cognitive/linguistic capa-
    bilities; Intellectual disabilities
Cognitive Linguistic Quick Test, 500
Cognitive/linguistic capabilities
    amyotrophic lateral sclerosis (ALS), 441–442
    aphasia, 467, 468, 472, 497, 500
    assessment, 186–187, 188*t*, 189, 190*t*, 191
    dementia, 508–515
    development of, 186–187
    Huntington's disease (HD), 516
    multiple sclerosis (ALS), 450
    Parkinson's disease (PD), 456–457
    primary progressive aphasia, 505–507
    screening for in acute medical settings, 539–540.
        540*f*
    symbol assessment
        advanced symbol use, 199, 201, 201*f*
        categorization and association, 201–203
        functional object use, 191, 192*f*, 193
        overview, 191, 197
        question-and-answer format, 197, 198*f*, 199
        receptive labeling and yes/no formats, 193, 194*f*
        requesting format, 199, 200*f*
        visual matching format, 193, 195*f*, 196, 196*f*
    traumatic brain injury (TBI), 519, 520*t*–522*t*,
        522–523, 526, 531
Collaborative teams, *see* Teams
Collections, as conversation starters, 315–316
College classes, peer support, 418–419
Color encoding systems, 73–74, 74*f*
Color perception, 215
Commenting, conversational, 291, 320–321
    see also Conversation skills
Communicating Partners approach, 278, 344

Communication
    among team members, 124, 126–127, 128f–129f,
        129–130
    assessing patterns in school settings, 421,
        422t–423t, 424–427
    changing nature of needs, 138, 223, 224f, 227,
        231, 503–504
    communicative intent, 187
    components of communicative competence,
        10–14, 136, 310–311
    current communication, assessing, 145–146, 146t,
        147f, 469–471
    development of, 82
    distinguishing nonintentional from intentional
        communication, 273–274, 274t
    layers of participation, 136
    purposes of, 8–10, 9t, 469–471
Communication Aid Users Society of Australia, 326
Communication and Symbolic Behavior Scales
        Developmental Profile, 188t, 189
Communication bill of rights, 220, 220t
Communication boards/displays
    aided language stimulation, 346f, 347f
    alphabet boards, 459, 460f, 524, 529, 544
    conversation displays, 318–319
    with conversational coaching, 313–314
    dual boards, 319
    Go Fish displays, 199, 201, 201f
    speech production and, 148
    topic boards, 459, 460f, 524
    for traumatic brain injury (TBI), 524
    for writing support, 386, 387f, 388
    see also Display devices
Communication breakdowns
    use of augmented comprehension (input) for, 476t,
        479–480, 480f, 483f
    see also Repair strategies, conversational
Communication cards, 492, 513
Communication diaries
    vocabulary assessment, 203
    vocabulary selection, 32
    see also Dictionaries
Communication disorders
    in acute medical settings, 534–536
    adults with acquired disabilities, 436–439
    aphasia, 467, 468–469
    autism, 244–245, 247–248
    brain-stem strokes, 460–461, 462–465
    dementia, 510t
    Guillain-Barré syndrome (GBS), 453–454
    Huntington's disease (HD), 516
    multiple sclerosis (MS), 448–449, 450, 451–452
    prevalence, 3, 5
    primary progressive aphasia (PPA), 505, 506, 507
    see also Language impairments; Speech disorders;
        Voice control
Communication displays, see Communication
        boards/displays
Communication Matrix, 145, 146t, 188t, 189
Communication needs, assessing
    in acute medical settings, 538–539
    adults with acquired disabilities, 436–438
    amyotrophic lateral sclerosis (ALS), 441
    aphasia, 466–471, 495–496

    brain-stem strokes, 461
    changing nature of needs, 138, 223, 224f, 227,
        231, 503–504
    multiple sclerosis (MS), 449
    overview, 137f, 138–139
    Parkinson's disease (PD), 456
Communication Needs Assessment Form for
        Aphasia, 496
Communication Needs Model of assessment,
        135–136, 538
Communication notebooks, 485, 485f, 507, 508f, 513
Communication opportunities
    choice making, 295–296
    importance of, 271–272
    for nonsymbolic communicators, 260–264, 260t,
        263f, 264t
    for school-age children, 265, 266
    through use of switches, 290–292
Communication partners
    of adults, 269
    assessing skills of, 500–501
    attitudes and preferences of, 151–155
    circles of communication partners (CCP), 404, 405f
    dementia and, 513–515
    partner-focused questions, 319–320
    perceptions of, 514–515
    skill levels of, 11–12, 156–157
    Social Networks approach, 267
    traumatic brain injury (TBI) and, 529
    in Tri-Focus Framework, 258f, 272
    unfamiliar partners, 155–156
    see also Facilitators; Partner-dependent
        communicators
Communication rates
    amyotrophic lateral sclerosis (ALS), 440, 441f, 446
    augmentative and alternative communication
        (AAC), 67, 79, 315, 321
    conversational speaking, 67
    enhancement techniques
        color encoding, 73–74
        message codes, 71–73
        message prediction, 75–80, 77f
        word codes, 69–71
    fingerspelling, 64
    manual sign systems, 50, 109
    Parkinson's disease (PD), 456, 458–459
    writing, 353, 383
Communication satisfaction, 230
Communication signal inventories, see Dictionaries
Communication skills, for kindergarten entry, 393t
Communication Supports Checklist for Programs
        Serving Individuals with Severe Disabili-
        ties, 220
Communication Survey, 230
Communicative Competence for Individuals Who Use
        AAC: From Research to Practice, 311
Communicative intent, role in cognitive/
        communication development, 187
Community-based programs
    importance of for adults, 268
    in less developed countries, 114
    trends, 114
    vocational internships, 396
    volunteer experiences, 396

Competitive educational participation, 398–399
COMPIC system, 60–61
Composition, *see* Writing
Comprehension, *see* Reading
Comprehension check procedure, 298–299
Comprehensive communicators, *see* Generative
    message communicators
Comprehensive Signed English Dictionary, 49
Comprehensive Test of Nonverbal Intelligence
    (CTONI), 190*t*
Computer screens
    glare, 215
    output displays, 107
    touch screens, 383*t*
Computer technologists, roles on intervention
    teams, 119, 125*t*
Conceptually Accurate Signed English (CASE), 48
Conditional requesting, 303
Consensus building, 437–438
Consequences, *see* Natural consequences
Consonant recognition, assessment, 209*t*
Constraints, assessing
    in acute medical settings, 545
    adults with acquired disabilities, 438–439
    amyotrophic lateral sclerosis (ALS), 444–445
    aphasia, 500–504
    constraints profile, overview, 151–157, 153*f*, 154*t*
    multiple sclerosis (MS), 451
    Parkinson's disease (PD), 457
    see also Barriers
Consumer satisfaction, evaluating, 229–230
Consumer Survey on Communicative Effective-
    ness, 230
Contact communication system, 79
Content-specific conversations, message selection, 21
Contextual choice communicators, 475–481, 477*f*,
    478*f*, 479*f*, 506
Contraction codes, 71
Controlled situation communicators, *see* Contextual
    choice communicators
Conventional literacy
    defined, 372
    reading instruction, 373–377
    writing instruction, 377–382
    see also Literacy
Conversation
    message management and selection, 17–22, 20*t*
    relevance, 315
    speaking rate, 67, 315
    structure of, 18–22
    written choice conversations, 476–478, 476*t*, 477*f*,
        478*f*, 479*f*
Conversation displays, 318–319
Conversation skills
    decision-making strategies, 253
    instructional techniques, 311–314
    introduction strategy, 314–315
    nonobligatory turn taking, 320–321
    partner-focused questions, 319–320
    regulatory phrases, 321
    repair strategies, 253, 321–323
    topic setting/initiating, 252–253, 315–319, 317*t*
Conversational coaching, 312–314, 313*f*
Cooperative learning groups, 422*t*–423*t*, 424–425

Core vocabulary lists, 29–30
Counseling, for parents, 253–254
Coverage vocabulary, 25–26, 27
Co:Writer 4000, 78, 492
Crayons, adaptations, 382, 383*f*
Creative Communicating, 262
Crime, 17
Criterion-based assessment, 160–161, 181
CTONI, *see* Comprehensive Test of Nonverbal
    Intelligence
Cued speech, 50–51
Cueing hierarchies, 512
Cultural considerations
    attitudes about technology, 152–154, 221
    nonverbal communication, 41
    perceptions of disability, 151–152
    Protocol for Culturally Inclusive Assessment of
        AAC, 153*f*, 154*t*
Cure Autism Now (CAN), 244
Current versus future interventions, *see* Today and
    tomorrow principle
Curriculum
    adaptations, 414, 416–417, 416*t*
    influence on educational participation, 397–398
Cursors
    adaptations, 383*t*
    control methods, 182, 184, 184*t*
Curved headrests, 177*f*

Daily living routines, 261
Danmar harness, 171*f*
Darci USB device, 70
DAS, *see* Developmental apraxia of speech
Deaf culture, use of manual sign systems, 47, 50
Deafblindness
    facilitator training programs, 278–279
    tactual reception of signing, 49–50
    see also Hearing impairments; Visual impairments
DEAL, *see* Dignity, Education, and Language
    Communication Center
DEAR, *see* Drop Everything and Read
Decision making
    in AAC intervention, 221–223, 226–227
    as conversation skill, 253, 489–490
    of intervention teams, 127
    see also Choice making
Decoding, 374–375
DECtalk, 103–104
Degenerative conditions, planning for,
    226–227, 438
Degenerative myopia, 215
Delayed assistance strategy, 304*t*
Dementia
    with amyotrophic lateral sclerosis (ALS), 442
    assessment, 191, 512
    intervention, 509–510, 511*f*, 512–515
    strengths and deficits, 508–509, 510*t*
    see also Huntington's disease (HD); Primary
        progressive aphasia
Demographic information
    AAC use, 4–5
    prevalence of communication disorders, 3, 5
Depression, multiple sclerosis (MS) and, 450

Developing countries
    challenges of, 154
    community-based programs, 114
    selection of AAC devices, 238
Development
    of children with autism, 247
    cognitive/communication development, 186–187
    language development, 327–341, 359–360
    see also Emergent literacy
Developmental apraxia of speech (DAS)
    AAC issues, 250–254
    described, 249
    manual sign systems, 43
    multimodal communication systems, 45
Developmental, Individual-Difference, Relationship-
        Based (DIR) model, 246
Developmental vocabulary, 26–27
Diaries
    vocabulary assessment, 203
    vocabulary selection, 32
Dictation, writing, 363–364, 363*t*
Dictionaries
    gesture, 283–285, 284*t*
    symbol, 318
DigiCom 2000, 85
Digitized speech, 105–106
Dignity, Education, and Language (DEAL) Com-
        munication Center, 324
DIR, *see* Developmental, Individual-Difference,
        Relationship-Based model
Direct selection methods
    in acute medical settings, 544
    assessment of motor skills for, 175–176, 177–178,
        179*f*, 180–181
    compared with scanning methods, 102–103
    overview, 93–97, 94*f*, 95*f*, 96*f*
Directed scanning
    overview, 100
    skill requirements, 184, 184*t*
Directions, *see* Procedural descriptions
Disabilities, individuals with
    attitudes about, 151–152
    changing roles of, 17, 231
    victimization of, 17
    see also specific disabilities and disorders
Disability Solutions (newsletter), 242, 250
Discrete trial teaching, 246
Display devices
    chart-based displays, 68*f*
    conversation displays, 318–319
    dynamic displays, 85, 86*f*–87*f*, 88, 338, 339*f*
    fixed displays, 84–85
    grid displays, 180*f*, 335–338, 337*f*, 339*f*
    hybrid displays, 85, 88
    physical characteristics
        display and item size, 90
        glare, 215
        number of items, 89
        organizing, 26, 84
        orientation of, 91–92
        output modes, 107, 108
        spacing and arrangement of items, 90, 91*f*, 92*f*
    tactile displays, 83, 90
    visual scene displays, 88, 89*f*, 335, 338, 482–483

    see also Communication boards/displays; Selection
        sets
Do2Learn, 262
Double vision, 214
Down syndrome
    intellectual disabilities, 240
    resources, 242
    total communication with, 45, 50–51
    vocabulary, 330
Down Syndrome Research and Practice, 242
Drawings
    aphasia and, 499
    of children, 38
    relationship to writing, 379
Drop Everything and Read (DEAR), 376
Dry-erase boards, 388*t*
Dual communication boards, 319
Dwell time of activation devices, 96
Dynamic displays, 85, 86*f*–87*f*, 88, 338, 339*f*
Dynamo device, 56
DynaSyms
    compared with other systems, 55
    language development and, 334
    need for instruction, 360
    overview, 56–57, 57*f*
DynaVox Series 4, 56, 88
Dysarthria
    amyotrophic lateral sclerosis (ALS), 440
    brain-stem strokes, 460
    cerebral palsy, 237
    Guillain-Barré syndrome (GBS), 453
    Huntington's disease (HD), 516
    multiple sclerosis (MS), 448–449
    Parkinson's disease (PD), 455–456
    traumatic brain injury (TBI), 519, 522
Dysgraphia, 354
Dyskinetic cerebral palsy, 236
Dystonic cerebral palsy, 236

Early childhood learning
    emergent literacy instruction, 367–368, 369*f*
    inclusion, 392
    see also Preschool children
Early intervention
    adaptive play, 261–264, 263*f*, 264*t*
    delivery of services, 259–260
    importance of for autism, 246–247
    inclusion, 392
    increasing communication opportunities,
        260–264, 260*t*, 263*f*, 264*t*
    participation analysis and intervention plan, 260,
        260*t*
    philosophy, 258–259
    routines, importance of, 261
*Early Use of Total Communication: Parents' Perspectives
        on Using Sign Language with Young Children
        with Down Syndrome*, 45
Easy Talk, 85
EBP, *see* Evidence-based practice
Echoes, message feedback, 102, 217
Ecological inventories
    for adult AAC users, 268–269, 270*f*–271*f*
    for vocabulary selection, 32

Education
   retention, 419
   separate schools, 396–397
   transitions, preschool to kindergarten, 392–394,
      393*t*
   see also Inclusion; Instruction
Educational participation
   active participation, 399–400
   competitive participation, 398–399
   involved participation, 400–401
   lack of, 397–398, 401
   prerequisites, 402
   see also Inclusion
Educational sign systems, *see* Parallel sign systems
Efficiency and response effectiveness, principle of, 256
Elearning Design Lab, 256
Electrolarynges, 454, 538, 542, 542*f*, 543*f*
Electronic communication, adults with acquired
      disabilities, 437, 466
Elementary school, *see* School-age children
Elicited choices, *see* Choice making
Elicited requests, *see* Requesting
Eligibility issues
   historical perspective, 133–135
   intellectual disabilities, 239
   verification testing, 160
E-mail, use of
   adults with acquired disabilities, 437, 466
   for augmented writing, 493
Emblems, 39
   see also Symbols
Emergent literacy
   assessment, 363–364, 363*t*
   instruction, 367–368, 369*f*
   see also Literacy
Emerging communicators, 472–475, 473*f*, 475*f*, 506
   see also Beginning communicators
*Emerging Literacy Success: Merging Whole Language
   and Technology for Students with Disabilities*, 370
Employment, adults with severe communication
      disorders, 436, 437
Encoding strategies
   chart-based codes, 68, 68*f*, 71–73, 73*f*
   color encoding, 73–74, 74*f*
   memory-based codes, 68
   message codes, 71–73, 73*f*
   message prediction, 75–80, 77*f*
   word codes, 69–70, 70*f*
Endemic iodine deficiency, 240–241
Endotracheal intubation, 534–535, 534*f*
Engineers, roles on intervention teams, 125*t*
English Braille–American Edition, 64
Enkidu Research, Inc., 76, 79
Environmental adaptations
   assessing, 150
   inclusive classrooms, 417
   physical structure, 225, 412, 417
   space/location, 225
Environmental inventories, for vocabulary selec-
      tion, 32
Episodic memory, 508
Errorless learning, 299
Ethnicity, *see* Cultural considerations
ETRAN system, 74*f*, 388*t*

Evaluation, *see* Assessment; Capability assessment;
      Outcomes
EvaluWare™, 164*t*, 216
Evidence-based practice (EBP), 222–223, 223*t*
Evoked potential tests, 212, 217
Expectant time delay strategy, 304*t*
Experiential skills, aphasia and, 500
Explicit requesting, *see* Requesting
Expressive language
   assessing, 497
   in AAC, 11
   of AAC users, 333
   Huntington's disease (HD), 516
   structured instructional approaches, 341–344, 343*f*
   traumatic brain injury (TBI), 520*t*–522*t*
Eye examinations, 211–213, 212*f*, 213*f*
Eye linking, 94*f*, 464, 544
Eye-pointing (gazing) systems
   in acute medical settings, 544
   assessment of motor skills for, 176, 178, 180, 180*f*
   brain-stem strokes and, 464
   case example, 81–82, 103
   chart-based displays, 68*f*
   color encoding, 73–74, 74*f*
   described, 93–95, 94*f*, 95*f*, 464
   ETRAN system, 74*f*, 388*t*
   eye-gaze vest, 95*f*
EZ Keys, 70, 78

Facial expressions, 40
Facilitated communication (FC), 323–326
Facilitated Communication Institute, 326
Facilitators
   defined, 157, 272
   feedback errors, 299–300
   gesture dictionaries, use of, 283–285, 284*t*
   for people with amyotrophic lateral sclerosis
      (ALS), 445
   role in facilitated communication (FC), 324–326
   scripted routines, 279, 280*t*, 281–283, 282*t*
   sensitizing to nonsymbolic communication,
      272–278, 274*t*
   skill levels of, 12, 143, 156–157
   support for, 439
   training for, 228, 273, 278–279, 394, 481–482,
      513–515
   training others, 503
   see also Instruction
FACS, *see* Functional Assessment of Communication
      Skills for Adults
Families
   aphasia assessment, role in, 496
   attitudes about AAC, 146, 148, 151–155, 224,
      438–439, 444, 503
   compromising with, 224–225
   consensus building, 437–438
   dementia and, 513–515
   as informants about vocabulary, 31
   involvement of on intervention teams, 111–112,
      114, 118
   needs of, 120*t*
   operational competence of, 12
   support for, 253–254

Families— *(continued)*
transition to kindergarten, role in, 393
see also Communication partners; Facilitators
"Families, Cultures, and AAC," 152
Farewell statements, message selection, 21–22
Fast mapping, 330–331
Fathers
needs of, 120*t*
see also Families; Parents
Fatigue
adults with acquired physical disabilities, 466
reducing, 28–29
FC, *see* Facilitated communication
FCMs, *see* Functional Communication Measures
FCT, *see* Functional communication training
Feature matching assessment method, 161
Feedback methods
activation feedback, 101
auditory feedback, 217
corrective feedback, 299–300
distinguished from input and output, 104
errors in, 299–300
message feedback, 102
verbal feedback, 280*t*, 281, 282*t*
Feet, positioning, 173*t*
"Female talk," 24
Fetal alcohol syndrome, 240
Field losses, vision, 214, 499
Filtered activation, 97, 451
Fingerspelling, 64
Finland, manual sign systems, 48
*First Things First: Early Communication for the Pre-
Symbolic Child with Severe Disabilities,* 277
First-letter-of-word spelling, 210
Fitzgerald key, 336
Fixed displays, 84–85
Floor sitters, 173–174, 174*f*
Follow-up
assessment, 138–139
intervention, 231
Forced-choice preferential looking (FPL) proce-
dures, 212–213, 213*f*
FPL, *see* Forced-choice preferential looking (FPL)
procedures
Fragile X syndrome, intellectual disabilities, 240
Frametalker, 79
Fringe vocabulary, 30–32
Frontotemporal dementia (FTD/ALS), 442
Frontotemporal lobar dementia syndrome (FTLD),
442
Functional Assessment of Communication Skills for
Adults (ASHA FACS), 191
Functional behavior assessment, 256
Functional Communication Measures (FCMs), 229
Functional communication training (FCT)
accept/reject behaviors, 277
attention-getting behaviors, 276
research reviews, 223*t*
Functional equivalence, principle of, 256
Functional goals, of communication, 9–10
Functional object use, assessment, 191, 192*f*, 193
Functional skills, evaluating, 229
*Functional Vision: A Bridge to Learning and Living—
Functional Vision Assessment* (videotape), 216

Functional visual competence, 216
Funding, as barrier, 157, 439, 545
Future communication needs, *see* Today and tomor-
row principle

GAS, *see* Goal Attainment Scaling
Gates-MacGinitie Reading Tests, 208*t*, 210
GBS, *see* Guillain-Barré syndrome
Gender
attitudes about AAC, 155
influence on message selection, 16
vocabulary and, 24–25
General case instruction, 305–306, 308
General education classrooms, *see* Classrooms
Generalization and maintenance, research reviews,
223*t*
Generalized requesting, *see* Requesting
Generative message communicators, 487–492, 488*t*,
489*f*, 491*f*, 506
Gestures
with developmental apraxia of speech (DAS),
250, 251
gesture dictionaries, 283–285, 284*t*, 318
nonsymbolic communicators, 273
as unaided symbols, 39–41, 108, 109
see also Manual sign systems
Glare, effect on displays, 215
Global aphasia, 468–469
Go Fish displays, 199, 201, 201*f*
Goal Attainment Scaling (GAS), 229
Goal/content matrix, 414, 415*t*
Goals
of communication, 8–10, 9*t*
for inclusion, 407, 410–414, 413*t*, 415*t*
of intervention teams, 120–121, 120*t*, 121
see also individual education programs (IEPs)
Goldman-Fristoe Test of Articulation, 149
Good-bye statements, *see* Farewell statements
Goodness-of-fit, principle of, 256–257
GRADE, *see* Group Reading Assessment and Diag-
nostic Evaluation
Graduated prompting, 314
Grammatical knowledge, 203–205
see also Morphology
Grapheme–phoneme correspondences, 361
Graphic symbols
audiovisual media, 422*t*–423*t*, 426–427
language development and, 359–360
literacy learning and, 360–362, 361*t*, 362*t*
orthographic symbol systems, 63–64
research reviews, 223*t*
in written choice conversation, 477, 477*f*, 478*f*
see also Symbols; Writing
Great Britain, manual sign systems, 47
Great Green Macaw device, 70
Greeting cards, 55
Greetings, 18, 291, 490
Grid displays, 180*f*, 335–338, 337*f*, 339*f*
Grocery list, sample, 492, 493*f*
Group instruction, 421, 422*t*–423*t*, 424
Group Reading Assessment and Diagnostic Evalua-
tion (GRADE), 208*t*
Group therapy, 502

Group–item scanning, 99, 100*f*
Guide to Child Nonverbal IQ Measures, 191
Guillain-Barré syndrome (GBS), 452–454
Gus! Communication Symbols, 62
Gus! Word Prediction software, 78

HAAT, *see* Human Activity Assistive Technology
    model
Hand Talk (Amer-Ind), 42–43
HandiCODE, 70
Hands, positioning, 173*t*
Handwriting
    fine motor skills and, 354
    see also Writing
Hanen curriculum, 283
Hanen Early Language Parent Program, 344
Hard copy output, 107
Hawking, Stephen, 7–8, 441, 447
Head
    positioning, 172*f*, 173*t*, 177*f*
    supports, 177*f*
Head injuries, *see* Traumatic brain injury (TBI)
Head mouse devices, 94–95
Head pointers, *see* Pointing methods
Headlights, *see* Pointing methods
HeadMouse, 95
HeadMouse Extreme, 95
Headrests, 177*f*
Headsticks
    for assessment of motor skills, 176, 178
    for direct pressure, 93
    illustration, 92*f*
    as writing adaptation, 382
    see also Pointing methods
Hearing impairments
    assessment, 217
    cerebral palsy, 237
    of communication partners, 457
    touch cues, use of, 279, 280*t*, 281, 282*t*
Hearing loss, cerebral palsy, 238
Hemiparesis, 468
Hemispheric losses, vision, 214
Hensinger head collars, 177*f*
High school
    inclusion, 396
    peer support, 418–419
    vocabulary, 23
Hips
    extensor thrust, 170*f*
    positioning, 170*f*, 173*t*
HIPSS, *see* Home Inventory of Problem-Solving
    Skills
Home
    as base for adults with acquired disabilities, 436, 441
    delivery of early intervention services, 259
    literacy experiences of children, 356–358, 367
    microswitch technology, 264*t*
    routines, importance of, 261
Home Inventory of Problem-Solving Skills
    (HIPSS), 188*t*
*Home Talk: A Family Assessment of Children Who
    are Deafblind*, 146*t*
Home talk, compared to school talk, 22–23

Hospitals
    "limited-use" policies, 142
    see also Acute medical settings
Human Activity Assistive Technology (HAAT)
    model, 136
Humor, 317–318
Hungary, prevalence of communication disorders, 5
Huntington's disease (HD), 516
Hybrid displays, 85, 88, 335
Hyperkinesia, 457
Hyperlexia, 245, 355
Hypertonia, 236

I-ASCC, *see* Index of Augmented Speech Compre-
    hensibility in Children
Iconic encoding
    assessment of, 202
    described, 72–73, 73*f*
    language development and, 334
    need for instruction in, 360
Iconicity of symbols
    defined, 36
    manual sign systems, 44
ICUs, *see* Acute medical settings
IDEA, *see* Individuals with Disabilities Education
    Act Amendments of 1997 (PL 105-17)
IEPs, *see* Individual education programs
Illustrator nonverbal behavior, 40
*Improving the Ability of Alzheimer's Patients to Commu-
    nicate*, 515
Incidental teaching, 246
Inclusion
    assessing instructional arrangements, 420–421,
        422*t*–423*t*, 424–429
    barriers and challenges, 142–143, 265–266,
        391–392, 420
    benefits of, 156, 265
    case examples, 397, 431
    components of
        educational participation, 397–402
        integration, 395–397
        overview, 394–395, 395*f*
        social participation, 403–404, 405*f*
        support, 405–406
    defined, 391
    inclusion maps, 408*f*, 409*f*
    models for facilitation, 266–268
    outcomes, evaluating, 429–431
    Participation Model
        adaptations, identifying, 414, 416–419, 416*t*
        goal/content matrix, 414, 415*t*
        individual education programs (IEPs),
            410–412, 412*t*
        participation and support patterns, 407, 408*f*,
            409*f*, 410
        student profiles, 410, 411*t*
        universal design for learning (UDL),
            412–414
Incomplete presentation strategy, 304*t*
Independence, importance of, 406
Independent communicators
    generative message communicators, 487–492,
        488*t*, 489*f*, 491*f*, 506

Independent communicators— *(continued)*
　specific-need communicators, 492–495, 493*f*,
　　494*f*, 495*t*, 506
　stored message communicators, 484–487, 485*f*,
　　486*f*, 486*t*
Independent reading, 376–377
The Index of Augmented Speech Comprehensibility
　in Children (I-ASCC), 149–150
Individual education programs (IEPs)
　in active educational participation, 399–400
　for AAC users, 189
　developing, 410–412, 412*t*
　influence on educational participation, 397–398
Individuals with Disabilities Education Act Amend-
　ments of 1997 (PL 105-17), 392
Infants, vision assessment, 216
Informal assessment, of language, 204–205
Information transfer, as goal of communication, 8,
　9*t*, 470–471
Infrared pointers, 94–95
Initiation of conversation, 252–253, 315–319, 317*t*
　see also Conversation skills
Input modes, 109–110
Instruction
　aided language stimulation, 344–348, 345*t*, 346*f*,
　　347*f*
　choice making, 295–301
　comprehension check procedure, 298–299
　conventional reading instruction, 373–377
　conversation skills, 311–314
　emergent literacy, 367–368, 369*f*
　general case instruction, 305–306, 308
　instructional arrangements, 421, 422*t*–423*t*,
　　424–427
　interactive model, 344
　naturalistic teaching interventions, 302–304, 304*t*
　Picture Exchange Communication System
　　(PECS), 304–305
　process writing, 378, 381
　rejection signals, 307–309
　requesting, 293, 301–307, 303*t*, 304*t*
　school literacy experiences, 358–359, 367–368
　strategy instruction, 378, 381
　structured approaches, 341–344, 343*f*
　System for Augmenting Language (SAL), 348–350
　writing, 377–382
　"yes" and "no" responses, 309–310
　see also Intervention
Insurance plans, 439
Integrated literacy experiences, 370
Integration
　levels of, 395–397, 395*f*
　of preschool children, 259–260
Integrative research reviews, 222, 223*t*
Intellectual disabilities
　AAC issues, 241–243
　autism, 244
　cerebral palsy, 237
　described, 239–241
　facilitators, assessing, 157
　literacy learning issues, 354–355
　manual sign systems, use of, 43, 49, 50
　see also Cognitive/linguistic capabilities; Dementia
Intelligent agents, 248

Intelligibility
　amyotrophic lateral sclerosis (ALS), 440, 441*f*, 446
　assessment, 149–150
　of manual sign systems, 44
　Parkinson's disease (PD), 456, 458–459
　traumatic brain injury (TBI), 522, 523, 524, 525*f*
　see also Repair strategies, conversational
Intensive care units (ICUs), *see* Acute medical settings
*InterAACtion Strategies for Intentional and Uninten-
　tional Communicators*, 269
Interaction Checklist for Augmentative Communi-
　cation, 146*t*
Interdependence of intervention teams, 119–124
Interdisciplinary teams
　defined, 113
　see also Teams
Internal dialogues, 9
International Council on English Braille, 64
International Society of Augmentative and Alterna-
　tive Communication (ISAAC), 111
Internet, and adults with acquired disabilities, 437, 466
Interpersonal skills
　assessment form, 128*f*–129*f*
　of intervention teams, 124, 126–127, 129–130
　types of, 126–127
Interrupted behavior chain intervention, *see* Beha-
　vior chain interruption strategy
Intervention
　aphasia, 469–471
　augmented writing approach, 443, 493–495, 494*f*
　behavior chain interruption strategy, 223*t*, 276
　cueing hierarchies, 512
　current versus future interventions, 223, 224*f*,
　　226–227
　decision making and planning, 221–223, 226–227
　dementia, 509–510, 511*f*, 512–515
　early intervention, 246–247
　environmental adaptations, 225, 412, 417
　evidence-based practice (EBP), 222–223, 223*t*
　language intervention methods
　　aided language stimulation, 344–348, 345*t*,
　　　346*f*, 347*f*
　　interactive model, 344
　　structured approaches, 341–344, 343*f*
　　System for Augmenting Language (SAL),
　　　348–350
　longitudinal nature of, 223, 224*f*, 226–227, 231
　natural abilities, increasing, 224–225
　naturalistic teaching interventions, 302–304, 304*t*
　opportunity barriers, 219–221
　primary progressive aphasia (PPA), 506–507
　school-age users of AAC, 266–268
　situation training, 485–486, 486*f*, 486*t*, 493–494,
　　495*t*
　spaced retrieval strategy, 512
　stimulation-type aphasia therapy, 469
　traumatic brain injury (TBI), 520–531, 523–525,
　　526–527, 528–529
　Tri-Focus Framework, 257–258, 258*f*
　when to begin, 254
　see also Instruction; Outcomes
Intervention teams, *see* Teams
Introduction strategy, 314–315
Intubation, 534–535, 534*f*

Invented spelling, 379
Inventory of Potential Communicative Acts
    (IPCA), 146*t*
Inverse scanning, 100
Involved educational participation, 400–401
Iodine deficiency, 240–241
Ireland, manual sign systems, 48
ISAAC, *see* International Society of Augmentative
    and Alternative Communication
Israel, AAC use, 238
ITalk2, 301

Japan, manual sign systems, 47
Joint action routines, 283
    see also Scripted routines
Joint visual attention, aphasia and, 473*t*
Joke cards, 317–318
Joysticks, 383*t*
Junior high school, peer support, 418–419

Keyboards
    adaptations, 383*t*
    ambiguous keyboards for letter selection, 76
    key echoes, 102
    keyguards, 457
Key-word signing (KWS), 47, 50
Kid Pix Studio software, 372
Kindergarten
    entry skills, 393*t*
    as goal for all preschool children, 259
    transition to, 392–394
Knock-knock jokes, 291, 317–318
Knowledge barriers, 143, 221, 539
Kochmeister, Sharisa, 323–324, 325
KWS, *see* Key-word signing

Labeling, attitudes about, 151, 152
Labeling skills
    receptive labeling, 193, 194*f*
    with speech-output technology, 248
    structured teaching approach, 342–343, 343*f*
LAM, *see* Language Activity Monitor
Lámh sign system, 48
Language
    assessment, 203–206
    asymmetry between input and output, 329, 333
    comprehension, supports for, 422*t*–423*t*,
        426–427
    intervention
        aided language stimulation, 344–348, 345*t*,
            346*f*, 347*f*
        interactive model, 344
        structured approaches, 341–344, 343*f*
        System for Augmenting Language (SAL),
            348–350
    language development
        of AAC users, 327–334
        message units, effect on, 334–341
        organizational strategies, effect on, 335–338
        symbol systems and, 334–335
Language Activity Monitor (LAM), 205, 229

Language impairments
    aphasia, 467, 468–469, 497
    autism, 244, 245, 248
    cerebral palsy, 237
    developmental apraxia of speech (DAS), 249, 251,
        252–253
    Huntington's disease (HD), 516
    multiple sclerosis (MS), 450
    primary progressive aphasia (PPA), 505, 506, 507
    traumatic brain injury (TBI), 519, 520*t*–522*t*,
        522–523, 526, 528, 531
    see also Speech disorders
Language maps, 427
Langue des Signes Québécoises (LSQ), 47
Lap trays, 172*f*
Large-group instruction, 421, 422*t*–423*t*
Laser pointers, 94, 96*f*, 464, 496
Learnability, of display devices, 85, 88
Learned helplessness, 187
Learning
    professionals as learners, 121–122
    universal design for learning, 412
*Learning Media Assessment of Students with Visual
    Impairments: A Resource Guide for Teachers*, 384
Learning stations/centers, 422*t*–423*t*, 424–425
Least dangerous assumption, principle of, 411–412
Legislation, as barrier to AAC use, 142
Leiter International Performance Scale, 190*t*
Let's Play!, 262
Letter writing, sample formats, 494*f*
Letter–category codes
    message coding, 71–72
    word coding, 69, 70–71
Letter-naming, assessment, 206, 208*t*, 363*t*
Letter-sound recognition, 209*t*, 361, 375
Levels of Cognitive Functioning scale, 519
Lexical processing, 361, 362*t*
Lexigrams, 62–63
Lifespace Access Profile, 164*t*
Light cueing, 345, 346–348
Light pointers, 94, 96*f*, 464, 496
Light sensitivity, 215
LightWRITER, 70, 78
Linear scanning, 98–99, 99*f*
Line-drawing symbols, as representational symbols, 53
Linguistic competence
    as component of communication, 11, 136, 310
    see also Cognitive/linguistic capabilities
LSQ, *see* Langue des Signes Québécoises
Listening comprehension, assessing, 364
Literacy
    adaptations, 376, 382–384, 383*f*, 383*t*
    assessing, 206–207, 208*t*, 209*t*, 210–211,
        362–366, 363*t*
    defined, 351
    importance of, 259, 351–352
    of individuals needing AAC support, 353–356
    learning
        challenges, 352, 357–358
        conventional literacy instruction, 372–382
        emergent literacy, 363–364, 363*t*, 366–372
        experiences of children who use AAC, 356–359
        language and, 359–362
        software, 371–372, 384–386, 385*t*, 386*t*

Literacy—*(continued)*
  skills, 359–362
  types of AAC support for, 352–353
Literate individuals, vocabulary selection, 28–29
LITTLEmack, 289
Loan banks, 115
Location adaptations, 225
Locked-in syndrome (LIS), 465–466
Longitudinal intervention, 223, 224*f*, 226–227, 231
Low-tech options
  activity displays, 337–338
  in acute medical settings, 538, 543
  for amyotrophic lateral sclerosis (ALS), 446
  for aphasia, 472, 485, 485*f*
  attitudes about, 156, 438–439
  compared with electronic devices, 156
  for developmental apraxia of speech (DAS),
    251–252
  for Huntington's disease (HD), 516
  for traumatic brain injury (TBI), 529
  see also Unaided symbols
LSQ, *see* Langue des Signes Québécoises
Lumbar supports, 175*f*

MacArthur-Bates Communicative Development
    Inventory: Words and Sentences, 32, 203
Macaw overlay (product), 85
Magic slates, 538, 541
Makaton Vocabulary program, 65–67, 66*f*
Making Action Plans (MAPs), 266–267, 271
"Male talk," 24
Manual sign systems
  combining signs with other techniques, 45, 47
  considerations for use, 44–45, 46*t*, 47
  with developmental apraxia of speech (DAS), 250
  guessability of, 43, 108
  input and output considerations, 108, 109
  language development and, 334
  memory impairments and, 108
  motor assessment for, 181
  national sign languages, 47
  parallel systems, 48–50
  reasons for use, 43–44
  research reviews, 223*t*
  selecting signs to teach, 45, 46*t*
  signing rates, 50, 64, 109
  speech production and, 148
  as supplements to spoken language, 50–51
  types of, 47–51
Manually coded English (MCE), 48–50
MAPs, *see* Making Action Plans
Maps, in written choice conversation, 477, 478*f*
Mastery learners, 121–222
Matching Assistive Technology & Child, 162*t*
Matching format, assessment, 193, 195*f*, 196, 196*f*
Matching Person and Technology, 229, 230
McDonald, Anne, 324
MCE, *see* Manually coded English
Meaningful Use of Speech Scale (MUSS), 148–149
Medicaid, 439
Medical facilities
  "limited-use" policies, 142
  see also Acute medical settings

Medicare, 210, 439, 502
Medicare Funding of AAC Technology Assessment/
    Application Protocol, 163*t*
Medications, adults with acquired physical disabili-
    ties, 455, 466
Melodic intonation therapy, 250–251
Membrane switches, *see* Touch pads
Memory
  dementia, 508–509
  Huntington's disease (HD), 516
  for making choices and requesting, 293
  multiple sclerosis (MS), 450
  requirements for use of AAC systems, 501
  role in cognitive/communication development, 187
  traumatic brain injury (TBI), 527, 528
Memory books, 510, 511*f*, 513, 515
Memory-based coding strategies, 68, 70–71
Mental retardation, *see* Intellectual disabilities
Message encoding strategies, 71–75, 73*f*, 74*f*
Message management
  conversational interactions, 17–22
  defined, 15
  factors affecting message selection, 16–17
  feedback, 102
  grammatically complete versus telegraphic
    messages, 321
  input modes, 109–110
  message acceleration, 28
  message units, length of, 320, 340–341
  output modes, 104–108
  preselecting messages, 83–84, 485
  vocabulary resources, 29–32
  vocabulary selection, 22–29
Message Mate, 85
Message prediction strategies, 75–80, 77*f*, 492
Message timing, *see* Rate enhancement techniques
Metacognitive skills
  aphasia and, 501
  role in cognitive/communication development, 187
  self-regulation, 375
Micrographia, 457
Microswitches, *see* Switches
Milieu teaching, 283, 302–304, 304*t*, 344
Miniature objects, 51–52
Minorities, *see* Cultural considerations
Minspeak
  association skills and, 202
  with Fitzgerald key, 336
  language development and, 334
  overview, 72–73
Missing item strategy, 304*t*
Modality instruction cards, 489–490, 489*f*
Modifications, *see* Adaptations
More than Words, 273, 344
Morphology
  capabilities of AAC users, 331
  morphosyntactic knowledge assessment, 203–205
Morse code
  overview, 69–70, 70*f*, 71
  spelling skills, 211
Mothers
  needs of, 120*t*
  see also Families; Parents
Motion-filtering software, 97, 451

Motivation, learned helplessness, 187
Motor impairments
    adaptations for, 262–263, 263*f*, 379, 382–383,
        383*f*, 383*t*
    amyotrophic lateral sclerosis (ALS), 442–443
    aphasia, 499
    brain-stem strokes, 462
    cerebral palsy, 236, 239
    choice-making adaptations, 300–301
    clinical illustrations, 184*t*, 185–186
    developmental apraxia of speech (DAS), 249
    Huntington's disease (HD), 516
    literacy learning issues, 353–356
    locked-in syndrome (LIS), 465
    multiple sclerosis (MS), 451
    Parkinson's disease (PD), 457
    toys for, 262–263, 263*f*
    traumatic brain injury (TBI), 519, 522,
        526–527, 528
Motor skills
    assessment
        for assessment tasks, 174–176
        for direct selection methods, 175–176,
            177–178, 179*f*, 180–181
        for switch control, 181–182, 183*f*, 184–185, 184*t*
    display sets and, 90–92, 91*f*, 92*f*
    manual signing and, 44–45, 181
Mouse devices, adaptations, 383*t*
Movement disorders, 166
Movement-based techniques, 279
MS, *see* Multiple sclerosis
Multicultural competence, 152, 153*f*, 154*t*
Multidisciplinary teams
    defined, 113
    see also Teams
Multimodal Communication Screening Task for
    Persons with Aphasia, 498
Multimodal systems
    amyotrophic lateral sclerosis (ALS), 446
    aphasia, 489–490, 489*f*
    autism, 355
    cerebral palsy, 239
    combining manual signs with other techniques,
        45, 47
    developmental apraxia of speech (DAS), 251–252
    effect on syntax development, 332
Multiple diagnoses, individuals with, 243
Multiple sclerosis (MS), 448–452
Muscle tone
    cerebral palsy, 236
    described, 165
    positioning methods, 169, 170*f*, 171*f*, 172*f*
Music, adaptations, 263–264
MUSS, *see* Meaningful Use of Speech Scale
Myopia, 215

NAAR, *see* National Alliance of Autism Research
Naglieri Nonverbal Ability Test–Individual, 190*t*
Narrative discourse, 362
    see also Storytelling
National Alliance of Autism Research (NAAR), 244
National Aphasia Association, survey, 467

National Center for Treatment Effectiveness in
    Communication Disorders, 229
National Center to Improve the Tools of Educators
    (NCITE), 414
National Institute of Neurological Disorders and
    Stroke, 516
National Joint Committee for the Communication
    Needs of Persons with Severe Disabilities
    (NJC), 134–135, 220
National sign languages, 47
Native Americans, use of Amer-Ind, 42–43
Natural consequences, in choice making, 299–300
Natural speech
    assessing potential for, 146, 148–150
    autism, 248–249
    brain-stem strokes, 464–465
    importance of supporting for preschool chil-
        dren, 259
    perceived effect of AAC on, 146, 148, 155,
        224–225, 250, 253–254
    traumatic brain injury (TBI), 523–524, 530
Naturalistic teaching interventions, 302–304, 304*t*
N3C, *see* Novel name–nameless category principle
NCITE, *see* National Center to Improve the Tools
    of Educators
Nebraska ALS Database, 440
Neck
    positioning, 172*f*, 173*t*
    supports, 177*f*
Neck-type electrolarynges, 538, 542, 542*f*
Needs First, 164*t*
Needs/wants, communicating
    aphasia and, 470
    assessment, 438
    coverage vocabulary, 25–26, 27
    as goal of communication, 8, 9*t*
Negation words, *see* Rejection signals
NJC, *see* National Joint Committee for the Com-
    munication Needs of Persons with Severe
    Disabilities
Nonconventional spelling, 379
Nonintentional signals, distinguishing from inten-
    tional communication, 273–274, 274*t*
Nonlinguistic communication, *see* Nonsymbolic
    communication; Nonverbal communication
Nonliterate individuals, vocabulary selection,
    27–28
Nonobligatory turn taking, 320–321
Nonsymbolic communication
    assessment of, 188–189, 190*t*, 191
    described, 255–256
    increasing communication opportunities,
        260–264, 260*t*, 263*f*, 264*t*
    intentional versus unintentional signals,
        273–275, 274*t*
    research reviews, 223*t*
    switches for, 296
    Tri-Focus Framework for intervention, 257–258,
        258*f*
Nonverbal communication
    with aphasia, 498
    assessment, 188–189, 190*t*, 191, 498
    with autism, 245
    cultural considerations, 41

Nonverbal communication—*(continued)*
  feedback, communicative competence and, 10
  gestures, 39–41
  nonverbal juncture cues, 346
  as unaided symbols, 38–39
  vocalizations, 41–42
Norm-referenced assessment, 159–160, 258
Norway, manual sign systems, 47
Note taking, 418–419
Notebooks, communication, 485, 485*f*, 507,
  508*f*, 513
Novel name–nameless category principle
  (N3C), 330
Numeric codes
  message coding, 72
  word coding, 69, 70–71
Nursing personnel, 537
Nystagmus, 214–215

Oakland Schools Picture Dictionary, 61
Object adaptor nonverbal behavior, 41
Objects as symbols, 51–52
Occupational therapists, roles on intervention teams,
  125*t*, 165, 174
Oculomotor functioning, 214–215
Older adults, *see* Adults
One-to-one instruction, 422*t*–423*t*, 425
Online Academy of Positive Behavioral Support, 404
Onscreen keyboards, 383*t*
Opaque symbols, 36
Operational competence
  amyotrophic lateral sclerosis (ALS) and, 444–445
  aphasia and, 501
  as component of communication, 11–12, 136, 310
Operational requirements profile, 150
Opportunity barriers
  in acute medical settings, 539
  defined, 141
  intellectual disabilities, individuals with, 241
  interventions, 219–221
  to literacy learning, 353
  types of, 142–144
Optic neuritis, 450
Optical pointers, 94, 96*f*, 383*t*
Oral-motor control for speech
  assessing in acute medical settings, 541–545
  see also Dysarthria
Oral-type electrolarynges, 454, 538, 542, 543*f*
Organizational strategies of AAC devices, effect on
  language learning, 335–338
Orthographic symbol systems, 63–64
Outcomes
  adults with acquired disabilities, 439
  consumer satisfaction, 229–230
  for educational participation levels, 398–401
  evaluations of, 228–229
  functional limitations, 229
  inclusive classrooms, evaluating, 429–431
  quality of life, 230–231
  universal design learning, 413
Output modes
  synthesized speech, 104–107

  visual output, 107–108
  see also Speech-generating devices (SGDs)

Pacer/Tally, 446
Parakeet 15 device, 85
Parallel sign systems, 48–50
Paraprofessionals
  facilitating classroom interactions, 429
  one-to-one instruction, 425
  role in transition to kindergarten, 394
Parents
  importance of intuition, 274
  as informants for fringe vocabulary, 31, 32
  needs of, 120*t*
  operational competence of, 12
  perspectives on literacy, 357
  support for, 253–254
  training programs for, 273, 278–279, 344
  see also Facilitators; Families
Parkinson's disease (PD)
  described, 455–456
  planning for, 226–227
Partial objects as symbols, 52
Participation, *see* Educational participation; Inclusion; Social considerations
Participation Inventory, 139, 140*f*, 141
Participation Model
  in acute medical settings, 538–545
  adults with acquired communication disorders,
  436–439
  aphasia, 469–471
  compared with Tri-Focus Framework, 257–258
  traumatic brain injury (TBI), 530
  see also Assessment; Inclusion
Participation patterns, identifying
  in acute medical settings, 538–539
  adults with acquired disabilities, 436–437
  amyotrophic lateral sclerosis (ALS), 441
  aphasia, 469
  early intervention, 260, 260*t*
  multiple sclerosis (MS), 449
  overview, 139, 140*f*, 141
  Parkinson's disease (PD), 456
  see also Assessment
Partner Attitudinal Survey, 157
Partner Rating Scale, 157
Partner reauditorization, 102, 321
Partner Skill Screening Form, 157
Partner-dependent communicators
  contextual choice communicators, 475–481, 477*f*,
  478*f*, 479*f*, 506
  emerging communicators, 472–475, 473*t*, 474*f*,
  475*f*, 506
  transitional communicators, 482–484, 483*t*,
  484*f*, 506
  see also Communication partners; Facilitators
Partner-focused questions, 319–320
Partner-perceived communication, *see* Nonsymbolic
  communication
PATH, *see* Planning Alternative Tomorrows with
  Hope
Pathfinder, 85

PCRs, *see* Photographic Communication Resources
PCS, *see* Picture Communication Symbols
PD, *see* Parkinson's disease
PDDs, *see* Pervasive developmental disorders
Peabody Individual Achievement Test, 208*t*, 211
Peabody Picture Vocabulary Test, 203
PECS, *see* Picture Exchange Communication System
Pedagogical sign systems, *see* Parallel sign systems
Peers
    buddy system, 429
    conversational coaching approach, 313–314
    influence on educational participation, 398
    instruction and support, 406, 418–419
    participation patterns as performance standards,
        139, 140*f*, 141, 257–258, 260*t*
    peer conferencing, 386
Pelvis
    positioning, 173*t*
    supports, 176*f*
Pencils, adaptations, 382, 383*f*, 383*t*
Perceptual skills
    aphasia, 499
    assessment, 211–218
    see also Sensory perceptual impairments
Performance learners, 222
Performance Report Tool (PeRT), 205
Perlocutionary communication, *see* Nonsymbolic
        communication
Personality disturbances, multiple sclerosis (MS), 450
Person-centered planning
    for adults, 269, 271
    Social Networks approach, 269, 404
PeRT, *see* Performance Report Tool
Pervasive developmental disorders (PDDs)
    AAC issues, 246–249
    described, 243–246
    see also Autism
Phonological processing
    assessment, 206–207, 208*t*, 209*t*
    capabilities of AAC users, 328–329
    as critical skill, 361, 362*t*
Photographic Communication Resources (PCRs), 62
Photographs
    as memory aid, 512
    as representational symbols, 53
    for writing instruction, 379
Physical structure adaptations, 225, 412
Physical therapists, roles on intervention teams,
        125*t*, 165, 174
Physicians
    in acute medical settings, 537–538
    resistance to AAC, 444
    roles on intervention teams, 125*t*
PIADS, *see* Psychological Impact of Assistive Devices
        Scale
Pick 'n Stick symbols, 61
Picsyms, 54, 55, 56–57
Pictogram symbol system, 57–59, 58*f*
Pictorial competence, preschool children, 37–38, 197
Pictorial Test of Intelligence, 190*t*
Picture Communication Symbols (PCS)
    compared with other systems, 44, 58, 330
    grammatical morphology and, 331

hard copy output, 107
    iconic codes, 73*f*
    language development and, 334
    need for instruction, 360
    overview, 54–55, 54*f*
Picture Exchange Communication System (PECS)
    speech production and, 148
    teaching self-initiated requesting, 304–305
Pictures, *see* Photographs; Symbols
Picture-to-print matching, 209*t*
Pidgin Sign English (PSE), 48
Pittsburgh Employment Conference for Augmented
        Communicators, 272
PL 101-336, *see* Americans with Disabilities Act of
        1990
PL 105-17, *see* Individuals with Disabilities Educa-
        tion Act Amendments of 1997
PL 105-394, *see* Assistive Technology Act Amend-
        ments of 2004
Planning Alternative Tomorrows with Hope
        (PATH), 266–267, 269, 271
Play
    adaptive, 261–264, 263*f*, 264*t*
    conversational coaching during, 313–314
    initiating, 315
Pointing methods
    in acute medical settings, 544
    adaptations using, 189
    assessment of motor skills for, 176, 178, 180, 180*f*
    case example, 81–82, 103
    chart-based displays, 68*f*
    color encoding, 73–74, 74*f*
    described, 93–95, 94*f*, 95*f*
    ETRAN system, 74*f*, 388*t*
    head pointers, 94–95, 96*f*, 383*t*, 464, 496
Policy
    as barrier to AAC use, 142, 160, 219
    "limited-use" policies, 142
    segregation policies, 142–143
Portable voice amplification, 458, 524
Positioning
    assessment, 171–174
    general principles and techniques, 166, 169–171
    need for assessment, 165
    neuromotor impairments, 165–166, 167*f*, 168*f*
    sitting, 166, 169–172, 170*f*, 171*f*, 172*f*, 173*t*
    supports, 173–174, 174*f*, 175*f*, 176*f*, 177*f*
    traumatic brain injury (TBI) and, 528
Positive interdependence, of intervention teams,
        119–124
PPA, *see* Primary progressive aphasia
PrAACtically Speaking, 319
Practice barriers, 143, 160, 220, 539
Pragmatics
    aphasia and, 500
    of AAC users, 327–328
Prediction strategies, 75–80, 77*f*, 492
Predictive assessment, 161
Preferences
    awareness of, 292
    see also Choice making
Prelinguistic communication, *see* Nonsymbolic com-
        munication

Prelinguistic Milieu Teaching, 283, 344
Preliterate individuals
    language and literacy development, 359–362,
        361t, 362t
    vocabulary selection, 25–27
    see also Beginning communicators; Nonsymbolic
        communication
Preschool children
    fantasy stories, 20
    inclusion mandate, 392
    increasing communication opportunities for,
        260–264, 260t, 263f, 264t
    integration of, 259–260
    pictorial competence, 37–38
    small talk, 20
    transition planning for, 392–394
    vocabulary, 23, 27
    see also Early intervention
Pressure-sensitive keys, 93
Presymbolic communication, research reviews, 223t
Pretend readings, 368
Primary motor impairments, see Motor impairments
Primary progressive aphasia (PPA), 505–507
    see also Aphasia
Primitive reflexes, 165–166, 167f, 168f
Print, learning about, 361, 363t
Print-to-print matching, 209t
Privacy issues, determining core vocabulary, 30
Problem behavior
    accept/reject signals, 277, 307
    attention-getting signals, 276
    as communication, 256
    communication breakdowns and, 322
    intellectual disabilities, individuals with, 242
    intervention principles, 256–257
    requesting behaviors, 301–302
    resources, 404
Problem-solving skills, 361
Procedural descriptions, message selection, 21
Procedural memory, 509, 512
Process writing, 378, 381
Processes, see Procedural descriptions
Professional practices, as barriers, 143, 160, 220, 539
Professionals
    operational competence of, 12
    training, 14
    see also Facilitators; Physicians; Teachers; Teams
Progress, measuring, see Outcomes
Project FACTT (Facilitating Augmentative Com-
    munication Through Technology), 350
PROMPT©, see Prompts for Restructuring Oral
    Muscular Phonetic Targets
Prompts
    in choice making, 299
    graduated prompting, 314
    stimulus-prompt-response instructional approach,
        341–344
Prompts for Restructuring Oral Muscular Phonetic
    Targets (PROMPT©), 250
Proprioceptive information, as activation feed-
    back, 101
    see also Tactile input
Protocol for Culturally Inclusive Assessment of
    AAC, 152, 153f, 154t, 163t

Protocol for Implementing Strategies Trials, 502
PSE, see Pidgin Sign English
P-switches, 443, 443f
Psychological Impact of Assistive Devices Scale
    (PIADS), 230
Psychologists, roles on intervention teams, 125t
Puppetry, play activities, 263–264

Quality Indicators for Assistive Technology (QIAT)
    Consortium, 220
Quality of Communication Life Scale, 230, 231
Quality of life, evaluating, 230–231
Quality of Life Profile: People with Physical and
    Sensory Disabilities (QOLP-PD), 230–231
Quebec User Evaluation of Satisfaction with Assis-
    tive Technology (QUEST 2.0), 229
Questions
    aphasia and, 476t, 478, 479f, 480f
    partner-focused questions, 319–320
    question-and-answer format, in assessment, 197,
        198f, 199
    yes/no questions, 193, 194f, 388t, 463
    see also Choice making

Rate enhancement techniques
    color encoding, 73–74
    message codes, 71–73
    message prediction, 75–80, 77f
    research, 70–71, 74–75, 79–80
    word codes, 69–71
    writing, 383
    see also Communication rates
Rating scales, in written choice conversation, 477, 477f
Readiness for AAC, see Assessment
Reading
    assistive software, 384–386, 386t
    comprehension
        assessment, 207, 208t, 210, 364
        literacy instruction, 375–376
    defined, 351
    independent reading, 376–377
    reading aloud, 356, 358, 369–370
    reading readiness, contrasted with emergent liter-
        acy, 366
    traumatic brain injury (TBI) and, 531
    see also Literacy
Real objects as symbols, 51
Reauditorization, 321
Rebus symbols, 55, 56f, 58
Recall memory, 509
Receptive language
    assessment, 193, 194f, 497
    of AAC users, 11, 333
    participation beyond knowledge level, 291
    receptive labeling, 193, 194f
    structured instructional approaches, 341–344, 343f
    traumatic brain injury (TBI) and, 520t–522t
    see also Language
Recognition learning, 412
Recognition memory, 509, 512
Recognition spelling, 210–211
Referential skills, 472, 473t, 498

Regulator nonverbal behavior, 40
Regulatory phrases, 321
Rehabilitation Engineering Research Center-
    Augmentative and Alternative Communica-
    tion (AAC-RERC)
    funding issues, 157, 439
    intelligent agents, 248
    letter prediction, 76
Rehabilitation Research and Training Center on
    Positive Behavior Support, 256, 404
Rejection signals
    aphasia and, 473, 473*t*
    nonsymbolic communicators, 274*t*, 275, 277
    scripted routines, 279, 280*t*, 281–283, 282*t*
    teaching, 307–309
    see also Acceptance signals; Yes/no questions
Related services, integrating, 267–268
Relationships, *see* Communication partners; Social
    considerations
Release activation, 96–97
Remnant books, as conversation starters, 316, 317*t*, 459
Repair strategies, conversational, 253, 321–323
Representational symbols, 53–62
Requesting
    in assessment, 199, 200*f*
    proportion of communicative interactions, 303–304
    teaching about, 293, 301–307, 303*t*, 304*t*
    see also Yes/no questions
Research
    effectiveness of alternative access options, 102–103
    integrative reviews, 222, 223*t*
Resource rooms, 396
Respiratory support, 534–536, 534*f*, 536*f*, 541–543
Respiratory therapists, 537
Response modes
    in inclusive classrooms, 422*t*–423*t*, 425–426
    of nonsymbolic communicators, 281
    supports and adaptations, 388*t*, 422*t*–423*t*,
        423*t*, 427
Response-recode (R-R) strategy, 320
Retention, 419
Retinitis pigmentosa, 216
Rett syndrome
    emergent literacy, 367
    planning for, 226–227
    speech-output technology with, 248
Rhymes, 209*t*, 375
Riddle cards, 317–318
Romet electrolarynges, 538, 542, 542*f*
Rooting reflex, 166
Routines, importance of, 261
Row–column scanning, 99, 100*f*
Royal Institute of Technology (Stockholm), 104
R-R, *see* Response-recode strategy
Rules of language, *see* Pragmatics

Sabotage routine, 347
Safe-laser head pointers, 96*f*, 464, 496
SAL, *see* System for Augmenting Language
Salient letter encoding, 71
Sampling, 205, 229
SCA, *see* Supported Conversation for Adults with
    Aphasia

Scaffolded formats, augmented writing, 493–494, 494*f*
Scanning techniques
    in acute medical settings, 545
    amyotrophic lateral sclerosis (ALS), 443
    assessment of motor skills for, 181–182,
        184–185, 184*t*
    auditory scanning, 41–42, 90, 98, 99
    brain-stem strokes, 464
    clinical illustrations, 184*t*, 185–186
    compared with direct selection methods, 102–103
    as response mode, 388*t*
    scanning patterns, 97–99, 98*f*, 99*f*, 100*f*
    selection control methods, 100–101
    timing and speed, 100
SCERTS™ (Social Communication, Emotional
    Regulation, and Transactional Support)
    Model, 246
Schedules, *see* Visual schedules
Schematic grid layouts, *see* Activity boards/displays
School Inventory of Problem-Solving Skills
    (SIPSS), 188*t*
School talk, vocabulary, 22–23
School-age children
    challenges, 265–266
    communication opportunities for, 265, 266
    intervention approaches for AAC users, 266–268
    vocabulary, 23
Schools
    emergent literacy instruction, 367–368, 369*f*
    guidelines for assistive technology, 220
    literacy experiences of children, 358–359
    see also Classrooms; Inclusion; Instruction
Scoliosis
    described, 166
    positioning methods, 169–170
Scotland, AAC use, 238
Screen messages, output displays, 107
ScripTalker, 79
Scripted routines
    with aphasia, 486, 486*f*
    overview, 279, 280*t*, 281–283, 282*t*
Seat work, 422*t*–423*t*, 425
Secondary school, *see* High school
SEE, *see* Signing Exact English
*See What We Say: Situational Vocabulary for Adults
    Who Use Augmentative and Alternative Com-
    munication*, 30
Segregation
    levels of, 396–397
    policies and practice, 142
    see also Inclusion
Seizures, 237
Selection sets
    direct selection techniques, 93–97, 94*f*, 95*f*, 96*f*
    physical characteristics, 88–92, 91*f*, 92*f*
    scanning techniques, 97–101, 98*f*, 99*f*, 100*f*
    types of displays, 83, 84–88, 86*f*–87*f*
Selective retention, 419
Self-adaptors, 40–41
Self-initiated requests, *see* Requesting
Self-injury, *see* Problem behavior
Self-perception, influence on educational participa-
    tion, 398
Self-regulation, 375

Self-stimulatory behavior, 277
    see also Problem behavior
Self-Talk symbols, compared with other systems, 54
Semantic compaction, *see* Iconic encoding
Semantics
    capabilities of AAC users, 329–331
    semantic knowledge, 362, 362*t*
    semantic memory, 508
    see also Vocabulary
Semantic-syntactic grid displays, 335–336
Sensory perceptual impairments
    in aphasia, 499
    assessment, 211–218
    brain-stem strokes, 462
    multiple sclerosis (MS), 450
    touch cues, use of, 279, 280*t*, 281, 282*t*
    see also Hearing impairments; Visual impairments
Sentence Intelligibility Test, 149, 446
Sequenced Inventory of Communication Develop-
        ment, 203
Severe speech and physical impairments (SSPI)
    language development, 335
    literacy learning issues, 353
    phonological processing skills, 206, 207, 329
    see also specific disorders
SGDs, *see* Speech-generating devices
Shadow light cueing, 345
Shaping, 274
Sharing time, 422*t*–423*t*, 424
Short Form of the Boston Diagnostic Aphasia
        Exam, 497
Short-term memory
    in dementia, 508–509
    for making choices and requesting, 293
    see also Memory
Shoulders
    positioning, 171*f*, 172*f*, 173*t*
    retractors, 171*f*
    supports, 175*f*
SHOUT, *see* Support Helps Others Use Technology
Sign It (game), 47
Sign language, *see* Manual sign systems
Signal inventories, *see* Dictionaries
Signed English, 49
Signing Exact English (SEE), 48
Signing Illustrated, 47
Signs, *see* Manual sign systems; Symbols
Signs of the Times, 48
Silent reading
    assessing, 364
    literacy instruction, 376–377
SIM, *see* Strategic Instruction Model
Simplified Technology, 262
SIPSS, *see* School Inventory of Problem-Solving Skills
Sitting, positioning, 166, 169–172, 170*f*, 171*f*,
        172*f*, 173*t*
Situation training, 485–486, 486*f*, 486*t*, 493–494, 495*t*
Skeletal deformities, 166
Skill barriers, 143, 221
Small talk, message selections, 19–20, 20*t*, 490
Small-group instruction, 422*t*–423*t*, 424
Smart access electronic communication systems, 490
Smart-Nav, 95

Social Communication, Emotional Regulation,
        and Transactional Support, *see* SCERTS™
        Model
Social considerations
    etiquette, 8–9, 9*t*, 471
    influence on message selection, 16–17, 18
    norms, for intervention teams, 126
    selective retention, 419
    skills for kindergarten entry, 393*t*
    social closeness
        aphasia and, 470
        as goal of communication, 8, 9*t*
    social competence
        autism and, 244–245, 247–248
        as component of communication, 12–13, 136,
            252–253, 310
        developmental apraxia of speech (DAS),
            252–253
    social participation
        circles of communication partners (CCP),
            404, 405*f*
        in educational settings, 403–404
Social learners, 222
Social Networks: A Communication Inventory for
        Individuals with Complex Communication
        Needs and their Communication Partners,
        146*t*, 404, 405, 410, 512
Social Networks approach, 267, 269
Social services workers, roles on intervention
        teams, 125*t*
Software
    capability assessment, 162*t*–164*t*, 205
    emergent literacy learning, 371–372
    generating communication displays, 54–55, 107
    literacy learning, 384–386, 385*t*, 386*t*
    motion-filtering software, 97, 451
    selection issues, 385–386
    for use with Blissymbolics, 60
    word prediction, 78
    see also specific programs
Sonar pointers, 94–95
South Africa, AAC use, 238
Spaced retrieval strategy, 512
Space/location adaptations, 225
Spasticity
    cerebral palsy, 236
    clinical illustration, 184*t*, 185–186
    described, 166
    positioning methods, 169, 170*f*, 171*f*, 172*f*
Speak Up, 272
Speaking Differently, 272
Speaking Dynamically, 86*f*–87*f*
Speaking Dynamically Pro, 78, 107
Special education classrooms, 396
Specific-need communicators, 492–495, 493*f*, 494*f*,
        495*t*, 506
Speech
    perceived interference of AAC on, 146, 148, 155,
        224–225, 250, 253–254
    tracheostomy and, 541–543
    vocabulary, 22
Speech disorders
    autism, 244

cerebral palsy (CP), 237
  developmental apraxia of speech (DAS), 249
  Huntington's disease (HD), 516
  Parkinson's disease (PD), 455–456, 458
  see also Communication disorders; Dysarthria;
    Language impairments
Speech intelligibility, *see* Intelligibility
Speech recognition technology, 95
Speech synthesis, *see* Speech-generating devices;
    Synthesized speech
Speech-generating devices (SGDs)
  in acute medical settings, 544
  adolescents, attitudes about, 156
  analysis of utterances, 205
  autism and, 248–249
  fixed displays, 84–85
  Medicare funding, 210
  research reviews, 223*t*
  speech production and, 148
  System for Augmenting Language (SAL) with,
    348–350
  visual scene displays with, 338
Speech-language pathologists
  as informants for vocabulary, 31
  professional practices, 143, 539
  roles on intervention teams, 121, 125*t*
  treatment of cerebral palsy, 238
Speech-to-print matching, 209*t*, 361
Speed
  of scanning, 100
  see also Communication rates; Rate enhancement
Spelling
  assessment, 208*t*, 209*t*, 210–211, 365, 365*t*
  nonconventional spelling, 379
  traumatic brain injury (TBI) and, 531
Splints with pencil attachments, 382, 383*f*
Spontaneous spelling, 210
Spouses, *see* Communication partners; Families
Springboard, 88
SSPI, *see* Severe speech and physical impairments
SSR, *see* Sustained silent reading
STAART, *see* Studies to Advance Autism Research
    and Treatment
Stages assessment tool, 188*t*
Standardized tests
  for individual education planning, 189
  language assessment, 204
  see also Norm-referenced assessment
Standing frames, environmental adaptations, 150
Step scanning, 101, 184–185, 184*t*
Step-by-Step Communicator, 291–292
Stimulation-type aphasia therapy, 469
Stimulus-prompt-response instructional approach,
    341–344
STNR, *see* Symmetrical tonic neck reflex
Stoelting Brief Nonverbal Intelligence Test, 190*t*
Storage capacity, of AAC devices, 17
Stored message communicators, 484–487, 485*f*,
    486*f*, 486*t*
Story maps, 430*f*
Story overlays, 368, 369*f*
StoryBliss, 107
Storybook reading, 369–370

Storytelling
  aphasia and, 470–471, 482, 484*f*
  message selections, 20–21
Strabismus, 214, 237
Strategic competence, as component of communica-
    tion, 13–14, 136, 310–311
Strategic Instruction Model (SIM), 311–312
Strategic learning, 412
Strategies trials, 502
Strategy instruction, 378, 381
Strokes, *see* Aphasia; Brain-stem strokes
Structured practice approach, 312
Student profiles, developing, 410, 411*t*
Student-led instruction, 422*t*–423*t*, 424–425
Studies to Advance Autism Research and Treatment
    (STAART), 244
Subasis bar, 170*f*
Supertalker, 301
Supplemented speech techniques, 149–150
Support
  enhancing language comprehension, 422*t*–423*t*,
    426–427
  for facilitators, 439
  for families, 253–254
  levels of classroom support, 405–406
  peer support, 418–419
  visual supports, initiating conversation, 315
  writing support, 386, 387*f*, 388
  see also Adaptations; Positioning
Support Helps Others Use Technology (SHOUT), 272
Supported Conversation for Adults with Aphasia
    (SCA), 481–482
Sustained silent reading (SSR), 376
Sweden, manual sign systems, 47, 48
Switches
  assessment of motor skills for, 181–182, 183*f*,
    184–185
  attention getting devices, 275–276
  for choice making, 296
  components of switch control, 181–182
  P-switches, 443, 443*f*
  scanning techniques, 100–101, 181–182, 184–185
  "talking switch" techniques, 289–292, 369
  with tape recorders, 527, 529
  for toys, 262–263, 264*t*
  use of with neuromotor disorders, 165–166,
    167*f*, 168*f*
Syllable chunks, 375
Symbol dictionaries, 283–285, 284*t*, 318
Symbols
  aided symbols
    abstract symbols, 62–63
    defined, 36
    input and output displays, 108, 109–110
    orthographic symbols, 63–64
    representational symbols, 53–62
    tangible symbols, 51–53
  categorization and association, assessment of,
    201–203
  in choice making, 297–298
  combined aided and unaided systems, 65–67
  effect on language learning, 334–335
  language development and, 359–360

Symbols— *(continued)*
    learning, 37–38, 70–71, 74–75
    literacy learning and, 360–362, 361*t*, 362*t*
    rate enhancement
        message encoding strategies, 71–75, 73*f*, 74*f*
        message prediction strategies, 75–80, 77*f*
        research, 70–71, 74–75, 79–80
        word encoding strategies, 69–71, 70*f*
    relationship to messages, 35
    research reviews, 223*t*
    role in cognitive/communication development, 187
    symbol assessment
        advanced symbol use, 199, 201, 201*f*
        categorization and association, 201–203
        functional object use, 191, 192*f*, 193
        overview, 191, 197
        question-and-answer format, 197, 198*f*, 199
        receptive labeling and yes/no formats, 193, 194*f*
        requesting format, 199, 200*f*
        visual matching format, 193, 195*f*, 196, 196*f*
    types of, 36
    unaided symbols
        defined, 36
        gestural codes, 42–43
        gestures, 39–41
        input and output modes, 108, 109
        manual sign systems, 43–51
        vocalizations, 41–42
    visual schedules, 287–289, 288*t*, 289*f*, 290*f*
    want symbols, 303*t*
Symmetrical tonic neck reflex (STNR), 166, 168*f*
Syntax
    capabilities of AAC users, 332–333
    syntactic awareness, 361, 362*t*
Synthesized speech
    advantages and disadvantages, 106–107
    audition and, 217
    overview, 104–106
    see also Speech-generating devices (SGDs)
System for Augmenting Language (SAL), 109–110,
        348–350

Tactile input
    symbol systems, 63–64, 63*f*
    tactile displays, 83, 90
    tactual reception of signing, 49–50, 64
Tagged questions, 476*t*, 478, 479*f*, 480*f*
TALK Boards, 79
Talking Pictures, 61
"Talking switch" techniques, 289–292, 369, 527, 529
Tangible Symbol Systems, Levels of Representation
        Pre-Test, 188*t*
Tangible symbols, 51–53, 148
Tantrums, *see* Problem behavior
Tape recorders
    switches with, 289–291, 369, 527, 529
    for telephone communication assistance, 492
Taxonomic grid displays, 336
TBI, *see* Traumatic brain injury
Teacher-led instruction, 421, 422*t*–423*t*, 424
Teachers
    attitudes about literacy instruction, 357
    influence on educational participation, 397–398

    as informants for fringe vocabulary, 31
    roles on intervention teams, 125*t*
"Teach–test" approach, 196
Teams
    accountability of team members, 130–131
    in acute medical settings, 536–538
    case examples, 117–118, 119, 121, 122–123, 124,
        126, 127, 131
    decision-making approaches, 127
    development, 111–113
    interpersonal skills, 124, 126–127, 128*f*–129*f*,
        129–130
    involvement of AAC users and families, 111–112,
        114, 118
    meetings and interactions, 117–118
    membership, 114–115, 118–119, 125*t*
    multicultural competence, 152, 153*f*, 154*t*
    positive interdependence, 119–124
    relational problems, 112–113, 116–117, 117*t*
    skill levels of members, 143
    structural/organizational issues, 112, 113–116, 116*t*
    types of, 113
Technology abandonment, 115
Technology, attitudes about, *see* Attitudes
TechSpeak, 85
TechTalk, 85
Telegraphic messages, 321, 340–341, 497
Telephone, adaptations, 446, 458, 492
*Tell Me a Story: A New Look at Real and Artificial
        Memory*, 20
Test for Auditory Comprehension of
        Language–Third Edition, 204
Test for Reception of Grammar–Version 2, 204
Test of Language Development, 204
Test of Nonverbal Intelligence (TONI-3), 190*t*
Test of Reading Comprehension, 208*t*
Text-to-speech devices, 105
Thematic curricula, 370
Thighs
    positioning, 170*f*, 173*t*
    supports, 176*f*
Thoracic supports, 175*f*
Time constraints, managing, 418–419
Timed activation, 96
Timing enhancement, 28
Today and tomorrow principle
    assessment and, 138
    changing nature of communication needs, 223,
        224*f*, 227, 231, 503–504
    in planning interventions, 223, 224*f*, 226–227
    in teaching choice making, 296
TONI-3, *see* Test of Nonverbal Intelligence
Topic boards, 459, 460*f*, 524
    see also Communication boards/displays
Topic-setting strategies, 252–253, 315–319, 317*t*
    see also Conversation skills
Total communication
    compared to aided language stimulation, 345
    with developmental apraxia of speech (DAS), 251
    with Down syndrome, 45, 50–51
    rate of speaking and signing, 109
Touch cue method, 250, 279, 280*t*, 281, 282*t*
Touch pads, 93
Touch screens, 383*t*

Toys, 261–263, 263f
Tracheostomy, 535–536, 536f, 541–543
Trackballs, 383t
Transcortical aphasia syndrome, 468
Transdisciplinary teams, defined, 113
    see also Teams
Transitional communicators, 482–484, 483t,
    484f, 506
Transitions, preschool to kindergarten, 392–394, 393t
Translucent symbols, 36
Transparent symbols, 36
Traumatic brain injury (TBI)
    assessment, 191, 526, 527–528, 530
    AAC use, 519, 524–525
    clinical illustration, 184t, 185–186
    described, 518–519, 520t–522t, 522–523
    interventions, 520–531, 523–525, 526–527,
        528–529
    professionals' shift in intervention focus, 517
Treatment approaches, see Intervention
Tremors
    multiple sclerosis (MS), 451
    Parkinson's disease (PD), 457
Tricare, 439
Tri-Focus Framework, 257–258, 258f
The Triple C (Checklist of Communication Compe-
    tencies), 188t
Truncation codes, 71
Trunk
    positioning, 171f, 172f, 173t
    supports, 175f
TTR, see Type-to-token ratio
Turn taking, 291, 320–321, 473, 473t
"20 questions" process, 42
Type-to-token ratio (TTR), 22
Typing, see Facilitated communication (FC)

UBC Research Project, see Unified Braille Code
    Research Project
UDL, see Universal design for learning
UKAT Toolkit, 163t
U-LAM, see Universal Language Activity Monitor
Unaided symbols
    Amer-Ind, 42–43
    defined, 36
    gestures, 39–41
    input and output modes, 108, 109
    manual sign systems, 43–51, 46t
    vocalizations, 41–42
Underdeveloped countries, see Developing countries
Understanding the Communication Problems of
    Alzheimer's Patients, 515
Unified Braille Code (UBC) Research Project, 64
UNIT, see Universal Nonverbal Intelligence Test
United Kingdom
    Makaton Vocabulary program, 65–67, 66f
    manual sign systems, 43
    prevalence of communication disorders, 5
Unity software, 73
Universal design for learning (UDL), 412–414,
    428–429
Universal Language Activity Monitor (U-LAM),
    205, 229

Universal Nonverbal Intelligence Test (UNIT), 190t
Universities and colleges, training programs, 14
User-initiated requests, see Requesting

Vanguard Plus, 78, 88
Vantage Plus, 78, 88
Velcro adaptations, 262, 263f
Ventilation support, 534–536, 534f, 536f, 541–543
Ventral pontine syndrome, see Locked-in syndrome
    (LIS)
Verbal cueing
    in aided language stimulation, 346–348
    in choice making, 299
    in scripted routines, 280t, 281, 282t
Verbal prompt-free strategy, 304t
Verification testing, see Norm-referenced assessment
Vermont Interdependent Services Team Approach
    (VISTA), 267–268
Vest, eye-gaze method, 95f
Victimization of individuals, 17
VISTA, see Vermont Interdependent Services Team
    Approach
Visual displays, see Display devices
Visual impairments
    with aphasia, 499
    assessment, 211–217, 212f, 213f
    auditory scanning, use of, 41–42
    with autism, 245
    with cerebral palsy, 237, 238, 356
    with intellectual disabilities, 356
    literacy learning issues, 356, 384
    with locked-in syndrome (LIS), 465
    with multiple sclerosis (MS), 450
    role in cognitive/communication development, 187
    tactual reception of signing, 49–50
    tangible symbols for, 51–52
    touch cues, use of, 279, 280t, 281, 282t
    with traumatic brain injury (TBI), 527, 528
Visual matching format, 193, 195f, 196, 196f
Visual scene displays, 88, 89f, 335, 338, 482–483
Visual schedules, 287–289, 288t, 289f, 290f
Vocabulary
    assessment, 203
    supports and adaptations, 422t–423t, 427
    see also Semantics
Vocabulary selection
    acceleration vocabulary, 28
    age variables, 23–24
    aided language stimulation, 345t
    core vocabulary lists, 28–30
    coverage vocabulary, 25–26, 27
    developmental vocabulary, 26–27
    fringe vocabulary, 30–32
    gender variables, 24–25
    school talk versus home talk, 22–23
    spoken versus written communication, 22
    use patterns, 29–30
Vocalizations
    of nonsymbolic communicators, 273
    as unaided symbols, 41–42
Vocational counselors, roles on intervention teams,
    125t
Vocational internships, 396

Voice banking, 544
Voice control
    Parkinson's disease (PD), 455–456, 458
    tracheostomy and, 541–543
Voice output options
    in acute medical settings, 544
    "talking switch" techniques, 289–292, 369
    technical advances, 17
    see also Speech-generating devices (SGDs)
Voice recognition technology, 95, 383*t*
VoicePal, 301
Volunteer experiences, high school students, 396

Wallets, communication, 485, 485*f*, 513
Want symbols, 303*t*
Wants and needs, *see* Needs/wants, communicating
W.A.T.I. Assistive Technology Assessment, 163*t*
Weakness
    brain-stem strokes, 464
    clinical illustration, 184*t*, 186
    Guillain-Barré syndrome (GBS), 453
    see also Motor impairments
Wernicke's aphasia, 468, 480–481
Western Aphasia Battery, 497
Wheelchairs
    environmental adaptations, 150
    positioning in, 170*f*, 171*f*, 172*f*, 173*t*
    supports, 175*f*, 176*f*, 177*f*
WHO, *see* World Health Organization
Wide Range Achievement Test, 210
Widgit Rebus Symbols, 55, 56*f*
Windswept position of the hip, described, 166
WiViK 3 on-screen keyboard, 78
Woodcock-Johnson III, 208*t*, 210
Word encoding strategies, 69–71, 70*f*
Word lists, core vocabulary lists, 29–30
Word prediction strategies, 75–80, 77*f*, 492
Word recognition
    assessment, 207, 208*t*, 210, 364

automatic word recognition, 373–374
    as critical skill, 361, 362*t*
"Word Walls," 374
WordPower software, 78
Work-related skills, for kindergarten entry, 393*t*
World Health Organization (WHO), prevalence of
        intellectual disabilities, 240
Wrap-up remarks, message selection, 21–22
Writers' Workshop, 380, 386
Writing
    aphasia and, 491–492, 493–495, 494*f*
    assessing, 363*t*, 365–366, 365*t*
    assistive software, 384–386, 385*t*
    augmented writing approach, 443, 493–495, 494*f*
    beginning writers, 379–380
    defined, 351
    emergent skills, 371
    motor impairments and, 353, 354
    options for individuals in acute medical settings, 543
    rate of production, 353
    skilled writers, 381
    for students who use AAC, 377–378, 386, 388
    supports and adaptations, 386, 387*f*, 388, 388*t*
    tools, adaptations to, 382, 383*f*, 383*t*
    vocabulary, 22
    see also Literacy
Writing with Symbols 2000 software, 372
Written choice conversation, 476–478, 476*t*, 477*f*,
        478*f*, 479*f*, 513
Wrong-item strategy, 304*t*

Yerkish lexigram symbols, 62–63
Yes/no questions
    aphasia and, 476*t*, 478, 479*f*, 480*f*
    in assessment, 193, 194*f*
    brain-stem strokes and, 463
    as response mode, 388*t*
    teaching about, 309–310
Yooralla Society of Victoria, Australia, 319